OXFORD MEDICAL PUBLICATIONS

Oxford Handbook of
Key Clinical
Evidence

Oxford Handbook of
Key Clinical Evidence

Edited by

James Harrison

Specialist Registrar in Cardiology,
London Deanery, UK

Kunal Kulkarni

Foundation Doctor,
Oxford Deanery, UK

Mohamed Baguneid

Consultant Vascular Surgeon,
Wythenshawe Hospital,
Manchester, UK

Bernard Prendergast

Consulant Cardiologist,
John Radcliffe Hospital,
Oxford, UK

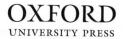

OXFORD
UNIVERSITY PRESS

OXFORD
UNIVERSITY PRESS

Great Clarendon Street, Oxford OX2 6DP

Oxford University Press is a department of the University of Oxford.
It furthers the University's objective of excellence in research, scholarship,
and education by publishing worldwide in

Oxford New York

Auckland Cape Town Dar es Salaam Hong Kong Karachi
Kuala Lumpur Madrid Melbourne Mexico City Nairobi
New Delhi Shanghai Taipei Toronto

with associated companies in Berlin Ibadan

Oxford is a registered trade mark of Oxford University Press
in the UK and in certain other countries

Published in the United States
by Oxford University Press Inc., New York

British Library Cataloguing in Publication Data

Data available

Library of Congress Cataloging in Publication Data

Data available

Typeset by Cepha Imaging Private Ltd., Bangalore, India
Printed in China
on acid-free paper through
Asia Pacific Offset

ISBN 978–0–19–923407–3

10 9 8 7 6 5 4 3 2 1

Foreword

If you have ever felt that you are drowning in an acronym soup of trials—HOT, CARDS, ADVANCE, and dozens of others—or that you have failed to keep up with the flood of research in journals, then you have picked up the right book. Herewith is a summary of many of the key clinical trials from the past few decades; some well known, some less known, and some unfortunately overlooked.

Since the 1960s when the US Food and Drug Administration began requiring clinical trials before approving new medications, there has been an exponential rise in the number of trials. While this plethora of evidence is good news for both patients and clinicians, it is all too easy to get lost in the maze. There are now at least 30,000 trials published each year (among the two million or so medical research articles per year). This means over 500 trials per week: enough to start a small bonfire. Of course, we don't want the important, high quality trials to go up in smoke. This book provides two key elements to help the busy clinician use the most important of these studies. First, it selects just the small fraction of key trials and reviews that have led, or should lead, to changes in clinical practice. Second, it provides a well-structured summary of the question, design, quality, and key findings of each trial selected.

Brian Haynes, Editor of *Evidence Based Medicine*, has suggested a '4S' taxonomy of medical research information which divides information resources into primary research studies, systematic reviews of those studies, synopses (of the studies or reviews), and systems—information accessible at the point of care. For those with limited time to read, the most important of these are the good synopses: the focus of this book. Sometimes we may want more detail from the original primary studies, and sometimes we will need a quick 'bottom line' while on the ward or in the clinic, and may turn to a pocket guideline. But for the majority of clinicians, the majority of reading time will be most usefully spent on synopses, which give sufficient detail to understand and interpret the evidence, but without overwhelming details.

For those wanting to improve their knowledge, and more importantly their care of patients, this book is a great start. After digesting this concentrated evidence, I would hope readers would be stimulated to continue pursuing new studies and reviews. In any case, if you find the information contained here novel and useful, I would hope you would discuss it with colleagues. Perhaps you doubt some of the findings? Well, discussion might lead to exploration of related evidence, checking for new work in the Cochrane Library, or perhaps even to initiating a new trial. No single study or textbook should be considered the last word. But if this book has taught you something new in the care of patients and sparked a desire to monitor new research, then it has served its purpose well.

Paul Glasziou
Professor of Evidence-Based Medicine
University of Oxford

Preface

If you are reading this book, then you have probably got at least a vague passing interest in EBM (evidence-based medicine). After all, it is an inescapable buzzword in modern medicine, and provokes an extreme range of reactions—from repulsion, to a belief in it as the panacea of sound clinical practice. Regardless of your preconceptions, our aim is simple: to demonstrate that EBM is an accessible and valuable tool when applied in the appropriate clinical context.

The greatest difficulty with EBM is that different readers will interpret a paper very differently; for example, an academic's or a statistician's view may well be quite markedly distinct from that of a clinician. Both parties may be correct in their analysis, but their differing backgrounds, experiences, and ultimate goals yield differences of opinion in their conclusions. In many cases it can simply be a lack of training that leads to avoidance of critique in certain aspects of a paper. For example, medical students receive little exposure to applied statistics during their training, making self-interpretation of the results section a frightening task. Not knowing how and where to look can make EBM seem an untameable beast best left for someone else to deal with. However, without rigorous scrutiny, EBM is meaningless. External factors such as cost and bureaucracy are inherent to all healthcare systems, but should not restrict the contribution of high quality evidence to clinical advances. Our hope is that this book will join the many resources that have sprung up in recent years to ensure that EBM remains free from undue influences and becomes a subject that is part-and-parcel of everyday clinical practice for healthcare workers of all levels and backgrounds.

We have attempted to strike the right balance between complexity and accessibility in ensuring that primary scientific and statistical facts are interpreted within a practical clinical context. The introductory chapters will hopefully provide the background and framework for this process, while the template-based interpretations of our expert clinicians demonstrate the process of critical analysis of papers that have made key changes to their clinical practice. This book will attract comments and, no doubt, criticism. It is not all-encompassing and there are unavoidable gaps and omissions. EBM itself is, ironically, an inexact science with opinion and, in particular, consensus forming a valuable component of its safe application to clinical practice. We welcome your feedback (please submit this via the book's page on the OUP website – http://www.oup.com). While we may not be able to respond to all emails individually, we do appreciate the opinions of our readers and will endeavour to incorporate suggested changes into future editions.

Acknowledgements

First and foremost, we owe our heartfelt thanks to all at Oxford University Press that have helped put this book together. In addition to the many behind-the-scenes team members (whom we apologise for not naming individually here), we would like to thank a number of key people.

We are indebted to our commissioning editor Liz Reeve, who together with Beth Womack saw traces of a book within the murky depths of our initial proposal. We would also like to thank our production editors Bethan Lee and Kate Wilson, who saw this project through to the end. We owe much to our many reviewers, both in and out of OUP, including Janet Peacock, Sally Kerry, Katy Oliver, Nick Nelson, and Sasha Abraham, who have all provided extremely valuable feedback; an extra thank-you to Joyce Cheung, who enjoyed her role as reviewer so much that she continued working with us in the unenviable role of copyeditor—a brave feat! We would like to thank Helen Hill for meticulously proofreading the final manuscript.

A special mention must go to Andrew Sandland, our development editor, for his tireless efforts in keeping this—at times overwhelming—project on track. Andrew has played a crucial role in helping coordinate all of the people involved in producing this book; without his help and advice, this book would not exist.

Finally, but most importantly, we would like to take this opportunity to thank our many expert contributors. This book is the product of our collaboration with over 50 clinicians and academics. It is through their knowledge and dedication that such a book has been possible, hopefully making EBM a more accessible subject for all.

JH, KK, MB, BP

Contents

Contributors

Sonya Abraham
Senior Lecturer in Rheumatology
and Medicine
Kennedy Institute of Rheumatology
Imperial College Healthcare
NHS Trust
London, UK

Sachin Agrawal
Specialist Registrar in Urology
St Peter's Hospital
Surrey, UK

Guruprasad Aithal
Consultant Hepatobiliary
Physician
Nottingham University
Hospitals NHS Trust
Nottingham, UK

Andrew Boulton
Professor of Medicine and
Consultant in Diabetes
Manchester Royal Infirmary
Manchester, UK

Andrew Bradley
Professor of Transplantation
Surgery
Addenbrooke's Hospital
Cambridge, UK

Ben Bridgewater
Consultant Cardiothoracic
Surgeon
Wythenshawe Hospital
Manchester, UK

Mike Brown
Honorary Consultant in Infectious
Diseases & Senior Lecturer
London School of Hygiene &
Tropical Medicine
London, UK

Nigel Bundred
Consultant Breast Surgeon
Wythenshawe Hospital
Manchester, UK

Stephen Bushby
Specialist Registrar in
Genitourinary Medicine
Newcastle General Hospital
Newcastle upon Tyne, UK

Harvinder Chahal
Specialist Registrar in
Endocrinology
St Bartholomew's Hospital
London, UK

Robert Chalmers
Consultant Dermatologist
Manchester Dermatology Centre
Salford, UK

Charles Crawley
Consultant Haematologist
Addenbrooke's Hospital
Cambridge, UK

Fiona Cuthbertson
Specialist Registrar in
Ophthalmology
Oxford Eye Hospital
Oxford, UK

Adam Dangoor
Specialist Registrar in Oncology
Christie Hospital NHS Trust
Manchester, UK

Thearina de Beer
Consultant Anaesthetist and
Intensivist
Nottingham University Hospitals
NHS Trust
Nottingham, UK

Bosko Dragovic
Consultant Obstetrician &
Gynaecologist
Northwick Park Hospital
Harrow, UK

William Drake
Consultant Endocrinologist
St Bartholomew's Hospital
London, UK

Richard Davenport
Consultant Neurologist
Western General Hospital
Edinburgh, UK

Andreas Fountoulakis
Specialist Registrar in General
Surgery
Wythenshawe Hospital
Manchester, UK

Simon Galloway
Consultant General Surgeon
Wythenshawe Hospital
Manchester, UK

Henk Giele
Consultant Plastic Reconstructive
and Hand Surgeon
Oxford Radcliffe Hospital and
Nuffield Orthopaedic Centre
Oxford, UK

Chris Griffiths
Professor of Dermatology
University of Manchester
Salford, UK

Richard Haynes
Clinical Research Fellow in
Renal Medicine
University of Oxford
Oxford, UK

Rob Henderson
Consultant Cardiologist
Nottingham City Hospital
Nottingham, UK

Oluseyi Hotonu
Specialist Registrar in
Genitourinary Medicine
Newcastle General Hospital
Newcastle upon Tyne, UK

Robin Illingworth
Consultant in Emergency
Medicine
St James's University Hospital
Leeds, UK

Philip Ind
Consultant Respiratory Physician
Faculty of Medicine
Imperial College
London, UK

James Kennedy
University Lecturer in Geratology
and Stroke Medicine
University of Oxford
Oxford, UK

Neil Kitchen
Consultant Neurosurgeon
National Hospital for Neurology &
Neurosurgery
London, UK

Ravi Kulkarni
Consultant Urological Surgeon
St Peter's Hospital,
Surrey, UK

George Laking
Consultant Oncologist
Auckland City Hospital
Auckland,
New Zealand

Michael Leahy
Consultant Medical Oncologist
Christie Hospital NHS Trust
Manchester, UK

Martin Lewis
Specialist Registrar in Haematology
Addenbrooke's Hospital
Cambridge, UK

Tim Littlewood
Consultant Haematologist
John Radcliffe Hospital
Oxford, UK

Diana Lockwood
Consultant Physician and
Professor of Tropical Medicine
University College London
Hospital and London School
of Hygiene & Tropical Medicine
London, UK

Robert Marcus
Consultant Haematologist
King's College Hospital
London, UK

Simon Milburn
Consultant Radiologist
James Cook University Hospital
Middlesbrough, UK

Jonathan Miles
Specialist Registrar in Orthopaedic
Surgery
Royal National Orthopaedic
Hospital
London, UK

Niall Moore
University Lecturer in Radiology
John Radcliffe Hospital
Oxford, UK

Neal Navani
Senior Clinical Fellow in
Respiratory Medicine
University College Hospital
London, UK

Agbor Ndip
Clinical Research Fellow in
Diabetes & Endocrinology
Manchester Royal Infirmary
Manchester, UK

Jane Ng
Specialist Registrar in Neurosurgery
National Hospital for Neurology &
Neurosurgery
London, UK

David O'Brien
Interventional Cardiology Fellow
Royal Alexandra Hospital
Alberta, Canada

James O'Hara
Specialist Registrar in
Otorhinolaryngology
The Freeman Hospital
Newcastle upon Tyne, UK

Vittorio Perricone
Consultant Vascular Surgeon
Blackpool Victoria Hospital
Blackpool, UK

Joan Pitkin
Consultant Obstetrician &
Gynaecologist
Northwick Park Hospital
Harrow, UK

James Price
Consultant in Community
Geriatrics and General
Internal Medicine
John Radcliffe Hospital
Oxford, UK

Jonathan Price
Clinical Tutor in Psychiatry
University of Oxford
Oxford, UK

John Salmon
Consultant Ophthalmologist
Oxford Eye Hospital
Oxford, UK

Nathan Sankar
Consultant in Genitourinary
Medicine
Newcastle Primary Care Trust
Newcastle upon Tyne, UK

John Sear
Nuffield Department of
Anaesthetics
John Radcliffe Hospital
Oxford, UK

John Senior
Faculty of History
Linacre College
Oxford, UK

David Simpson
Specialist Registrar in
Neurology
Western General Hospital
Edinburgh, UK

John Skinner
Senior Lecturer and Consultant
Orthopaedic Surgeon
Institute of Orthopaedics
Middlesex, UK

Neil Soni
Consultant in Intensive Care and
Anaesthesia
Chelsea and Westminster
Hospital
London, UK

Sarah Stirling
Specialist Registrar in Intensive
Care & Anaesthesia
London, UK

Julian Sutton
Consultant in Medical Microbiology
& Infectious Diseases
South East Regional HPA Laboratory
Southampton General Hospital
Southampton, UK

Matthew Taylor
Wellcome Trust Research
Training Fellow
University Department of
Psychiatry
Oxford, UK

Peter Taylor
Professor of Experimental
Rheumatology
Kennedy Institute of Rheumatology
Imperial College Healthcare NHS
Trust
London, UK

Lyndal Trevena
Senior Lecturer and General
Practitioner
The University of Sydney
Sydney, Australia

Clare van Halsema
Specialist Registrar in Infectious
Diseases
North Manchester General
Hospital
Manchester, UK

Richard Warren
Clinical Lecturer in
Dermatology
Manchester Dermatology
Centre
Salford, UK

Chris Watson
Reader in Transplantation Surgery
Addenbrooke's Hospital
Cambridge, UK

Ed Wilkins
Consultant Physician in Infectious
Diseases
North Manchester General
Hospital
Manchester, UK

Janet Wilson
Professor of Otolaryngology &
Head and Neck Surgery
University of Newcastle
Newcastle upon Tyne, UK

Christopher Winearls
Consultant Renal Physician
Oxford Kidney Unit
Oxford Radcliffe Hospital
NHS Trust
Oxford, UK

Sing Yang Soon
Specialist Registrar in
Cardiothoracic Surgery
Wythenshawe Hospital
Manchester, UK

Symbols and abbreviations

+ve	positive
−ve	negative
°	degree
%	percentage
±	with or without
=	equal to
>	greater than
<	less than
≥	equal to or greater than
≤	equal to or less than
α	alpha
β	beta
γ	gamma
®	registered
™	trademark symbol
A&E	accident and emergency
AAA	abdominal aortic aneurysm
ABG	arterial blood gas
ABPI	ankle–brachial pressure index
ABVD	adriamycin, bleomycin, vinblastine, dacarbazine
ACBM	doxoubicin, carmustine, cyclophosphamide, melphalan
ACC	American College of Cardiology
ACE	angiotensin-converting enzyme
ACL	anterior cruciate ligament
ACR	American College of Rheumatology
ACS	acute coronary syndrome
ACT	abstinence contingent treatment
ADL	activities of daily living
AED	anti-epileptic drug; automatic external defibrillator
AHA	American Heart Association
AHI	apnoea/hypopnoea index
AI	aromatase inhibitor
ALI	acute lung injury
ALL	acute lymphoblastic leukaemia

ALS	amyotrophic lateral sclerosis
ALT	alanine transaminase
AMD	age-related macular degeneration
AML	acute myeloblastic leukaemia
ANCA	anti-neutrophil cytoplasmic antigen
AOM	acute otitis media
APACHE	acute physiology and chronic health evaluation
APC	activated protein C
APTT	activated partial thromboplastin time
ARDS	acute respiratory distress syndrome
ARF	acute renal failure
ART	antiretroviral therapy
ASA	acetylsalicylic acid
AST	aspartate transaminase
ASTRO	American Society for Therapeutic Oncology and Radiology
ATRA	all transretinoic acid
AUA	American Urological Association
AUC	area under curve
AUR	acute urinary retention
AZA	azathioprine
BAS	brief anxiety scale
BASDAI	Bath ankylosing spondylitis disease activity index
BASFI	Bath ankylosing spondylitis functional index
BASMI	Bath ankylosing spondylitis metrology index
bd	*bis in die* (twice daily)
BDP	beclomethasone diproprionate
BIS	bispectral index
BMI	body mass index
BMS	bare metal stent
BMT	bone marrow transplant
BP	blood pressure; bullous pemphigoid
BPH	benign prostatic hyperplasia
BSA	body surface area
BSCVA	best spectacle-corrected visual acuity
CABG	coronary artery bypass graft
CAD	coronary artery disease
CAPD	chronic ambulatory peritoneal dialysis
CBD	common bile duct
CBT	cognitive behavioural therapy

CCF	congestive cardiac failure
CD	cluster of differentiation
CDRQ	chronic respiratory disease questionnaire
CEA	carotid endarterectomy
CFS	chronic fatigue syndrome
cfu	colony forming units
CHOP	cyclophosphamide, doxorubicin, vincristine, prednisolone
CI	confidence interval
CKD	chronic kidney disease
cm	centimetre
CML	chronic myeloid leukaemia
CNI	calcineurin inhibitor
CNVM	choroidal neovascular membranes
CO_2	carbon dioxide
COPD	chronic obstructive pulmonary disease
COX	cyclooxygenase
CPAP	continuous positive airways pressure
CPRS	comprehensive psychiatric rating scale
CRC	colorectal cancer
CRP	C-reactive protein
CRS	chronic rhinosinusitis
CS	caesarean section
CSF	cerebrospinal fluid
CSM	Committee on Safety of Medicines
CSMO	clinically significant macular oedema
CSS	clinical severity score
CSU	catheter-sampled urine
CT	computed tomography
CTA	CT angiography
CTPA	CT pulmonary angiogram
C-VAMP	cyclophosphamide, vincristine, doxorubicin, and methylpred
CVC	central venous catheter/catheterisation
d	day(s)
3D	three-dimensional
DAS	disease activity score
DAS-28	28 joint disease activity score
dB	decibel
DCIS	ductal carcinoma *in situ*
DDH	developmental dysplasia of the hip

D-HAQ	Dutch version of the health assessment questionnaire
DHP	Dix–Hallpike
DIC	disseminated intravascular coagulation
DKH	diskhaler
dL	decilitre
DLBCL	diffuse large B-cell lymphoma
DM	diabetes mellitus
DMSA	dimercaptosuccinic acid
DNA	deoxyribonucleic acid
DO_2	O_2 delivery
DP	dipyridamole
DRE	digital rectal examination
DSA	digital subtraction angiography
DSM	diagnostic and statistical manual of mental disorders
DTG	double Tubigrip® bandage
DVT	deep vein thrombosis
EBM	evidence-based medicine
EBP	epidural blood patch
EBRT	external beam radiotherapy
ECG	electrocardiogram
ECOG	Eastern Cooperative Oncology Group
ECT	electroconvulsive therapy
ED	emergency department
EDTA	ethylenediamine-tetraacetic acid
EEG	electroencephalogram
EFS	event-free survival
e.g	for example
EGDT	early goal-directed therapy
EGFR	estimated glomerular filtration rate
ELISA	enzyme-linked immunosorbant assay
EM	Epley's manoeuvre
EMS	emergency medical services
ENT	ear, nose, and throat
Epo	erythropoietin
ERCP	endoscopic retrograde cholangio-pancreatography
ES	early stabilisation
ESR	erythrocyte sedimentation rate
ESRD	end-stage renal disease
ESRF	end-stage renal failure
ESS	endoscopic sinus surgery
ESWL	extracorporeal shock wave lithotripsy

EVAR	endovascular aneurysm repair
FDA	(US) Food and Drug Administration
FDP	flexor digitorum profundus
FDS	flexor digitorum superficialis
FEV_1	forced expiratory volume in 1 second
FFS	failure-free survival
FISH	fluorescent *in situ* hybridisation
FOB	faecal occult blood
F/U	follow-up
FVC	forced vital capacity
GCS	Glasgow coma score
G-CSF	granulocyte-colony stimulating factor
GFR	glomerular filtration rate
GI	gastrointestinal
GP	general practitioner
Gy	gray
h	hour
HA	hydroxyapatite
HAART	highly active antiretroviral therapy
HAD	hospital anxiety and depression
HAQ	health assessment questionnaire
Hb	haemoglobin
HBC	hepatitis B virus
HbF	foetal haemoglobin
HCV	hepatitis C virus
HDL	high-density lipoprotein
HDU	high dependency unit
HFSS	heart failure survival score
Hg	mercury
HHD	handheld Doppler
HIFU	high intensity focused ultrasound
HIV	human immunodeficiency virus
HR	hazard ratio
HRQOL	health-related quality of life
HRT	hormone replacement therapy
HSV	herpes simplex virus
HZV	herpes zoster virus
ICA	internal carotid artery
ICS	inhaled corticosteroid
ICU	intensive care unit
IDDM	insulin-dependent diabetes mellitus

IIEF	international index of erectile function
IL-2	interleukin-2
IL-2R	interleukin-2 receptor
IM	intramuscular
IMA	internal mammary artery
INR	international normalised ratio
IOP	intra-ocular pressure
IPD	individual patient data
IPI	international prognostic index
IPSS	international prostate symptom score
ISS	injury severity score
IV	intravenous
IVC	inferior vena cava
IVU	intravenous urography
kg	kilogram
KPS	Karnofsky performance score
KUB	kidney, ureter, and bladder
L	litre
LABA	long-acting β-agonist
LAD	left axis deviation
LASIK	laser-assisted in situ keratomileusis
LDH	lactate dehydrogenase
LDL	low-density lipoprotein
LFA-3	leucocyte function associated antigen-type 3
LHRH	luteinising hormone releasing hormone
LMWH	low molecular weight heparin
LOC	loss of consciousness
LOCM	low osmolality contrast media
LS	late stabilisation
LSCS	lower segment caesarean section
LTOT	long-term oxygen therapy
LUTS	lower urinary tract symptoms
LV	left ventricle
LVRS	lung volume reduction surgery
MADRS	Mattis dementia rating scale
MAP	mean arterial pressure
MARP	maximum anal resting pressure
MCA	minimum cross-sectional area
mcg	microgram
MCV	mean cell volume
MDI	metre dose inhaler

MDR	multi-drug resistance
MDRD	modification of diet in renal disease
mg	milligram
MGMT	O^6-methylguanine DNA methyltransferase
MHI	minimal head injury
MI	myocardial infarction
MIC	minimal inhibitory concentration
min	minute
miu	million international unit
mL	milliliter
mm	millimeter
MMF	mycophenolate mofetil
mmHg	millimeter of mercury
mmol	millimole
MOD	multiple organ dysfunction
MOF	multi-organ failure
MOPP	mechlorethamine, vincristine, procarbazine, prednisolone
MRC	Medical Research Council
MRI	magnetic resonance imaging
MRS	mandibular repositioning splints
MRSA	methicillin-resistant *Staphylococcus aureus*
MS	multiple sclerosis
MSU	midstream urine
MU	million units
MUGA	multiple-gated acquisition
6MWD	6 minute walk distance
MWT	maintenance of wakefulness test
NAPSI	nail psoriasis severity index
NCC	neurocysticercosis
nCPAP	nasal continuous positive airways pressure
ng	nanogram
NHL	non-Hodgkin's lymphoma
NHS	National Health Service
NICE	National Institute for Health and Clinical Excellence
NIV	non-invasive ventilation
NNT	number needed to treat
NO	nitric oxide
NPV	negative predictive value
NRT	nicotine replacement therapy
ns	not significant

NSAID	non-steroidal anti-inflammatory drug
NSCLC	non-small cell lung cancer
NSTEMI	non-ST elevation myocardial infarction
NYHA	New York Heart Association
O_2	oxygen
od	*omni die* (once daily)
ODI	Oswestry disability index
OE	otitis externa
OHS	ocular histoplasmosis
OHT	ocular hypertension
OME	otitis media with effusion
OR	odds ratio
OS	overall survival
OSA	obstructive sleep apnoea
PAC	pulmonary artery catheter
P_aCO_2	arterial pressure of carbon dioxide
PAH	pulmonary arterial hypertension
PAP	pulmonary artery pressure
PASI	psoriasis area severity index
PC	primary care
PC-BPPV	posterior canal benign paroxysmal positional vertigo
PCI	percutaneous coronary intervention
PCOS	polycystic ovary syndrome
PD	Parkinson's disease; peritoneal dialysis
PDE	phosphodiesterase
PDPH	post-dural puncture headache
PDQ	Parkinson's disease questionnaire
PE	pulmonary embolism
PEEP	positive end expiratory pressure
PEF	peak expiratory flow
PI	protease inhibitor
PO	*per os* (by mouth)
POAG	primary open angle glaucoma
PONV	postoperative nausea and vomiting
PPI	proton pump inhibitor
pProm	preterm prelabour rupture of membranes
PPV	positive predictive value
PRK	photorefractive keratectomy
PRP	pan-retinal photocoagulation
PSA	prostate specific antigen
PUVA	psoralen UVA

PVP	photo-selective vaporisation
qds	*quater die sumendus* (four times daily)
RBBB	right bundle branch block
RCC	renal cell carcinoma
RCM	red cell mass
RCT	randomised controlled trial
RICE	rest, ice, compression, elevation
ROSC	return of spontaneous circulation
RPA	recursive partitioning analysis
RR	relative risk
RRR	relative risk reduction
RRT	renal replacement therapy
RT	radiotherapy
rTPA	recombinant tissue plasminogen activator
RV	residual volume
s	second
SAHS	sleep apnoea/hypopnoea syndrome
SaO_2	arterial oxygen saturation
SASSAD	six area six sign atopic eczema score
SC	subcutaneous
SCT	saccharine clearance test
SF	sapheno-femoral junction
SF36	short form-36
SFA	superficial femoral artery
SGRQ	St George's Respiratory Questionnaire
SIGN	Scottish Intercollegiate Guideline Network
SIRS	systemic inflammatory response syndrome
SMG	self-management group
SNOT 20	Sinonasal Outcome Test-20
SPL	spontaneous preterm labour
SRS	stereotactic radiosurgery
SSI	surgical site infection
SSIH	spontaneous supratentorial intracerebral haemorrhage
SSRI	selective serotonin reuptake inhibitor
SST	short synacthen test
STEMI	ST elevation myocardial infarction
STN	subthalamic nucleus
SVR	sustained virological response
SWOG	Southwest Oncology Group
TAD	tip-apex distance
TAT	traditional asthma treatment

TB	tuberculosis
Tc99m	technetium 99m
TDI	transition dyspnoea index
tds	*ter die sumendus* (three times daily)
TIA	transient ischaemic attack
TIVA	total IV anaesthesia
TLC	total lung capacity
TME	total mesorectal excision
TPMT	thiopurine methyl transferase
TRUS	transrectal ultrasound
TTGA	tissue transglutaminase antibody
TURP	transurethral resection of the prostate
TVT	tension-free vaginal tape
U	unit
UCVA	uncorrected visual acuity
UFH	unfractionated heparin
UK	United Kingdom
UPDRS	unified Parkinson's disease rating scale
US	ultrasonography
USA	United States of America
UTI	urinary tract infection
UVPP	uvulopalatopharyngoplasty
VA	visual acuity
VAC	vacuum-assisted closure
VAS	visual analogue score
VEGF	vascular endothelial growth factor
VF	ventricular fibrillation; visual field
VL	viral load
VLDL	very low density lipoprotein
V/Q	ventilation/perfusion
VR	vestibular rehabilitation
VT	ventricular tachycardia
VTE	venous thromboembolism
VUR	vesicoureteral reflux
WBC	white blood cells
WBRT	whole brain radiation therapy
WCC	white cell count
WHO	World Health Organisation
wk	week
y	year

How to use this book

Introduction

With growing emphasis on evidence-based medicine (EBM), there is a need for all healthcare professionals to be aware of the important evidence that shapes their clinical practice. While several sources (ranging from internet databases to journals) exist to house the vast number of articles published everyday, approaching these can be daunting. For the uninitiated, literature searching is a tiresome and complex process, especially as it can be difficult to determine which studies are significant and clinically relevant without prerequisite specialist knowledge. Furthermore, even if the reader is aware of the importance of a particular study, navigating the complexities of its methodology and accurately evaluating its results to arrive at the correct conclusions can be an equally frustrating task. In the modern era, time constraints make this an even greater challenge, leaving many just 'reading the abstract' and at times inappropriately applying the authors' conclusions into their clinical practice.

This book has been written by experts in each specialty to provide a simple and fast search tool for locating relevant key clinical evidence. A brief critique of the important and salient points of each trial is also provided. This serves as a 'rapid learning aid' for those who want to understand more about the landmark clinical trials in a specialty without having to trawl through vast amounts of material. There will be those who gasp in horror at this unashamedly simple stripping down of evidence. Others may question the selection of certain studies. However, making EBM amenable to all requires a degree of ruthlessness in the selection and presentation of trials and their data. We hope that the reader will gain an understanding of the underlying process behind EBM through analysis of the trial methodologies and outcomes of the notable studies considered in this book, allowing future research to be conducted and scrutinised at a similarly high level.

Layout and formatting

This book is divided into two sections, medicine and surgery, each incorporating their respective sub-specialties. Individual chapters contain landmark trials that have influenced practice in that specialty, and are subdivided according to conventional disease groupings. Allocation of trials to individual chapters has not been an easy task, in particular due to considerable overlap between topics. Thus, although we have grouped similarly themed trials where possible, in some cases topics have been placed within the specialty most relevant to daily clinical practice (e.g. deep vein thrombosis in Emergency Medicine).

In order to maintain consistency, we have applied a broadly standardised two-page template for the analysis of individual trials. All spellings are in British English, with internationally agreed nomenclature whenever multiple variations have arisen (e.g. names of drugs). Country of origin-specific references, e.g. to the UK's National Institute for Health and Clinical Excellence (NICE) or Royal Colleges, have only been included when necessary to convey the impact of a study.

Trial selection

In a book of this nature, the personal preferences of our expert contributors are inherent in the selection of studies. However, in order to ensure a consistent approach and to minimise selection bias, we presented several criteria:

- *Need for impact:* a paper must have made (or must have the future potential to make) a significant impact on clinical practice.
- *Important topics:* trials should relate to the key issues/diseases in the specialty and not to more esoteric and/or less clinically relevant topics, particularly those less relevant to non-specialist audiences.
- *Sound methodology:* level 1b evidence (randomised controlled trials (RCTs) from peer-reviewed journals) whenever possible. Lower quality evidence permitted if it is influential.
- *Number of trials:* maximum of 25 trials per chapter (with some understandable variation between different specialties).
- *Discussion with peers:* authors were requested to consult with colleagues when selecting and interpreting trials.

It is important to note that this book is not intended to be a collection of evidence-based protocols for guiding all aspects of clinical management; textbooks such as the *Oxford Handbook of Clinical Medicine* already serve this purpose. Furthermore, with the aim of focusing upon therapeutic intervention, there are a number of notable exclusions. These include standalone scientific discoveries (the discovery of penicillin did not come about as a result of a methodologically sound trial!), epidemiological associations (e.g. Sir Richard Doll's pioneering work establishing the relationship between smoking and lung cancer), and scoring systems/severity criteria (e.g. development of Wells' criteria for deep vein thrombosis or the CURB-65 prognostic score for pneumonia).

The primary focus of this book is the RCT. There are several other important resources that focus on meta-analysis, as it is these that largely drive treatment decisions. However, with meta-analyses relying upon high quality RCTs to drive them, the increasing focus often placed upon level 1a evidence can often leave the RCT to fall by the wayside. RCTs with rigorous methodology that are sufficiently powered to detect statistical differences in clearly defined outcomes are vital in ensuring bias limitation and appropriate application of evidence to practice. This book serves as a 'Who's Who' of those RCTs that have stood the test of scrutiny and time, and have led to an evidence-based change in clinical practice. These trials are presented with a brief discussion of a much wider context; isolated application of the result of individual RCTs to clinical practice is not recommended. For a treatment-related approach to clinical evidence, resources such as the *Cochrane Collaboration* and the *British Medical Journal's Clinical Evidence* are to be commended for bringing EBM from the academic to the clinician. Direct applicability of evidence to diagnostic and therapeutic practices is increasingly supported by excellent guidelines from national bodies, e.g. the American Heart Association or the British Thoracic Society. In the UK, evidence-based 'best practice' guidelines are also presented by the various Royal Colleges. However, overcoming financial hurdles and time constraints is often required before these translate to the guidelines recommended by individual centres.

Although our contributors have had the entirety of the vast clinical literature from which to select their trials (over 3,000 medical journals exist with over 17 million citations on Medline), it is no surprise that a considerable number of those featured in this book hail from journals such as the *Lancet*, *New England Journal of Medicine*, *Journal of the American Medical Association* or the *British Medical Journal*. It is possible that their wide readership and high impact factor (a measure based upon citations, first proposed in the 1960s) have in themselves led to a selection bias, both for the purposes of this book as well as for literature reviews undertaken beyond the confines of this text. This places an important responsibility upon the shoulders of their editors with regard to the maintenance of high standards. Interestingly, although citations are a useful tool for tracking the progress of research, studies have shown little correlation between highly cited papers and their ranking by experts decades later, perhaps due to poor papers being cited repeatedly for their notorious flaws. Extrapolation of clinical evidence to clinical practice must therefore be undertaken with care and only applied to relevant populations; independent review of the results, alongside the various indices for rating the quality and strength of evidence-based recommendations (e.g. GRADE system), are helpful practical tools.

Limitations

Recognition of the remit and limitation of a study is an important attribute to be considered when interpreting its results. In this regard, our book is no exception, with some understandable limitations of its own. Foremost, perhaps, is space; we have, at times, had to be somewhat brutal in our selection of trials in order to allow space for the range of specialties encompassed within this book. This is, therefore, far from an exhaustive selection of all the important trials that exist in the literature. Furthermore, studies are usually reported as medium length articles in the medical literature (typically around 3,000–4,000 words); this book only provides a two-page summary of each paper, not the complete picture.

Our many contributors have provided their interpretation of published data in good faith, and in keeping with their understanding of best practice within their specialty. However, the medical literature is not perfect. At times, the quality of evidence is limited through no fault of the researchers. This is particularly the case for some surgical topics, where RCTs cannot always be conducted and may sometimes be inappropriate. Therefore, the onus is on all evidence-based practitioners to critically appraise the available literature. Clinical research is not infallible and errors of judgement are often made. The correction of errors and the withdrawal of both papers themselves and the therapeutic agents they test are not unheard of.

Evidence is nothing without its interpretation in the appropriate context. We therefore recommend that readers who wish to consider the results of individual studies use the analysis in the book not in isolation, but as an adjunct to the original literature. The summaries will highlight the key aspects of the findings, while the original papers will provide a fuller understanding of the context and any further analysis/limitations. The interpretation of medical statistics is an art as well as a science. This is often the aspect of EBM that frightens most casual observers; in this regard, the statistical significance of the results presented in this book has been presented in a simplified form for clarity. Readers should consider the summaries in conjunction with the more detailed statistical analysis presented in the original paper. In an era of cost cutting, the financial implications of any findings should also be considered.

Of final note is an understandable concern that the book could rapidly become out of date. While there may have been some important studies published between editing and publication, we feel that our selection criterion requiring a study to have made notable impact upon practice will have minimised this; while new research emerges daily, only a very small percentage achieves landmark status. Indeed, it is often only several years later that the relative clinical importance of a trial becomes established.

What makes a good study?

Our other introductory chapters answer this question from a more historical and technical perspective. However, after review of the 1,000+ trials considered for this book, a number of more basic attributes have emerged that make the study of EBM considerably more palatable from a reader's perspective. In particular, we applaud those that exude intrinsic simplicity from the outset, for example, by using consistency of layout; and straightforward and concise wording to explain concepts; and clear diagrams, tables, and flow charts to show participant progression and results. Furthermore, all data must be accounted for; for example, the reasons for participant withdrawal must be explicitly stated. Perplexing one's readers is not a mark of scientific prowess, and it is surprising how many studies have chosen to hide their findings behind a guise of complexity. One wonders whether this is in order to mask poor methodology or simply due to poor author understanding. It is precisely this unnecessary complexity and poor presentation that makes EBM an unapproachable subject for many. The editorial efforts of leading journals to standardise and simplify their formats have been a welcome stride in incorporating EBM into everyday practice. It is our hope that this book will take this process a step further.

With a need to focus on the methodology of individual studies, and through space constraints, we have made limited consideration of the ethical and conflict of interest issues that surround scientific research. Consent and ethical approval are key areas that must underlie all research, the principles of which are now established in various international guidelines (Nuremberg code, Declaration of Helsinki), as well as through the work of various bodies (e.g. UK's Nuffield Council on Bioethics). Despite guidelines, some claim that research conveying favourable outcomes (particularly when influenced by those with a conflict of interest, such as association with a pharmaceutical company) is more likely to be published than a study reporting negative findings. Furthermore, there is not always correlation between the actual results of trials/meta-analysis and the conclusions drawn by the authors. The source of such bias is unclear, but must be overcome. Similarly, a solution is not easy; restriction of corporate funding may lead to a significant decrease in research activity.

Controversy is inherent to scientific study, and both the media and researchers have a moral obligation to ensure that the public are reminded that snippets of discussion do not necessarily translate to straightforward conclusions. Deliberate reporting of misleading and biased information in order to produce attention-grabbing headlines is a dangerous game and serves only to yield unrealistic expectations; public scandals should not deter research. The studies presented in this book serve as a reminder of the overall victory of balanced scientific endeavour and of the evolving practice of EBM.

Chapter 1

The history of evidence-based medicine

The nature of evidence

'The words of a dialectician are like a spider's web: of no practical value but a triumph of ingenuity' (Aristotle)

The pursuit of tests for therapeutic interventions has been a characteristic of Western medicine since ancient times. Whereas Eastern medical systems centred on wisdom and tradition, the West centred on the known, how it was constituted (methodology), and expertise. The 'stasis' of Chinese and Hindu medical systems reflected the civil and moral orders of their respective cosmologies. However, 'physis', the Greek for 'nature' or 'change' from which we get the term 'physics', reflected the West's.[1]

Nature could be in hiding or personify the essence of things as in the veiled Egyptian goddess, Isis, or the Roman goddess of Nature, Diana. In a world of constant change, the veil of Isis could be lifted or Diana's secrets discovered by the arts ('techne') and the sciences.[2]

Such attitudes towards Nature characterised the founding of modern experimental science in the 17th century in which Nature was a laboratory and could be brought to court, interrogated, and if necessary, tortured. However, during the Romantic era, an opposing vision of Nature arose. Nature had her secrets but she was not veiled. The shutters were in our eyes for not seeing Nature outright.

Overview of the history of clinical trials

Historical accounts of the clinical trial are usually expressed through the lens of presentism: how the various components of the first modern randomised controlled trial (RCT)—the comparison, blinding, and randomisation—culminated in Austin Bradford Hill's 1946 trial of streptomycin for tuberculosis. Accounts include the first references to comparative approaches; therapeutic assessments, e.g. (rich vs plain diet in the Bible); James Lind's 18th century controlled trial of citrus fruit for scurvy; the recognition of the importance of suggestion or confidence in the treatment effect in both patient and practitioner, with subsequent adoption of blinding and placebos in trials of animal magnetism and homeopathy in the 18th and 19th centuries; and later quantification and randomisation to remove bias in the 19th and 20th centuries.[3]

The factual context of the development of the RCT is important if only to emphasise the historicity of contemporary research methodology. However, the adoption of the various components of the trial at any one time has as much to do with changing socio-political and ethical contexts as the 'objective' scientific standards of evidence. Evidence is not just scientific data floating in some ethereal medium, but is linked to facts and beliefs of the various members of diverse medical communities who interpret evidence and deploy it to legitimise various strategies.

References

1. Bates D (ed.) (1995). Knowledge and the Scholarly Tradition (Cambridge University Press) p. xvii.
2. Hacking I (2007). 'Almost zero' - Review of Hadot P, The Veil of Isis: An Essay on the History of the Ideas of Nature. Translated by M Chase (Harvard 2006) - LRB 29, p.29–30.
3. Bull J (1959). The Historical Development of Clinical Therapeutic Trials. *Journal of Chronic Disease* 19: 218–258.

Making comparisons

From physic to medicine

The terms 'physic' and 'medicine' denote two separate traditions in medicine: one based on learning and preservation of health, the other based on experience and curing.[1]

The ancient notion of 'physic' (meaning 'nature') characterised the physician's art. The aim was to advise right living in accordance with nature, based upon Galen's humoral principles of blood, phlegm, black and yellow bile. A balance of these denoted health, and an imbalance, 'dyscrasis' (ill health). The focus was on regulating the six non-naturals— food and drink, the environment, evacuations, sleep, exercise, and state of mind—in order to maintain natural body balance. Herbal concoctions and bloodletting practices restored the humoral imbalance. Ancient pharmacology could boast some 760 medicinal plants and herbs as well as rules to adjudicate their effectiveness. A drug needed to be pure and work in all cases of the disease, with its effectiveness corresponding to dose and strength. Testing a drug's effectiveness in humans under different conditions was a 'final trial'.[2]

'Medico', derived from the Latin 'to drug' or 'dye', emphasised the ability to treat disease with drugs. Its adoption coincided with the rise of the new experimental philosophy in the 17th century associated with Isaac Newton, Robert Boyle, Francis Bacon, and René Descartes.

New remedies, such as the cinchona bark from South America, and the new chemical remedies introduced earlier by Paracelsus, (including mercury, arsenic, iron, lead, and sulphur) challenged traditional medicine. William Withering's discovery of foxglove (digitalis) for dropsy and Edward Jenner's vaccination against smallpox in the 18th century reinforced the curative aspect of medicine. Indeed, in his utopian fantasy, New Atlantis (1627), were not Francis Bacon's 'Compilers' and 'Lamps' the forerunners of the UK's National Institute for Health and Clinical Excellence (NICE)? He wrote:

> 'We have three [practitioners] that draw the experiments of the former four [the 'Pioneers' or 'Miners'] into titles and tables to give better light for the drawing of observations and axioms out of them [and] Lamps [who] direct new experiments of a higher light.'

Primacy of clinical experience

What was crucial to good practice in both traditions was 'clinical experience'—whether using countless remedies associated with 'empirics', or those conforming to Galen's experiences. The great Muslim physician, Rhazes (AD 865–925) believed the experience of one wise doctor was worth more than all of what was written in books:

> 'So when you see these symptoms, then proceed with bloodletting. For I once saved one group [of patients] by it, while I intentionally neglected [to bleed] another group. By doing that, I wished to reach a conclusion.'

Making comparisons was essential to assessing the efficacy of treatment. In his 1364 'Letter to Bocaccio', the humanist, Petrarch, went one step further in his critique of Galenic depletive remedies:

> 'I solemnly affirm and believe, if a hundred or a thousand men of the same age, same temperament and habits, together with the same surroundings,

were attacked at the same time by the same disease, that if one half followed the prescriptions of the doctors of the variety of those practising at the present day, and that the other half took no medicine but relied on Nature's instincts, I have no doubt as to which half would escape.'

The first reference to randomisation

Several hundred years later, in 1662, the iatrochemist, JB Van Helmont, upped the rhetorical stakes in attacks on orthodox medicine, urging the use of lots in order to make fair comparisons:

'Let us take out of the Hospitals … 200 or 500 poor People, that have Fevers, Pleurisies, etc. Let us divide them in halfes, let us cast lots, that one half of them may fall to my share, and the other to yours; I will cure them without bloodletting and sensible evacuation; but do as you do, as ye know (for neither do I tye you up to the boasting, or of Phlebotomy, or the abstinence from a solutive Medicine) we shall see how many Funerals both of us shall have.'

The outcomes of lotteries or the roll of dice were keenly debated by Puritan divines in the 17th century; were they direct signs of God's will or determined by natural law? Van Helmont's use of lots ensured that bias was avoided in assembling the two groups. Whether he actually meant to conduct the experiment remains debatable.

Ambrose Paré: comparison in surgery

With the shift in emphasis to the curative component of medicine, surgeons too eschewed old practices and put their faith in personal observation and experience. The renowned French surgeon, Ambrose Paré, made this within patient comparison in 1575:

'A German guard was very drunk and his flask caught fire and caused great damage to his hands and face, and I was called to dress him. I applied onions to one half of his face and the usual remedies to the other. At the second dressing I found the side where I had applied the onions to have no blisters nor scarring and the other side to be all blistered.'

More famously, Paré determined that the use of cautery was otiose to the outcome of gunshot wounds—much to the relief of the victims:

'At last I ran out of oil and was constrained to apply a digestive made of egg yolk, oil of roses and turpentine. That night I could not sleep easily thinking that by the default in cautery I would find the wounded to whom I had failed to apply the said oil dead of poisoning; and this made me get up at first light to visit them. Beyond my hopes I found those on whom I had put the digestive dressing feeling little pain from their wounds, which were not swollen or inflamed, and having spent quite a restful night. But the others, to whom the said oil had been applied, I found fevered, with great pain and swelling around their wounds.'

References

1. Cook H (1990). The New Philosophy and Medicine in Seventeenth Century England (in Lindberg D and Westman R (Eds.) - Reappraisals of the Scientfic Revolution) (Cambridge University Press) - p.397–436.
2. Darmani N Avicenna. *Journal of Islamic Medical Association of North America* 1995; 26: 78–81.

The first prospective controlled trial

In 1747, the naval surgeon, James Lind, used comparative groups to assess the correct treatment for scurvy while on board his ship, the Salisbury. He published his 'A treatise on the scurvy' in 1753 and is rightly considered to be the pioneer of the first prospective, controlled clinical trial.

Scurvy was considered to be a putrid disease of the blood associated with moist air that blocked perspiration, and had long plagued long sea voyages. The practice of doling out citrus fruit as an anti-inflammatory potion had been adopted by the Portuguese since the 16th century. Sir Captain James Lancaster, working for the East India Co., conducted a quasi-controlled trial as early as 1601, when the diet of one of the four ships under his command was supplemented with two teaspoons of lemon juice. It seems unlikely that this was a deliberately designed experiment— rather a situation forced by a shortage of supplies, in the tradition of Paré. Towards completion of the journey, it was noted:

'Very many of our men were fallen sicke of the scurvey in all our ships and unlesse it were in the generals ship only, the other three were so weake of men that they could hardly handle the sayles.'[1]

The three ships had acted as unintentional controls.

James Lind was well aware of the literature on scurvy when he published his own investigations. He had, in fact, conducted a systematic review. The trial was deliberately prospective in assessing the merits of six treatments:

'I took twelve patients … Their cases were as similar as I could have them. They … had putrid gums, the spots and lassitude, with weakness of the knees … They had one diet common to all … Two of them were ordered each a quarter of cider a day, Two others took twenty-five gutts of elixir of vitriol, three times a day, Two others took spoonfuls of vinegar, three times a day … Two of the worst patients were put under a course of sea water … Two others had had each two oranges and one lemon … They continued but six days under this course… The two remaining patients took … nutmeg … and an electuary … and purged three times a-day.'[2]

The pair given the citrus fruit were fit for duty six days later and put to taking care of the others who remained sick. In the face of good evidence about the effectiveness of oranges and lemons in scurvy, why did it take some 43 years before the Navy Board regularly stocked the ships with citrus fruit? The uncertain explanation of scurvy certainly played a role in its slow uptake allowing other remedies such as 'McBride's malt wort' and sauerkraut to be given equal consideration. Cumulative clinical experience and numerical record keeping in the fleet and in its hospitals during the ensuing decades allowed the clinical features of scurvy and its treatment to be better assessed. Largely through the efforts of Sir Gilbert Blane, the general issue of lemon juice finally occurred in 1795.

References

1. Anon (1601–1606). The Voyages of Sir James Lancaster to the East Indies and the Voyage of Captain John Knight (1606) to seek the North-West passage. (Hakluyt Society Publications, London, 1877).
2. Lind J (1753). A treatise of the Scurvy. (Edinburgh: Sands, Murray & Cochrane) p.192–4.

The enlightenment

Smallpox and the arithmetic tradition

An analytical approach to assessing interventions in the 18th century was taken up by the inoculators of smallpox. They stood in line with the arithmetic tradition that stemmed from numerical analysis of the London Bills of Mortality; this was initiated in the 17th century by two London tradesmen who created the notion of 'political arithmetic' or social statistics. Such bills set out the numbers and causes of death in each parish. A century later, innovative inoculators such as the Yorkshire doctor, Thomas Nettleton, published calculations of ratios of mortality to morbidity and inoculated smallpox in a number of towns. For the preceding year, Nettleton recorded a total of 3,405 cases, with 636 deaths. The 18.8% mortality rate was compared to 0% for the inoculated groups![1]

The Near and Far Eastern practice of inoculation had been introduced by Lady Mary Montagu and others a decade or so earlier. It was the first widespread intervention not only to inspire numerical assessments, but also to raise widespread concerns about safety and efficacy. Human experimentation was the test of choice. Persuaded by his daughter, Caroline, Princess of Wales, George I agreed to pardon six convicts in Newgate Prison if they agreed to volunteer for a trial of inoculation. Three men were matched with three women for age. All six survived and were subsequently pardoned. As a quasi-test of efficacy, Maitland, the doctor in charge, also arranged for one of the inoculated women in the trial to sleep next to a young smallpox victim. After six weeks of exposure, she had not fallen sick.

Smallpox inoculation became widespread by the 1750s, largely due to Princess Caroline having had her own children inoculated. However, much religious opposition accompanied the practice. From today's perspective, the data collected by Nettleton and others were imperfect, as they did not know the exposure period or the rate of the inoculated patients. Given the high incidence of natural smallpox in the 18th century, efficacy did seem to have been reasonably well established and the data gathered did represent numerical evidence for the efficacy of inoculation.[2]

References

1. Nettleton T (1724). Part of a letter from Dr Nettleton, physician at Halifax, to Dr R Jurin. 'Sec concerning the inoculation of the small pox, and the mortality of that distemper'. Transactions of the Royal Society of London (1722–1723). 32, 209–12.
2. Huth E (2005). Quantitative evidence for judgements on the efficacy of inoculation for the prevention of smallpox. England and the New England in the 1700s. The James Lind Library.

The importance of case studies

The reporting of individual case studies characterised much of 18th century medical literature in which new procedures and cures were introduced to an increasingly consumer-focused medical marketplace. William Withering was exceptional in resisting the pressures of the market and rushing to publish his first successes of treating dropsy with foxglove (digitalis). Caution prevailed until he had assembled enough evidence—156 cases over a ten-year period in 1785, he wrote:

'It would have been an easy task to have given select cases, whose successful treatment would have spoken strongly in favour of the medicine, and perhaps been flattering to my own reputation. But Truth and Science would condemn the procedure. I have therefore mentioned every case ... proper or improper, successful or otherwise.'

With equal circumspection, the Revd William Stone waited five years to announce the results of his studies on the successful treatment of rheumatic fever with willow bark (*Salix alba*).[1]

Withering was aware that factors such as age affected the outcome of his patients treated with foxglove, but it was in the work of the surgeon, William Cheselden—famous for his lithotomy operation—that a more sophisticated appreciation was realised. In an appendix to the 4th edition of 'The anatomy of the human body (1740)', he wrote:

'But what is of most consequence to be known is the ages of those who recovered, and those who died.'[2]

He grouped his 213 patients in ten-year age groups and reported the number of deaths for each group, thus showing the substantially lower mortality among children than in adults.

References

1. Stone W (1764). An account of the success of the bark of the willow in the cure of agues. Philosophical transactions of the Royal Society, 54, 195–200.
2. Quoted in: Tröhler U (2003). Cheselden's 1740 presentation of data on age-specific mortality after lithotomy. p.333. The James Lind Library.

The 19th century

Pierre Louis and 'La méthode numérique'

The 19th century Parisian physician, Pierre Louis, is credited as the founder of modern epidemiology by emphasising group comparison and population thinking in therapeutic assessments.[1]

Louis's quantitative approach was based upon a form of medical empiricism called 'sensualism', developed by the 18th century philosophers, Condillac and Cabanis. The patron saint of this cult of observation was Hippocrates—a mythical Hippocrates that had revolted against the philosophers' hypotheses and theories. Cabanis held that true causes could never be known—only relations between objects. The work of Condorcet and Laplace on probability provided the other platform for Louis's numerical method. For Louis, facts had no value unless they were enumerated. To test therapies, only groups of patients 'blindly selected' and undergoing different treatments (rather than individual cases) could yield sufficient evidence to adduce the significance of differential mortality rates.

In his own investigations, Louis found that bloodletting made no difference to the outcome of pneumonia, whether it was performed early or late, or whether large amounts were taken or not. In 1835 he wrote:

'What was to be done in order to know whether bloodletting had any favourable influence on pneumonitis, and the extent of that influence? Evidently to ascertain whether, other things being equal, the patients who were bled on the first, second, third or fourth day of their illness, recovered more readily than those bled at a later period. In the same manner, it was necessary to estimate the influence of age, or, more generally, any other circumstance, on the appreciable effects of bloodletting.'

Concerning populations, he wrote:

'For example, in any particular epidemic, let us suppose five hundred of the sick, taken indiscriminately, are subjected to one kind of treatment, and five hundred others, taken in the same manner, are treated in a different mode; if the mortality is greater among the first than among the second, must we not conclude that the treatment was less appropriate, or less efficacious in the first class than in the second? It is unavoidable; for among so large a collection, similarities of conditions will necessarily be met with, and all things being equal, the conclusion will be rigorous.'

Louis did not advocate randomised allocation of the intervention in his bloodletting study. Therefore, there remains the question of whether the early and late bloodletting groups were really comparable, given the late group had already survived the early disease stages and were subsequently more likely to have a better prognosis than those receiving the intervention in the earlier, acute stages of the disease.

References

1. Morabia A. PCA Lewis and the Birth of Clincial Epidermiology. *Journal of Clinical Epidemiology* 1996; 49: 1327–33.

Statistical developments

Size matters and confidence intervals

The numerical method linked both hospital medicine and the rise of public health in the early decades of the 19th century, and became a tool for social analysis and reform. The concept of the 'average man' was coined at the time by Adolphe Quetelet and provided a means for detached clinical judgement that only the surety of statistics could provide.

Thomas Graham Balfour's 1854 report of a clinical trial of homeopathic belladonna for scarlet fever was an early acknowledgement of the importance of sample size in the assessment of an intervention.[1] In the Royal Military Asylum at Chelsea, Balfour conducted a trial on soldiers' orphans by giving them belladonna alternatively. He noted little difference in morbidity between those who received the belladonna (2/26) and those who did not (2/75), concluding 'the numbers are too small to justify deductions as to the prophylactic power of belladonna.' Since only four boys came down with scarlet fever, no confident conclusion could be reached, thus avoiding what today would be a 'type 2' error, i.e. assumption of no difference when one exists (a false negative).

The concept of confidence interval also arose during this period, allowing chance effects to be reduced if a range of treatment differences were calculated within which real differences were likely to lie. The French physician, Gavarret, applied Poisson's probability calculation to Louis's mortality data on bloodletting, and demonstrated the weakness of the numerical method. By calculating 'the limit of possible errors', one was able to judge whether a difference between two average mortality rates in two groups of patients (each group having received different treatments) represented a true difference between the treatments. It took over 100 years for Gavarret's ideas to catch on![2]

Statistics and discontents

The rise of the Paris Hospital during the French revolutionary period provided fertile ground to develop a new theory of disease in which the clinical gaze shifted from the bedside and patient self-reporting of symptoms to the correlation of symptoms with anatomico-pathological changes. Mass observation and autopsies of the poor in Parisian hospitals increasingly confirmed this ontological trend in which disease was perceived as a real entity. Laennec used his stethoscope to observe the signs of disease, and the reification of the patient gathered momentum during the ensuing decades as technology encroached upon the doctor–patient relationship. The rise of laboratory medicine in Germany from the 1830s hastened this trend and introduced another notion of disease: a physico-chemical process explained by the blind inexorable laws of natural science. Physiological phenomena—chemicals in the blood and urine, temperature, the ratio of red and white cells, blood pressure, nerve conduction, etc.—were to be observed, measured, and defined, according to definitions of normal and abnormal.

Claude Bernard's seminal work, '*An introduction to the study of experimental medicine*' (1865), was a paean to positivism, placing physiology among the exact sciences. In reference to his own discoveries—the concept of the 'milieu intérieur' (homeostasis), the glycogenic function of the liver, the discovery of vasomotor nerves, the action of curare, and the function of the pancreatic juices, Bernard urged a strict determinism in studying disease that focused on real and effective causes. In this regard, statistics, with its use of averages, was too conjectural and indeterministic—as if a physiologist who:

> 'took urine from a railroad station urinal where people of all nations passed, and who believed he could thus present an analysis of an average European urine!'

The spectre of vitalism hovered over medicine and biology in mid-century France, and for Bernard, the future path of scientific medicine lay in 'discovering new facts, instead of trying to reduce to equations the facts which science already possesses'. Bernard provided another example of the inutility of statistics in surgery:

> 'A great surgeon performs operations for stone by a single method; later he makes a statistical summary of deaths and recoveries, and he concludes from these statistics that the mortality law for this operation is two out of five. Well, I say that this ratio means literally nothing scientifically and gives us no certainty in performing the next operation; for we do not know whether the next case will be among the recoveries or the deaths. What really should be done, instead of gathering facts empirically, is to study them more accurately, each in its special determinism … to discover in them the cause of mortal accidents so as to master the cause and avoid the accidents.'

Physiology thus provided the experimental foundations of scientific medicine—not the hospital wards where natural histories of pathological lesions were classified, nor at the sick bed where too many imponderables prevented strict scientific understanding of disease. Bernard's experimental method pointed the way to future pharmacological research, but few therapeutic spin-offs arose until the advent of Pasteurism, and later chemotherapy, in the latter half of the 19th century.

Statistics and sanitarians

In comparison to scientific medicine's promise to cure, the 'sanitary idea' had already produced dividends by the 1860s in preventing disease, especially in crowded cities. In the summer of 1854, believing an outbreak of cholera was due to contaminated water supply, the London doctor, John Snow, urged the Parish guardians in Soho to remove the handle of the Broad Street pump. The number of cases plummeted, thus confirming his theory that cholera was due to a waterborne organism. A pioneer in medical cartography, Snow's work proved seminal in promoting public health measures to ensure healthier lives for Londoners through efficient waste disposal and clean water supplies.[3]

Snow's dramatic evidence contrasted sharply with Semmelweis, a Hungarian physician, who demonstrated the principle of antisepsis prior to Joseph Lister's landmark 1867 publication on the use of carbolic acid in surgery. Semmelweis, attached to the Vienna Krankenhaus (the largest maternity hospital in the world), proved that puerperal fever could be reduced in the maternity wards if medical teams washed their hands between the autopsy and delivery rooms. His evidence was based upon a retrospective, accidentally controlled trial. Between 1840 and 1846,

Semmelweis noted mortality rates from childbed fever were 98/1,000 in the ward staffed by doctors and medical students, but only 36/1,000 in the ward staffed by midwives. With large numbers involved (nearly 43,000 births and some 300 deaths), he knew these findings were not due to chance. The explanation? Simple hand hygiene. As midwives did not conduct autopsies, Semmelweis insisted medical men washed their hands before examining patients on the maternity wards. The chloride of lime hand wash cut the death rate to 13/1,000.[4]

Semmelweis was not the ideal publicist of his findings. Mentally unstable, he ended up in an asylum. He was insensitive to professional etiquette and polemic in his dealings with colleagues who viewed his major work '*Etiology, concept and prophylaxis of childbed fever*' (1860) as good, sound, practical advice in the sanitary tradition, but nothing extraordinary.[5]

References

1. Chalmers I, Toth B (2002). Thomas Graham Balfour's 1854 report of a clinical trial of belladonna given to prevent scarlet fever. The James Lind Library.
2. Gavarret L (1840). Principes généraux de statistique médicale: ou développement des règales qui doivent présider à son emploi. Paris: Bechet Jeune and Labé.
3. Snow J (1855). On the mode of the Communication of the Cholera. WH Frost (ed Snow on Cholera) (New York 1936).
4. Semmelweiss I (1860). Etiology, Concept and Prophylaxis of Childbed Fever. Trans Murphy F. (Medical Classics 1941).
5. Loudon I (2002). Ignaz Philip Semmelweiss' studies of Death in Childbirth. The James Lind Library.

Of placebos and the mind in 18ᵗʰ and 19ᵗʰ century healing

Doctors had long recognised that much illness was self-limiting. Moreover, a patient's psychology was often crucial in determining therapeutic outcomes. The renowned Edinburgh physician and lecturer, William Cullen, gave substance to such thoughts when he referred in his 1772 lectures to the use of placebos in medicine.[1]

Placebo, from the Latin 'to please', was originally used in the context of religious ritual and flattery. It metamorphosed into a medical term in Cullen's lexicon when, in prescribing a mustard plaster without any curative intent, he said:

> 'I own that I did not trust much to it, but I gave it because it is necessary to give a medicine, and as what I call a placebo. If I had thought of any internal medicine it would have been a dose of the Dover's powders.'[2]

For Cullen, all illness arose from irritability of the nervous system, and his promulgation of an active placebo (as compared with a more familiar inert one, such as a bread pill) to please a difficult patient, showed how such notions as 'sympathy' and 'vitalism' informed his mind-body therapeutics and psychosomatic theory of illness.

Testing mesmerism

The idea of inducing a hypnotic trance in patients by the action of a universal fluid, 'animal magnetism', was called mesmerism after the famous Viennese physician, Franz Anton Mesmer. He stood accused in 1780 of making fraudulent claims about his discovery of animal magnetism and its therapeutic effects. In a series of trials undertaken by members of the Academy of Sciences and Medicine, women were blindfolded and asked to either locate the source of the 'mesmerism' or were deceived into thinking they were subject to mesmeric influences when this was not the case. In others, sham or decoy assessments were part of the investigations in which trees were mesmerised or plain water was used. All tests revealed that unblinding removed the effects and that the evinced effects were due to the imagination.[3]

One trial proposed by the Mesmerists, yet never undertaken, seemed quite reasonable:

> '24 patients are to be chosen of whom 12 will be reserved to the Faculté to be treated by the ordinary methods: the other 12 will be assigned to the Author who will treat them according to his particular method. The Author excludes from the selection all Venereal diseases.
>
> In the first instance, written reports will be made of the condition of each patient: each report will be signed by the Commissioners of the Faculté, by the Author and by the persons appointed by the government.
>
> The selection of patients will be made by the Faculté or by the Faculté and the Author together. In order to avoid any later argument and all the questions that could be raised about differences in age, in temperament, in diseases, in their symptoms etc. the assignment of the patients shall be made by the method of lots.'[4]

The Faculty would have no truck with this early formulation of an RCT. Nevertheless, mesmerism's popularity was only temporarily blunted by the Royal Commission's negative conclusions. Throughout the 19th century, the magnetic movement waxed and waned.

Policing the allopathy-homeopathy boundary

Blind assessment acted as a method to police the boundaries between conventional and irregular medicine, and to guard against potential quackery. Dr John Haygarth used a sham device to investigate Perkins's tractors, small metal rods that purportedly cured all ailments through 'electrophysical force'. Five patients with rheumatism, unaware of the evaluation, were chosen from Bath General Hospital and treated with either real or wooden tractors in a cross-over study. Patients in both groups reported significant improvements. Haygarth concluded:

> 'The whole effect undoubtedly depends upon the impression which can be made upon the patient's imagination.'[5]

Homeopathy particularly attracted the ire of orthodox physicians. In Trousseau's investigations at the Hôtel Dieu in 1834, bread pills were used as a placebo, supposedly the first reference to the use of an inert substance. A series of ten patients were given the sham pills (there was no comparison arm using genuine homeopathic remedies), and Trousseau and his students concluded that the observed results were due solely to patient expectation. Further studies by John Forbes and the Milwaukee Academy of Medicine improved upon Trousseau's method by including a concurrent placebo and homeopathic remedy arm as well as double-blinding of genuine homeopathic and sugar pills.

References

1. Kerr C, Milne I, Kaptchuk T (2007). William Cullen and a missing mind-body link in the early history of placebos. The James Lind Library.
2. Cullen W (1722). Lectures: Edinburgh, February–April, p.218–9.
3. Kaptchuk T (1998). International Ignorance: A History of Blind Assessment and Placebo Controls. Bull. History of Medicine 72, 389–33.
4. Mesmer's proposals for a trial of the curative results of his treatment of patients by 'Animal Magnetism' read to an assembly of the Faculté de Médecine de Paris by Delson, on behalf of Mesmer on 18th September 1870 and of the Facultés response (from Mesmer (1781)) - Précis historique des fairs relatifs au magnétisme animal jusques en avril 1781.
5. Haygarth J (1800). Of the imagination as a cause and as a cure of disorders of the body: exemplified by fictitious tractors, and epidemical convulsions. Bath: R, Crutwell - p.4.

Problems of design: the clinical trial in the 19th and 20th centuries

The idea of a placebo as both an inert and physiologically active substance persisted throughout the 19th century. Therapeutic nihilists like the American of heart murmur fame, Austin Flint, and leading Guy's Hospital physician, Withey Gull, used active placebos such as tincture of quassia or mint water in their respective assessments of rheumatism remedies. They concluded that the conventional remedies had no effect on the natural course of the disease and that patients could get well by themselves.[1] However, in step with the growth of the pharmaceutical industry, the placebo as an inert substance gained purchase as a control in the pharmacological testing of drugs and vaccines whose 'active' molecular constituents were of central interest.

Vaccination and antisera production for typhoid, diphtheria, and other infectious diseases reached industrial proportions by the end of the 19th century. In Germany, Adolf Bingel performed one of the first large-scale clinical trials to assess the new diphtheria antitoxin. Between 1911 and 1914, he assigned over 900 patients alternatively to either the antitoxin serum or normal horse serum. Both patients and doctors were blinded to the intervention.[2]

The ethics of placebos

More pragmatic concerns about how to attract patients to a no-treatment comparison arm of a trial rather than concerns about countering suggestions, governed Anglo-American attitudes towards the adoption of blind assessment and placebos in clinical trials.[3] Informed consent was not an ethical norm until after World War II and dummy treatment became a legitimate concurrent control. Tuberculosis trials of sanocrysin (sodium and gold thiosulphate) in Michigan used a single, blind assessment, and distilled water as a control.[4]

At the London Hospital, a variety of 16 drugs (nitrates, narcotics, and digitalis, among them) were used in a placebo-controlled, cross-over design to assess their efficacy in the treatment of angina. No tested drug was better than placebo.[5]

Gold's influential trial of methylxanthines for angina provided the acknowledgement that suggestion could also be the rationale behind placebo use. 'Spontaneous variation' was the usual explanation for improvements in both treatment and placebo arms. Though avoiding the word 'suggestion', Gold and his Harvard colleagues referred to 'confidence of the treatment' to explain the effects:

> 'Some expressed definite conviction at times that it was the drug which was responsible for the relief. That the drug was often the lactulose placebo, and some patients insisted upon its efficacy ... justifies all the circumspection one can exercise.'[6]

The idea that the mind and its beliefs could affect medical outcomes had been well established in the previous century. The benefits of electrotherapy, for example, in the treatment of nervous ailments, were often ascribed to the numinous quality of the latest electrical gadgetry.[7]

Anti-quackery investigations often used sham controls.[8] There was growing evidence from the science of endocrinology that biology and psychology were linked. However, adoption of blind assessment was not a major feature of mainstream medicine until after World War II.

Therapeutic perspectives in the progressive era

During the interwar period, uptake of the controlled trial was determined by factors such as how dramatic the effects of the intervention were. In the 1930s, with the introduction of sulphonamides saving lives, Colebrook and colleagues at St Mary's Hospital dispensed with concurrent controls in their studies on puerperal fever, instead utilising historical controls- i.e. comparing the mortality rates over a four-year period, before and after the introduction of Prontosil. These were sufficient to show a convincing effect of the intervention.[9]

Where the effects of Prontosil were less obvious in the treatment of other infections, more carefully designed trials were proposed using alternation of patients to control and treatment groups.[10] Sporadic references to randomisation to avoid allocation bias in clinical trials did occur before Fisher's influential 'Design of experiments' was published in 1935. In 1928, Dora Colebrook used the drawing of lots to avoid allocation bias in studying the effects of screened and unscreened ultraviolet light on schoolchildren.[11]

Nevertheless, allocation through alternation remained in vogue throughout the interwar period in spite of growing awareness of its limitations. A key milestone in methodological sophistication was reached in 1934 when Austin Bradford Hill, Professor of Medical Statistics and Epidemiology at the London School of Hygiene and Tropical Medicine, criticised the Medical Research Council's (MRC's) multicentre serum therapy trial in pneumonia for its relatively small numbers and the mixture of ways in which control groups were allocated.[12]

Hill had learnt his statistics from Karl Pearson and Major Greenwood, two pioneering figures in modern statistics and epidemiology. Greenwood was the first Professor of Epidemiology and Vital Statistics at the London School of Hygiene and Tropical Medicine. In his 1934 textbook 'Epidemics and crowd-diseases', Greenwood discussed the need to consider both the play of chance and differences between the individuals compared in order to assess a treatment-in this case, vaccination.

Karl Pearson, building on the work of Francis Galton and Quetelet's earlier theory of probabilities, consolidated the discipline of biometrics and opened up the field of vital and medical statistics. Pearson grasped the significance of correlations, and produced one of the first meta-analyses (the mainstay of EBM) when asked to analyse the relative infection and mortality rates among soldiers who had volunteered for inoculation against typhoid fever and those who had not.[13] After consolidating the disparate studies into one, Pearson presented tables of the observed outcomes, each study being assigned its own line showing a measure of effect. Interestingly, Pearson's analysis took issue with the effect of anti-typhoid vaccination, thereby delaying its widespread adoption by the army for almost a decade.

References

1. Flint A (1863). A contribution toward the natural history of articular rheumatism; consisting of a report of thirteen cases treated solely with palliative measures. *American Journal of the Medical Sciences* 46, 17–36.

2. Bingel A (1918). Über Behandlung der Diphtherie mit gewöhnlichem Pferdeserum. Deutsches Archiv für Kluimsche Medizin. 125, 284–332.

3. Kaptchuk op cit - p.423–7.

4. Amberson J, McMahon B, Pinner M. A clinical trial of sanocrysin in pulmonary tuberculosis. *American Review of Tuberculosis* 1931; 24, 401–35.

5. Evans W, Hoyle C. The comparative value of drugs used in the continuous treatment of angina pectoris. *Quarterly Journal of Medicine* 1933; 7, 311–38.

6. Gold H, Kwit N, Otto H. The xanthines (theobromine and aminophyllin) in the treatment of cardiac pain. *J. American Medical Association*. 1937; 108, 2173–9.

7. Senior J (1994). Rationalising electrotherapy in neurology, 1860–1920. (Oxford-D. Phil Thesis).

8. Anon. Two Electronic Diagnoses: The Reactions of a Guinea Pig and Sheep to the Reaction of Abrams. *Journal of the American Medical Association* 1922; 79, 2244–8.

9. Colebrook L, Kenny M. Treatment of human puerperal infections, and of experimental infections in mice, with Prontosil. *Lancet* 1936; 1, 1279–86. *See also* Loudon I, (2002). The use of historical controls and concurrent controls to assess the effects of sulphonamides, 1936–1945. The James Lind Library.

10. Schwentker F, Waghelstein J. A note on the use of Sulfanilamide in scarlet fever, *Baltimore Health News* 1938; 15, 41–44.

11. Doull J, Hardy M, Clark J et al. The effect of irradiation with ultra-violet light on the frequency of attacks of upper respiratory disease (common colds) *American J of Hygiene* 1931; 13, 460–77.

12. See Chalmers I (2002). Medical Research Council Therapeutic Trials Committee (1934). The serum treatment of lobar pneumonia. *British Medical Journal* 1, 241–245. In: The James Lind Library.

13. Pearson K. Report on certain enteric fever inoculation statistics. *British Medical Journal* 1904; 3: 1243–6. *See also* O' Rourke K (2006). A historical perspective on meta-analysis dealing quantitatively with varying study results. The James Lind Library.

The rise of the randomised controlled trial

AB Hill and the first RCT

Both AB Hill and Major Greenwood were responsible for applying medical statistics to epidemiological problems of wider social significance—occupational and public health. During the interwar period, Hill's collaboration with Richard Doll on smoking was groundbreaking. Hill published widely on the topic of medicine and statistics in the Lancet, and in the early 1930s, grew to appreciate the benefit of randomisation. Not for purely statistical reasons did he include randomisation in the design of the MRC's 1946 clinical trial of streptomycin in tuberculosis—the first double-blinded RCT.[1]

Although the importance of randomisation lay in being able to stochastically measure degrees of uncertainty and variance that allowed null hypothesis testing and causal inferences to be made, evidence suggests that such important mathematical rationalisations had little to do with the MRC's design. In the 1946 study, patients with tuberculosis were randomised using random sampling numbers and sealed envelopes, to either streptomycin and bed rest or bed rest alone.[2] As Hill later reflected, words like 'random samples' were left out of the protocols at that time as they might have scared off collaborating physicians who did not want their clinical autonomy curtailed. Streptomycin was in short supply in post-war Britain and evidence of its dramatic effects was well known. Randomisation in the guise of concealed allocation was thus adopted to counter accusations of favouritism.

What turned the double-blinded RCT into a universally accepted tool was its promise of 'scientificity' by replacing clinical judgement with statistics and standardised protocols, and also taking into account the effects of bias. The placebo effect, associated with the older idea of 'suggestion' that had once been the province of the quacks, was now viewed as a confounder in medical decision-making. This appealed to the medical elite and by the 1960s, the RCT became a powerful tool by which organisational and social problems could be fixed. Come the early 1990s, EBM advocates held the RCT as a gold standard in medical evidence, together with the systematic review.[3]

'All treatment must be proved to be effective'

Archie Cochrane's '*Effectiveness and efficiency*' (1972) was particularly influential in disseminating the gospel of the RCT in Britain.[4] Shaped by his wartime experiences as a prisoner of war doctor in Salonica, the book highlighted his motto 'all treatment must be proved to be effective', especially in light of the healing power of nature:

> *'There were about 11,000 POWs … The diet was about 600 calories per day … we all had diarrhoea. In addition we had epidemics of typhoid, diphtheria, infections, jaundice and cases of pitting oedema above the knee … We had some aspirin, some antacid and some antiseptic … I had expected 100s to die … in fact there were only 4 deaths [over 6 months]. This excellent result had nothing to do with the therapy nor my clinical skill. It demonstrated … the importance of the recuperative powers of the body.'*

Pitting oedema proved to be of particular concern, as it was originally thought to be an epidemic of 'wet beriberi' caused by vitamin B deficiency.

Cochrane decided to do an experiment in line with his medical hero, James Lind:

'I chose 20 men all emaciated and with oedema above the knee. I put 10 in each of 2 wards. They all received the standard rations but those in 1 ward were given supplements of yeast, 3 times a day [paid for by himself]. In the other ward they got vitamin C. By the 4th day most of the men in the yeast room were feeling better unlike those in the vitamin C.'

The obvious inference was that the diet was improved for the prisoners. But, as Cochrane later reminisced, the quality of the trial had a lot to answer for, despite a successful outcome:

'I was testing the wrong hypothesis [now thought to be hypoproteinaemic oedema caused by famine not beriberi], the numbers too small and they were not randomised. The outcome measure was pitiful [frequency of urine output] and the trial did not go on long enough.'

Cochrane speculated that it was the protein in the yeast that did the trick. After the war, Cochrane joined the staff at the MRC Pneumoconiosis Research Unit in South Wales, later becoming Director of the MRC Epidemiology Unit in Cardiff and Professor of Medicine at the Welsh National School of Medicine. At that time, he developed interests in health service research in the National Health Service (NHS) and became an ardent proponent of the RCT.

The RCT and discontents

Since Archie Cochrane's day, the methodological integrity of the RCT has been called into question. Concomitant with the growth of the industrial-academic-governmental complex, the RCT has proven not to be an inflexible mathematical model, but an agent subject to accommodations and compromises that serve medical and socio-economic ends. In the hands of 'Big Pharma' (the global pharmaceutical corporations), the RCT became a market tool enabling questionable drugs like interferon to penetrate the market place in the 1980s.[5] Whistle-blowing books on the pharmaceutical industry point out that it is neither a model of free enterprise nor one of innovation. Moreover, what industry-sponsored research yields is often subject to bias due to conduct and reporting methods.[6]

Currently, the RCT acts as a lightning rod in debates about whether EBM is a gift horse or a Trojan horse in health care.[7] Anthropologists and ethnographers argue its spectre of positivism adumbrates other forms of purportedly valid evidence and ignores patient perspectives. Others see EBM as a managerial tool reinforcing the NHS's bureaucratic top-down approach to regulating the entire health service through 'quality assurance' systems that lead to inappropriate cost cutting and loss of clinical autonomy.[8] Does EBM lead to surveillance medicine or is it a revolutionary phase in medical progress providing increased transparency of professional knowledge and expertise? The debates rumble on.

Historical perspectives show that the clinical trial did not spring *ex machina* out of Zeus's head, but evolved in response to a host of socio-economic factors that shaped the medical profession and its overriding concerns—not least being 'to prove that all treatment must be effective'. In the current climate of contestable evidence about what constitutes effective therapy, the controlled clinical trial is but an epiphenomenon of deeper underlying unease about the art and science of medicine and the ever increasing gap between the natural and 'techne'.

Ethics and experimentation

The disempowered patient: ethics and choice

Jettisoning natural histories of disease (based on external symptoms that made sense to the patient) and delving into the unexplored interior of the body, the so-called 'clinical gaze', severed the links with the past and the doctor–patient relationship. The hospital became the scene of death and of the disempowered charity patient in Eugène Sue's 'Les mystères de Paris' (1844):

'If Dr Griffon wanted to test the comparative effect of a new and quite dangerous medication in order to be able to ascertain its favourable impact on one organ or another, he would take a certain number of patients, treat one group by the new method, another by the old, and leave others solely to the forces of nature … He went on without pity making his patients swallow iodine, strychnine or arsenic to the extreme limits of physiological tolerance or, to put it plainly, to the extinction of life.'

More carefully construed ethical scenarios appeared when the transformation of modern medicine in the late 19th and early 20th centuries (by bacteriology, new technologies and surgical procedures, pharmaceuticals, and the reorganisation of the hospital), became increasingly associated with clinical research and human experimentation.

GB Shaw's drama, 'The doctor's dilemma' (1906), considered the rationing of scarce resources—in this case, a vaccine against tuberculosis, and raised the question 'what is the value of different human lives?' In Lewis's 'Arrowsmith' (1925), the scientific ideals of the medical researcher vs the needs of the experimental population posed the central dilemma. Ordered to the plague-infested West Indies to conduct a controlled trial of his newly discovered 'phage' serum, the defining moment came when, succumbing to humanitarian concerns, Martin Arrowsmith gave the serum to all those affected, leaving no control arm.

Nuremberg and all that

Old paternalistic notions about 'doctor knows best' came under increasing strain during the interwar period. The normative ethical framework finally became otiose under the racial policies of Nazi Germany when medical researchers committed crimes against humanity. Voluntary and informed consent headed the list of guidelines for research workers enshrined in the Nuremberg Code after World War II. Later amendments, such as the Declaration of Helsinki (1964), clarified the differences between therapeutic and non-therapeutic experiments. But guidelines and self-policing were insufficient to instil ethical conduct among researchers. The ubiquitous ethical committees that now dominate the landscape of modern research arose after abuses uncovered by MH Pappworth in the UK and HK Beecher in the USA. They revealed the routine use of mental defectives and prisoners as human guinea pigs in prestigious medical schools and hospitals, and of cancer patients in risky treatments.[9,10]

Obvious legal loopholes have been tightened over the years to protect vulnerable groups in clinical research. But in an age of dependence upon pharmaceutical industry-funded research, the problem has not gone away. John Le Carré's film, 'The constant gardener' (2001), is a timely tale set in Kenya about a cover-up of the testing of a tuberculosis drug that had severe side effects on trial subjects. In fact, drug disasters have been a major public concern since thalidomide was withdrawn in 1961 due to horrendous foetal defects. Recent research on drug company-funded RCT drug trials has revealed how the concept of 'equipoise' is violated through comparator bias (making inappropriate comparisons with a placebo, or with too little or too high a dose of the comparator drug).[11] The events that unfolded at London's Northwick Park Hospital (2006-7), in which a disastrous drug trial left six healthy volunteers with multi-organ failure and little compensation, are poignant reminders that even in the highly regulated climate of Data and Safety Committees and government guidelines, rules can be bent, conflicts of interest can arise, and public trust can be jeopardised, especially when basic issues such as safety and informed consent in clinical research remain ethically refractory.[12]

References

1. Hill A. Suspended judgement: Memories of the British Streptomycin trial in Tuberculosis. The First Randomised Trial. *Controlled Clinical Trials* 1990; 11, 77–9.
2. Medical Research Council. Streptomycin treatment of pulmonary tuberculosis *British Medical Journal* 1948; 2, 769–82.
3. Devereaux P, Yusuf S. The evolution of the randomized controlled trial and its role in evidence-based decision making. *Journal of Internal Medicine* 2003; 254, 105–13.
4. Cochrane A (1972). Effectiveness and efficiency: random reflections on health services. Nuffield Provincial Trust, as quoted in Cochrane A and Blythe M. One Man's Medicine: An Autobiography of Professor Archie Cochrane, British Medical Journal 1989 p. xiii.
5. Pieters T. 'Marketing Medicines through Randomised Controlled Trials: the Case of Interferon, British Medical Journal 1998; 347, 1231–3.
6. Djulbegovic B, Lacevic M, Cantor A et al. The uncertainty principle and industry-sponsored research. *Lancet* 2000; 356, 635–8.
7. Lambert H, Gordon E, Bogdon-Lewis E. Introduction: Gift horse or Trojan horse? Social Science perspectives on evidence-based health care. *Social Science and Medicine* 2006; 62, 2613–20.
8. Charlton B, Miles A. The rise and fall of EBM. *Quarterly Journal of Medicine* 1998; 91, 371–4.
9. Pappworth M (1967). Human Guinea Pigs, London, Routledge.
10. Beecher H. Ethics and clinical research. *New England Journal of Medicine* 1966; 274, 1354–60.
11. Mann H, Djulbegovic B (2007). Why comparisons must address genuine uncertainties. The James Lind Library.
12. Hattenstone S (2007). Everbody thought we were toxic waste. *The Guardian.* Feb 17 p.20–4.

Further reading

Davis M, Stark A, eds (2001). *Conflict of interest in the professions.* Oxford University Press, Oxford.

Dopson S, Fitzgerald L, eds (2005). *Knowledge to action? Evidence-based health care in context.* Oxford University Press, Oxford.

Hacking I (1975). *The emergence of probability.* Cambridge University Press, Cambridge.

Illich I (1975). *Medical nemesis: the expropriation of health.* Trinity Press, London.

Moynihan R, Cassel A (2005). *Selling sickness: how the world's biggest pharmaceutical companies are turning us all into patients.* Nation Press, New York.

Porter R (1989). *Health for sale: quackery in England, 1660–1850.* Manchester University Press, Manchester.

Rosser Matthews J (1995). *Quantification and the quest for medical certainty.* Princeton University Press, Princeton.

Shapin S (1996). *A social history of truth: civility and science in seventeeth-century England.* University of Chicago Press, Chicago.

The James Lind Library. Available from: http://www.Jameslindlibrary.org.

Chronology

Below is a chronological summary of references discussed in this chapter:

Pre-1700s

BC Daniel. *Ch1:1–16:* comparison of diets.

c.900 al-Razi. *The comprehensive book of medicine:* comparison of bloodletting with no treatment group.

1364 Petrarch F. *Letter to Bocaccio, Rerum Senilium V.3:* comparing like with like.

1575 Paré A. *Les oeuvres de M. Ambroise Paré, conseiller et premier chirurgien du Roy:* within group comparison of wound salve.

1662 Van Helmont JB. *Oriatrike or physics refined:* use of lots in making comparisons.

1700s

1724 Nettleton T. *Part of a letter from Dr. Nettleton, physician at Halifax, to Dr. Jurin:* arithmetic analysis of small pox inoculation.

1726 Swift J. *Gulliver's travels:* satire on morals and the new mechanical philosphy.

1740 Cheselden W. *The anatomy of the human body:* importance of age specific outcomes.

1753 Lind J. *A treatise of the scurvy:* first prospective controlled trial of citrus fruit against scurvy.

1764 Stone E. *An account of the success of the bark of the willow in the cure of agues:* dramatic effects in sufficient number of case studies.

1772 Cullen W. *Clinical lectures:* first medical context of 'placebo' to please.

1780 Academy of Medicine, Paris: trials on Mesmer's animal magnetism using blind assessment.

1800s

1834 Trousseau A, Gouraud H. *Répertoire clinique: expériences homeopathiques tentées à l'Hôtel-Dieu de Paris. J des Connaissances Médico-Chirurgicales:* first use of inert placebo, bread pill in homeopathy trials.

1835 Louis P. *Recherches sur les effets de la saignée … —la méthode numérique:* founder of modern epidemiology, emphasising group comparison and population thinking.

1840 Gavarret J. *Principes généraux de statistique médicale ou developpement des règles qui doivent présider à son emploi:* first use of confidence intervals.

1846 Forbes J. *Homeopathy, allopathy and 'young physic':* use of concurrent arm and blind assessment.

1854 Balfour T, quoted in West C. *Lectures on the diseases of infancy and childhood:* trial of belladonna against scarlet fever—importance of sample size.

1860 Semmelweis I. *Etiology, concept and prophylaxis of childbed fever:* accidentally controlled trial—unacknowledged pioneers of antisepsis.

1865 Sutton H. *Cases of rheumatic fever treated for the most part by mint water:* therapeutic nihilistic use of active placebos.

1900–45

1904 Pearson K. *Report on certain enteric fever inoculation statistics:* first meta-analysis of typhoid vaccination.
1918 Bingel A. *Über Behandlung der Diphtherie mit gewöhnlichem Pferdeserum:* first large-scale, double-blinded trial using alternation.
1923 Fisher R: discovery of notion of randomisation.
1931 Doull J, Hardy M, Clark J, et al. *The effect of irradiation with ultra-violet light on the frequency of attacks of upper respiratory disease (common colds):* adoption of random sampling machine to create treatment and control groups.
1934 Greenwood M. *Epidemics and crowd-diseases.* Medical Research Council Therapeutic Trials Committee. *The serum treatment of lobar pneumonia:* AB Hill's critique of trial design especially of alternation and small numbers.
1935 Fisher R, *The design of experiments:* influential text of experimental design using randomisation.
1937 Gold H, Kwit N, Otto H. *The xanthines (theobromine and aminophyllin) in the treatment of cardiac pain:* first recognition of countering 'suggestion' in controlled trial in Anglo-North America.

1945–2000

1948 Medical Research Council. *Streptomycin treatment of pulmonary tuberculosis:* first RCT designed by AB Hill.
1948 *Nuremberg Code:* voluntary consent plus nine other principles governing human experimentation.
1964 *Declaration of Helsinki:* clarification between therapeutic and non-therapeutic experimentation.
1966 Beecher HK. *Ethics and clinical research:* whistle-blowing unethical human experimentation in USA.
1967 Pappworth MH. *Human guinea pigs:* whistle-blowing in the UK about abuses in routine clinical research.
1972 Cochrane AL. *Effectiveness and efficiency: random reflections on health services:* clarion call for the RCT in health research —'All treatments must be proved effective'.
1995 Moore T. *Deadly medicine: why tens of thousands of patients died in America's worst drug disaster:* RCTs implicated in 1980s anti-arrhythmic drug disaster.
1998 Pieters T. *Marketing medicines through randomised controlled trials: the case of interferon:* rise of Big Pharma—the RCT as a marketing tool.

2000s

2000 Djulbegovic B, Lacevic M, Cantor A, et al. *The uncertainty principle and industry-sponsored research:* 'Big Pharma' and comparator bias in RCTs.
2008 *The creation of the prozac myth, The Guardian:* publication bias.

An introduction to evidence-based medicine

How did EBM develop?

Throughout the history of the practice of medicine clinicians have used 'evidence' from their own clinical experiences, such as the clinical findings from individual patients, to inform decisions about health care. However, with the emergence of new technologies, treatment modalities, and epidemiological methods in the latter half of the 20th century, some began to question whether we might be doing more harm than good in our attempts to 'cure' disease.

Alvan Feinstein is thought by many to be the founding father of clinical epidemiology, the science underpinning EBM. His seminal book urged clinicians to be more scientific about the practice of clinical medicine, and was published two decades after the end of World War II, during an era of new large-scale epidemiologic studies such as the Framingham Heart Study (1949), the Salk vaccine trial (1954), and the Surgeon General's report on 'Smoking and health' (1964).

In 1971, Archie Cochrane also wrote an important and controversial book suggesting that clinicians were perhaps overly devoted to their patients, with many overtreating in an effort to do everything possible to 'cure'. He argued that the systematic application of medical research, in particular evidence from randomised controlled trials (RCTs), should be encouraged so as to maximise the use of therapies proven to be safe and effective and to minimise the impact of ineffective and unsafe ones.

David Sackett and colleagues developed these concepts further when they wrote about clinical epidemiology and the 'science of the art of medicine'. Their book described ways in which the principles of population epidemiology might be applied to individual patients' care decisions and, in particular, the appraisal of research for quality.

As this book will highlight, there are many 'key' clinical trials that have had a profound impact on the effective practice of medicine in the manner that Feinstein, Cochrane, and Sackett proposed. In the wider medical literature, one will unfortunately find many examples of poorly conducted trials, which could do harm if their results were applied to clinical practice. There are also examples of simple and effective treatments that have not been adopted into practice and perhaps should be. This book, as we have explained, is not a comprehensive summary of evidence-based clinical practice; it simply highlights some of the many key clinical trials of effective treatments that are relevant to clinical practice today.

What is the process of EBM?

'The practice of evidence-based medicine means integrating clinical expertise (proficiency, judgement acquired through clinical practice and use of individual patient's right, predicaments, preferences) with the best available expert evidence from systematic research.'

This definition, from Sackett's seminal paper in 1996, has been translated into five steps, which we shall refer to in this chapter as the '5 A's'. These were designed to help clinicians find the best available expert evidence from a systematic search. Most clinicians would practice at least the first four of these steps, as outlined below.

The development of the EBM process has been an important step towards helping clinicians keep up-to-date at a time where clinical medicine is advancing rapidly and patients are becoming more involved in health care decisions. It is impossible for a single clinician to be familiar with all of the best evidence they might need for their daily clinical practice. It has been estimated that approximately 560,000 new medical articles are published every year and 20,000 new randomised trials are registered. That is equivalent to 1,500 new articles and 55 new trials per day.

A recent analysis of 100 of the best quality systematic reviews published in the journal *ACP Journal Club* between 1995 and 2005 showed that the median survival time before new and important evidence was found on a particular topic was 5½ years. Almost 25% were out of date within two years and a further 7% before the article had even been published.

Books like this, which summarise some of the highest quality evidence, may simplify part of the process for busy clinicians; however, they alone will not always be able to answer the question that faces a clinician or their patient. Therefore, the following five steps provide a framework for clinicians who wish to incorporate the best scientific evidence into their clinical decisions.

STEP 1—Asking

Some would argue this to be the most important step in the EBM process. Before rushing onto the Internet to search for an answer, it is important to pause and think about what your precise question is. There are two aspects to this:

A. Refining your question

Refining a question into several parts using the PICO (**P**opulation/**P**atient problem, **I**ntervention, **C**omparison, **O**utcome) framework can help identify useful key words for a search and will increase the chances of finding an appropriate answer to the question. Most of us have experienced the frustration of typing ill-defined keywords into a general search engine such as *Google*, and ending up with countless irrelevant 'hits'. Therefore, using a framework such as PICO to develop the best keywords can save a considerable amount of time. The components of the PICO framework, are:

The **PICO** framework for refining a clinical question

*i. **P**opulation/**P**atient problem*

Describe who the question pertains to (e.g. elderly men with prostate cancer or toddlers with pharyngitis).

*ii. **I**ntervention*

Define what treatment, test, or exposure is being considered in this case (e.g. oral penicillin, back exercises, smoking exposure). It is also useful to define some of the details (e.g. duration, dose), i.e. the 'when' and 'where'.

*iii. **C**omparison*

Define what the intervention would be compared against (e.g. oral vs topical therapy, proposed intervention vs placebo/gold standard intervention or criteria). Note that this section may not always be relevant.

*iv. **O**utcome*

Define the outcomes that are important and relevant for the patient (e.g. pain relief, return to work). We often focus exclusively on the beneficial outcomes of treatment, but we should also consider the importance of minimising the associated risks or harm (e.g. side effects, long-term complications).

B. Defining the question type

The second part of 'asking' is to define the *type* of question that is being asked. A number of researchers have systematically analysed the types of questions that clinicians ask. The most frequent questions pertain to treatment, with questions about the cause or 'aetiology' of a condition and 'diagnosis' questions also being common.

It is important to consider the type of question, so that the best source of evidence can be used to find the answer. To illustrate this first step of the EBM process, let us consider a hypothetical case:

David, a 37 year-old male, comes to see you with a 24-hour history of fever, myalgia, and sore throat. On examination, he has a temperature of 38°C and an erythematous throat with no exudate but enlarged cervical lymph nodes. The rest of the physical examination is normal. He has important meetings at work during the following week and wants to get better as quickly as possible.

The unstructured or 'raw' question that our hypothetical practitioner first asks, is:

'Should this patient be prescribed an antibiotic?'

The **P**opulation/**P**atient problem in this case would be 'adult with acute sore throat', the **I**ntervention is 'antibiotics', the **C**omparator is 'watch and wait', and the **O**utcomes are 'symptom relief' and 'return to work'. This is a question about treatment. Having 'asked' an answerable question, the next step in the process of EBM is to 'access' the evidence to search for an answer.

STEP 2—Accessing

It is impossible to cover this issue comprehensively in this introductory chapter. With an ever-increasing number of evidence-based resources, accessibility and costs need to be considered; some resources are only available for a subscription fee to which not all institutions will subscribe. This section will focus on the generic principles of searching that should be applicable in a wide range of contexts, at minimal or no cost.

A. Selecting and combining keywords for the search strategy

Generally speaking, the PICO framework can be used as the basis of a search strategy, with, in the first instance, a combined **P**roblem AND **I**ntervention. If this remains too broad, then one or more of the **O**utcomes can always be added. Referring back to our case example about David, we might consider 'sore throat' AND 'antibiotic'. If that yields more results than are manageable, then 'sore throat' AND 'antibiotic' AND 'symptom relief' may be tried to further refine the results. For a more comprehensive searching, 'medical subject headings' (MeSH) alongside more detailed searching strategies should be applied.

B. Matching the question type against the best study design, taking into account the levels of evidence

Research involves measurement of various outcomes, including the effects of treatment and the accuracy of tests. All measurements have some random error, attributable to chance. However, measurements can also be subject to systematic error or bias. The best evidence avoids these pitfalls. This book deliberately focuses on well-conducted RCTs, wherever possible, because they are the best type of study to answer questions about treatment.

The list on p.33 shows study designs that answer treatment questions. The further down the list (or levels of evidence), the greater the risk of bias. Randomising participants in a study reduces bias because confounding factors (such as age, gender, smoking status, etc.) are evenly distributed between the intervention and control arms of the study. In other words, the only difference between the groups is whether or not they receive the intervention since their allocation to a particular arm of the study is purely by chance. Expert opinion or clinical experience is more open to bias. However, in some cases, particularly for rare events and conditions, this might be the only evidence available.

Levels of evidence

Level	Type of evidence
1a	Evidence from systematic reviews or meta analysis of RCTs
1b	Evidence from at least one RCT
2a	Evidence from at least one controlled study without randomisation
2b	Evidence from at least one other type of quasi-experimental study
3	Evidence from non-experimental descriptive studies, such as comparative studies, correlation studies, and case control studies
4	Evidence from expert committee reports or opinions and/or clinical experience of respected authorities

While it is important to consider using level-1 evidence if at all possible, it is not always feasible to randomise people in a study. The reasons for this may be both practical and ethical. This will be the case particularly for studies that look at prognosis or aetiology. It is clearly impossible to randomise someone to 'get breast cancer' or to 'not get breast cancer'. However, it *is* possible to follow-up women who have breast cancer and compare them with a similar group of women who do not have breast cancer, and to then look for associated factors.

C. Identifying the best source for accessing this study type
Studies published in peer-reviewed journals can usually be accessed through electronic databases, usually based around particular content areas. Journals and their articles may be contained within more than one database if they are applicable to more than one content area. *Medline* is the most commonly encountered database of medical journals. Other examples include *Cinahl* (includes many nursing and allied health journals) and *PsychInfo* (contains many psychology journals).

Medline: *Medline* is the US National Library of Medicine's (NLM's) premier bibliographic database. It contains about 13 million references to journal articles in life sciences, with a concentration in biomedicine dating back to 1966. A technical committee selects which journals are included and participating journals submit their citations every time a new issue is published. Since 2002, 1500–3500 citations have been added each day from Tuesday to Saturday. More information about the NLM can be found at http://www.nlm.nih.gov/nlmhome.html.

Searching the electronic databases can be done via a search engine. A single search engine might be able to access several indexes, websites, or databases. Equally, a single database might be accessible via several search engines. For example, *Medline* can be searched using *Entrez PubMed* (http://www.pubmed.org or http://www.ncbi.nlm.nih.gov/sites/entrez), *Ovid* (http://www.ovid.com), *Silver Platter* software, or even *Google* (http://www.google.com).

Although some search engines and databases are available free of charge, others require a subscription and limit free access to the abstract only. Therefore your ability to access some evidence will be restricted by your local employer or library's subscriptions. This can be a problem for those in remote settings, low-income countries, or for self-employed practitioners. In the UK, an *Athens* login is sometimes required to procure access to certain resources (http://www.athens.ac.uk). Universal free access to *Medline* via *PubMed* provides free access to all abstracts as well as to some full text versions of journals. It can be accessed by either typing '*PubMed*' into any web search engine or by using the links above.

Applying these principles to our case study example gives the following result:

> Typing 'antibiotics AND pharyngitis' into PubMed provides over 2000 journal articles, which cover a whole range of study types.

In routine practice, 2000 hits is an impractical number to review. Therefore, some search engines such as *Ovid* and *Entrez PubMed* have pre-programmed 'filters' that can be applied to limit the search to particular study types. In this example, it would be useful to limit the search to systematic reviews of RCTs since these will provide the highest level of evidence for answering a treatment question (level-1a):

> Limiting the search to systematic reviews using the filter section called 'clinical queries' on PubMed or 'Limits' on Ovid provides 70 'hits'.

The Cochrane Library: We now find a *Cochrane* review on 'Antibiotics for sore throats' (containing a summary of the results of 27 RCTs on this topic) within the first couple of hits. The Cochrane Library's database of systematic reviews (level-1a evidence) is perhaps one of the most useful resources for therapy-related questions. It is available through http://www.thecochranelibrary.org.

British Medical Journal's Clinical Evidence: Another helpful resource for addressing treatment and management-related questions. It can be found at http://clinicalevidence.bmj.com/ceweb/index.jsp.

STEP 3—Appraising critically

This step involves assessing the quality of a study. A poorly conducted systematic review or RCT may not be worth considering, as the results may be misleading due to methodological flaws and sources of bias. Numerous checklists have been developed to help clinicians decide whether a study is valid or not. In the next sections of this chapter, we will look at the appraisal process for RCTs in much greater detail, as this study type is the focus of this book. The table opposite summarises a number of widely used checklists for appraising and reporting on a broader range of study types that will not be covered in further detail here, but may be useful for readers in other contexts:

Common appraisal and reporting checklists

Checklist source	Study types	Location
JAMA Users' Guide Series	All	Centre for Health Evidence http://www.cche.net/usersguides/main.asp
QUORUM	Systematic reviews	Moher D *et al.* Lancet 1999;354:1896–1900
AGREE	Clinical Practice Guideline	http://www.agreecollaboration.org
CONSORT	RCTs	http://www.consort-statement.org
MOOSE	Non-randomised observational studies	Stroup D *et al.* JAMA 2000;283:2008–12

Questions to consider when appraising systematic reviews (meta-analysis):

1. Has a focused question been asked and answered?
2. Were the search criteria well defined and was the search process rigorous?
3. Were the individual study methodologies rigorous and consistent?
4. Were the combined study results analysed using the appropriate statistical tools?

STEP 4—Applying

This step remains one of the most challenging, yet most important, steps within the EBM process. One may argue that this embodies the true art of medicine as it requires the 'integration of best evidence with clinical expertise, the patient's circumstances, and their personal preferences.' A recent study of general practitioners found that being able to tailor evidence appropriately to individual patient decisions remained a major barrier to the use of evidence in practice. By contrast, access to the Internet and attitudes towards EBM had improved. Most practitioners in this study also expressed a preference for involving their patients in making decisions, yet useful tools to facilitate this remained largely under-utilised. We will explore this in greater detail later in the chapter.

STEP 5—Assessing

This is not always practiced by clinicians, but is a potentially useful step that requires the clinician to reflect upon the previous four steps and consider ways in which they might be improved in subsequent efforts.

How do you assess the quality of an RCT?

Given the focus of this book, this section will discuss the appraisal of RCTs only. As mentioned in the previous section, there are many well-developed and frequently used checklists for appraising the quality of a study. Here, we will focus on the JAMA (Journal of the American Medical Association) checklist. As you develop your EBM skills, you may find that a different checklist suits your needs. While not developed specifically for critical appraisal, the CONSORT checklist was developed in the early 1990s by a group of journal editors, trialists, and methodologists who wanted to improve the quality of reporting on clinical trials. The outcome was the CONSORT statement (**CON**solidated **S**tandards **O**f **R**eporting **T**rials), a useful point of reference (see link on previous page).

The JAMA quality assessment checklist for RCTs

*I. Are the results of this single preventive or therapeutic trial valid?**

Main questions to answer:

1. Was the assignment of patients to treatments randomised? Was the randomisation list concealed?
2. Were all patients who entered the trial accounted for at its conclusion? Were they analysed in the groups to which they were randomised?

Finer points to address:

3. Were patients and clinicians kept 'blind' to which treatment was being received?
4. Aside from the experimental treatment, were the groups treated equally?
5. Were the groups similar at the start of the trial?

II. Are the valid results of this study important?

III. Can you apply this valid, important evidence about a treatment in caring for your patient?

1. Do these results apply to your patients?
   a. Is your patient so different from those in the trial that its results cannot help you?
   b. How great would the potential benefit of therapy actually be for your individual patient?
2. Are your patient's values and preferences satisfied by the regimen and its consequences?
   a. Do you and your patient have a clear assessment of their values and preferences?
   b. Are these met by this regimen and its consequences?

* Adapted From Sackett, Richardson, Rosenberg and Haynes (1997) Evidence-Based Medicine: How to Practice and Teach EBM. Churchill Livingstone, London.

Methodology: will the RCT design produce valid results?

Null hypothesis and errors: The null hypothesis is a hypothesis formed at the outset of a study involving a treatment vs control, which is presumed true unless nullified or refuted by statistical evidence. For example, when comparing a drug with placebo, the null hypothesis would be 'the new drug is of equal efficacy to the placebo'. Statistically significant analysis of the data would then be required in order to prove that the new drug was more effective. Two types of errors can subsequently arise:

- Type 1 or α: rejecting a hypothesis that should have been accepted (false positive), i.e. stating that a difference was observed when this was not actually the case.
- Type 2 or β: accepting a hypothesis that should have been rejected (false negative), i.e. stating that no difference was observed when in fact a difference was present.

Bias: Bias, the systematic over or underestimation of the true effect, can be introduced at a number of stages. The main sources of bias in RCTs come from either poor randomisation and/or through loss to follow-up after randomisation.

Randomisation: The method of randomisation is very important in a trial. Where possible, it should be done independently so that the researchers are 'blinded' to the allocation of participants. Randomly allocating participants to treatment or control groups is a highly effective way of reducing bias as it ensures both groups are likely to be very similar (i.e. similar baseline characteristics) to begin with. Any differences between the two groups are then most likely to be attributable to the intervention itself.

Blinding: Blinding participants (and/or researchers), when measuring the outcomes of interest, is a method by which studies can attempt to reduce the unwanted influences of bias and improve internal validity. This can take several forms: *single-blind* (patient is unaware which intervention they have been allocated), *double-blind* (both researcher (clinician) and patient are unaware which intervention the patient has been allocated); *triple-blind* (when the researcher, patient, and outcome assessor do not know which intervention the patient has been allocated to). There are a number of types of bias, some of which can be found in the Figure below:*

Types of Bias

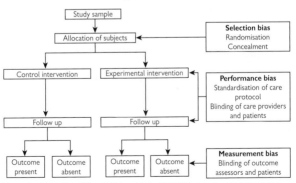

* Reproduced from: Khan K, Kunz R, Kleijnen J, Antes G. (2003) Systematic reviews to support evidence-based medicine: How to review and apply findings of systematic reviews. Royal Society of Medicine, London.

Follow-up: Another important factor to check is whether or not patients have been adequately followed up. In particular, this should be to ensure that there has not been a high drop-out rate in one arm of the trial, compared with the other. Participants should not be swapped from one group to the other. If this does unavoidably occur for ethical or other reasons, then the analysis should consider what would have happened had they stayed in their original group (sometimes called 'intention-to-treat' analysis). Omitting the patients who withdrew may overestimate treatment effects.

Are the valid results of this study important?

There are a range of statistical tools available to quantitatively assess the relative importance and significance of study data. It is crucial to select the appropriate test for the particular data in a study. Although there is no single algorithm that can be applied to determine which test is best in every case, a decision tree can help. Further discussion of this is well beyond the scope of this book, but there are a number of helpful Internet-based resources, such as:

- Which Test: http://www.whichtest.info

the treatment group compared with the probability of a hazard at time 't in the control group, i.e. the effect of a variable upon the risk of an event. Sometimes, the hazard ratio is simply referred to as the 'relative risk'.

H. 95% Confidence interval (CI)

The terms outlined above (RR, OR, HR, and difference of the means) are all estimates of the effect of the study factor on the population in question. However, there will always be some error associated with this, particularly if there are only a small number of people participating in the study (i.e. a small sample size). The 95% CI is the range within which we are 95% confident that the true estimate of effect lies. Note, that if the 95% CI for an OR or RR value crosses 1.0 (the point of no effect), then it is possible that the true effect is none, i.e. the effect is not statistically significant.

I. P-values and statistical significance

A p-value is the probability of the observed difference being due to chance. Traditionally, if the p value is <0.05, then the result is considered statistically significant.

Statistical terms

The size and direction of the effect of a treatment (i.e. dichotomous data) is often reported as an 'Odds Ratio' (OR), 'Relative Risk' (RR), 'Hazard Ratio' (HR), or the 'difference in means'. To see if there is much error around this estimate, the '95% confidence interval' can be calculated to ensure that it does not cross the null value (the point of no effect). Whether or not there is a statistically significant effect can be determined by seeing whether the 'p-value' is <0.05. We will now examine some of the key terminology in more detail:

A. Difference between group means

Used for continuous data, e.g. the mean reading score in treatment group A minus the mean reading score in the control group B.

B. Relative risk (RR)

This is the risk of outcome in the treatment group relative to the other (usually control) group. It is a ratio. For example, using hypothetical values for our antibiotics and sore throat case study, the proportion of people who took antibiotics and still had a sore throat after three days (30%) is divided by the proportion of people in the control group with a sore throat persisting at three days (60%) to give a RR=0.50. A RR=1.0 means that there is no effect of the treatment. In other words, this implies that there was no difference between treatment and control groups (i.e. the null value). If the RR is >1.0 for an adverse outcome such as death, this generally means the effect is harmful. If the RR is <1.0, then the treatment is protective. To use our example, a RR=0.5 means that people in the treatment group are half as likely to have sore throat symptoms at three days compared with controls. The further away the RR is from the null value, the greater is the effect of the treatment.

Outcome and exposure status

	Outcome present	Outcome not present	
Exposed to treatment: Treatment group	A	B	Number exposed (A+B)
Not exposed to treatment: Control group	C	D	Number not exposed (C+D)
	Number with outcome (A+C)	Number without outcome (B+D)	

$$RR = \frac{\text{proportion with outcome in treatment group}}{\text{proportion with outcome in control group}}$$

$$= \frac{A/(A+B)}{C/(C+D)}$$

$$= \frac{\text{exposure event rate (EER)}}{\text{control event rate (CER)}}$$

Hopefully you can now see how important it is to consider whether you are using a *relative* or an *absolute* risk reduction. The ARR in this example shows that using this hypothetical drug in the high risk population will prevent many more cases than in the low risk population. This is a point that might be very relevant when considering the trade-off between the benefits and harms or the costs of treatment.

E. Number needed to treat (NNT)

This is the number of patients who need to be treated with the studied intervention in order to prevent one event. It is calculated as the inverse of the ARR:

$$NNT = \frac{1}{ARR}$$

In our hypothetical sore throat example, we would find that the NNT for the 'high strep risk' population would be 1/0.30 or 3.33. This means that we would need to treat just over three patients to prevent persistent sore throat. In the 'low strep risk population', the NNT would be 1/0.05

C. Relative risk reduction (RRR)

Rather than trying to discuss the effect of a treatment as a ratio, it is often more clinically relevant to express the effect as a difference. This can be done in relative (i.e. in relation to the effect on controls) or absolute terms (which shows the actual size of the effect on that particular population—see the next section). The RRR will be the same regardless of the population. It can be calculated using the following formula:

$$** \text{ RRR} = \frac{(CER - EER)}{CER}$$

If we consider this for our case study example, the RRR would be (60%-30%)/60% = a 50% reduction in sore throat symptoms at day 3.

D. Absolute risk reduction (ARR)

In contrast to the RRR, the absolute risk reduction (ARR) is simply the difference between the event/outcome rate in the treatment group and that of the control group:

$$** \text{ ARR} = CER - EER$$

The ARR is said to be a much more clinically relevant estimate of effect because it takes into account the prevalence of an outcome in that particular population. In our hypothetical sore throat study, the symptom rate at day 3 in the control population is quite high at 60%. This may be because the study has been conducted in a population with high rates of Group A *Streptococcus*. The ARR for this study would be 60%–30%, which is a 30% reduction in sore throat by using antibiotics. However, if the study was conducted in a lower risk population where the prevalence of Group A *Streptococcus* in the control group was only 10%, then the ARR would be much less. You may recall that, in this hypothetical study, the RR was 0.5, so we would expect the treatment group in this low risk population to have a symptom rate of around 5%. In other words, the ARR for this low risk population is only 10%–5%, which is 5% (compared to 30% in the high risk population).

which is 20. In other words, in the lower risk population, we need to treat 20 people with antibiotics to prevent one persistent sore throat.

It is important to note that the NNT is only applicable when the study population is similar to the target patient population for whom the tested intervention is intended. When the treatment increases the risk of the harmful outcome, then the inverse of the risk difference is called the 'number needed to harm' (NNH).

F. Odds ratio (OR)

We often talk about the 'odds' of an event occurring. The 'odds'—or chance—of us winning the lottery is small. This seems obvious, but how do we measure the odds of a clinical event occurring? The odds ratio is the ratio of the odds of a disease occurring in the presence of an exposure relative to the odds of the disease occurring in the absence of the exposure. The odds ratio is commonly used in case-control studies.

Looking back to the 'outcome and exposure status' table, the odds ratio can be defined by the following formula:

$$OR = \frac{\text{odds of disease in the presence of exposure}}{\text{odds of disease in the absence of exposure}}$$

$$= A/B \text{ divided by } C/D$$

$$= AD/BC$$

Therefore, this is the odds of the outcome in the treatment group relative to the odds of the outcome in controls. Again, an OR of 1.0 means that there is no difference between the treatment and control groups. An OR >1.0 for an adverse outcome such as death means an increased risk. In some studies, the OR is a reasonable estimate of the RR, but only if the outcome is uncommon.

G. Hazard ratio (HR)

Used in survival analysis, this is the probability of a hazard at time 't' in

J. Tools applicable to diagnostic studies

These studies investigate the ability of a particular diagnostic or screening test to detect a disorder in the sample population. The performance of the test can then be evaluated:

- Sensitivity: proportion of people with a disorder that are correctly diagnosed as positive by the test. The higher the sensitivity of a test, the more likely a negative result will rule out presence of the disorder (high **SeN**sitivity rules **OUT** = SNOUT).
- Specificity: proportion of people without the disorder that are correctly excluded as negative by the test. The higher the specificity of a test, the more likely a positive result will rule in presence of the disorder (high **SP**ecificity rules **IN** = SPIN).
- Positive predictive value (PPV): proportion of people with a positive test who actually have the disorder.
- Negative predictive value (NPV): proportion of people with a negative test who do not have the disorder.
- Likelihood ratio (LR): provides a direct estimate of how much a test result will change the odds of having a disease. The likelihood ratio for a positive result (LR+) is how much the odds of the disease increase when a test is positive. The likelihood ratio for a negative result (LR-) is how much the odds of the disease decrease when a test is negative.

	Disorder present	Disorder absent
Positive test	a	b
Negative test	c	d

Sensitivity = $a/(a+c)$ PPV = $a/(a+b)$

Specificity = $c/(b+d)$ NPV = $d/(c+d)$

LR = Probability of test result in someone with the disease/Probability of test result in someone without the disease

LR+ (+ve test) = sensitivity/(1−specificity)

LR− (−ve test) = (1−sensitivity)/specificity

Can you apply this evidence about a treatment in caring for your patient?

Several issues need to be considered when generalising the results of an RCT for a particular patient population. This is often a sticking point for practitioners, who frequently find themselves trying to apply either hospital-based studies or studies conducted in other countries with different health care systems and patterns of disease to their own community-based populations. Trials conducted in hospital clinics may include higher proportions of patients with more serious disease than community-based samples, a factor that needs to be considered. The following questions should be considered:

What is the role of the patient in applying evidence?

Sackett's definition of EBM, quoted at the beginning of this chapter, clearly includes patient preference as an important component. However, to what extent do patients want to be involved in health care decisions? A recent survey of over 8,000 people in eight European countries showed that the majority of people do want some active role. The extent to which patients want to be involved may vary with culture, age, and socioeconomic group, as well as with the disease and its severity.

However, a direct link between patient involvement in decision-making and improved health and well-being is poorly documented. McNutt succinctly argues that patient involvement in decision-making is concerned with two things: 1) informing them of the consequences of the available options, including the probabilities of these where available, and 2) the opportunity to trade-off the benefits and risks for them. This may not result in the patient actually making the final decision, but does describe a process of involvement.

There has been increasing interest in 'decision aids' as effective tools for increasing patient involvement in decision-making. A *Cochrane* review of 32 RCTs concluded that decision aids increased patient knowledge of the options, compared to usual care, with gains ranging from 9% to 30% (weighted mean difference 19%, 95% CI = 13 to 24). Decision aids also increased realistic expectations of the benefits and harms of different options (as measured by patients' perception of the probability of outcomes), resulting in improved patient satisfaction with the decision-making process and greater agreement between patient values and actual choice.

Beyond this book: what is the role of systematic reviews and clinical practice guidelines?

For some clinical questions, there have been a number of good quality RCTs conducted across different populations and these are often summarised in systematic reviews. Clearly, if a good quality systematic review summarises and pools the results of several RCTs, then that source of evidence should be considered. The *Cochrane* database of systematic reviews is an excellent source of such evidence. If results from several trials can be pooled quantitatively (into a meta-analysis), this will provide a summary estimate of the effect of the treatment. Clinical practice guidelines are often a locally derived summary of systematically derived evidence, which has taken into account local application and health system contexts. They may also be an excellent source of evidence. However, it is important to note that not every clinical condition or topic will necessarily have a simple, accurate, up-to-date, and unbiased research-based answer. As an adjunct to clinical expertise, EBM has become increasingly central to medical practice, providing the impetus for ensuring health care professionals remain up-to-date with advances.

Further reading

Feinstein A. (1967) *Clinical Judgement*. The Williams and Wilkins Company, Baltimore.

Cochrane A. (1971) *Effectiveness and efficiency: Random reflections on health services*. Abingdon: Burgess and Son Ltd, Abingdon.

Sackett D, Haynes B, Tugwell P. (1985) *Clinical Epidemiology: A basic science for clinical medicine*. Little, Brown and Company, Toronto.

Sackett D, Rosenberg W, Muir Gray J et al. (1996) Evidence based medicine: what it is and what it isn't. *BMJ* 312, 71–2.

Del Mar C, Glasziou P, Mayer D. (2004) Teaching evidence-based medicine. *BMJ* 329, 989–90.

Glasziou P, Haynes B. (2005) The paths from research to improved health outcomes. *ACP Journal Club*. 142, 8–10.

Shojania K, Sampson M, Ansan M et al. (2007) How quickly do systematic reviews go out of date? A survival analysis. *Arch Intern Med* 147.

Del Mar C, Silagy C, Glasziou P et al. (2001) Feasibility of an evidence-based literature search service for general practitioners. *Med J Austr* 175, 134–7.

Gonzalez-Gonzalez AI, Sanchez-Mateos J et al. (2007) Information needs and information-seeking behaviour of primary care physicians. *Ann Fam Med* 345–352.

Ely V, Osheroff J, Gorman P et al. (2000) A taxonomy of generic clinical questions: classification study. *BMJ* 321, 429–32.

Del Mar C, Glasziou PP, Spinks A. (2006) *Antibiotics for sore throat*. Cochrane Database of Systematic Reviews 18, CD000023.

Trevena LJ, Irwig L, Isaacs A et al. (2007) General practitioners want simpler formats and tools for individualising evidence within clinical decisions: a cross sectional study in New South Wales, Australia. *Austr Fam Phys* 36(12); 1065–69.

Sackett DL, Scott Richardson W, Rosenberg W et al. (1998) *Evidence-based medicine: How to practice and teach EBM*. Churchill Livingstone.

Altman D, Schulz K, Moher D et al. (2001) The revised CONSORT statement for reporting randomized trials: Explanation and elaboration. *Ann Intern Med* 134, 663–94.

Coulter A, Jenkinson C. (2005) European patients' views on the responsiveness of health systems and healthcare providers. *Eur J Public Health* 15, 355–360.

McKinstry B. (2000) Do patients wish to be involved in decision making in the consultation? A cross sectional survey with video vignettes. *BMJ* 321, 867–71.

Beaver K, Jones D, Susnerwala S, Craven O et al. (2005) Exploring the decision-making preferences of people with colorectal cancer. *Health Expectations* 8, 103–113.

McNutt R. (2004) Shared Medical Decision Making: Problems, Process, Progress. *JAMA* 292, 2516–8.

Part 1

Medical specialties

Cardiology

Introduction

'After all, in spite of opinion, prejudice or error, Time will fix the real value upon this discovery, and determine whether I have imposed upon myself and others, or contributed to the benefit of science and mankind.' (William Withering, 1785)

So said William Withering in his *Account of the Foxglove and some of its Medical Uses*, in which he described the therapeutic effects of fox-glove extract in a series of patients with dropsy. His seminal observations sparked a debate about the benefit of digitalis, the active ingredient of foxglove, which was to continue for over two centuries. Controversy was only finally resolved in 1997 with the publication of a randomised, placebo-controlled trial in over 7,000 patients with heart failure.

To date, several thousand randomised trials of cardiac treatments have been published, and over the past few decades clinical cardiology has grad-ually evolved from an experience-based towards an evidence-based spe-cialty. Cardiologists, once revered for their prowess with a stethoscope, are now as likely to be discussing the results of the latest randomised trial as the nuances of cardiac auscultation. The current generation of cardi-ologists often refer to themselves as 'plumbers', 'electricians', or 'imagers', depending on their subspecialty interest, but all have access to an exten-sive and growing therapeutic armamentarium, increasingly supported by the results of randomised clinical trials.

Selecting a small number of trials for a chapter on evidence-based car-diology is therefore challenging. We have attempted to make an eclectic selection and to provide a balanced interpretation of the trial results. All of the trials have influenced cardiological practice, but integration of the evidence from them into routine patient management is not easy. Randomised trials recruit selected patients and the results may not be applicable to the generality of patients with cardiac disease. Women and the elderly are, for instance, often under-represented. Moreover, analyses of clinical trials often emphasise sub-group analyses, but the pitfalls of this approach were illustrated by the ISIS-2 investigators who reported that patients with acute myocardial infarction born under astrological star signs Gemini and Libra seem not to benefit from aspirin!

Astute clinicians will also recognise that there are other valuable sources of evidence apart from randomised trials: some years ago proponents of evidence-based practice were invited to volunteer for a randomised clin-ical trial of parachute use during gravitational challenge—not surprisingly there were few takers!

We hope this chapter may help to familiarise clinicians with some of the evidence underpinning contemporary cardiological practice and encourage interest in the future development of the cardiological evidence-base.

Coronary artery disease: statins

4S (Scandinavian Simvastatin Survival Study): Randomised trial of cholesterol lowering in 4,444 patients with coronary heart disease.

AUTHORS: Pedersen T, Kjekshus J, Berg K, *et al.*
REFERENCE: Lancet (1994) 344, 1383–9.
STUDY DESIGN: RCT
EVIDENCE LEVEL: 1b

Key message

In patients with established coronary artery disease and total cholesterol levels of 5.5–8.0mmol/L, the addition of simvastatin to regular medical therapy results in a 30% reduction in total mortality relative to placebo, with no effect on non-cardiac mortality.

Impact

Lipid-lowering therapy with a statin is now part of the standard treatment of patients with coronary heart disease (CHD).

Aims

Epidemiological evidence demonstrates a powerful association between hypercholesterolaemia and CHD, with early studies of cholesterol lowering for both primary and secondary prevention demonstrating reduced CHD events. Nevertheless, drug treatment for hypercholesterolaemia remained controversial as no mortality outcome data were available, and an increase in the risk of non-cardiac death from cancer or violence had been reported. This trial was designed to study the effects of long-term treatment with simvastatin (a 3-hydroxy-3-methylglutaryl coenzyme A [HMGCoA] reductase inhibitor) on mortality and morbidity in patients with CHD.

Methods

Patients: 4,444 patients at 94 Scandinavian centres.

Inclusion criteria: Compliance with 2-wk placebo run-in, and:
- Age 35–70y, with previous myocardial infarction (MI) or angina;
- Fasting cholesterol level 5.5–8.0mmol/L after dietary advice;
- Fasting triglyceride level <2.5mmol/L after dietary advice.

Groups:
- Dietary advice and simvastatin 20mg daily, increased to 40mg daily if total cholesterol exceeded 5.2mmol/L (n=2221);
- Dietary advice and matching placebo (n=2223).

Primary endpoint: Total mortality.

Secondary endpoint: 'Major coronary events'—coronary deaths, definite or probable hospital-verified non-fatal MI, resuscitated cardiac arrest, definite silent MI verified by ECG.

Other endpoints: Myocardial revascularisation (coronary artery bypass graft—CABG, or percutaneous coronary intervention—PCI).

Follow-up: Mean F/U=5.6y.

Results

Treatment with simvastatin was associated with reductions in serum total cholesterol, LDL cholesterol, and triglycerides, but a significant increase in HDL cholesterol.

	Simvastatin	Placebo	RRR (95% CI)	p
Mean change in total cholesterol	25% decrease	1% increase	Not reported	Not reported
Mean change in LDL	35% decrease	1% increase	Not reported	Not reported
Mean change in HDL	8% increase	1% increase	Not reported	Not reported
Mean change in trigs	10% decrease	7% increase	Not reported	Not reported
Primary endpoint: death	182 (8%)	256 (12%)	0.70 (0.58 to 0.85)	0.0003
Secondary endpoint: 'major coronary events'	431 (19%)	622 (28%)	0.66 (0.52 to 0.8)	0.00001
All coronary deaths	111 (5%)	189 (8.5%)	0.58 (0.46 to 0.73)	Not reported
All non-cardiovascular deaths	46 (2.1%)	49 (2.2%)	Not reported	ns
Coronary surgery or angioplasty	252 (11.3%)	383 (17.2%)	0.63 (0.54 to 0.74)	<0.00001
Fatal and non-fatal cerebrovascular events	70 (3.2%)	98 (4.4%)	0.70 (0.52 to 0.96)	0.02

Discussion

This trial demonstrated for the first time that in patients with overt CHD, the addition of simvastatin to standard medical therapy significantly reduced mortality and morbidity. The 10-y F/U data is now available for this study, and, although >80% of the two groups were ultimately on open label statin therapy, the survival benefit of an initial 5-y statin treatment persisted, with no increase in cancer deaths up to a median F/U of 10.4y. Subsequent trials (e.g. LIPID: *N Engl J Med (1998) 339, 1349–57*; CARE: *N Engl J Med (1996) 335, 1001–9*; HPS: *Lancet (2002) 360, 7–22*) have confirmed the beneficial effects of statin therapy. In a meta-analysis of 14 such trials (including >90,000 patients), statin therapy reduced the 5-y incidence of major coronary events, myocardial revascularisation, and stroke by about one fifth per mmol/L reduction in LDL cholesterol. The absolute benefits of statin therapy were largely independent of initial lipid profile, but were determined by the absolute risk of adverse vascular events and the absolute reduction in LDL achieved.

Problems

• Only 19% of patients were women, and the mortality rate for women in the placebo group was half that of men. Nevertheless, simvastatin reduced the risk of major adverse events in women to roughly the same extent as in men, and the benefits of treating women have been confirmed in meta-analyses.

Coronary artery disease: statins in primary prevention

WOSCOPS (West of Scotland Coronary Prevention Study): Prevention of coronary heart disease with pravastatin in men with hypercholesterolaemia.

AUTHORS: Shepherd J, Cobbe S, Ford I *et al.*
REFERENCE: N Engl J Med (1995) 333, 1301–7.
STUDY DESIGN: RCT
EVIDENCE LEVEL: 1b

Key message

Treatment with pravastatin (a 3-HMGCoA reductase inhibitor) in middle-aged men with hypercholesterolaemia (mean cholesterol 7.0mmol/L) significantly reduces the risk of myocardial infarction (MI) or death from cardiovascular (CV) causes with no excess risk of non-cardiac death.

Impact

Lipid-lowering therapy with pravastatin is effective in the primary prevention of coronary heart disease (CHD) in middle-aged men with hypercholesterolaemia. More recent studies also suggest that statin therapy may be indicated for all patients at high risk of CV events, even if LDL cholesterol is within or below the current normal range.

Aims

RCTs had shown that using lipid-lowering therapy with 3-hydroxy-3-methylglutaryl coenzyme A (HMGCoA) reductase inhibitors in patients with established CHD reduced all-cause mortality and death from CHD. Early evidence also suggested that lipid-lowering therapy for primary prevention might reduce CHD mortality, but increase the risk of death due to non-CV causes. The aim of WOSCOPS was to study the effectiveness of pravastatin in preventing coronary events in men with hypercholesterolaemia and no history of prior MI.

Methods

Patients: 6595 patients from primary care facilities in West Scotland.

Inclusion criteria:
- Age 45–64y;
- Fasting low density lipoprotein (LDL) cholesterol levels following dietary advice of ≥4mmol/L (with at least one value >4.5mmol/L and <6mmol/L on previous screening visits).

Exclusion criteria:
- No serious ECG abnormalities (pathological Q waves or arrhythmias);
- No history of prior MI.

Groups:
- Dietary advice + placebo (n=3293);
- Dietary advice + pravastatin 40mg daily (n=3302).

Primary endpoint: Combined endpoint of definite non-fatal MI and death from CHD.

Secondary endpoints:
- Definite non-fatal MI;
- Death definitely from CHD;
- Death from all CV causes;
- Death from non-CV causes;
- All deaths.

Follow-up: Mean F/U=4.9y.

Results

Primary endpoint	Placebo	Pravastatin	RRR (95% CI)	p
Death or non-fatal MI	248 (7.9%)	174 (5.5%)	31% (17 to 43)	<0.001
Secondary endpoints				
Definite non-fatal MI	204 (6.5%)	143 (4.6%)	31% (15 to 45)	<0.001
Death from definite CHD	52 (1.7%)	38 (1.2%)	28% (10 to 52)	0.1
Death from CV causes	73 (2.3%)	50 (1.6%)	32% (3 to 553)	0.03
Death from non-CV causes	62 (1.9%)	56 (1.7%)	11% (−28 to 38)	0.5
All deaths	135 (4.1%)	106 (3.2%)	22% (0 to 40)	0.05

- Baseline mean serum chol = 7.0±0.6mmol/L; LDL = 5.0±0.5mmol/L.
- Pravastatin lowered serum cholesterol by 20% and LDL by 26%, but increased HDL by 5%; reduced the requirement for coronary angiography or myocardial revascularisation by 31% and 37%, respectively; was well tolerated with no significant differences in myalgia, muscle aches, or elevation of muscle enzymes.

Discussion

Treatment with pravastatin (40mg od) in men with moderate hypercholesterolaemia and no history of MI reduced the risk of MI and death from cardiac causes without influencing death from non-CV causes. The benefit of treatment started to appear within 6 months and pravastatin was well tolerated. These data suggest giving pravastatin to 1000 middle-aged men with hypercholesterolaemia and no evidence of previous MI for 5y would prevent seven CV deaths, 20 non-fatal MIs, 14 coronary angiograms, and eight myocardial revascularisation procedures. Data from additional RCTs suggest a beneficial effect of statin treatment in primary prevention in patients with average cholesterol levels *(AFCAPS/TexCAPS, JAMA (1998) 279, 1615–22)* or even irrespective of baseline cholesterol levels *(HPS. Lancet (2002) 360, 7–22)*.

Problems

- WOSCOPS recruited middle-aged white men in Scotland, and the trial did not provide evidence to support the use of lipid-lowering therapy for primary prevention therapy in women or in other ethnic groups.
- The widespread use of statin therapy for primary prevention is controversial, partly because of its high cost. In an economic analysis based on WOSCOPS, lipid-lowering in men with hypercholesterolaemia was considered cost-effective, particularly when targeted at individuals with additional risk factors.

Hypertension: optimal treatment

> **ASCOT–BPLA** (**A**nglo-**S**candinavian **C**ardiac **O**utcomes **T**rial— **B**lood **P**ressure **L**owering **A**rm): Prevention of cardiovascular events with an antihypertensive regimen of amlodipine adding perindopril as required vs atenolol adding bendroflumethiazide as required.
>
> **AUTHORS:** Dahlof B, Sever P, Wedel H *et al.*
> **REFERENCE:** Lancet (2005) 366, 895–906.
> **STUDY DESIGN:** RCT
> **EVIDENCE LEVEL:** 1b

Key message

ASCOT–BPLA compared amlodipine + perindopril vs atenolol + ben-droflumethiazide (BFZ) in the treatment of patients with hypertension (HTN). The trial was stopped early because of reductions in all-cause mortality, fatal and non-fatal stroke, total cardiovascular (CV) events and procedures, and risk of developing diabetes—all in favour of the 'newer' regime.

Impact

In the absence of compelling reasons to prescribe β-blockers or thiazide diuretics, first-line antihypertensive therapy should now be based on the newer agents.

Aims

Treatment of HTN with antihypertensive drugs significantly reduces the risk of both CV and cerebrovascular events. ASCOT–BPLA was designed to assess whether newer blood pressure (BP)-lowering agents with meta-bolically favourable profiles would have a greater effect on outcome than older/conventional therapy.

Methods

Patients: 19,342 patients at multiple centres in the UK and Nordic countries.

Inclusion criteria:
- Age 40–79y;
- Untreated HTN with systolic BP (SBP) ≥160mmHg ± diastolic BP (DBP) ≥100mmHg, or treated HTN with SBP ≥140mmHg ± DBP ≥90mmHg;
- ≥3 of: left ventricular hypertrophy, type 2 diabetes mellitus, peripheral vascular disease, previous stroke or transient ischaemic attack (TIA), male gender, age ≥55y, proteinuria or microalbuminuria, smoking, total cholesterol:HDL >6, *or* family history of premature coronary heart disease (CHD).

Exclusion criteria: Previous MI, current angina, cerebrovascular accident (CVA) within 3 months, fasting triglycerides >4.5mmol/L, heart failure, uncontrolled arrhythmias, clinically important biochemical/haematological abnormality.

Groups:
- Amlodipine-based regime: amlodipine (5mg then 10mg od)+ perindo-pril (4mg then 8mg od)+ doxazosin (4mg then 8mg od) (n=9639).

- Atenolol-based regime: atenolol (50mg then 100mg od)+ BFZ (1.25mg then 2.5mg od)+ doxazosin (4mg then 8mg od) (n=9618).

Follow-up: Median F/U=5.5y (0.3% lost to F/U).

Primary endpoint	Secondary endpoints	Tertiary endpoints
Non-fatal MI, including silent MI + fatal CHD	All-cause mortality	Unstable angina
	Total stroke	New diabetes mellitus
	Primary endpoint minus silent infarction	New renal failure
	Coronary events and procedures	
	CV mortality	
	Non-fatal and fatal heart failure	

Results

	Amlodipine	Atenolol	Mean difference (mmHg)	p
Final SBP (SD)	136.1 (15.4)	137.7 (17.9)	2.7	<0.0001
Final DBP (SD)	77.4 (9.5)	79.2 (10.0)	1.9	<0.0001

Primary endpoint	Amlodipine	Atenolol	HR (95% CI)	p
Non-fatal MI + fatal CHD	429 (5%)	474 (5%)	0.90 (0.79 to 1.02)	0.1
Secondary endpoints				
All-cause mortality	738 (8%)	820 (9%)	0.89 (0.81 to 0.99)	0.02
Total stroke	327 (3%)	422 (4%)	0.77 (0.66 to 0.89)	0.0003
Tertiary endpoints				
Development of diabetes	567 (6%)	799 (8%)	0.70 (0.63 to 0.78)	<0.0001

Discussion

Earlier trials had shown β-blockers and thiazide diuretics (either together or as single agents) to reduce significantly the risk of CV events in hypertensive populations, and guidelines had recommended their use as first-line therapy. ASCOT–BPLA showed that treatment of moderate risk hypertensive patients with amlodipine (plus perindopril, if required) improved significantly CV outcomes and risk of new onset diabetes compared with atenolol (plus BFZ, if required).

Problems

- ASCOT–BPLA did not reach its primary endpoint, and was terminated early because of a mortality difference between the two groups.
- The trial included predominantly white male subjects. Female patients also benefited from the amlodipine-based regime, but caution should be exercised in extrapolating the data to other ethnic groups.

Myocardial infarction: thrombolysis

ISIS-2 (2nd International Study of Infarct Survival): Randomised trial of intravenous streptokinase, oral aspirin, both, or neither among 17,187 cases of suspected acute myocardial infarction.

AUTHORS: ISIS-2 collaborative group.
REFERENCE: Lancet (1988) 2, 349–60.
STUDY DESIGN: RCT
EVIDENCE LEVEL: 1b

Key message

IV streptokinase and oral aspirin reduce 5-wk mortality in patients with suspected acute myocardial infarction (AMI).

Impact

ISIS-2 was one of the first 'mega-trials' to have a major influence on the practice of clinical cardiology, and led to the widespread use of thrombolytic therapy and aspirin in the treatment of patients with AMI.

Aims

In 1985, an overview of several small trials had suggested that thrombolytic therapy reduced mortality by about 25% in patients with AMI. Similarly, an overview of trials of long-term antiplatelet therapy suggested benefit in patients with previous AMI, but limited evidence for aspirin during the acute phase. Therefore, this study was designed to test the efficacy of thrombolytic therapy and aspirin during the acute phase of AMI.

Methods

Patients: 17,187 patients at 417 hospitals in 17 countries.

Inclusion criteria: Suitable for thrombolytic therapy:
- Within 24h of onset of suspected AMI;
- No definite contraindications to streptokinase or aspirin.

Exclusion criteria:
- Absolute: Previous stroke, gastrointestinal haemorrhage, or ulcer;
- Relative: Recent arterial puncture or severe trauma, severe persistent hypertension, known allergy to streptokinase, or aspirin.

Groups: 2x2 factorial design. Streptokinase alone (n=4300), aspirin alone (n=4295), streptokinase and aspirin (n=4292), and neither (n=4300):
- IV streptokinase (1.5MU administered over 1h) (n=8592) or matching IV placebo (n=8595);
- Enteric-coated aspirin (162.5mg daily) (n=8587) or matching placebo (n=8600) for 1 month.

Primary endpoint: Vascular mortality at 5wk (long-term mortality also reported).

Results

Vascular mortality at 35d	Treatment	Placebo	RRR (95% CI)	p
Streptokinase vs placebo	9.2%	12.0%	25% (18 to 32%)	<0.00001
Aspirin vs placebo	9.4%	11.8%	23% (15 to 30%)	<0.00001
Streptokinase + aspirin vs placebo	8.0%	13.2%	42% (34 to 50%)	<0.00001

- Streptokinase was associated with a small excess of minor (3.5% vs 1.0%) and major (0.5% vs 0.2%) bleeds.
- Streptokinase produced a small excess risk of early stroke due to intracranial haemorrhage, but this was offset by a lower risk of stroke during later F/U. Hence, there was no overall difference in the rate of stroke between the streptokinase and placebo groups (0.7% vs 0.8%, respectively).
- Aspirin was associated with significant reductions in the risk of re-infarction and non-fatal stroke, but no increase in bleeding. These benefits were independent of the delay from symptom onset to treatment.

Discussion

ISIS-2 confirmed that fibrinolysis and short-term aspirin were beneficial in patients with suspected AMI; it was one of the first large RCTs in cardiology to have a major clinical impact. In this study, IV streptokinase prevented 28 vascular deaths per 1000 patients treated. This benefit was greatest among patients presenting within 4h of symptom onset. Short-term treatment with aspirin also prevented 24 vascular deaths per 1000 patients, but this benefit was not influenced by time from symptom onset. Aspirin and streptokinase had additive effects, and together prevented 52 vascular deaths per 1000 patients treated. Since ISIS-2 was published, several other RCTs have tested the use of newer 'fibrin-specific' agents (e.g. alteplase, reteplase) and support the use of fibrinolysis in patients with suspected AMI. Meta-analysis (50,000 patients) demonstrates benefit in patients presenting with ST elevation or left bundle branch block (LBBB), but a trend towards harm in those with ST depression. Treatment within the first hour of symptoms ('the golden hour') may prevent 65 deaths per 1000 patients treated. Guidelines now recommend fibrinolysis for patients presenting within 12h of symptom onset and ST elevation, new (or presumed new) LBBB, or evidence of posterior MI. It may also be reasonable to administer later fibrinolysis to patients with continuing ischaemic symptoms.

Problems

- Fibrinolysis is widely used in the treatment of AMI but has several important limitations. First, around half of all patients admitted to hospital with ST segment elevation AMI are ineligible for treatment. Second, treatment restores normal flow in the infarct-related artery in only 50%, and 25% of these patients re-occlude the vessel within 3 months. Primary angioplasty is an alternative treatment strategy for patients with ST elevation AMI and restores normal flow in the infarct-related artery in 90% of cases.

Myocardial infarction: primary angioplasty vs thrombolysis

Primary angioplasty vs intravenous thrombolytic therapy for acute myocardial infarction: a quantitative review of 23 randomised trials.

AUTHORS: Keeley E, Boura J, Grines C.
REFERENCE: Lancet (2003) 361, 13–20.
STUDY DESIGN: Meta-analysis
EVIDENCE LEVEL: 1a

Key message

This meta-analysis combined the results of several RCTs of fibrinolysis vs primary angioplasty in the management of patients with acute myocardial infarction (AMI). It provides compelling evidence that primary angioplasty is superior to fibrinolytic therapy in reducing mortality, non-fatal re-infarction, and stroke in patients eligible for reperfusion.

Impact

Primary angioplasty is the preferred treatment strategy for patients with reperfusion-eligible AMI, provided that experienced personnel and an appropriate catheter laboratory environment are available, and that the procedure can be carried out within 90min of presentation.

Aims

Fibrinolytic therapy reduces mortality in patients with acute myocardial infarction (AMI) associated with ST segment elevation or new (or presumably new) left bundle branch block (LBBB). Numerous small RCTs had also demonstrated that primary angioplasty (coronary balloon angioplasty without previous or concomitant fibrinolytic therapy) could re-open occluded arteries in these patients, although these trials had limited individual statistical power. This quantitative meta-analysis aimed to assess the impact of primary angioplasty on mortality and other important clinical outcomes.

Methods

A literature search identified 23 RCTs which assigned a total of 7739 patients with AMI to fibrinolytic therapy or primary angioplasty.

Inclusion criteria: Varied between trials. Most enrolled patients with ischaemic symptoms and ST segment elevation (≥1mm in two contiguous leads) or LBBB, and no contraindication to thrombolytic therapy.

Groups: Fibrinolytic agent: streptokinase in eight trials (n=1837) and a fibrin-specific agent in 15 trials (n=5902). Overall, 3,872 patients treated by primary angioplasty and 3867 patients given fibrinolysis. Stents were used in 12 trials and glycoprotein IIb/IIIa receptor inhibitors in eight.

Primary endpoints: Included short-term (4–6wk) and long-term (6–18 months) mortality, non-fatal re-infarction, and stroke.

Results

Endpoint	Thrombolysis	Primary PCI	p
Short-term mortality	9%	7%	0.0002
Non-fatal re-infarction	7%	3%	<0.0001
Stroke	2%	1%	0.0004
Death, non-fatal re-infarction, and stroke	14%	8%	<0.0001
Major bleeding	5%	7%	0.03

Short-term benefits of primary angioplasty maintained during F/U over 6–18mo.

Discussion

Previous angiographic studies had suggested that fibrinolytic therapy in patients with ST elevation AMI restored normal flow in the infarct-related artery in around 50% of cases. By contrast, primary angioplasty had been shown to restore normal coronary flow in over 90% of patients. However, transfer of patients with AMI to a catheter laboratory can lead to a delay in achieving myocardial reperfusion.

This meta-analysis provided evidence that primary angioplasty was superior to thrombolysis in the treatment of AMI with lower rates of mortality, non-fatal re-infarction, and stroke. Several of the trials were conducted before the widespread use of coronary stents or glycoprotein IIb/IIIa receptor antagonists; as these are known to improve outcome, the benefit of primary angioplasty may have been underestimated.

On the other hand, the trials of primary angioplasty vs fibrinolysis only enrolled a total of 7,739 patients. Most of the trials were small (<200 patients) and designed with surrogate endpoints such as infarct-artery patency or infarct size. Moreover, the SHOCK trial (*N Engl J Med* (1999) 341, 625–34), enrolled a high-risk group of patients in cardiogenic shock and compared a direct invasive strategy with initial medical stabilisation. When this trial was excluded and the analysis restricted to trials using a fibrin-specific fibrinolytic agent, the difference in mortality was no longer significant.

Problems

- The evidence favouring primary angioplasty over fibrinolysis for patients with AMI is modest and should be interpreted with caution. Nevertheless, this meta-analysis had a profound influence on guidelines and clinical practice—in many countries, primary angioplasty is the default management strategy for patients with ST elevation AMI.
- Provision of a primary angioplasty service to a large community is logistically challenging and requires close collaboration between ambulance services, emergency care departments, and interventional cardiology teams.
- Pre-hospital thrombolysis may be as effective as primary angioplasty. Further research is required to determine the optimal reperfusion strategy, particularly for patients presenting early after symptom onset or those in geographically remote locations.

Myocardial infarction: rescue angioplasty

> **REACT (REscue Angioplasty vs Conservative treatment or repeat Thrombolysis) study:** Rescue angioplasty after failed thrombolytic therapy for acute myocardial infarction.
>
> **AUTHORS:** Gershlick A, Stephens-Lloyd A, Hughes S *et al.*
> **REFERENCE:** N Engl J Med (2005) 353, 2758–68.
> **STUDY DESIGN:** RCT
> **EVIDENCE LEVEL:** 1b

Key message

In patients with ECG evidence of failed reperfusion after fibrinolytic treatment for acute myocardial infarction (AMI), rescue angioplasty is associated with lower adverse event rates than conservative care or repeat fibrinolysis.

Impact

Rescue angioplasty may be considered for patients in whom reperfusion fails to occur after fibrinolytic therapy. There is no evidence to support repeat fibrinolysis in this setting.

Aims

Fibrinolytic therapy in patients with ST segment elevation AMI results in reperfusion of the infarct-related artery in around 50% of patients. Appropriate treatment for those in whom reperfusion fails to occur is uncertain. This study aimed to compare three different treatment strategies for patients with failed reperfusion: conservative care, repeat thrombolysis, and 'rescue' angioplasty.

Methods

Patients: 427 patients at 35 centres in the UK.

Inclusion criteria:
- Age 21–85y;
- Failed reperfusion 90min after commencing fibrinolytic therapy (defined as <50% resolution of ST segment elevation ± chest pain).

Exclusion criteria:
- LBBB;
- Contraindication to repeat fibrinolysis;
- Estimated body weight <75kg;
- Persistent hypertension;
- Cardiogenic shock.

Groups:
- Repeat fibrinolysis (n=142);
- Conservative therapy (n=141);
- Rescue angioplasty (n=144).

Primary endpoint: Combined rate of death, recurrent AMI, cerebrovascular event, or severe heart failure at 6 months.

Secondary endpoints:
- Individual components of the primary endpoint;
- Rates of bleeding and revascularisation at 6 months.

Follow-up: F/U at 1, 6, and 12 months.

Results

Event rates at 6 months	Repeat fibrinolysis	Conservative	Rescue PCI	*p*
Primary endpoint	31.0%	29.8%	15.3%	0.003
Death	12.7%	12.8%	6.2%	0.12
Re-infarction	10.6%	8.5%	2.1%	<0.01
Cerebrovascular event	0.7%	0.7%	2.1%	0.6
Severe heart failure	7.0%	7.8%	4.9%	0.6
Major bleed	4.9%	3.5%	2.8%	0.7
Minor bleed	7.0%	5.7%	22.9%	<0.001
Revascularisation	23.2%	20.6%	13.2%	0.08

Discussion

This study showed that rescue angioplasty was associated with a better outcome than repeat fibrinolysis or conservative care in patients with failed reperfusion after initial fibrinolytic treatment for AMI. There was a significant reduction in the rate of re-infarction and trends towards lower rates of death and severe heart failure. The excess risk of minor bleeding in the rescue group was due to arterial puncture and may have been exacerbated by concomitant glycoprotein IIb/IIIa receptor inhibition. Meta-analysis of six trials (908 patients) (*J Am Coll Cardiol* (2007) *49*, 422–30) of rescue angioplasty demonstrated significant reductions in re-infarction and heart failure, a non-significant trend to lower all-cause mortality, and an increased risk of stroke and minor bleeding. The absolute reduction in the composite endpoint of death, re-infarction, and heart failure was 11%, indicating that only nine patients need to be treated by rescue angioplasty to avoid one such event. In three trials (410 patients) of repeat fibrinolysis, there was no effect on mortality or re-infarction, but an increased risk of minor bleeding. Thus, rescue angioplasty is a reasonable strategy for patients with failed reperfusion, but there is no evidence to support repeat fibrinolytic therapy.

Problems

- Although this was the largest study of rescue angioplasty, it only included 427 patients and had limited statistical power. Fewer than 1,000 patients have been randomised in trials of rescue angioplasty and the evidence base to support this strategy is modest.
- Provision of effective rescue angioplasty services for large populations is difficult and requires systems for rapid transfer of patients with failed reperfusion to hospitals with emergency catheter laboratory facilities.

Myocardial infarction: clopidogrel and metoprolol

COMMIT (ClOpidogrel and Metoprolol in Myocardial Infarction Trial): Addition of clopidogrel to aspirin in 45,852 patients with acute myocardial infarction.

AUTHORS: COMMIT collaborative group.
REFERENCE: Lancet (2005) 366, 1607–21; (2005) 366, 1622–32.
STUDY DESIGN: RCT
EVIDENCE LEVEL: 1b

Key message

In patients with acute myocardial infarction (AMI), the addition of clopidogrel to standard therapy, including aspirin, reduces mortality and the combined endpoint of death, re-infarction, and stroke. Early administration of beta (β)-blocker after AMI reduces the risk of re-infarction and ventricular fibrillation, but increases the risk of cardiogenic shock during the first day after hospital admission.

Impact

Clopidogrel (75mg od) is indicated for up to 4wk following AMI. β-blockers should be started after AMI once the haemodynamic condition of the patient is stable.

Aims

Administration of aspirin within a few hours of the onset of AMI reduces mortality as well as the risk of re-infarction and stroke. This study aimed to test whether the addition of clopidogrel to aspirin in patients with suspected AMI would be beneficial. The role of β-blockade after AMI is established, but the use of early IV treatment is controversial, particularly as most previous studies were done before fibrinolytic and antiplatelet therapy became routine. Therefore, COMMIT also aimed to assess whether early β-blockade in AMI offered benefit, in addition to standard treatment.

Methods

Patients: 45,852 patients admitted to 1,250 hospitals in China.

Inclusion criteria: ST segment elevation, left bundle branch block, or ST segment depression within 24h of onset of symptoms of suspected AMI.

Exclusion criteria:
- Clear indications for *or* contraindications to the study treatments;
- Patients treated by primary percutaneous coronary intervention.

Groups: All patients given aspirin (162mg od). 2x2 factorial design:
- Clopidogrel (75mg od) (n=22961) or placebo (n=22891) for 4wk.
- IV, then oral metoprolol (n=22929) or placebo (n=22923)

Primary endpoints:
- Composite of death, re-infarction, or stroke (clopidogrel analysis);
- Composite of death, re-infarction, or cardiac arrest (metoprolol analysis);
- Death from any cause.

Secondary endpoints:
- Re-infarction;
- Ventricular fibrillation or other cardiac arrest;
- Cardiogenic shock;
- Bleeding.

Follow-up: F/U to hospital discharge or for 28d.

Results

Primary endpoint	Clopidogrel	Placebo	p
Death, re-infarction, or stoke	9.2%	10.1%	0.002
Death from any cause	7.5%	8.1%	0.03

- The risk of bleeding (all fatal, transfused, or cerebral bleeds) was not influenced by clopidogrel—either overall in patients aged >70y or in those given fibrinolytic therapy.

Primary endpoint	Metoprolol	Placebo	p
Death, re-infarction, or cardiac arrest	9.4%	9.9%	0.1
Death from any cause	7.7%	7.8%	0.7
Secondary endpoint			
Re-infarction	2.0%	2.5%	0.001
Ventricular fibrillation	2.5%	3.0%	0.001
Cardiogenic shock	2.2%	1.7%	0.0002

Discussion

COMMIT demonstrated that addition of clopidogrel to aspirin in patients with AMI reduced mortality and the rate of major adverse cardiovascular events. Treatment with clopidogrel for about 2wk prevented six deaths or nine adverse events (death, re-infarction, or stroke) per 1000 patients treated without increasing bleeding risk. The benefit was seen across a wide range of patients and was not influenced by the use of other treatments (including fibrinolysis). The study recruited patients in China, but it is likely that the results can be applied to other populations. Although the absolute benefit of adding clopidogrel to aspirin was modest, it is now part of the standard management of AMI.

The study also demonstrated that early β-blockade does not reduce in-hospital mortality or the composite endpoint of death, re-infarction, or cardiac arrest. Treatment with metoprolol did reduce the risk of re-infarction and ventricular fibrillation, but this was balanced by increased risk of early cardiogenic shock. Thus, it is reasonable to delay β-blockade until the haemodynamic condition of the patient is stable. Continued β-blockade as secondary prevention following hospital discharge will further increase the benefit of treatment.

Problems

- A standard dose of clopidogrel was used; an initial loading dose might have had greater benefit.
- Duration of clopidogrel treatment was only 2wk; further study is required to determine whether longer term treatment is beneficial.

Non-ST elevation acute coronary syndrome: enoxaparin

ESSENCE (**E**fficacy and **S**afety of **S**ubcutaneous **E**noxaparin in **N**on-Q-wave **C**oronary **E**vents) **study:** A comparison of low molecular weight heparin with unfractionated heparin for unstable coronary artery disease.

AUTHORS: Cohen M, Demers C, Gurfinkel E et al.
REFERENCE: N Engl J Med (1997) 337, 447–52.
STUDY DESIGN: RCT
EVIDENCE LEVEL: 1b

Key message

Antithrombotic therapy with subcutaneous enoxaparin and aspirin is more effective than continuous IV unfractionated heparin (UFH) and aspirin at reducing ischaemic events in patients with non-ST elevation acute coronary syndrome (ACS).

Impact

Enoxaparin is administered routinely in the acute management of patients with non-ST elevation ACS.

Aims

Several small trials had suggested that IV UFH reduced the risk of ischaemic events in patients with non-ST elevation ACS. Low molecular weight heparins (LMWH) have several potential advantages over UFH, including predictable anticoagulant effect and no requirement for anticoagulant monitoring. This study was designed to compare the efficacy and safety of enoxaparin and UFH in patients with non-ST elevation ACS.

Methods

Patients: 3171 patients at 176 hospitals in ten countries.

Inclusion criteria: Eligible patients had angina within the previous 24h associated with one of the following:
- ST segment depression of ≥ 0.1mV, transient ST segment elevation, or T wave changes in two contiguous leads;
- Previous myocardial infarction (MI) or revascularisation;
- Previous invasive/non-invasive investigations suggesting coronary artery disease.

Exclusion criteria:
- Left bundle branch block or persistent ST elevation;
- Contraindication to anticoagulation;
- Creatinine clearance <30mL/min.

Groups:
- Enoxaparin: 1mg/kg body weight enoxaparin SC every 12h with an IV placebo bolus and infusion (n=1607);

- UFH: Subcutaneous placebo injections and an IV bolus of UFH (usually 5000U) followed by continuous heparin infusion at a dose determined by the activated partial thromboplastin time (APTT) (n=1564).

Primary endpoint:
- Composite of death, non-fatal MI, and recurrent angina at 48h, 14d, and 30d.

Secondary endpoints:
- Rate of death and non-fatal MI at 48h, 14d, and 30d;
- Major and minor haemorrhage.

Results

Primary endpoint	UFH	Enoxaparin	*p*
Composite primary endpoint	**19.8%**	**16.6%**	**0.02**
Death (at 14d)	2.3%	2.2%	0.9
MI (at 14d)	3.8%	2.7%	0.06
Recurrent angina (at 14d)	15.5%	12.9%	0.03
Primary endpoint (at 30d)	23.3%	19.8%	0.02
Death/MI (at 30d)	7.7%	6.2%	0.08
Revascularisation (at 30d)	32.2%	27.0%	0.001
Bleeding			
Any bleeding (at 30d)	14.2%	18.4%	0.001
Major bleeding (at 30d)	7.0%	6.5%	0.6

Discussion

ESSENCE demonstrated that enoxaparin was more effective than UFH in reducing ischaemic events at 14d (sustained at 30d) in patients with non-ST elevation ACS. The difference in the composite endpoint was driven mainly by a reduction in the risk of recurrent angina, but at 30d, there was a trend for a lower rate of death or MI in the enoxaparin group. Enoxaparin was associated with an increased risk of minor but not major bleeding. Meta-analysis of trials of enoxaparin vs UFH included 21,946 patients with non-ST elevation ACS—enoxaparin prevented ten deaths or non-fatal MI per 1,000 patients without increasing bleeding risk (*Eur Heart J* (2007) 28, 2077–86).

Problems

- The beneficial effects of enoxaparin in non-ST elevation ACS cannot be translated to other LMWHs with different pharmacological profiles.
- Most of the trials of LMWH were conducted before widespread use of thienopyridines (ticlopidine or clopidogrel) or glycoprotein IIb/IIIa receptor antagonists.
- Although enoxaparin is widely used in the management of patients with non-ST elevation ACS, novel antithrombins (including bivalirudin and fondaparinux) may be associated with a lower risk of bleeding.

Non-ST elevation acute coronary syndrome: glycoprotein IIb/IIIa antagonists

> **PURSUIT** (**P**latelet glycoprotein IIb/IIIa in **U**nstable angina: **R**eceptor **S**uppression **U**sing **I**ntegrilin **T**herapy) **trial:** Inhibition of platelet glycoprotein IIb/IIIa with eptifibatide in patients with acute coronary syndromes.
>
> **AUTHORS:** The PURSUIT Trial Investigators.
> **REFERENCE:** N Engl J Med (1998) 339, 436–43.
> **STUDY DESIGN:** RCT
> **EVIDENCE LEVEL:** 1b

Key message

Treatment with eptifibatide reduces the risk of death or myocardial infarction (MI) in patients with non-ST segment elevation acute coronary syndromes (ACS), particularly among those at high risk of recurrent events.

Impact

Small molecule glycoprotein (GP) IIb/IIIa receptor antagonists are recommended for patients with non-ST segment elevation ACS at high risk of recurrent events, including patients with raised serum troponin or recurrent ischaemia, and those scheduled for an invasive strategy.

Aims

ACS is caused by the disruption of an atherosclerotic plaque, which leads to platelet aggregation and intra-coronary thrombus formation. Patients presenting with non-ST segment elevation ACS are at high risk of ischaemic complications, and standard treatment includes antiplatelet and antithrombin medication to prevent progression to death or non-fatal MI. Eptifibatide reversibly blocks the platelet GP IIb/IIIa receptor and inhibits platelet aggregation. This study was designed to assess whether eptifibatide offered incremental benefit over standard treatment with aspirin and IV unfractionated heparin (UFH) in patients with non-ST elevation ACS.

Methods

Patients: 10,948 patients at 726 hospitals in 28 countries.

Inclusion criteria:
- Ischaemic chest pain at rest for ≥10min within previous 24h;
- Transient ST segment deviation *or* T wave inversion or an elevated serum creatine kinase-MB.

Exclusion criteria:
- Persistent ST segment elevation;
- Active or recent bleeding, bleeding diathesis, recent major surgery;
- Systolic BP >200mmHg or diastolic BP >110mmHg;
- Stroke within previous 30d or any haemorrhagic stroke;
- Renal failure;
- Pregnancy;
- Thrombolytic therapy.

Groups:
- Eptifibatide: high-dose regimen included an IV bolus dose (200mcg/kg), followed by an infusion (2.0mcg/kg/min) (n=4722);

- Placebo: given as a matching IV bolus and infusion (n=4739).

Primary endpoint: Combined rate of death and non-fatal MI at 30d.

Secondary endpoints:
- Components of the composite primary endpoint;
- Efficacy in patients undergoing percutaneous coronary intervention;
- Bleeding complications and platelet counts;
- Major bleeding, defined as intracranial haemorrhage or bleeding associated with a drop in haematocrit of ≥15% or a drop in haemoglobin concentration of ≥5g/dL.

Results

Primary endpoint	Eptifibatide	Placebo	*p*
Death or non-fatal MI			
at 96h	7.6%	9.1%	0.01
at 7d	10.1%	11.6%	0.02
at 30d	14.2%	15.7%	0.04
Secondary endpoints			
Death at 30d	3.5%	3.7%	0.5
MI at 30d	12.6%	13.5%	0.1
Blood transfusion	11.6%	9.2%	RR 1.3 (95% CI 1.1 to 1.4)
Major bleeding	10.6%	9.1%	0.02
Thrombocytopaenia	6.8%	6.7%	ns
Stroke	0.7%	0.8%	0.4

Discussion

In PURSUIT a GP IIb/IIIa receptor antagonist (in addition to standard treatment with aspirin and UFH) reduced the risk of death or non-fatal MI at 30d. This benefit appeared within 4d of randomisation. The absolute reduction in the primary endpoint was small (1.5%), but substantially greater (5.1%) among patients undergoing percutaneous revascularisation within 72h. This benefit has to be balanced against the 1.5% absolute excess of major bleeds. Meta-analysis of six RCTs of IIb/IIIa inhibitors included 31,402 patients with ACS, not scheduled to undergo early coronary revascularisation. IIb/IIIa indibitors reduced the occurrence of death or MI, the greatest benefit being in patients with the highest risk of thrombotic complications. Guidelines now recommend GP IIb/IIIa inhibitors in high-risk patients, including those with elevated serum troponin or recurrent ischaemia, and those selected for an invasive management strategy.

Problems

- PURSUIT and other trials of IIb/IIIa receptor antagonists were conducted before thienopyridines (e.g. clopidogrel) and low molecular weight heparins were used routinely in patients with non-ST segment elevation ACS. Integrating evidence from these trials into contemporary practice is challenging, and the role of triple antiplatelet therapy with aspirin, thienopyridines, and IIb/IIIa receptor antagonists is uncertain.

Non-ST elevation acute coronary syndrome: clopidogrel

CURE (**C**lopidogrel in **U**nstable angina to prevent **R**ecurrent **E**vents): Effects of clopidogrel in addition to aspirin in patients with acute coronary syndrome without ST segment elevation.

AUTHORS: CURE Trial Investigators.
REFERENCE: N Engl J Med (2001) 345, 494–502.
STUDY DESIGN: RCT
EVIDENCE LEVEL: 1b

Key message

Clopidogrel, in addition to aspirin, confers cardiovascular (CV) benefits in patients with acute coronary syndrome (ACS) without ST segment elevation, but increases the risk of major bleeding.

Impact

Clopidogrel (75mg od) is prescribed routinely in patients with non-ST segment elevation ACS.

Aims

ACS is caused by erosion or rupture of an atherosclerotic plaque with subsequent platelet-mediated coronary thrombosis. Aspirin irreversibly inhibits cyclooxygenase-dependent platelet aggregation and reduces the risk of death, myocardial infarction (MI), and recurrent ischaemia in patients with unstable coronary artery disease. Clopidogrel is a thienopyridine derivative which inhibits adenosine diphosphate-induced platelet aggregation. This study aimed to test whether the addition of clopidogrel to aspirin could improve outcome in patients with non-ST segment elevation ACS.

Methods

Patients: 12,562 patients at 482 centres in 28 countries.

Inclusion criteria:
- Patients presenting within 24h of onset of symptoms of ACS without ST segment elevation;
- The protocol was amended after the first 3,000 patients had been recruited. Thereafter, patients were only enrolled if they had ECG changes or elevation of a serum cardiac marker or enzyme.

Exclusion criteria:
- Contraindication to antithrombotic treatment;
- High risk of bleeding;
- Severe heart failure;
- Oral anticoagulant therapy;
- Coronary revascularisation within previous 3 months;
- Glycoprotein IIb/IIIa receptor antagonists in previous 3d.

Groups: Mean duration of therapy 9 months. Aspirin (75–325mg od) was given to all patients:
- Clopidogrel (300mg loading, then 75mg od) (n=6259);
- Placebo (n=6303).

Primary endpoint:
- CV death, non-fatal MI or stroke;
- CV death, MI, stroke, or refractory ischaemia.

Secondary endpoint: Major bleeding.

Follow-up: At 3 monthly intervals for a mean of 9 months.

Results

Endpoint	Clopidogrel	Placebo	*p*
CV death, MI, or stroke	9.3%	11.4%	<0.001
CV death, MI, stroke, refractory ischaemia	16.5%	18.8%	<0.001
CV death	5.1%	5.5%	ns
MI	5.2%	6.7%	<0.05
Stroke	1.2%	1.4%	ns
Refractory ischaemia	8.7%	9.3%	ns
Minor bleeding	5.1%	2.4%	<0.001
Major bleeding	3.7%	2.7%	0.001
Life-threatening bleeding	2.2%	1.8%	0.1

Discussion

Addition of clopidogrel to aspirin in patients with non-ST segment elevation ACS reduced the risk of MI, with a trend towards lower rates of stroke and CV death. Clopidogrel also reduced the risk of recurrent ischaemia, during initial hospitalisation. These benefits emerged within 24h of starting treatment but should be balanced against increased risk of minor and major bleeding. Treatment of 1000 patients with clopidogrel for 9 months will prevent 28 adverse CV events (CV death, MI, or stroke) in 22 patients, but will cause an additional ten major bleeds (of which six will require transfusion and four may be life-threatening). Overall, treatment with clopidogrel results in net clinical benefit, and is now part of the standard management of patients with non-ST elevation ACS.

Problems

- The loading dose of clopidogrel was 300mg, but higher loading doses (600mg) have been shown to have more rapid antiplatelet effect and possible additional clinical benefit.
- Although clopidogrel was continued for a mean of 9 months, most benefit accrued within the first 3 months. Further research is required to ascertain the optimal duration of treatment.
- Treating all patients with non-ST segment elevation ACS with clopidogrel is expensive but economic analyses confirm that dual antiplatelet therapy for 9 months after presentation is cost-effective.

Non-ST elevation acute coronary syndrome: invasive vs conservative treatment

RITA-3 (British Heart Foundation Randomised Intervention Trial of unstable Angina): Invasive vs conservative treatment for patients with unstable angina or non-ST elevation myocardial infarction.

AUTHORS: Fox K, Poole-Wilson P, Henderson R et al.
REFERENCE: Lancet (2002) 360, 743–51.
STUDY DESIGN: RCT
EVIDENCE LEVEL: 1b

Key message

An early invasive strategy (percutaneous coronary intervention, PCI) in patients with non-ST segment elevation acute coronary syndrome (ACS) is superior to a conservative strategy. Benefit is greatest in patients with the highest baseline risk.

Impact

International guidelines recommend an early invasive strategy in patients with non-ST elevation ACS: (i) who have refractory angina or haemodynamic or electrical instability, or (ii) who have an elevated risk for further clinical events.

Aims

Patients with non-ST elevation ACS are at risk of recurrent episodes of myocardial ischaemia and injury. An early invasive strategy (PCI) may stabilise the acute ischaemic syndrome and reduce the risk of further myocardial injury. On the other hand, a conservative 'ischaemia-driven' strategy with a period of intensive medical treatment may prevent recurrent myocardial ischaemia and avoid procedural complications. This study was designed to compare these two strategies.

Methods

Patients: 1810 patients at 45 hospitals in England and Scotland.

Inclusion criteria: Cardiac chest pain at rest within previous 48h and at least one of:
- ECG evidence of myocardial ischaemia (ST segment depression, transient ST segment elevation, left bundle branch block, or T wave invertion);
- Pathological Q waves suggesting previous myocardial infarction (MI);
- Coronary artery disease on a previous angiogram.

Exclusion criteria:
- Reperfusion eligible MI or MI within previous month;
- PCI (in previous 12 months) or coronary artery bypass surgery (at any time);
- Haemodynamically significant valve disease;
- Cardiomyopathy.

Groups: All patients were treated with aspirin and enoxaparin
- Conservative care (n=915): anti-anginal and additional antithrombotic medication determined by the supervising clinician. Coronary angiography reserved for recurrent ischaemia;

- Invasive care (n=895): coronary angiography within 72h of randomisation and subsequent myocardial revascularisation as clinically indicated.

Primary endpoints: Combined rate of death, MI, or refractory angina at 4 months; combined rate of death and MI at 1y.

Secondary endpoints:
- Angina and quality-of-life (QoL) scores;
- Health economic evaluation;
- Combined rates of death and MI at 5y.

Results

Primary endpoint	Invasive care	Conservative care	Risk ratio (95% CI)	*p*
Death, MI, and refractory angina at 4 months	9.6%	14.5%	0.66 (0.51 to 0.85)	0.001
Death and MI at 1y	7.6%	8.3%	0.91 (0.67 to 1.25)	0.6

- At 4 months and 1y, patients in the invasive group had less angina, took less anti-anginal medication, and had greater gains in QoL scores.
- In a F/U report (*Lancet* (2008) 366, 914–20), the combined rate of death or MI after 5y was lower in the invasive strategy group (16.6% vs 20.0%; odds ratio 0.78; 95%CI 0.61 to 0.99, p=0.044).

Discussion

In this study, an early invasive strategy in patients with non-ST elevation ACS was superior to a conservative strategy. The main early benefit was a reduction in the risk of refractory angina, but during later F/U, additional benefit emerged with a lower rate of death and non-fatal MI. The benefits of the invasive strategy were greatest in patients with highest baseline risk. Other trials of early invasive vs conservative treatment strategies have reported similar results. In a meta-analysis of seven trials involving >9000 patients with non-ST segment elevation ACS (*JAMA* (2005) 293, 2908–17), a routine invasive strategy was associated with a higher risk of death or MI during the initial hospital admission, but an overall reduction in MI, severe angina, and repeat hospital admission over 17 months F/U.

Problems

- The early invasive strategy resulted in a beneficial effect in men but not in women. This finding must be interpreted cautiously as there were significant differences in risk factor profiles and revascularisation policies between men and women, which were not explained by disease severity. Further research is needed to evaluate the impact of the early invasive strategy in women.
- A myocardial revascularisation procedure was eventually performed in 38% of the conservative group. The mechanism of the progressive benefit over time in the early invasive group is unclear.
- The optimal timing of the early invasive strategy remains uncertain. A single trial (ISAR-COOL: *JAMA* (2003) 290, 1593–99) has suggested that very early invasive treatment confers additional benefit; further evidence is required.

Coronary artery disease: percutaneous intervention

> **COURAGE** (**C**linical **O**utcomes **U**tilising **R**evascularisation and **AG**gressive drug **E**valuation) trial: Optimal medical therapy with or without percutaneous coronary intervention for stable coronary disease.
>
> **AUTHORS:** Boden W, O'Rourke R, Teo K *et al.*
> **REFERENCE:** New Engl J Med (2007) 356,1503–16.
> **STUDY DESIGN:** RCT
> **EVIDENCE LEVEL:** 1b

Key message

COURAGE assessed the impact of percutaneous coronary intervention (PCI) (including the use of bare metal coronary stents) on prognosis in patients with stable coronary artery disease. In patients on optimal medical therapy, an initial strategy of routine PCI does not reduce the risk of death, myocardial infarction (MI), or other cardiovascular (CV) events when compared with a strategy of selective PCI for angina.

Impact

PCI with bare metal coronary stents does not influence the risk of death or MI in patients with stable coronary artery disease who are on optimal medical therapy. PCI should be reserved for patients with limiting angina and is not indicated in patients with asymptomatic or mildly symptomatic coronary artery disease.

Aims

Although coronary balloon angioplasty is an effective treatment for chronic stable angina, it has never been shown to improve mortality or risk of MI in these patients. This trial aimed to compare an initial strategy of optimal medical therapy and routine PCI (including coronary stents), with an initial strategy of optimal medical therapy alone.

Methods

Patients: 2287 patients at 50 centres in the USA.

Inclusion criteria:
- Stable coronary artery disease;
- Canadian Cardiovascular Society class I–III angina;
- Significant stenosis in ≥1 proximal epicardial coronary artery with objective evidence of myocardial ischaemia or typical angina;
- Coronary anatomy suitable for PCI;
- Ejection fraction ≥30%.

Exclusion criteria:
- Persistent Canadian Cardiovascular Society class IV angina;
- Markedly positive exercise test (within stage 1 of the Bruce protocol);
- Revascularisation within the previous 6 months.

Groups: All patients given angiotensin-converting enzyme inhibitors, anti-ischaemic, antiplatelet and lipid-lowering therapy:
- Optimal medical therapy (n=1138);
- Optimal medical therapy and PCI (n=1149).

Follow-up: Mean F/U 4.6y.

Primary endpoint: Composite of death from any cause and non-fatal MI.

Secondary endpoints:
- Composite of death, MI, and stroke;
- Hospitalisation for unstable angina (with negative biomarkers);
- Canadian Cardiovascular Society Angina class.

Results

Primary endpoint	Optimal medical and PCI	Optimal medical	*p*
Death or non-fatal MI	19.0%	18.5%	0.6
Secondary endpoints			
Death	7.6%	8.3%	
MI	13.2%	12.3%	0.3
Death, MI, stroke	20.0%	19.5%	0.6
Hospitalisation for unstable angina	12.4%	11.8%	0.6
Additional revascularisation	21.1%	32.6%	<0.001
Angina-free at 3y	72%	67%	0.02
Angina-free at 5y	74%	72%	ns

Discussion

Previous trials had shown that coronary balloon angioplasty was an effective treatment for stable angina, but did not influence risk of death or MI. COURAGE confirmed these findings for PCI with bare metal coronary stents. More patients in the PCI group were free from angina with lower use of anti-anginal medications, but this difference reduced over time, probably because of additional revascularisation and intensive control of vascular risk factors in the optimal medical therapy arm.

Problems

- The trial compared two initial treatment strategies, but following assignment, 32.6% of the medical group underwent a revascularisation procedure (for severe or unstable symptoms), and 21.1% of the PCI group had a repeat revascularisation procedure (probably for restenosis).
- Patients were enrolled over a period of 4.5y. During this time, there were advances in both medical and interventional treatments for coronary artery disease. Importantly, COURAGE was conducted before the introduction of drug-eluting stents, but available data indicate that these do not confer prognostic benefit when compared with bare metal stents.

Coronary artery disease: stents vs balloon angioplasty

BENESTENT (**BE**lgium **NE**therlands **STENT**) study: A comparison of balloon-expandable-stent implantation with balloon angioplasty in patients with coronary artery disease.

AUTHORS: Serruys P, de Jaegere P, Kiemeneij F et al.
REFERENCE: N Engl J Med (1994) 331, 489–95.
STUDY DESIGN: RCT
EVIDENCE LEVEL: 1b

Key message
This study demonstrates better outcomes in patients who receive a bare metal coronary stent compared with those treated with balloon angioplasty alone.

Impact
Coronary stents have now been implanted in millions of patients worldwide and are a standard component of percutaneous coronary intervention procedures.

Aims
Balloon-expandable metallic coronary stents were initially developed to treat coronary dissection and occlusion occurring during percutaneous coronary balloon angioplasty. Coronary stents may also reduce the risk of recurrence of the treated stenosis ('restenosis'). BENESTENT was designed to assess whether routine coronary stent placement would improve angiographic and clinical outcome as compared with standard balloon angioplasty.

Methods
Patients: 520 patients at multiple European centres.

Inclusion criteria:
- Single, *de novo* coronary lesions supplying normal myocardium;
- Target lesion length <15mm;
- Target vessel >3mm diameter;
- No contraindication to anticoagulant or antiplatelet therapy.

Exclusion criteria:
- Ostial or bifurcation stenosis;
- Previously grafted vessel;
- Suspected intra-coronary thrombus.

Groups:
- Bare metal stent (n=259 oral anticoagulation for 3 months);
- Balloon angioplasty (n=257).

Primary endpoints:
- **Clinical**: Composite of death, cerebrovascular accident, myocardial infarction (MI), coronary artery bypass surgery, repeat angioplasty of the target stenosis at 6 months;
- **Angiographic**: Minimal luminal diameter in target stenosis at 6 months.

Secondary endpoints:
- Angiographic success rate;
- Procedural success rate;
- Restenosis rate.

Follow-up: Quantitative coronary angiography and clinical F/U at 6 months.

Results

Event rates at 7 months	Balloon angioplasty (n=257)	Stent (n=259)	p
Death	0.4%	0.8%	ns
Stroke	0.8%	0%	ns
MI	4.6%	4.2%	ns
Coronary bypass surgery	4.2%	6.2%	ns
Repeat angioplasty	23.3%	13.5%	<0.05
Any event	29.6%	20.1%	<0.05

At 6 months the mean minimal luminal diameter in the target stenosis was 1.73mm in the balloon angioplasty group and 1.82mm in the stent group ($p=0.09$), with restenosis rates of 32% and 22%, respectively ($p=0.02$).

Discussion

This study demonstrated that routine deployment of a bare metal coronary stent improves clinical and angiographic outcomes when compared with simple balloon angioplasty alone. This benefit was obtained at the cost of an increased risk of arterial access site complications and a longer hospital stay (8.1d vs 3.5d, $p=0.001$). Subsequent RCTs have shown that coronary stents can be implanted safely with high pressure balloon dilatation and antiplatelet treatment (aspirin plus ticlopidine or clopidogrel), obviating the need for anticoagulation and greatly reducing the risk of arterial access site bleeding.

Problems
- BENESTENT confirmed that routine use of a bare metal stent was beneficial in a highly selected population with simple coronary lesions. Other RCTs have shown that stents are also beneficial in patients with more complex coronary anatomy.
- Late F/U data for patients treated with bare metal stents are very limited.
- Drug-eluting stents are now available which further reduce the risk of restenosis (see RAVEL).

Coronary artery disease: percutaneous intervention vs surgery

ARTS (**A**rterial **R**evascularisation **T**herapies **S**tudy): Comparison of coronary artery bypass surgery and stenting for the treatment of multi-vessel coronary disease.

AUTHORS: Serruys P, Unger F, Sousa J et al.
REFERENCE: N Engl J Med (2001) 344, 1117–24.
STUDY DESIGN: RCT
EVIDENCE LEVEL: 1b

Key message

In patients with multi-vessel disease, coronary stenting and coronary artery bypass surgery are associated with comparable rates of mortality, stroke, and myocardial infarction (MI). However, coronary stenting is associated with a greater requirement for repeat revascularisation.

Impact

The results of this study suggest that selected patients with multi-vessel coronary artery disease can be treated safely with either coronary stenting or coronary artery bypass surgery. Coronary stenting is associated with a higher risk of additional revascularisation procedures and less relief of angina, but has a lower cost over 3-y F/U.

Aims

Previous trials comparing coronary balloon angioplasty and coronary artery bypass surgery in patients with single and multi-vessel disease had demonstrated similar rates of death and MI, but a much higher rate of repeat revascularisation after percutaneous treatment. ARTS was designed to compare the long-term effects of percutaneous coronary intervention using bare metal stents with coronary artery bypass surgery in patients with multi-vessel coronary artery disease.

Methods

Patients: 1205 patients from 67 international centres.

Inclusion criteria:

- Stable angina, unstable angina, or silent ischaemia, with ≥2 coronary lesions in different major vessels considered amenable to stenting; one vessel could be occluded if occlusion judged to be <1 month old;
- Left ventricular ejection fraction >30%.

Exclusion criteria:

- MI within the previous week or overt congestive cardiac failure;
- Previous cerebrovascular accident;
- Severe hepatic or renal disease;
- Diseased saphenous veins;
- Neutro/thrombocytopaenia or intolerance to aspirin or ticlopidine;
- Requirement for other major surgery.

Groups:
- Percutaneous coronary intervention (n=600);
- Coronary artery bypass surgery (n=605).

Primary endpoint: Major adverse cardiac or cerebrovascular events within 1y, including death, stroke, transient ischaemic attack (TIA), reversible ischaemic neurological deficit, non-fatal MI, and repeat revascularisation by percutaneous intervention or surgery.

Secondary endpoints:
- Angina;
- Use of medication;
- Cost and cost effectiveness, quality of life measures.

Follow-up: At 1 and 6 months, then at 1 and 5y.

Results

	Stent	Surgery	*p*
Primary endpoint (at 1y)			
Any adverse cardiac or cerebrovascular event	26.2%	12.2%	<0.001
Secondary endpoints (at 1y)			
Death	2.5%	2.8%	ns
MI	6.2%	4.8%	ns
Stroke	1.7%	2.1%	ns
Composite of death, MI, or stroke	9.3%	8.8%	ns
Any repeat revascularisation	21.0%	3.8%	<0.001
Angina at 1y	21.1%	10.5%	<0.001

These results were maintained at 5y.

Discussion

Patients with multi-vessel disease treated by coronary stenting or bypass surgery had comparable rates of death, stroke, and MI over 5-y F/U. The stent strategy was associated with the need for more repeat revascularisation and resulted in less effective relief of angina. However, it did have a lower total cost.

Problems

- ARTS enrolled a highly selected population suitable for either myocardial revascularisation procedure. The results may not be applicable to the wider population of patients undergoing these procedures.
- ARTS was conducted before drug-eluting stents became available. Trials of percutaneous coronary intervention in multi-vessel disease using this new technology (e.g. SYNTAX) are ongoing.

Coronary artery disease: drug-eluting vs bare metal stents

RAVEL (RAndomised study with the sirolimus coated BX VELocity balloon expandable stent): A randomised comparison of a sirolimus-eluting stent with a bare metal stent for coronary revascularisation.

AUTHORS: Morice M, Serruys P, Sousa J et al (RAVEL study group).
REFERENCE: New Engl J Med (2002) 346,1773–80.
STUDY DESIGN: RCT
EVIDENCE LEVEL: 1b

Key message
Drug-eluting stents (DES) greatly reduce restenosis compared with bare metal stents.

Impact
A DES is the stent of choice in patients at high risk of restenosis undergoing percutaneous coronary intervention (PCI). These patients include those with diabetes mellitus, previous in-stent restenosis, and coronary artery lesions >16mm in length or in vessels <3mm in diameter.

Aims
Recurrent stenosis (restenosis) in the segment of vessel treated with either a stent or balloon angioplasty is the Achilles heel of percutaneous coronary intervention (PCI). Sirolimus inhibits smooth muscle cell migration and proliferation following vascular balloon injury. This trial was designed to ascertain whether sirolimus-eluting stents could reduce in-stent restenosis when compared with bare metal stents.

Methods
Patients: 238 patients at 19 European and Latin American centres.

Inclusion criteria:
- Age >18y;
- Single, *de novo* coronary lesions;
- Maximum lesion length 18mm;
- Target vessel 2.5–3.5mm diameter.

Groups: Both groups received 2 months of clopidogrel and aspirin:
- Bare metal stent (n=118);
- Drug-eluting (sirolimus-eluting) stent (n=120).

Primary endpoint: In-stent late luminal loss (difference between minimal luminal diameter at time of stent implant and at 6 months F/U).

Secondary endpoints:
- Rate of restenosis (>50% luminal narrowing at 6 months);
- Major adverse cardiac events (MACE): death, MI, and need for further target vessel revascularisation;
- In-stent neointimal volume assessed by intravascular ultrasound.

Follow-up: At 1, 6, and 12 months with simultaneous coronary angiography.

Results

Primary endpoint	Bare metal stent	Drug-eluting stent	p
Mean late luminal loss*	0.8±90.53mm	−0.1±90.33mm	<0.001
Secondary endpoints			
In-stent restenosis	26.6%	0%	<0.001
MACE	28.8%	5.8%	<0.001
In-stent neointimal volume*	37±928mm^3	2±95mm^3	<0.001
Stent thrombosis	None	None	—

*Means±SD

Discussion

Previous trials had demonstrated bare metal stents to be associated with in-stent restenosis in up to 30% of patients, often leading to further revascularisation (either with another PCI or bypass surgery). This study demonstrated, for the first time, that a stent coated with sirolimus could reduce this risk substantially. Numerous trials have since confirmed the efficacy of several different drug-eluting stents in reducing the risk of restenosis and repeat target lesion revascularisation.

Problems

- Although there were no episodes of stent thrombosis in RAVEL, it has become apparent that this dangerous phenomenon can occur following DES implantation, especially if clopidogrel and aspirin are discontinued prematurely.
- DES generally require prolonged treatment with aspirin and clopidogrel which increases the risk of bleeding.
- This study only confirmed the benefit of DES in simple lesions, although subsequent studies have confirmed benefits in patients with more complex coronary anatomy.
- DES are approximately three times more expensive than conventional bare metal stents and their cost-effectiveness is the subject of debate.

Heart failure: β-blockers

CIBIS II (**C**ardiac **I**nsufficiency **BI**soprolol **S**tudy).

AUTHORS: CIBIS-II Investigators and Committees.
REFERENCE: Lancet (1999) 353, 9–13.
STUDY DESIGN: RCT
EVIDENCE LEVEL: 1b

Key message

Bisoprolol (in addition to conventional medical therapy with angiotensin-converting enzyme (ACE) inhibition and diuretics) significantly reduces all-cause mortality, cardiovascular (CV) mortality, and hospitalisation, in patients with New York Heart Association (NYHA) Class III or IV chronic heart failure (CHF).

Impact

β-blockade is now considered standard treatment in contemporary management of CHF; the choice of agent remains controversial.

Aims

Previous small studies and meta-analyses had suggested that β-blockers reduce mortality in patients with CHF. The initial CIBIS trial also suggested such benefits, but did not reach statistical significance. CIBIS II was designed to investigate the effects of bisoprolol (a highly selective β_1 adrenoceptor antagonist) on mortality and morbidity in patients with CHF.

Methods

Patients: 2647 patients from 18 European countries.

Inclusion criteria: CHF NYHA Class III or IV:
- Age 18–80y;
- Ejection fraction (EF) ≤35%;
- Treatment with diuretic and ACE inhibitor (ACE-I) (or other vasodilators if intolerant of ACE-I).

Exclusion criteria:
- Uncontrolled hypertension;
- Myocardial infarction (MI) or unstable angina in preceding 3 months;
- Percutaneous transluminal coronary angioplasty (PTCA) or coronary artery bypass graft (CABG) in previous 6 months;
- Previous or scheduled cardiac transplantation;
- Atrioventricular block (>1st degree) without permanent pacemaker;
- Resting HR <60 beats per min or systolic BP at rest <100mmHg;
- Serum creatinine >300mc/L;
- Reversible obstructive airways disease;
- Pre-existing or planned β-blocker therapy.

Groups:
- Optimal medical therapy and placebo (n=1320);
- Optimal medical therapy and bisoprolol (1.25–10mg od) titrated according to tolerance (n=1327).

Primary endpoint: All-cause mortality.

Secondary endpoints:
- All-cause hospital admissions;
- CV mortality;
- CV mortality and CV hospital admissions;
- Permanent premature treatment withdrawals.

Follow-up: Mean F/U 1.3y.

Results

Primary endpoint	Placebo	Bisoprolol	HR (95% CI)	p
All-cause mortality	228 (17%)	156 (12%)	0.66 (0.54 to 0.81)	<0.0001
Secondary endpoints				
All-cause hospital admissions	513 (39%)	440 (33%)	0.80 (0.71 to 0.91)	0.0006
CV mortality	161 (12%)	119 (9%)	0.71 (0.56 to 0.90)	0.005
CV mortality and CV hospital admissions	463 (35%)	388 (29%)	0.79 (0.69 to 0.90)	0.0004
Permanent premature treatment withdrawals	192 (15%)	194 (15%)	1.00 (0.82 to 1.22)	1.0

Discussion

This study provided convincing evidence that addition of bisoprolol to standard therapy is beneficial in patients with NYHA class III and IV CHF. The precise mechanism of benefit was unclear, but may include an anti-arrhythmic effect interaction with neuroendocrine activation seen in CHF, protection against the toxic effect of catecholamines, and favourable left ventricular remodelling. To date, metoprolol, bisoprolol, and carvedilol have all been shown to have mortality benefits in the treatment of CHF. The use of β-blockers in severe (NYHA Class IV) CHF has been contro-versial, and such patients were under-represented in CIBIS II and other clinical trials. The COPERNICUS trial (*N Engl J Med* (2001) 344, 1651–58) addressed this issue, and showed that carvedilol was well tolerated and improved survival by 35% relative to placebo.

Problems

- Despite proven benefit of β-blockade after MI, the role of these agents in patients with CHF immediately post-MI has been uncertain. The CAPRICORN (*Lancet* (2001) 357, 1385–90) study confirmed that carvedilol reduced all-cause mortality in patients with recent MI and EF <40%.
- Debate regarding the choice of β-blocker for patients with CHF continues. Carvedilol conferred greater benefit than metoprolol in the COMET trial (*Lancet* (2003) 362, 7–13), although the long-acting meto-prolol preparation previously associated with mortality benefit was not used in this study.

Heart failure: spironolactone

RALES (**R**andomised **AL**dactone **E**valuation **S**tudy): The effect of spironolactone on morbidity and mortality in patients with severe heart failure.

AUTHORS: Pitt B, Zannad F, Remme W *et al.*
REFERENCE: N Engl J Med (1999) 341, 709–17.
STUDY DESIGN: RCT
EVIDENCE LEVEL: 1b

Key message

The addition of spironolactone to standard therapy results in significant mortality and morbidity benefit in patients with severe heart failure (HF).

Impact

The addition of spironolactone to standard therapy is now recommended practice in the management of severe HF.

Aims

The role of aldosterone in the pathophysiology of HF is well recognised. Its effects are wide-ranging, including salt and water retention, vascular and cardiac fibrosis, and activation of the sympathetic and parasympathetic nervous systems. Angiotensin-converting enzyme inhibitors (ACE-Is) do not completely inhibit the renin-angiotensin-aldosterone system, and adding an aldosterone receptor blocker may provide incremental benefit. However, co-prescription of these agents can cause hyperkalaemia. This study was designed to assess the efficacy and safety of aldosterone receptor blockade with spironolactone in patients with severe HF already receiving standard therapy (with ACE-I and loop diuretic).

Methods

Patients: 1663 patients at multiple centres in 15 countries worldwide.

Inclusion criteria: HF diagnosis ≥6wk pre-enrolment:
• New York Heart Association (NYHA) Class III or IV heart failure;
• Treatment with an ACE-I and a loop diuretic;
• Ejection fraction ≤35% within 6 months of enrolment.

Exclusion criteria:
• Primary operable valvular heart disease or congenital heart disease;
• Unstable angina;
• Heart transplantation;
• Primary hepatic failure, active cancer, or any life-threatening disease;
• Serum creatinine >221micromol/L or potassium >5mmol/L.

Groups:
• Standard therapy and spironolactone (25mg od, up-titrated to 50mg od or down-titrated to 25mg on alternate days, according to symptoms and serum potassium level) (n=822);
• Standard therapy and placebo (n=841).

Primary endpoint: Death from any cause.

Secondary endpoints:
- Death from cardiac causes;
- Hospital admission from cardiac causes;
- Combined incidence of death from or hospital admission for cardiac causes.

Follow-up: Mean 24 months.

Results

Primary endpoint	Spiro	Placebo	RR (95% CI)	*p*
Death	284 (35%)	386 (46%)	0.70 (0.59 to 0.82)	<0.001
Secondary endpoints				
Death from cardiac causes	226 (27%)	314 (37%)	0.69 (0.58 to 0.82)	<0.001
Hospn–cardiac causes	260/515*	336/753*	0.70 (0.59 to 0.82)	<0.001
Change in NYHA class:				<0.001
Improved	41%	33%		between
Unchanged	21%	18%		groups
Worsened	38%	48%		

* Number of events/number of patients.

- Study stopped early when interim analysis showed spironolactone reduced overall risk of death by 30% and risk of death attributable to cardiac causes by 31%. This benefit appeared to be due to a lower risk of sudden cardiac death or death from progressive HF.
- Spironolactone was well tolerated. Although statistically significant increases in serum creatinine (4–9micromol/L) and potassium (0.3mmol/L) were seen with spironolactone, these were not considered clinically significant.

Discussion

Addition of spironolactone to standard therapy in patients with severe HF significantly reduced the risk of death from any cause, death from cardiac causes, combined risk of death and hospital admission for cardiac causes, and deterioration of symptoms, when compared with placebo. The mechanism underlying these beneficial effects remains unclear, but is unlikely to be related to diuresis.

Problems

- Only 10% of patients were taking a β-blocker at the start of the study, although the benefits of spironolactone were not influenced by concurrent β-blockade.
- Gynaecomastia and breast pain were relatively common side effects of spironolactone. Eplerenone is a more selective aldosterone receptor antagonist with an improved side effect profile; its benefits have been demonstrated in the EPHESUS trial (N Engl J Med (2003) 348, 1309–21).
- Serious hyperkalaemia was infrequent, possibly because of the relatively low dose of spironolactone, and the exclusion of patients with elevated serum creatinine or potassium at baseline. Hyperkalaemia may be more frequent in everyday practice.

Heart failure: angiotensin-II receptor antagonists

> **CHARM (C**andesartan in **H**eart failure **A**ssessment of **R**eduction in **M**ortality and **M**orbidity) trial: Effects of candesartan in patients with chronic heart failure and reduced left ventricular systolic function.
>
> **AUTHORS:** Pfeffer M, Swedburg K, Granger C et al.
> **REFERENCE:** Lancet (2003) 362, 759–66.
> **STUDY DESIGN:** RCT
> **EVIDENCE LEVEL:** 1b

Key message

Fewer all-cause deaths are seen in patients treated with candesartan, in addition to fewer cardiovascular (CV) deaths or hospital admissions for heart failure (HF).

Impact

The CHARM programme supports the use of candesartan irrespective of concurrent treatment or ejection fraction in patients with chronic heart failure (CHF).

Aims

Previous studies had shown angiotensin-converting enzyme inhibitors (ACE-I), β-blockers, and aldosterone antagonists to reduce mortality and morbidity independently in patients with CHF. Despite these treatments, mortality rates had remained high. The CHARM programme aimed to study the effects of an angiotensin receptor antagonist (candesartan) in patients with CHF, including those previously intolerant of an ACE-I (CHARM Alternative), those already taking an ACE-I (CHARM Added), and those with clinical HF but preserved left ventricular (LV) function (CHARM Preserved).

Methods

Patients: 7601 patients from 618 centres worldwide.

Inclusion criteria:
- NYHA class II-IV HF, of ≥4wk duration;
- Men and women aged ≥18y.

Exclusion criteria:
- Serum creatinine >265micromol/L or serum potassium >5.5mmol/L;
- Known bilateral renal artery stenosis;
- Symptomatic hypotension;
- Women of childbearing potential not taking adequate contraception;
- Critical aortic or mitral stenosis;
- Myocardial infarction, stroke, open heart surgery in previous 4wk;
- Use of an angiotensin receptor antagonist in previous 2wk.

Component trials: Patients randomised to candesartan or matching placebo in a double-blind fashion, in all three arms:

- CHARM Preserved: LV ejection fraction (EF) >40% (n=3032);
- CHARM Added: LVEF ≤40% and already treated with ACE-I (n=2548);
- CHARM Alternative: LVEF ≤40% and previously intolerant of ACE-I (n=2028).

Primary endpoint:

- CHARM overall: All-cause mortality;
- CHARM component trials: composite of cardiovascular (CV) death or hospitalisation for CHF.

Secondary endpoints: CV deaths and hospitalisation for CHF.

Follow-up: Mean: CHARM overall=37.7 months;
CHARM Preserved=36.6 months; CHARM Added=41 months;
CHARM Alternative=33.7 months.

Results

Primary endpoint	Candesartan (n=3803)	Placebo (n=3796)	Covariate adjusted HR (95% CI)	p
Death any cause	886 (23%)	945 (25%)	0.90 (0.82 to 0.99)	0.032
Secondary endpoints				
CV death	691 (18%)	769 (20%)	0.87 (0.78 to 0.96)	0.006
Hospitalisation for HF	757 (20%)	918 (24%)	0.77 (0.70 to 0.84)	<0.0001

Results shown for CHARM overall.

- Similar statistically significant results were seen in CHARM Added and CHARM Alternative, but not in CHARM Preserved.

Discussion

The theoretical benefit of selective angiotensin II receptor blockade was supported by the results of the programme, demonstrating overall mortality benefit in these high-risk patients with CHF. Candesartan conferred benefit in those already taking current best medical therapy, including an ACE-I, β-blocker, digoxin, loop diuretic, and spironolactone. Component trials showed that the best predictor of mortality was reduction in LVEF <40%, both arms of *CHARM Preserved* having significantly better prognosis than the other groups.

CHARM Alternative suggested that candesartan conferred similar benefits to ACE-I and supported the use of candesartan in individuals with CHF who are intolerant of ACE-I. Concerns that excessive renin-angiotensin blockade might be detrimental were not borne out in *CHARM Added*, which suggested that this practice was safe and reduced CV death and hospitalisation for CHF.

Heart failure: implantable cardioverter-defibrillator vs amiodarone

> **SCD HeFT** (**S**udden **C**ardiac **D**eath in **HEA**rt **F**ailure **T**rial):
> Amiodarone or an implantable cardioverter-defibrillator for congestive heart failure.
>
> **AUTHORS:** Bardy G, Lee KL, Mark DB, *et al.*
> **REFERENCE:** N Engl J Med (2005) 352, 225–37.
> **STUDY DESIGN:** RCT
> **EVIDENCE LEVEL:** 1b

Key message

In patients with New York Heart Association (NYHA) Class II or III heart failure (HF) and a left ventricular ejection fraction (LVEF) of ≤35%, implantation of a single lead cardioverter-defibrillator reduces mortality by 23%. Amiodarone has no effect on survival.

Impact

Implantation of a cardioverter-defibrillator should be considered in the management of patients with NYHA Class II or III HF and LVEF of ≤35%.

Aims

Sudden cardiac death is a leading cause of death in patients with HF. Treatment options to prevent sudden death include amiodarone and an implantable cardioverter-defibrillator (ICD). This study was designed to determine whether amiodarone or a single lead ICD could reduce mortality in patients with mild to moderate HF.

Methods

Patients: 2,521 patients from multiple centres in the USA and Canada.

Inclusion criteria:
- Age >18y;
- NYHA Class II or III chronic stable HF of ischaemic or non-ischaemic aetiology;
- LVEF ≤35%.

Groups: All patients treated with standard therapies including angiotensin-converting enzyme inhibitor (ACE-I), β-adrenoceptor blocker, aldosterone receptor blocker, aspirin, and statin, when appropriate:
- Amiodarone: Loading dose (800mg od for 1wk), followed by 200mg, 300mg, or 400mg od (depending upon weight) for 3wk followed by a maintenance dose of 200–400 mg daily (n = 845);
- Placebo: Double-blinded to identical regime as amiodarone (n = 847);
- Single chamber ICD: Implanted a median of 3d after randomisation. Shock-only mode—programmed to deliver a shock for ventricular rates >187 per min. Antitachycardia pacing was not permitted and antibradycardia pacing was only used if the intrinsic heart rate fell to <34 per min (n=829).

Primary endpoint: All-cause mortality.

Follow-up: Median 45.5 months.

Results

	Mortality at 5y				
	Placebo (n = 847)	Amiodarone (n = 845)	ICD (n = 829)	*p* (amiodarone vs placebo)	*p* (ICD vs placebo)
All patients	36.1%	34.0%	28.9%	0.5	0.007
Ischaemic HF	43.2%	41.7%	35.9%	0.7	0.05
Non-ischaemic HF	27.9%	25.8%	21.4%	0.7	0.06
NYHA class II	32.0%	26.4%	20.1%	0.2	<0.001
NYHA class III	45.6%	52.8%	48.4%	0.01	0.3

Discussion

This study demonstrated that a single lead implantable defibrillator reduces the risk of death over 5y by 23% in patients with NYHA class II or III HF and an ejection fraction ≤35%. By contrast, amiodarone did not influence survival. The benefit of ICD therapy was evident in patients with ischaemic and non-ischaemic HF. Unexpectedly, a prespecified subgroup analysis suggested that patients with more severe HF did not benefit from ICD therapy and may be harmed by amiodarone. However, these findings have not been reproduced in other trials. In a subsequent meta-analysis of 12 RCTs, including 8516 patients with LV systolic dysfunction *(Ann Intern Med* (2007) 147, 251–62), ICD therapy reduced mortality by 20%. This benefit was mainly driven by a 54% relative reduction in the risk of sudden cardiac death.

Problems

- Single chamber ICDs were used; the results cannot be extrapolated to the use of dual chamber or biventricular devices.
- Over two thirds of ICD recipients never received a therapeutic ICD shock, and 10% received an inappropriate shock. Further research is required to identify patients most likely to benefit from an ICD.
- The trials of ICD therapy enrolled selected patients; the safety and efficacy of ICD therapy in the wider HF population is unknown.
- Longer term risks and costs of ICD implantation are also unknown.
- Although ICD therapy improves life expectancy in patients with HF, impact on overall quality of life remains controversial.

Heart failure: cardiac resynchronisation therapy

> **CARE-HF (<u>CA</u>rdiac <u>RE</u>synchronisation – <u>H</u>eart <u>F</u>ailure) study:**
> The effect of cardiac resynchronisation on morbidity and mortality in heart failure
>
> **AUTHORS:** Cleland J, Daubert J, Erdmann E *et al.*
> **REFERENCE:** N Engl J Med (2005) 352, 1539–49.
> **STUDY DESIGN:** RCT
> **EVIDENCE LEVEL:** 1b

Key message

In patients with NYHA Class III or IV heart failure receiving optimal pharmacological therapy cardiac resynchronisation therapy (CRT) confers additional mortality and morbidity benefit.

Impact

CRT is indicated in patients with NYHA Class III or IV HF and evidence of left ventricular (LV) dyssynchrony.

Aims

Patients with HF commonly have regions of delayed myocardial activation and contraction leading to so-called cardiac dyssynchrony. CRT (implantation of an atrio-biventricular pacing system to resynchronise right ventricular and LV activation and contraction) improves symptoms, quality of life (QoL), and exercise capacity in these patients. This study aimed to assess whether the addition of CRT to standard medical therapy reduced mortality in patients with NYHA Class III–IV HF and cardiac dyssynchrony.

Methods

Patients: 813 patients from 82 European centres.

Inclusion criteria: HF diagnosis ≥6wk before enrolment:
- NYHA Class III or IV (at time of enrolment);
- Ejection fraction ≤35%;
- LV end diastolic dimension of ≥30mm;
- ECG: QRS complex duration of ≥120ms. If the QRS duration was <149ms, two additional echo criteria for LV dyssynchrony were required.

Exclusion criteria:
- Major cardiovascular (CV) event in previous 6wk;
- Other indications for pacemaker or implantable defibrillator;
- HF requiring continuous intravenous therapy;
- Atrial arrhythmias.

Groups:
- Medical therapy alone (n=404);
- Medical therapy and CRT (n=409).

Primary endpoint: Composite of death from any cause or unplanned hospitalisation for a major CV event.

Secondary endpoints:
- Death from any cause;
- Composite of death and unplanned hospitalisation for HF;
- NYHA and QoL score at 90d;
- Echo assessment of dyssynchrony, LV function, and mitral regurgitation;
- N-terminal pro-brain natriuretic peptide.

Follow-up: Mean 29.4 months.

Results

Primary endpoint	Medical alone	Medical + CRT	HR (95% CI)	*p*
Death + hospitalisation for major CV event	224 (55%)	159 (39%)	0.63 (0.51 to 0.77)	<0.001
Secondary endpoints				
Death (any cause)	120 (30%)	82 (20%)	0.64 (0.48 to 0.85)	<0.002
Death or hospitalisation (HF)	191 (47%)	118 (29%)	0.54 (0.43 to 0.68)	<0.001
QoL scores (mean ± SD)			**Difference (95% CI)**	*p*
NYHA class (at 90d)	2.7 (±0.9)	2.1 (±1.0)	0.6 (0.4 to 0.7)	<0.001
Minnesota score	40 (±22)	31 (±22)	−10 (−8 to −12)	<0.001
EuroQoL EQ-5D	0.63 (±0.29)	0.7 (±0.28)	0.08 (0.04 to 0.12)	<0.001

Discussion

This was the first trial to show that CRT alone (without defibrillator capability) improved mortality in patients with HF and LV dyssynchrony. Benefits of CRT were seen in addition to standard medical therapy and irrespective of the aetiology of HF. Use of contemporary medication (angiotensin-converting enzyme inhibitors, β-blockers, and spironolactone) was high in both groups.

Problems

- Patients with less severe (NYHA class I–II) HF have been poorly represented in clinical trials of CRT, and little evidence exists to guide their treatment, even in the presence of LV dyssynchrony. CRT may impact on the natural history of HF, if used earlier in the disease process.
- Identification of patients who benefit most from CRT remains problematic. Patients with QRS prolongation do not necessarily have echocardiographic evidence of dyssynchrony and vice versa. New parameters such as tissue Doppler imaging are currently being evaluated to optimise patient selection and device programming.

Atrial fibrillation: stroke prevention

ACTIVE W (**A**trial fibrillation **C**lopidogrel **T**rial with **I**rbesartan for prevention of **V**ascular **E**vents): Clopidogrel plus aspirin vs oral anticoagulation for atrial fibrillation.

AUTHORS: ACTIVE Writing Group.
REFERENCE: Lancet (2006) 367, 1903–12.
STUDY DESIGN: RCT
EVIDENCE LEVEL: 1b

Key message
Oral anticoagulation is superior to aspirin and clopidogrel in preventing vascular events in patients with atrial fibrillation (AF) at high risk of stroke.

Impact
Oral anticoagulation remains the optimal antithrombotic strategy for prevention of vascular events in patients with AF at high risk of stroke.

Aims
Patients with AF are at increased risk of stroke and other systemic embolic events. Oral anticoagulation reduces the risk of stroke by two thirds compared with no treatment, but also increases the risk of bleeding. Aspirin is less effective, reducing the risk of stroke by about 22%, but the additional benefit of adding clopidogrel to aspirin is unknown. The ACTIVE W trial was designed to test whether clopidogrel and aspirin in combination are non-inferior to oral anticoagulation.

Methods
Patients: 6706 patients from 522 centres in 31 countries (mean age 70.2y).

Inclusion criteria: ECG evidence of AF and ≥1 of the following:
- Treatment for systemic hypertension;
- Previous cerebrovascular accident (CVA), transient ischaemic attack (TIA), or other systemic embolism;
- Ejection fraction <45%;
- Peripheral arterial disease;
- Age 55–74y, and diabetes mellitus or coronary artery disease.

Exclusion criteria:
- Contraindication to clopidogrel or oral anticoagulation;
- Peptic ulcer disease within the previous 6 months;
- Previous intracerebral haemorrhage;
- Significant thrombocytopaenia (platelet count <50x10^9/L);
- Mitral stenosis.

Groups:
- Clopidogrel (75mg od) plus aspirin (75–100mg od, recommended) (n=3335);
- Oral anticoagulation (target INR 2.0–3.0) (n=3371).

Primary endpoint: The composite of stroke, other systemic embolism, myocardial infarction (MI), or vascular death.
Secondary endpoints: Bleeding categorised according to severity.
Follow-up: The trial was stopped prematurely after a median of 1.3y F/U.

Results

AF was permanent in >30% of patients, and 77% were receiving antico-agulation before randomisation. During the study, 64% of INR values in patients on oral anticoagulation therapy were in the therapeutic range.

	Clopidogrel and aspirin (% per y)	Oral anticoagulation (% per y)	p
Composite primary endpoint	5.60%	3.93%	0.0003
Non-central nervous system embolism	0.43%	0.10%	0.005
MI	0.86%	0.55%	0.09
Stroke	2.39%	1.40%	0.001
Vascular death	2.87%	2.52%	0.3
Major bleeding	2.42%	2.21%	0.5
Primary outcome and major bleeding	7.56%	5.45%	<0.0001

Discussion

Oral anticoagulation was superior to aspirin and clopidogrel for prevention of vascular events in patients with AF at high risk of stroke. This difference was driven mainly by higher rates of stroke and other systemic embolism amongst patients treated with aspirin and clopidogrel. The majority of patients recruited had previously taken oral anticoagulation, and selection bias in favour of oral anticoagulation therapy might have influenced the results. Therefore, the results of ACTIVE W apply mainly to patients previously taking oral anticoagulation. For patients with no previous exposure to either treatment, the relative benefits are not well defined.

Problems

- Patients in this trial were at high risk of systemic embolism; additional research is required to elucidate the relative benefits of anticoagulation and dual antiplatelet therapy in patients at lower risk.
- Whether clopidogrel provides additional benefit when added to aspirin is unknown. This question is being addressed by the ACTIVE A study.

Atrial fibrillation: rate vs rhythm control

AFFIRM (**A**trial **F**ibrillation **F**ollow-up **I**nvestigation of **R**hythm **M**anagement) study: A comparison of rate control and rhythm control in patients with atrial fibrillation.

AUTHORS: AFFIRM Investigators.
REFERENCE: N Engl J Med (2002) 347, 1825–33.
STUDY DESIGN: RCT
EVIDENCE LEVEL: 1b

Key message

In patients with atrial fibrillation (AF), a rhythm control strategy to maintain sinus rhythm is associated with a higher risk of adverse drug effects and confers no survival or other advantage over a rate control strategy.

Impact

The majority of patients with AF can be managed safely with a rate control strategy coupled with appropriate anticoagulation. A rhythm control strategy using anti-arrhythmic drugs and electrical cardioversion to maintain sinus rhythm may be appropriate for patients at low risk of stroke and recurrent atrial arrhythmia.

Aims

Treatment of AF may be directed towards maintenance of sinus rhythm ('rhythm control') using anti-arrhythmic medication and cardioversion. The objective of this strategy is the reduction of symptoms, need for anti-coagulation and risk of stroke, and improvement of exercise tolerance and quality of life (QoL). In the alternative 'rate control' strategy, the ventricular rate can be controlled using drugs that block atrioventricular conduction, coupled with oral anticoagulation to reduce the risk of systemic embolism. This study was designed to compare the long-term effects of these alternative strategies.

Methods

Patients: 4060 patients from 213 US centres.

Inclusion criteria: AF plus:
- ≥65y of age or other risk factors for stroke;
- AF likely to be recurrent;
- AF likely to cause illness or death;
- Long-term treatment warranted;
- Anticoagulation not contraindicated.

Groups:
- Rate control (n = 2027);
- Rhythm control (n = 2033).

Primary endpoint: All-cause mortality.

Secondary endpoints:
- Composite of death, disabling stroke, disabling anoxic encephalopathy, major bleeding, or cardiac arrest;
- Hospitalisation;
- Adverse drug reactions.

Follow-up: Median=3.5y (maximum 6y).

Results

- At 5y, 35% of the rate control group were in sinus rhythm, and over 80% of patients in AF had adequate rate control.
- At each F/U assessment during the trial, approximately 85% of the rate control group and 70% of the rhythm control group were anticoagulated.

	Rhythm control	Rate control	*p*
Death	26.7%	25.9%	0.08
Composite secondary endpoint	32.7%	32.2%	0.3
Hospitalisation	80.1%	73.0%	<0.001
Adverse drug reaction	0.8%	0.2%	0.007

Discussion

In patients with AF and risk factors for stroke, rhythm control offered no advantage over rate control. The rhythm control strategy was associated with a trend towards a higher mortality, but risk of stroke was similar in the two groups. Most strokes occurred in patients in whom anticoagulation had been discontinued or was sub-therapeutic, emphasising the importance of anticoagulation for the prevention of stroke in patients with AF. The rhythm control group had a higher risk of adverse drug effects and admission to hospital.

Problems

- Patients recruited were over 65y of age or had other risk factors for stroke. The results may not be applicable to younger patients without risk factors, including patients with 'lone' AF.
- In AFFIRM, rhythm control did not improve measures of QoL relative to rate control. The impact of AF on exercise tolerance requires further evaluation.
- Since AFFIRM was reported, there has been considerable interest in surgical and catheter-based procedures to treat AF. These strategies require further evaluation in RCTs.

Pacing: dual chamber vs ventricular

> **CTOPP** (**C**anadian **T**rial **O**f **P**hysiologic **P**acing): Effects of physiologic pacing vs ventricular pacing on the risk of stroke and death due to cardiovascular causes.
>
> **AUTHORS:** Connolly S, Kerr C, Gent M et al.
> **REFERENCE:** N Engl J Med (2000) 342, 1385–91.
> **STUDY DESIGN:** RCT
> **EVIDENCE LEVEL:** 1b

Key message

Physiological (dual chamber) pacing is associated with a higher complication rate at implantation and a modest reduction in the long-term risk of atrial fibrillation (AF). However, there is no beneficial effect on mortality, risk of stroke, or hospitalisation for heart failure (HF).

Impact

For many patients with symptomatic bradycardia, the risks and benefits of dual chamber pacing are finely balanced, and single lead pacing is a reasonable alternative strategy.

Aims

Early pacemakers used a single lead to pace a single cardiac chamber (usually the right ventricle) at a fixed rate. Dual chamber pacemakers use two leads to sense and pace both the right atrium and right ventricle, and are capable of maintaining atrioventricular synchrony and increasing heart rate during stress. In a small trial of atrial vs ventricular pacing in patients with sick sinus syndrome, atrial pacing was associated with improved survival, fewer thromboembolic complications, and less AF and HF. This study assessed the benefit of dual chamber pacing over ventricular pacing in a large cohort of patients.

Methods

Patients: 2568 patients at 32 Canadian hospitals.

Inclusion criteria:
- Age ≥18y;
- Symptomatic bradycardia requiring treatment with a pacemaker.

Exclusion criteria:
- Chronic AF;
- Complete heart block due to atrioventricular nodal ablation;
- Life expectancy <2y due to a non-cardiac condition.

Groups:
- Single lead ventricular pacing (n=1474);
- Dual chamber pacing (n=1094).

Primary endpoint: Composite of stroke and cardiovascular (CV) death.

Secondary endpoint: Composite of death (any cause), AF (for ≥15min) or admission to hospital with HF.

Follow-up: Mean 3y.

Results

Outcomes	Ventricular pacing	Physiologic pacing	p
Annual rate of stroke or CV death	5.5%	4.9%	0.3
Annual rate of death	6.6%	6.3%	0.9
Annual rate of AF	6.6%	5.3%	0.05
Annual rate of hospitalisation with HF	3.5%	3.1%	0.5
Annual rate of stroke	1.1%	1.0%	Not reported
Complication of implantation	3.8%	9.0%	<0.001

Discussion

In this large trial of two different pacing modes, physiological pacing was associated with a modest (18%) relative reduction in the risk of AF, which appeared after 2y and was maintained over 6.4y F/U (*circulation* (2004) 109, 357–62). This reduced risk of AF did not translate into altered risk of death, stroke, or hospitalisation with HF. Since the results were published, several other trials of different pacing modes have been reported. In the UK-PACE trial (*Heart* (1997) 78, 221–3), single chamber ventricular pacing in elderly patients with high-grade atrioventricular block did not influence mortality or the incidence of CV events when compared with dual chamber pacing.

Problems

- In this study, subgroup analysis suggested that physiological pacing is beneficial in patients with unpaced heart rates <60 beats per min; further research is required to confirm this observation.
- Dual chamber pacemakers are more expensive with higher risk of minor complications. Evidence that preservation of atrioventricular synchrony maintains quality of life requires further assessment.
- Conventional right ventricular pacing is associated with abnormal ventricular activation. The long-term effects of pacing techniques that synchronise ventricular activation (including biventricular and septal pacing) also require further evaluation in randomised trials.

Dermatology

Introduction

The ability to diagnose and treat skin disease is a matter which non-dermatologist physicians have long regarded as akin to sorcery, involving the use of long Latin names and an array of bizarre topical concoctions and obscure systemic medications. The enormous number of disease entities encountered by dermatologists gives rise to the paradox that they commonly encounter rarities; for many of these, there is scant evidence of efficacy of any intervention. On the other hand, great advances in the management of some of the more common skin diseases have been made over the past century.

One of the pioneers in the scientific investigation of skin disease was the Faeroese physician and Nobel laureate, Niels Finsen. In the late 19th century, he hypothesised that ultraviolet light might be beneficial for lupus vulgaris—a once common and disfiguring form of tuberculosis of the skin, developed a lamp to produce it, and then set about methodically demonstrating its efficacy. Antibiotics and corticosteroids, introduced in the middle of the last century, have made an enormous impact on relieving suffering from skin disease.

Over the past forty years, the most spectacular advances have been in the understanding and treatment of inflammatory skin disease. Isotretinoin has revolutionised the management of severe acne. Fifty years ago, arsenic was virtually the only available systemic therapy for severe psoriasis; dermatologists have long abandoned arsenic, but have a whole range of drugs, from methotrexate and cyclosporin to designer biological drugs such as infliximab and efalizumab, to offer their patients. With the increasing number of therapeutic options for many skin diseases has come the need for better evidence of relative efficacy, acceptability, and safety. This need has been only in part fulfilled. Furthermore, depressingly, there has been little progress in the management of advanced malignant melanoma or, more trivially, of viral warts. This chapter considers the highlights of the evidence base behind some of these advances.

Atopic eczema: tacrolimus

A short-term trial of tacrolimus ointment for atopic dermatitis.

AUTHORS: Ruzicka T, Bieber T, Schöpf E *et al.*
REFERENCE: N Engl J Med (1997) 337, 816–21.
STUDY DESIGN: RCT
EVIDENCE LEVEL: 1b

Key message

The first RCT to show the efficacy of topical tacrolimus in the treatment of atopic eczema.

Impact

Topical tacrolimus has been a significant addition to the therapeutic armamentarium for the treatment of atopic eczema. Topical steroid application has the potential to cause skin atrophy. This is not the case with topical tacrolimus, and its use is widespread in those patients who have had significant previous exposure to topical steroids, especially at sites prone to skin atrophy such as the face and flexures.

Aims

This study aimed to evaluate the efficacy and safety of 0.03%, 0.1%, and 0.3% topical tacrolimus ointment in the treatment of atopic eczema in a randomised double-blind study.

Methods

Patients: 213 patients at 16 European centres (age range 13–60y).

Inclusion criteria:
- Moderate to severe atopic eczema;
- Washout period of 3wk for other topicals (other than emollients);
- Symptomatic area 200cm^2 of skin on trunk and/or extremities.

Groups:
- Topical tacrolimus: 0.03% (n=54), 0.1% (n=54), 0.3% (n=51);
- Inactive vehicle cream (n=54).

Primary endpoint: Change in score (sum of scores for erythema, oedema, and pruritus in the treated area) from baseline to completion of treatment.

Secondary endpoints: Other parameters (scored by investigator and patients) added to primary endpoint score.

Follow-up: Assessment performed at baseline, at day 3 of treatment, then at weeks 1, 2, and 3. Final review 1wk after completion of treatment. *Investigator:* scored on a 0–3 scale for severity of erythema, oedema, oozing or crusting, excoriation, and lichenification of involved skin. *Patient:* graded pruritus, which was converted to a score of 0–3.

Results

		Vehicle cream	Tacrolimus (strength)			p (each tacrolimus group vs vehicle)
			(0.03%)	(0.1%)	(0.3%)	
% decrease in summary score	Trunk	22.5	66.7	83.3	75.0	<0.001
	Face	25.0	71.4	83.3	83.3	<0.001

Discussion

This study demonstrated the efficacy of topical tacrolimus in the treatment of atopic eczema. There was no statistically significant difference between the active treatments, although there was a trend of advantage with increasing concentration. There were no significant differences between the treatment groups in the overall incidence of adverse events, and burning sensation at the site of application was the only reported problem. Absorption of the drug was minimal, with the majority of patients having undetectable levels of tacrolimus at all intervals of the study.

Problems

- This study was performed over 3wk. Clearly, the longer term efficacy and safety of topical tacrolimus must be key areas for future studies.
- The number of patients involved in the study was small. This issue is the likely explanation for the lack of observed differences between the 0.03% and 0.1% tacrolimus treatment groups; the trend was towards an advantage for the 0.1% group.

Atopic eczema: azathioprine

Azathioprine dosed by thiopurine methyltransferase activity for moderate to severe atopic eczema: a double-blind, randomised controlled trial.

AUTHORS: Meggitt S, Gray J, Reynolds N.
REFERENCE: Lancet (2006) 367, 839–46.
STUDY DESIGN: RCT
EVIDENCE LEVEL: 1b

Key message

The largest RCT to show that azathioprine is an effective treatment for moderate to severe atopic eczema, highlighting how genetic polymorphisms in the enzyme, thiopurine methyl transferase (TPMT), can be used to optimise individual treatment doses with the aims of increasing safety, efficacy, and tolerability.

Impact

Azathioprine had been used for selected patients with severe atopic eczema for many years, but had previously been evaluated in only one small controlled study. With the utilisation of TPMT activity to determine individual doses, the investigators observed a much lower dropout rate than in the previous study.

Aims

Standard topical therapy is often only partly effective for atopic eczema. The efficacy of second-line therapies such as cyclosporin and ultraviolet B light has been demonstrated, although there are risks of toxicity associated with long-term use. Open studies had shown azathioprine to be effective in moderate to severe eczema, although evidence from RCTs was lacking. This study aimed to evaluate the efficacy and safety of azathioprine in moderate to severe atopic eczema. As individual differences in azathioprine toxicity had been associated with TPMT enzyme activity, this study also investigated the role of a dosing schedule based on this assessment.

Methods

Patients: 63 patients from four centres in the UK (age range 16–65y).

Inclusion criteria: Moderate to severe atopic eczema.

Exclusion criteria:
- Admitted to hospital;
- Treated with ciclosporin, systemic steroids, topical tacrolimus, Chinese herbal medicine, or evening primrose oil in the preceding 3 months;
- Unstable atopic eczema in previous 2wk;
- Very low TPMT activity (<2.5nmol/h/mL red blood cells);
- Serious illness.

Groups: Parallel groups in a ratio of 2:1:
- Azathioprine: dosing dependent on bodyweight and TPMT activity (either normal or low) (n=42);
- Placebo (n=21).

Evaluations: Six area six sign atopic eczema score (SASSAD): graded six key physical signs of atopic eczema (erythema, dryness, lichenification, exudation, excoriation, and cracking). Assessed by single investigator at: 2wk pre-treatment, and 0, 4, 8, 12wk and at 3 and 6 months post-treatment.

Primary endpoint: Change in disease activity score (SASSAD) from baseline to 12wk.

Secondary endpoints: Included:
- Reduction in % body surface area (BSA) involved;
- Improvement in quality of life (QoL).

Results

Endpoint	Azathioprine	Placebo	Difference (95% CI)
Reduction in SASSAD	12.0	6.6	5.4 (1.4 to 9.3)
Reduction in % BSA	25.8	14.6	11.2 (1.6 to 21.0)
Improvement in QoL	5.9	2.4	3.5 (0.3 to 6.7)

Discussion

This study confirmed the efficacy of azathioprine as a second-line treatment for moderate to severe atopic eczema, albeit in a relatively small group of patients. A total of 11% of the general population have low TPMT activity, as a consequence of genetic variation within the gene coding for the TPMT enzyme, and are vulnerable to myelosuppression when treated with azathioprine. Fear of inducing this serious complication may also result in underdosing of patients with normal TPMT activity. This tailored approach to the dosing of azathioprine is novel and may be applicable to other therapies and treatment areas in the future.

Problems

- This study was in a small group of patients with moderate to severe atopic eczema. Although statistical significance was seen between the groups for the primary endpoint, the 95% CIs were wide, and there was no significant difference in some of the other secondary endpoints (not shown).
- TPMT activity is currently assessed by enzyme activity rather than genotype and recorded as 'normal', 'low', or 'very low'. Although none of the patients with low TPMT activity developed myelosuppression, the number studied was small (n=5). Therefore, the contribution of TPMT testing to the outcome of this study cannot be readily quantified.

Psoriasis: photochemotherapy vs dithranol

Comparison of photochemotherapy and dithranol in the treatment of chronic plaque psoriasis.

AUTHORS: Rogers S, Marks J, Shuster S, Hillyard C.
REFERENCE: Lancet (1979) 1, 455–8.
STUDY DESIGN: RCT
EVIDENCE LEVEL: 1b

Key message
The first RCT to show the effectiveness of 8-methoxypsoralen combined with long-wave ultraviolet light (PUVA).

Impact
Photochemotherapy is a very effective treatment for moderate to severe psoriasis, but cumulative exposure causes a significant increase in skin cancer, which now limits its use.

Aims
Topical dithranol and ultraviolet B therapy (Ingram regimen) was a well-established therapy for psoriasis when psoralen and long-wave ultraviolet light (PUVA) therapy was introduced in the 1970s. This study aimed to compare the Ingram regimen with PUVA in patients with at least 10% body surface are a (excluding sclap) psoriasis involvement.

Methods
Patients: 224 patients at two centres in the UK (age range 35–70y).

Inclusion criteria:
- Age >18y;
- ≥10% of body surface area (excluding the scalp) involved;
- No cytotoxic drugs/oral corticosteroids in the previous month.

Groups:
- Ingram regimen: daily dithranol at maximal dose tolerated (0.01%–0.4%). Removed 24h later then incremental exposure to UVB (n=111);
- PUVA regimen: 8-methoxypsoralen in combination with UVA administered on Monday, Wednesday, and Friday (n=113).

Follow-up:
- Dithranol: Daily evaluation. If no response by 6wk, then deemed a therapeutic failure.
- PUVA: Three times a week. Up to 30 treatments permitted.

Primary endpoint: Psoriasis clearance.

Secondary endpoints:
- Time to clearance;
- Side effects of PUVA.

Results

Primary endpoint	PUVA	Dithranol and UVB	p
Psoriasis clearance (%)	103/113 (91)	91/111 (82)	<0.05
Time to clearance (d)	34.4	20.4	<0.001

Discussion

In this study, PUVA proved to be an effective therapy for the treatment of chronic plaque psoriasis. Each treatment course was cheaper, took less nurse and patient time, and was well tolerated. Concerns expressed in this paper regarding the potential increased risk of skin cancer were well founded with an increased incidence of squamous cell carcinoma proven soon after.[*] Narrow band UVB appears to be safer than PUVA in this regard, and is now the standard form of phototherapy used for chronic plaque psoriasis. PUVA continues to be used in resistant cases of chronic plaque psoriasis and a number of other dermatological conditions.

Problems

- Although patient baseline characteristics were provided, it would have been useful to know that the two groups were well balanced in terms of their treatment history. It is possible that patients who have had multiple courses of intensive topical therapy and/or systemic treatments such as methotrexate may be more resistant to future therapy.

---

[*] Stern RS, Laird N, Melski J et al. (1984) Cutaneous squamous-cell carcinoma in patients treated with PUVA. N Engl J Med **310,** 1156–61.

Psoriasis: topical calcipotriol

Systematic review of comparative efficacy and tolerability of calcipotriol in treating chronic plaque psoriasis.

AUTHORS: Ashcroft D, Li Wan Po A, Williams H *et al.*
REFERENCE: BMJ (2000) 320, 963–7.
STUDY DESIGN: Systematic review
EVIDENCE LEVEL: 1a

Key message

Topical calcipotriol is effective in treating mild to moderate chronic plaque psoriasis, but is associated with a high frequency of skin irritation.

Impact

Topical calcipotriol is now established as the first-line topical therapy for mild to moderate chronic plaque psoriasis. Its efficacy is superior to most other topical agents and is comparable to potent topical corticosteroids. Although calcipotriol causes more skin irritation than topical corticosteroids, it does not carry the same long-term risks (such as skin atrophy).

Aims

Despite many available agents, a sporadic course and variable response to treatment make psoriasis difficult to treat. Calcipotriol, a synthetic vitamin D3 analogue, had become an increasingly popular therapy. This systematic review aimed to evaluate the comparative efficacy and tolerability of topical calcipotriol in the treatment of mild to moderate chronic plaque psoriasis.

Methods

Patients: 6038 patients with plaque psoriasis reported from 37 trials.

Studies included:

RCTs of 0.005% calcipotriol (cream or ointment) used to treat patients with chronic plaque psoriasis were found using a systematic search (1987–99) of Medline, EMBASE, the Cochrane controlled trials register as well as a BIDS index search for studies on calcipotriol and its various names. Studies included:

- Calcipotriol vs placebo;
- Calcipotriol vs potent topical corticosteroids;
- Calcipotriol vs very potent topical corticosteroids;
- Calcipotriol vs moderate topical corticosteroids plus calcipotriol;
- Calcipotriol vs potent topical corticosteroids plus calcipotriol;
- Calcipotriol administered bd vs od;
- Calcipotriol vs calcitriol;
- Calcipotriol vs coal tar;
- Calcipotriol vs 'short contact' dithranol;
- Calcipotriol vs ultraviolet B phototherapy plus calcipotriol.

Outcomes:
- Efficacy;
- Adverse effects.

Results

Differences in % score on Psoriasis Area and Severity Index from baseline (selected results only; (95% CL))

Calcipotriol vs placebo	44.1% (27.8 to 60.4)
Calcipotriol vs potent topical corticosteroids	6.5% (2.4 to 10.6)
Calcipotriol vs very potent topical corticosteroids	10.2% (−0.7 to 21.1)
Calcipotriol vs calcitriol	50.9% (30.6 to 71.2)
Calcipotriol vs coal tar	38.9% (26.9 to 50.9)
Calcipotriol vs 'short contact' dithranol	15.4% (10.1 to 20.7)

- Calcipotriol was shown to be significantly more irritant than both potent and very potent topical corticosteroids. In contrast, short contact dithranol was significantly more irritant than calcipotriol.

Discussion

This systematic review demonstrated that topical calcipotriol was more effective than calcitriol, coal tar, short contact dithranol, and tacalcitol in the treatment of mild to moderate chronic plaque psoriasis. Comparable efficacy was seen with potent topical steroids at 8wk of treatment. Although potent topical steroids have fewer short-term side effects than calcipotriol, their use is limited by the induction of skin atrophy, rebound of psoriasis after breaks in treatment, and the potential for systemic absorption. Therefore, despite the skin irritation caused by calcipotriol (which rarely leads to withdrawal of treatment), it should be a first-line therapy in patients with mild to moderate chronic plaque psoriasis.

Problems

- Psoriasis causes significant psychosocial morbidity. This systematic review highlighted that only one in 37 trials included within this review measured quality of life.
- Potent topical steroids showed comparable efficacy with less short-term side effects than calcipotriol. It would have been useful to have comparative data beyond 8wk of therapy.
- Away from clinical trials, patients will often switch between different topical regimens. Trials focusing on the risk to benefit ratios of combined regimens of calcipotriol with other antipsoriatic agents would be desirable.

Psoriasis: targeted biological therapy

Treatment of chronic plaque psoriasis by selective targeting of memory effector T lymphocytes.

AUTHORS: Ellis C, Krueger G (for Alefacept Clinical Study Group)
REFERENCE: N Engl J Med (2001) 345, 248–55.
STUDY DESIGN: RCT
EVIDENCE LEVEL: 1b

Key message
The first multicentre, placebo-controlled, double-blind RCT to demonstrate the efficacy of a targeted biological therapy in suppressing chronic plaque psoriasis.

Impact
Although alefacept is not licensed for use in the European Union, biological therapy using other agents has become an important part of the management of moderate and severe chronic plaque psoriasis since this study, particularly when more standard systemic therapies have failed. In contrast to traditional systemic agents, biological therapies do not appear to cause kidney or liver damage. However, long-term efficacy and safety data are still required.

Aims
Although mild psoriasis can often be controlled with topical agents, more severe forms of the condition often require systemic immunosuppression or ultraviolet therapy. The former carries toxic side effects, the latter risk and inconvenience. Furthermore, disease recurrence can occur after immunosuppression is withdrawn. T lymphocytes are implicated in many chronic autoimmune/inflammatory diseases, with the interaction between CD2 and its ligand, LFA-3 (leucocyte function associated antigen-type 3), being necessary for memory T lymphocyte activation. The LFA-3-IgG recombinant fusion protein, alefacept, was designed to prevent CD2 and LFA-3 interaction. This study aimed to assess the short-term efficacy and safety of alefacept in the treatment of psoriasis.

Methods
Patients: 426 patients at 22 centres in the USA (age range 18–70y).

Inclusion criteria:
- Diagnosis of chronic plaque psoriasis;
- ≥10% body surface area involvement;
- Previously received systemic treatment and/or phototherapy.

Exclusions included:
- Serious hepatic or renal disease;
- History of cancer (except basal cell carcinoma);
- Serious infection in previous 3 months.

Groups:
Four parallel groups received weekly IV infusions for 12wk of:
- Alefacept: 0.025mg/kg (n=57) or 0.075mg/kg (n=55) or 0.15mg/kg (n=58);
- Placebo (n=59).

Primary endpoint: Mean overall % decrease in clinical severity (as assessed by Psoriasis Area Severity Index (PASI) from baseline to 2wk after study completion).

Secondary endpoints: Those who achieved ≥75% reduction in PASI from baseline to 2wk after completion of therapy (PASI 75).

Follow-up: Performed every 2wk during treatment, and at wk 1, 2, 4, 8 and 12, for a total of 24wk.

Results

	Alefacept dose (mg/kg)			Placebo	p
	0.025	0.075	0.15		
Mean PASI decrease (%)	38	53	53	21	<0.001
% achieving PASI 75	2	33	31	10	0.02

Discussion

This study demonstrated the efficacy of targeted biological therapy for psoriasis. It is clear that psoriasis is in part an immune-mediated disease. By specifically targeting memory effector T lymphocytes with a recombinant protein, a reduction in the levels of these circulating T cells was seen, correlating with clinical improvement. Since this study, an increasing number of 'biological therapies' have been introduced for use in psoriasis, with data on their efficacy and safety extending to 1y (see *EXPRESS study*). Novel agents targeting various parts of the immune cascade involved in psoriasis are in development.

Problems

- Psoriasis causes significant psychosocial morbidity; there was no end-point to assess whether treatment led to improved quality of life.
- PASI 75 improvement seen with this biological agent was not significantly better than many existing systemic treatments. Formal comparisons between biological and standard therapies are urgently required.
- Clearly, long-term data from all biological agents are desirable. This should be possible as UK registries are in place to document a minimum of 5-y F/U on patients who start such therapy.

Psoriasis: methotrexate vs ciclosporin

Methotrexate vs ciclosporin in moderate to severe chronic plaque psoriasis.

AUTHORS: Heydendael V, Spuls P, Opmeer B *et al.*
REFERENCE: N Engl J Med (2003) 349, 658–65.
STUDY DESIGN: RCT
EVIDENCE LEVEL: 1b

Key message
There is no significant difference in efficacy between methotrexate and ciclosporin for the treatment of moderate to severe psoriasis.

Impact
One of the very few good quality evidence-based studies to have been performed comparing commonly used systemic agents for the treatment of moderate to severe psoriasis. This study has allowed clinicians to select the most suitable therapy on a case-to-case basis in the knowledge that the efficacy of both agents is comparable.

Aims
Numerous topical treatments exist for psoriasis. For more refractory disease, the systemic immunosuppressive agents, ciclosporin and methotrexate, can be used. With no consensus as to which is superior, this study aimed to compare methotrexate and ciclosporin in terms of their efficacy and side effects, and the improvement in quality of life in patients with moderate to severe psoriasis.

Methods
Patients: 88 patients at one centre in the Netherlands (age range 35–70y).

Inclusion criteria:
- Age >18y;
- Moderate to severe chronic plaque psoriasis as defined by Psoriasis Area Severity Index (PASI) ≥8;
- Insufficient response to topical or UVB therapy; no prior treatment with methotrexate or ciclosporin.

Exclusion criteria:
- Hepatic/renal impairment;
- Uncontrolled hypertension;
- History of cancer;
- Acute infection.

Groups:
- Methotrexate: initial dose 15mg per wk (n=44);
- Ciclosporin: initial dose 3mg/kg/d (n=44).

Primary endpoint: Difference between the groups in PASI after 16wk of treatment.

Secondary endpoints:
• Quality of life (QoL) after 16wk;
• Reported side effects.

Follow-up: Efficacy: PASI performed at baseline, and monthly thereafter to 1y. QoL: assessed using Dutch version of the Medical Outcomes Study 36-item Short-Form General Health Survey (SF36) at baseline, then every 8wk thereafter to 1y.

Results

Primary endpoints	Methotrexate	Ciclosporin
Baseline PASI (mean ± SE)	13.4 ± 3.6	14.0 ± 6.6
Week 16 PASI (mean ± SE)	5.0 ± 0.7	3.8 ± 0.5

• After adjustment for baseline values, the mean absolute difference in values at 16wk was 1.3 (95% CI –0.2 to 2.8; $p=0.09$).

Secondary endpoints:
• No significant difference after 16wk treatment in SF36;
• No serious or irreversible side effects observed. Therapy discontinued in 12 patients (methotrexate group) due to elevated liver enzymes. Only one patient discontinued ciclosporin (due to elevated bilirubin).

Discussion

These two systemic therapies have been used for many years in the treatment of moderate to severe psoriasis. They had never been directly compared before. Although the study was useful in determining the relative efficacy and short-term toxicity of each treatment, in practice they are often used in different settings. Ciclosporin is licensed as a short-term therapy for psoriasis due to the risk of renal toxicity in the medium to long term. Methotrexate can be used in the long term and, unlike ciclosporin, is useful in the treatment of psoriatic arthritis. Furthermore, a rotational approach to therapy is often adopted such that in time, a significant number of patients will have used both treatments.

Problems

• The dosing schedule in this study, particularly that of methotrexate, may not be representative of that used in day-to-day practice in the UK, where dose escalation is slower and from a lower baseline. There is no clear consensus on the optimal induction and maintenance regimen for methotrexate.
• Although the study design in this trial was randomised and double-blinded, the number of patients involved was small and may not have been sufficient to detect differences between the two therapies.

Psoriasis: infliximab therapy

EXPRESS (Evaluation of infliXimab For PsoRiasis Efficacy and Safety Study): Infliximab induction and maintenance therapy for moderate to severe psoriasis, a phase III, multicentre, double-blind trial.

AUTHORS: Reich K, Nestle F, Papp K et al.
REFERENCE: Lancet (2005) 366, 1367–74.
STUDY DESIGN: RCT
EVIDENCE LEVEL: 1b

Key message
The first double-blind RCT to show the sustained efficacy of the biological therapy, infliximab, for moderate to severe psoriasis through 1y of therapy.

Impact
This study has established infliximab as one of the most effective therapies currently available for the treatment of patients with moderate to severe psoriasis.

Aims
Therapies which neutralise the biological activity of tumour necrosis factor-α (TNFα) such as infliximab are novel in the treatment of psoriasis. As psoriasis is a chronic disease that usually requires long-term treatment, the aim of this study was to assess the efficacy (on skin and nail disease) and safety of continuous therapy (50wk) with infliximab in patients with moderate to severe psoriasis.

Methods
Patients: 378 patients at 32 dermatology centres in Europe and North America.

Inclusion criteria:
• Moderate to severe psoriasis for ≥6 months;
• Candidate for systemic or phototherapy;
• Psoriasis Area and Severity Index (PASI) ≥12 and affected body surface area ≥10%.

Exclusions:
• History of serious infection;
• Active tuberculosis;
• Lymphoproliferative disease.

Groups: 4:1 ratio of infusions of either:
• Infliximab: 5mg/kg at wk 0, 2, and 6, then every 8wk to wk46 (with evaluation at each visit and at wk50) (n=301);
• Placebo → infliximab: placebo at wk 0, 2, and 6, then every 8wk; at wk24, placebo-treated patients crossed to infliximab treatment (given at wk24, 26, and 30, and every 8wk to wk46; evaluation at each visit and at wk50) (n=77).

Primary endpoint: The proportion of patients achieving ≥75% improvement in PASI from baseline to wk10.

Secondary endpoints/measures:
- Proportion achieving PASI 75 improvement from baseline at wk24;
- Proportion achieving a physician's global assessment (PGA) score of cleared (0) or minimal (1) for their psoriasis at wk 10, 24, and 50;
- Proportion achieving 50% improvement from baseline (PASI 50) and 90% improvement from baseline (PASI 90) at wk24 and 50;
- % improvement in the Nail Psoriasis Severity Index (NAPSI) at wk10, 24, and 50.

Results

	Wk10			Wk24			Wk50	
	Plac	Inf	*p*	Plac	Inf	*p*	Plac/ Inf	Inf
PASI 75	3%	80%	<0.0001	4%	82%	<0.0001	77%	61%
PASI 90	1%	57%	<0.0001	1%	58%	<0.0001	50%	45%

Plac: Placebo

Inf: Infliximab

Discussion

These data demonstrated that infliximab monotherapy was highly effective in the treatment of moderate to severe psoriasis. Improvement in skin and nail disease was rapid and sustained in the majority of responders for up to 50wk of treatment. The treatment was well tolerated, with 80% of patients completing all infusions.

Problems

- Although this study had efficacy and safety data extending to 1y, concerns remain over the long-term effects of immunosuppression by TNF blockers and their potential for inducing serious long-term complications such as skin cancer and lymphoproliferative disorders.
- In the UK, the annual drug costs of biological therapies such as infliximab are around £10,000. Traditional systemic agents such as methotrexate are much cheaper with annual drug costs of £55.
- Although highly effective, infliximab must be given to patients via an IV infusion in a day care or similar unit. Other biological therapies such as efalizumab, etanercept and adalimumab are available as subcutaneous injections which can be self-administered.

Acne: systemic retinoids

Isotretinoin vs placebo in the treatment of cystic acne. A randomised double-blind study.

AUTHORS: Peck G, Olsen T, Butkus D *et al.*
REFERENCE: J Am Acad Dermatol (1982) 6, 735–45.
STUDY DESIGN: RCT
EVIDENCE LEVEL: 1b

Key message
The first placebo-controlled RCT to show the efficacy of oral isotretinoin in the treatment of cystic acne.

Impact
Isotretinoin revolutionised therapy for patients with severe scarring acne. Its efficacy is high and long-lasting in a significant proportion of acne patients. Prescribers need to be fully aware of its teratogenicity and possible link with severe mood disturbance.

Aims
A significant proportion of patients with cystic acne do not respond to standard acne treatments such as topical and/or oral antibiotics. Isotretinoin, an oral retinoid, derived from vitamin A, acts by reducing the production of sebum from sebaceous glands, possibly through a mechanism involving alteration of their DNA transcription. This study aimed to compare the efficacy of oral isotretinoin with placebo in cystic acne.

Methods
Patients: 33 patients.

Inclusion criteria:
- ≥10 inflamed deep dermal or subcutaneous acne cysts or nodules ≥4mm diameter;
- Minimal response to previous acne therapies;
- Discontinued all other acne therapies >1 month before study entry.

Groups:
- Isotretinoin: 0.5mg/kg/d, for up to 4 months (n=16);
- Placebo: for up to 4 months (n=17).
- If there was no improvement in cystic acne at the time of each monthly F/U, the dose of isotretinoin or placebo could be increased by 0.5mg/kg/d. If there was worsening, the double-blind code could be broken with cross-over to the active drug.

Primary endpoint: Nodules and cysts counted and measured.

Secondary endpoints:
- Biopsies of forehead skin to assess sebaceous gland size;
- Quantitative analysis of forehead sebum production.

Follow-up: Performed at baseline, then monthly to 4 months.

Results

	Isotretinoin	Placebo	*p*
1 month % change in cysts	17% decrease	33% increase	0.001
2 month % change in cysts	32% decrease	58% increase	0.008

- At the 1-month F/U, eight patients in the placebo group were switched to isotretinoin as their acne was worse. After 2 months, a further six were switched to isotretinoin.
- 32 of 33 patients had at least one 4 months course of isotretinoin. 27 of the 32 patients had complete disease clearance to at least 38 months post-treatment.

Discussion

This study demonstrated the impressive efficacy of oral isotretinoin in the treatment of cystic acne. It also highlighted the need for some patients to have prolonged courses of isotretinoin beyond 4 months duration. The secondary endpoints assessed sebaceous gland size in skin biopsies and quantitative sebum production from forehead skin, both of which were reduced (the latter by approximately 93%, confirming the mechanism of action of isotretinoin). No patients dropped out of the study due to adverse events, although most had dose-dependent dryness of mucous membranes. Laboratory abnormalities were limited to small elevations of liver enzymes and triglyceride levels, these returning to normal after completion of therapy.

Problems

- Although this study was performed in a very small cohort of patients, the dramatic efficacy of isotretinoin was clearly demonstrated. On the other hand, the study was not sufficiently large to detect important adverse events. The prescription of isotretinoin is currently tightly regulated due to its teratogenic effects and the potential for mood related adverse events.
- It would have been useful to trial isotretinoin against a systemic antibiotic so that the gold standard therapy at that time could have been directly compared.

Bullous pemphigoid: corticosteroids

A comparison of oral and topical corticosteroids in patients with bullous pemphigoid.

AUTHORS: Joly P, Roujeau J, Benichou J *et al.*
REFERENCE: N Engl J Med (2002) 346, 321–7.
STUDY DESIGN: RCT
EVIDENCE LEVEL: 1b

Key message

Topical corticosteroid therapy is effective for both moderate and extensive bullous pemphigoid (BP), and has superior safety to oral corticosteroid therapy for extensive disease.

Impact

Systemic corticosteroids were previously considered the standard treatment for BP. This trial brought this practice into question. BP is classically a disease of the elderly; the superior safety of topical corticosteroids means that they should now be considered as first-line therapy for patients who develop this condition.

Aims

Systemic corticosteroids had been the mainstay of treatment for BP, the most common autoimmune blistering disease of the skin. The elderly are particularly affected, and this group of patients often poorly tolerates this treatment with consequent high mortality rates. Previous studies have failed to support the use of alternative immunosuppressive drugs. Therefore, this study aimed to assess whether topical corticosteroids increased the rate of survival among patients with BP and whether they provided effective control of the disease.

Methods

Patients: 324 patients at 27 dermatology centres in France.

Inclusion criteria:
- Clinical features suggestive of BP;
- Histological findings consistent with BP (sub-epidermal blisters; linear deposits of IgG and C3 along the basement membrane zone).

Exclusion criteria:
- Predominant or exclusive mucosal involvement;
- Treatment with oral or topical corticosteroids, dapsone or immunosuppressive drugs during the previous 6 months.

Groups: Stratified by disease severity: moderate (≤10) or extensive (>10) new bullae (blisters) daily, over previous 3d:
- Topical application: of 0.05% clobetasol propionate cream (*moderate:* n=77; *extensive:* n=93);
- Oral prednisolone: 0.5mg/kg/d for moderate disease and 1mg/kg/d for extensive disease (*moderate:* n=76; *extensive:* n=95).

Evaluations: At baseline, then at F/U visits (d 7, 14, 21, 30, 90, 180, and 360). Patients assessed for the number of new bullae, time to relapse, and any side effects.

Primary endpoint: Overall survival during the first year after BP onset.

Secondary endpoints: Control of disease at 21d.

Results

Primary endpoint	Topical	Oral	p
% survival (moderate disease)	70	70	1.0
% survival (extensive disease)	76	59	0.02
Secondary endpoint			
% control at d21 (moderate disease)	100	95	0.06
% control at d21 (severe disease)	99	91	0.02

Discussion

This study confirmed the poor prognosis (mortality rate 41%) of patients with extensive BP who were treated with oral prednisolone at a dose of 1mg/kg/d. For this specific subgroup of patients, the study showed a statistically significant advantage for the use of potent topical steroids. It was suggested that this regimen should be considered as the standard therapy for patients with extensive BP. Control of BP and 1-y survival in patients with moderate disease were similar for oral and topical corticosteroids.

Problems

- The study was non-blinded. The authors argue that this was acceptable as it could not influence the primary endpoint, mortality at 1y. However, it is possible that the open nature of the study could have influenced the secondary endpoints, which involved a degree of subjective assessment of patients.
- The number in each of the four groups was small. This is reflected in the statistical differences between the groups and the trial endpoints, where significant differences were only just $p<0.05$.
- In many cases of BP, patients are switched onto non-steroid-based therapies (e.g. azathioprine) after short-term disease control is gained with steroids. Therefore, many patients may not require steroids for as long as 12 months, which was the time period assessed in this study.

Treatment of cutaneous warts

Local treatments for cutaneous warts: systematic review

AUTHORS: Gibbs S, Harvey I, Sterling J, Stark R.
REFERENCE: BMJ (2002) 325, 461.
STUDY DESIGN: Systematic review
EVIDENCE LEVEL: 1a

Key message
The evidence for the efficacy of treatment for cutaneous warts is weak; the best available is for topical treatments containing salicylic acid.

Impact
This review highlighted the very poor evidence base for the treatment of cutaneous warts. In particular, the widely employed technique of cryotherapy does not appear to be an effective option.

Aims
Viral warts on the hands and feet are common, benign, and usually self-limiting in the immunocompetent. For this reason, they are usually not treated. However, some patients—for pain or cosmesis—prefer treatment. Although a number of options are available, no evidence-based consensus exists as to what treatment is optimal. This systematic review aimed to assess the evidence for the efficacy of local treatments for cutaneous warts.

Methods
Study selection: RCTs of any local treatment for uncomplicated cutaneous warts.

Trials included:
- Salicylic acid (n=13);
- Cryotherapy (n=15);
- Intralesional bleomycin (n=5);
- Fluorouracil (n=4);
- Intralesional interferons (n=6);
- Dinitrochlorobenzene (n=2);
- Photodynamic therapy (n=4);
- Pulsed dye laser (n=1).

Evaluations: Trial quality was classified as 'high', 'medium', and 'low' and, where possible, data pooled to allow assessment of the primary endpoint.

Primary endpoint: Complete clearance of warts.

Results
82% of trials assessed classified as 'low' quality. Key findings:
- Salicylic acid:
  - Pooled data from six placebo-controlled trials;
  - Cure rate 75% cases vs 48% controls (OR 3.91; 95% CI 2.40 to 6.36).

- Dinitrochlorobenzene:
  - Pooled data from two trials;
  - Cure rate 80% cases vs 38% controls (OR 6.67; 95% CI 2.44 to 18.23).
- Cryotherapy:
  - Pooled data from four trials of 'aggressive' vs 'gentle' applications;
  - Cure rate 52% vs 31%, respectively (OR 1.45–9.41).
- No benefit was shown in pooled data from two small trials of cryotherapy vs placebo.

Discussion

The authors of this systematic review had great difficulty reviewing the research in a systematic fashion due to the heterogeneity of study design, methods, and outcome. The only conclusion that could be drawn was that there was very little high quality research on the efficacy of various local treatments for warts. Treatment with both salicylic acid and contact immunotherapy with dinitrochlorobenzene appeared to be beneficial, although the latter had the potential for significant adverse events. Interestingly, cryotherapy, which is widely employed in the treatment of cutaneous warts, had little evidence to support its use.

Problems

- Due to the poor quality of study design, it was impossible to draw any meaningful conclusions about most of the cutaneous therapies employed in the treatment of warts.
- Cryotherapy is one of the most commonly employed treatment modalities for cutaneous warts. Of the 16 trials included in the systematic review, most studied different treatment regimens rather than comparing cryotherapy with other treatments or placebo. The effectiveness of cryotherapy remains uncertain.

Onychomycosis: antifungals

Double-blind, randomised study of continuous terbinafine compared with intermittent itraconazole in the treatment of toenail onychomycosis.

AUTHORS: Evans E, Sigurgeirsson B (for the LION study group).
REFERENCE: BMJ (1999) 318, 1031–5.
STUDY DESIGN: RCT
EVIDENCE LEVEL: 1b

Key message
Continuous terbinafine is significantly more effective than intermittent itraconazole in the treatment of patients with toenail onychomycosis.

Impact
Terbinafine is the gold standard therapy for the treatment of toenail onychomycosis. Rarely, oral terbinafine can cause significant hepatic and/or cutaneous adverse events such that patients still require appropriate counselling before embarking on a potentially curative course of therapy.

Aims
Onychomycosis is one of the most common curable nail diseases. Terbinafine (a fungicidal allylamine) and itraconazole (a fungistatic triazole) are two of the commonly used treatments. As therapeutic concentrations of itraconazole persist after discontinuation of therapy, intermittent treatment is widely used. This study aimed to compare the efficacy and safety of continuous terbinafine with intermittent itraconazole in the treatment of toenail onychomycosis.

Methods
Patients: 496 patients at 35 centres in six European countries.

Inclusion criteria:
• Age 18–75y.
• Clinical diagnosis of onychomycosis of the great toenail confirmed by positive results on mycological culture or microscopy.

Exclusion criteria:
• Use of a systemic antifungal agent in the previous 12 months;
• Use of a topical antifungal agent within 4wk of screening.

Groups: Four parallel groups:
• Terbinafine (250mg daily) for 12wk (group 1) or 16wk (group 2);
• Itraconazole (400mg daily) for 1wk in every month for 12 (group 3) or 16wk (group 4).

Evaluations: Assessed at wk 4, 8, 12, 16, and then F/U (blinded) at wk 24, 36, 48, and 72.

Primary endpoint: Assessment of mycological cure rates at wk 72.

Secondary endpoints: Clinical cure (100% toenail clearing).

Results

Endpoint	Terbinafine 12wk	Terbinafine 16wk	Itraconazole 3 cycles	Itraconazole 4 cycles
Mycological cure	81/107 (76%)	80/99 (81%)	41/107 (38%)	53/108 (49%)
Clinical cure	59/110 (54%)	59/98 (60%)	34/107 (32%)	35/109 (32%)

- Differences in mycological cure and clinical cure significantly favoured terbinafine ($p<0.0001$ and <0.002, respectively).

Discussion

The study demonstrated that terbinafine 250mg od, over 12 or 16wk produced better mycological and clinical cure rates at wk72 than intermittent itraconazole given over the same periods. The safety profiles of both drugs were similar. It is likely that the superior efficacy of terbinafine is related to its primary fungicidal actions as opposed to the fungistatic actions of itraconazole.

Problems

- The paper stated that most side effects in both groups were considered by investigators to be mild or moderate and unrelated to study medications. They do not list any serious adverse events. Clearly, it is important to be aware of any potentially significant adverse events as many patients with toenail onychomycosis may have asymptomatic disease, and there is a balance to be made between risk and benefit of any treatment, particularly if systemic.
- Mycological culture and microscopy are not sensitive tests for detecting fungal infections of the nails. In clinical practice, it may be necessary to take serial clippings for microscopy and culture to prove the presence of an infection.
- It would be useful to know about relapse and/or reinfection of treated patients over a longer period of time (e.g. 2–5y).

Photoageing: topical tretinoin

Topical tretinoin improves photoaged skin: a double-blind vehicle-controlled study.

AUTHORS: Weiss J, Elliss C, Headington J, Voorhees J.
REFERENCE: JAMA (1988) 259, 527–32.
STUDY DESIGN: RCT
EVIDENCE LEVEL: 1b

Key message
The first double-blind, placebo-controlled RCT to show that a topical retinoid improves photoaged skin.

Impact
The holy grail of preventing and/or reversing the skin ageing process remains an area of active research. However, topical retinoids remain the only form of therapy to demonstrate improvement in clinical features of photoaged skin.

Aims
Skin ageing can be divided into intrinsic ageing (largely due to endogenous/genetic factors) and photoageing (caused principally by ultraviolet (UV) light-based chronic sun exposure). Photoageing is characterised by changes, including epidermal dysplasia with cellular atypia, loss of keratinocyte polarity, dermal damage with elastosis, loss of collagen, an increase in glycosaminoglycans, and a modest inflammatory infiltrate. With topical tretinoin (all-*trans*-retinoic acid) having been shown to enhance repair of UV-damaged skin in mouse models, it had been suggested that some of the changes associated with photoageing were reversible. Although some structural improvement with tretinoin cream had also been reported in humans, these findings had not been substantiated by RCTs. This study aimed to evaluate the efficacy of 0.1% tretinoin cream in the treatment of photoageing, assessing clinical and histological improvement.

Methods
Patients: 40 patients at one centre in the USA (age range 35–70y).

Inclusion criteria:
- Clinically diagnosed with photoageing of the face and forearms;
- Stopped all topical medications 2wk prior to the study;
- Good general health.

Groups:
- 0.1% tretinoin: daily applications to face and left forearm; vehicle cream applied to the right forearm (n=20);
- Vehicle cream: daily application to the face and left forearm; 0.1% tretinoin applied to the right forearm (n=20).

Primary endpoint: Patients' faces and forearms graded compared with pre-therapy (worse, no change, slightly improved, or much improved).

Secondary endpoints: 4mm full-thickness punch biopsy for histological analysis; pre-therapy and at wk16.

Follow-up: Evaluations pre-therapy, and at wk2, 4, 8, 12, and 16.

Results

Primary endpoint: global response	Vehicle cream	Tretinoin cream	p
Much improved	0 (0%)	9 (30%)	<0.001
Improved	0 (0%)	12 (40%)	<0.001
Slightly improved	0 (0%)	9 (30%)	<0.001
No change or worse	30 (100%)	0 (0%)	<0.001

- 30 of 40 randomised patients completed the study. Three withdrew due to severe tretinoin-induced dermatitis, the other seven for issues unrelated to treatment.

Histological data:
- Obtained from 28 patients;
- Demonstrated a mean increase in epidermal thickness ($p=0.02$) with diminished melanocytic hypertrophy and hyperplasia in the tretinoin treatment group. Essentially, smoother more evenly pigmented skin with histology confirming the clinical findings.

Discussion

It is clear that an agent that could prevent and/or reverse any part of the ageing process would have far wider therapeutic applications than simply being of 'cosmetic' value. Work in this area continues. Most individuals in this study suffered from tretinoin-induced dermatitis, in some cases lasting for the whole treatment course. This involved irritation, dryness, and reddening of the skin; in practice, this may prove unacceptable, particularly for those using this as a 'cosmetic' treatment.

Problems

- There was no comparison of differing strengths of topical tretinoin.
- It is hard to perform a blinded study with an agent such as topical tretinoin as nearly all patients treated with this therapy develop signs of skin irritation, potentially unblinding investigators.
- Only Caucasian patients studied.

Diabetes

Introduction

Arateus, the 2nd century Alexandrian physician, first coined the term 'diabetes' when he encountered a case of a patient complaining of excessive urination. For many centuries, this prominent symptom (polyuria) led to diabetes being considered as a disease solely of the kidneys. This theory has since been refuted by research uncovering its multifactorial aetio-pathogenesis, with complications affecting multiple organ systems; it goes far beyond being an endocrine disorder of the pancreas, and requires consideration of other systems, including cardiovascular (cerebrovascular and peripheral vascular disease), renal (nephropathy), ophthalmic (retinopathy), neurological (neuropathy—both peripheral and autonomic), orthopaedic (diabetic foot, Charcot neuroarthropathy), psychiatric (depression, anxiety), infectious (respiratory, skin, urinary tract), dermatological (ulcers, dermopathy, necrobiosis lipoidica diabeticorum, bullosa diabeticorum) … the list goes on. Indeed, it is fair to say that 'if you fully understand diabetes and its complications, then you truly understand medicine!'

Although this assertion may appear slightly exaggerated, there remains a substantial truth in its central thesis. In fact, it can be suggested that diabetes has become modern medicine's equivalent of syphilis, the multi-system nature of which took some time to be fully appreciated. In Western practice, about one in four patients admitted to hospital have diabetes. Its high prevalence and incidence, coupled with costly multi-organ complications, have been reflected by an unparalleled surge in diabetes-related research over the last decade. In this era of evidence-based medical practice, one may have to dedicate a considerable amount of time to keep abreast with new knowledge, concepts, and innovation. With this wealth of available resources, it can, unfortunately, be frustratingly arduous for a clinician to find the time to understand the most reliable evidence that underpins the practice of diabetology. This chapter will focus on key clinical trials that have had a significant impact on our understanding and/or treatment over the past decade.

Primary prevention: lifestyle intervention

> **DPS** (Finnish Diabetes Prevention Study): Prevention of type 2 diabetes mellitus by changes in lifestyle among subjects with impaired glucose tolerance.
>
> **AUTHORS:** Tuomilehto J, Lindstrom J, Eriksson J *et al.*
> **REFERENCE:** N Engl J Med (2001) 344, 1343–50.
> **STUDY DESIGN:** RCT
> **EVIDENCE LEVEL:** 1b

Key message

This landmark RCT study shows that type 2 diabetes mellitus (DM) can be prevented in high-risk patients through lifestyle changes.

Impact

In view of the rising incidence of type 2 DM, lifestyle changes are currently advocated to reduce the burden of diabetes. Today, healthy diet, weight reduction in overweight people, and regular moderate physical exercise are important lifestyle measures in diabetes prevention.

Aims

Lifestyle factors are key determinants in the development of type 2 DM, especially in those at high risk. People with impaired glucose tolerance (IGT) have derangements in glucose metabolism, and are thus at high risk of developing type 2 DM. This study was conducted to determine the feasibility and effect of lifestyle changes designed to prevent or delay the onset of type 2 DM in people with IGT.

Methods

Patients: 522 patients at five centres in Finland.

Inclusion criteria:
- IGT (defined as fasting blood glucose <7.8mmol/L and 7.8–11.1mmol/L, 2h after a 75g glucose load in an oral glucose tolerance test, OGTT);
- Overweight (defined as BMI ≥25);
- Age 40–65y.

Exclusion criteria:
- Diagnosis of DM;
- Chronic disease and unlikely to survive >6y;
- Psychological and physical impairments deemed likely to interfere with the study.

Groups:
- Control: oral advice and written information on diet and exercise;
- Intervention: detailed individualised dietary and exercise advice with preset goals and guidance on how these can be achieved.

Primary endpoint: Development of DM (according to 1985 World Health Organisation criteria).

Follow-up: Control group: Annually. *Intervention group:* Seven sessions in the first year, then three sessions annually for the rest of the study period, for nutritional advice. Study started in 1993, last patient assigned in 1998. Initially planned to run for 6y after this, but was terminated in 2000 when an interim analysis showed that the intervention was clearly beneficial.

Results

Primary endpoint	Intervention	Control	p
Cumulative incidence of DM	11%	23%	<0.001

Discussion

Previous studies, notably the Da Qing trial *(Diabetes Care* (1997) 20, 537–44) and the Malmo 6-year feasibility study *(Diabetologia* (1991) 34, 891–8), had shown that lifestyle interventions prevented or delayed the onset of type 2 DM in people with IGT. However, neither of these studies were randomised. The DPS, a carefully designed RCT, also showed that lifestyle intervention was clearly beneficial. The NNT by lifestyle intervention for 1y to prevent one case of incident type 2 DM in people with IGT was 22. In an extended F/U of the study participants for 7y, the authors subsequently showed that the benefits of this intervention were maintained. These results have been confirmed on a larger scale by an equivalent USA-based study, the Diabetes Prevention Program (DPP).

Problems

- The staff involved in this trial were not blinded to the intervention/control groups.
- The glucose levels used to define IGT in this study included subjects who today would be classified as having type 2 DM. This raises the question as to whether this could be truly classified as a 'prevention' (as opposed to a 'delayed onset') study.

Primary prevention: metformin vs lifestyle intervention

> **DPP** (**D**iabetes **P**revention **P**rogram): Reduction in the incidence of
> type 2 diabetes with lifestyle intervention or metformin.
>
> **AUTHORS:** The diabetes prevention research group.
> **REFERENCE:** N Engl J Med (2002) 346, 393–402.
> **STUDY DESIGN:** RCT
> **EVIDENCE LEVEL:** 1b

Key message

In patients with impaired glucose tolerance (IGT), intensive lifestyle
modification and to a lesser extent, metformin, significantly reduce the
incidence of type 2 diabetes mellitus (DM).

Impact

Lifestyle changes are now universally recommended not only to prevent
the development of DM, but also to improve overall cardiovascular
health, particularly in those at high risk.

Aims

Other studies, such as the Da Qing trial and the almost contemporary
Finnish Diabetes Prevention Study, had shown lifestyle interventions to
be effective in preventing or delaying the onset of DM in high-risk subjects. This larger study aimed to test the veracity of these findings across
varied ethnic groups in the USA, using newly defined American Diabetes
Association (ADA) 1997 criteria for the diagnosis of DM and IGT. It specifically sought to determine whether lifestyle intervention and the bigua-
nide, metformin, were both effective in preventing DM and which of them
was more effective.

Methods

Patients: 3234 non-diabetic subjects at 27 centres in the USA.

Inclusion criteria:
- Age ≥25y;
- BMI ≥24 (22 in Asians);
- IGT: fasting plasma glucose (FPG) 5.3–6.9mmol/L and 7.8–11.0 at 2h
  post-75g glucose load in an oral glucose tolerance test (OGTT).

Groups:
- Metformin (850mg bd) plus standard lifestyle recommendations (n=1073);
- Placebo (bd) plus standard lifestyle recommendations (n=1082);
- Individualised intensive programme of lifestyle modification: target being to
  lose 7% body weight and to do 150min of exercise per wk (n=1079).

Primary endpoint: Diabetes (FPG ≥7.8mmol/L; *or* ≥11.0mmol/L, 2h post-
75g OGTT).

Follow-up: Quarterly in metformin and placebo groups to assess adherence; monthly in the intensive lifestyle group. All groups had F/U for 2y.

Results

Primary endpoint	Lifestyle	Metformin	Placebo
Incidence of DM per 100 person-years	4.8	7.8	11.0

- $p < 0.001$ for each comparison;
- Risk reduction: lifestyle vs placebo 58%; metformin vs placebo 31%; lifestyle vs metformin 39%.

Discussion

This trial confirmed that lifestyle modification in a large and high-risk multiracial cohort with IGT effectively prevented or delayed the onset of type 2 DM. The oral antidiabetic agent, metformin, was also effective in preventing DM in people with IGT, but was inferior to lifestyle modification; its effect was most marked in people with higher baseline BMI and blood glucose levels. The benefits of various pharmacological agents have been examined in other studies. In the STOP-NIDDM study (*Diabetes Care* (1998) 21, 1720–5), arcabose was shown to reduce the incidence of DM (number to treat (NNT) 22), while in the TRIPOD study (*Controlled Clinical Trials* (1998) 19, 217–31), troglitazone reduced the incidence of DM in high-risk Hispanic women with gestational diabetes (NNT 6). However, this agent was noted to be hepatotoxic in an abandoned fourth arm of the DPP. The recent DREAM trial (*Diabetes Care* (2008) 31, 1007–14) used rosiglitazone/ramipril in people with IGT and/or impaired fasting glucose (IFG), concluding that for every 1000 people treated with rosiglitazone for about 3y, 144 cases of DM would be prevented at the expense of about four cases of congestive heart failure. In summary, whereas the evidence for lifestyle intervention in reducing the incidence of type 2 DM is striking, the same cannot be said of pharmacological interventions, with studies having produced mixed results.

Problems

- This study investigated the preventive effect of a drug that is used to treat DM, and this raises the question as to whether the benefits observed in those on metformin were simply due to this drug's glucose-lowering effect.

Preventing complications: intensive treatment

> **DCCT** (Diabetes Control and Complications Trial): The effect of intensive treatment of diabetes on the development and progression of long-term complications in insulin-dependent diabetes mellitus.
>
> **AUTHORS:** Diabetes Control and Complications Trial Research Group.
> **REFERENCE:** N Engl J Med (1993) 329, 977–86.
> **STUDY DESIGN:** RCT
> **EVIDENCE LEVEL:** 1b

Key message

'Tight control' of blood sugar levels with intensive insulin treatment delays the onset and slows the progression of diabetes-related complications.

Impact

It is now accepted that blood glucose control in type 1 DM should be optimised towards attaining DCCT targets: HbA_{1C} <7.5% (or <6.5% for those at increased risk of arterial disease).

Aims

Long-term microvascular and neurological complications cause major morbidity and mortality in type 1 diabetes mellitus (DM). The aim of this study was to compare the effects of two treatment regimes—intensive vs conventional—with regard to their effects on the development and progression of the early vascular and neurological complications.

Methods

Patients: 1441 teenagers/young adults at 29 centres in the USA and Canada.

Inclusion criteria: Age 13–39y, with type 1 DM for 1–15y; insulin dependence as defined by deficient C-peptide secretion.

Exclusion criteria: Hypertension, hypercholesterolaemia, or other significant medical conditions; severe diabetes-related complications.

Groups:
- *Primary prevention cohort (n=726):* Type 1 DM for 1–5y, with no complications (no retinopathy and urinary albumin excretion <40mg/24h)
- *Secondary prevention cohort (n=715):* Type 1 DM for 1–15y, with mild to moderate non-proliferative retinopathy and urinary albumin excretion <200mg/24h.
- *Conventional therapy (CT):* with urine or blood sugar tests and 1–2 insulin injections per d (n=378 primary, 342 secondary);
- *Intensive treatment (IT):* initial hospitalisation for education and stabilisation, ≥4 blood sugar tests per d, insulin ≥3 per d by pump or injections (n=348 primary, 363 secondary).

Primary endpoints
- Rate of onset of retinopathy in the primary prevention cohort;
- Rate of progression of retinopathy in the secondary intervention cohort.

Follow-up: CT group: three monthly F/U (target HbA$_{1C}$ <9.0%). *IT group:* monthly visits, frequent telephone calls by diabetes nurse educators (target HbA$_{1C}$ <6.0%). Care team comprised physician, nurse, dietician, and behavioural therapist. Mean F/U=6.5y (range 3–9y).

Results

	Conventional	Intensive	*p*
Primary prevention group			
Total incidence of retinopathy	91	23	<0.001
Reduction in retinopathy	–	76% (95% CI 62 to 85%)	–
Secondary prevention group			
Total incidence of retinopathy	77	43	0.002
Slowed progression of retinopathy	–	54% (95% CI 39 to 66%)	–
Combined cohort: Mean HbA1c	231±55mg/dL	155±30mg/dL	<0.001

The intensively treated group (combined cohort) showed reduction in occurrence of three major microvascular complications in all subgroups:
- 76% reduction in diabetic retinopathy;
- 57% reduction in progression of kidney disease;
- 60% reduction in progression of neuropathy.

Discussion

This study found differences between the intensive and conventional groups to be apparent within 3y. The curves showing the rate of development of complications between the two groups progressively diverged as the years went by, suggesting an overtly beneficial effect of intensive insulin therapy in type 1 DM. The chief adverse events associated with the intensively treated group were a 2–3 fold increase in severe hypoglycaemia and an average small weight gain (1kg).

Problems

- Mean F/U was only 6.5y—short when considering long-term complications such as retinopathy. However, DCCT patients subsequently had >10y F/U in the EDIC study, which confirmed these findings.
- Retinopathy: too few patients were affected by severe retinopathy or macular oedema or required laser treatment to notice a significant difference between groups. In the secondary prevention group, the incidence of progression of retinopathy in the first year was higher in the intensive group. This suggests patients who have suddenly improved glycaemic control should be watched carefully as they are at risk of initial worsening before benefit is obtained.

Preventing complications: intensive glycaemic control

UKPDS (United Kingdom Prospective Diabetes Study) 33: Intensive blood glucose control with sulphonylureas or insulin compared with conventional treatment and risk of complications in patients with type 2 diabetes.

AUTHORS: UKPDS Group.
REFERENCE: Lancet (1998) 352, 837–53.
STUDY DESIGN: RCT
EVIDENCE LEVEL: 1b

Key message

HbA_{1C} level and the life-threatening complications of DM can be reduced by more intensive management using existing treatments (UKPDS 33 and 34). Reducing blood pressure in these patients reduces the risk of fatal and non-fatal complications (UKPDS 38 and 39).

Impact

As perhaps the single most important study ever conducted in type 2 DM, this underpinned the need for aggressive treatment in maintaining good glycaemic control. It has been the most important driving force behind many international guidelines, including those of the UK's National Institute of Health and Clinical Excellence (NICE), in setting targets for tight glycaemic control (HbA_{1C} between 6.5% and 7.5%), based on the risk of microvascular and macrovascular complications.

Aims

Patients with type 2 DM are at risk of developing both microvascular and macrovascular complications in the setting of chronic hyperglycaemia. The aims of UKPDS were to determine whether: (a) intensive use of pharmacological therapy to lower blood sugar would result in clinical benefits (reduced cardiovascular and microvascular complications), and (b) the use of sulphonylureas, metformin, or insulin had specific therapeutic advantages or disadvantages (UKPDS 33 and 34).

Methods

Patients: 5102 recruited (randomised: 3867 UKPDS 33; 753 UKPDS 34), from 23 clinics in the UK (82% Caucasian; 10% Asian; 8% Afro-Caribbean).

Inclusion criteria: Age 25–65y, with newly diagnosed type 2 DM and fasting plasma glucose (FPG) >6mmol/L on two mornings, 1–3wk apart.

Exclusion criteria: Ketonuria >3mmol/L *or* serum creatinine >175μmol/L; myocardial infarction (MI) in last y, angina, heart failure, major vascular event, malignant hypertension, contraindication to insulin treatment; retinopathy requiring laser treatment.

Groups:
Non-overweight patients (UKPDS 33): After 3 months dietary run-in:
Intensive (target FPG <6.0mmol/L): received insulin (30%) or sulphonylurea (40%)
(n=2729); Conventional (target FPG <15.0mmol/L): diet only (30%) (n=1138).

NB. It became clear that no oral agent could maintain the intensive group goal. Thus, combination
therapy was used, mixing insulin or metformin with sulphonylureas. Those in the conventional group
developing FPG >15mmol/L were secondarily randomised to sulphonylurea or insulin therapy.

Overweight patients (UKPDS 34):
Intensive: treatment with metformin (n=342); conventional: diet only (n=411).

NB. A secondary analysis compared 342 patients in metformin group with 951 patients allocated
intensive control with chlorpropamide (n=265), glibenclamide (n=277), or insulin (n=409).

Primary endpoints: 21 endpoints defined, including: any DM–related
complications, DM-related deaths, and all-cause mortality.

Follow-up: 3–4 monthly for the duration of the study (10y).

Results

Primary endpoints	Intensive	Conventional	p	RR (95% CI)
Any DM-related	35.3%	38.5%	0.03	0.88 (0.79 to 0.99)
DM-related death	10.4%	11.3%	0.3	0.90 (0.73 to 1.11)
All-cause mortality	17.9%	18.7%	0.4	0.94 (0.80 to 1.10)
Median HbA$_{1C}$	7.0%	7.9%	<0.0001	–
MI	14.2%	16.3%	0.05	0.84 (0.71 to 1.00)
Microvascular	8.2%	10.6%	0.01	0.75 (0.60 to 0.93)
Single endpoints				
Retinal photocoagulation	7.6%	10.3%	0.003	0.71 (0.53 to 0.96)
Vitreous haemorrhage	0.7%	0.9%	0.5	0.77 (0.28 to 2.11)
Blindness in one eye	2.9%	3.3%	0.4	0.84 (0.51- to 1.40)
Cataract extraction	5.5%	7.0%	0.05	0.76 (0.53 to 1.08)

Intensive metformin treatment decreased the risks of DM-related endpoints in overweight patients (32%, p=0.0023); DM-related death and all-
cause mortality (36%, p=0.011); and MI (39%, p=0.010) vs conventional
treatment. Oddly, the supplementary analysis of UKPDS 34 showed
sulphonylurea-treated patients given metformin had significant increases
in DM-related (96%) and all-cause deaths (60%) vs conventional therapy.

Discussion
This study showed the importance of good blood glucose control in
reducing the incidence of microvascular complications. The method of
control seemed less important.

Problems
- The endpoints related to eye disease (diabetic retinopathy) were
  indicators of late disease, and a F/U of only 10y may not be sufficient to
  get an accurate idea of patients' risk of developing these complications.

Preventing complications: perindopril and indapamide

> **ADVANCE (Action in Diabetes and VAscular disease: preterax and diamicroN MR Controlled Evaluation) study:** Effects of a fixed combination of perindopril and indapamide on macrovascular and microvascular outcomes in patients with type 2 diabetes mellitus.
>
> **AUTHORS:** ADVANCE collaborative group.
> **REFERENCE:** Lancet (2007) 370, 829–40.
> **STUDY DESIGN:** RCT
> **EVIDENCE LEVEL:** 1b

Key message

In patients with diabetes mellitus (DM), a fixed combination of perindopril-indapamide reduces the risk of death and macrovascular or microvascular events, independent of initial blood pressure (BP) level or concomitant medication.

Impact

The population sampled in this study was large and involved various ethnic groups, thus providing strong evidence for the use of this fixed combination in different settings across the world. The BP-lowering arm of this study ended in June 2007, and the blood glucose-lowering arm (the largest ever to date) in December 2007. Although the results of the latter have not yet been published, interim results have suggested no change in the risk of death from intensive blood glucose lowering. These results do not support those of the ACCORD study, which suggested increased mortality with intensive control. Action to Control Cardiovascular Risk in Diabetes (http://www.accordtrial.org/

Aims

Current recommendations for treating BP in patients with DM are based on arbitrary targets. This target-driven approach is usually resource-intensive, and may miss out patients who are not hypertensive by current definitions but who may still benefit from BP reduction. The BP arm of the ADVANCE trial was designed to verify whether 'blind' addition of a fixed combination of perindopril-indapamide to a diverse group of people with type 2 DM, irrespective of their initial BP or other treatment (including BP medication), was safe and effective in reducing vascular events. The blood glucose-lowering arm aimed to determine whether intensive blood glucose-lowering treatment would alter outcomes such as mortality (not yet published).

Methods

Patients: 11,140 patients at 215 centres across 20 countries in Asia, Australasia, Europe, and North America.

Inclusion criteria:
- Age ≥55y;
- Diagnosed with type 2 DM after the age of 30;
- EITHER history of major cardiovascular (CV) disease OR one risk factor for CV disease.

Groups: 2×2 factorial design comparing:
- Double-blind comparison of perindopril-indapamide (2mg/0.625mg, increased to 4mg/1.25mg to achieve target BP) vs matching placebo: (n=5569 vs 5571);
- Open-label comparison of modified release gliclazide (30–120mg od) in an intensive regime vs standard glucose control guidelines.

Primary endpoint: Composite of major macrovascular (CV death, non-fatal MI, non-fatal stroke) and microvascular events (nephropathy, retinopathy).

Secondary endpoints: All-cause mortality; CV death; total coronary events; major cerebrovascular events; total cerebrovascular events; heart failure; and peripheral vascular disease.

Follow-up: At 3, 4, and 6 months, then every 6 months until study end.

Results
- After mean of 4.3y F/U, 73% of those assigned active treatment and 74% of those assigned control remained in the study.
- Significant reduction in primary endpoint; separate reductions in macrovascular and microvascular complications were not independently significant.

	Perindopril-indapamide (n=5569)	Placebo (n=5571)	RRR (95% CI)	*p*
Primary endpoint	861	938	9% (0 to 17)	0.04
Macrovascular	480	520	8% (−4 to 19)	0.2
Microvascular	439	477	9% (−4 to 20)	0.2

Discussion
This study showed that adding a fixed combination of perindopril-indapamide to a wide variety of people with type 2 DM reduced major vascular events (including death), independent of initial BP levels. In fact, for every 66 patients started on such combination over a 5y period, one would avoid at least one major vascular event, and for every 79 patients, one death would be averted. This may be of importance in the primary care setting as general practitioners may find this a better way of achieving target coronary heart disease reduction without needing specialist input. Many experts argue that it is the BP reduction that is important and not necessarily the particular agent(s) used.

Problem
- The cost-effectiveness of such a strategy has yet to be established, and this must be taken into consideration before large-scale prescription of this fixed drug combination is widely accepted.

Preventing complications: control of blood pressure

> **HOT** (**H**ypertension **O**ptimal **T**reatment) trial: Effects of intensive blood pressure-lowering and low-dose aspirin in patients with hypertension.
>
> **AUTHORS:** Hansson L, Zanchetti A, Carruthers S *et al.*
> **REFERENCE:** Lancet (1998) 351, 1755–62.
> **STUDY DESIGN:** RCT
> **EVIDENCE LEVEL:** 1b

Key message

Patients with diabetes mellitus (DM) and hypertension benefit from active optimal reduction of their BP to normotensive levels.

Impact

The recommended target diastolic BP (DBP) in patients with DM has been reduced to <80mmHg without any major concern about risk. Before this study, it was debated that BP reduction to normotensive levels was associated with excess cardiovascular (CV) risk. The HOT trial was the first RCT to dispel this misconception.

Aims

The CV effect of BP reduction in hypertensive individuals is a J-shaped relationship—there is a level below which subsequent BP reduction results in adverse CV events. It was generally assumed from observational studies that <140/90mmHg was the optimal threshold. However, this BP level is still above the normotensive range. This trial was designed to assess the risk/benefit of further BP reduction (towards normotensive levels) on CV events. Although this study was primarily aimed at the general hypertensive population, the greatest benefits had previously been observed amongst those with DM; this subgroup will be the main focus of this analysis.

Methods

Patients: 19,193 patients (1,501 with DM) from 26 countries in Europe, North and South America, and Asia.

Inclusion criteria:
- Age 50–80y;
- Diagnosis of hypertension;
- DBP between 100–115mmHg.

Groups: All three groups received 5mg long-acting calcium channel blocker (felodipine) with subsequent dose adjustments and addition of angiotensin-converting enzyme inhibitors (ACE-Is), beta (β)-blockers or diuretics, as per predefined protocol, to achieve target BP:
- DBP target ≤ 90mmHg (n=6264; 501 with DM);
- DBP target ≤ 85mmHg (n=6264; 501 with DM);
- DBP target ≤ 80mmHg (n=6262; 499 with DM).

Primary endpoint: Major CV events:
- Fatal and non fatal MI;
- Fatal and non-fatal stroke;
- Other CV deaths.

Follow-up: At baseline, then at 3 and 6 months; and subsequently every 6 months.

Results

	Number of events in patients with DM		
	DBP ≤90mmHg	≤85mmHg	≤80mmHg
Major CV events	45	34	22
Major CV events, including silent MI	48	42	30
	RR (95 % CI)		
Major CV events	1.32 (0.84 to 2.06)	1.56 (0.91 to 2.67)	2.06 (1.24 to 3.44)
Major CV events, including silent MI	1.13 (0.75 to 1.71)	1.42 (0.89 to 2.26)	1.60 (1.02 to 2.53)

Discussion

These data clarified the need to reduce BP (especially diastolic) to optimal targets in patients with hypertension. The greatest benefits were observed in patients with DM. This study demonstrated that targets as low as <80mmHg could be achieved with no significant risk. This has been confirmed by subsequent controlled studies and has resulted in lowered BP targets for people with DM. The current National Institute of Health and Clinical Excellence (NICE) guidelines recommend a target of <140/80mmHg in the general population and even lower values in people with DM (depending on the presence or absence of proteinuria).

Problems

- Renal endpoints were not examined in this study despite the fact that DM remains the commonest cause of end-stage renal disease in the Western world, and microalbuminuria (frequent in DM) is an independent risk factor for coronary heart disease.
- More recent trials have shown that apart from BP lowering, ACE-Is and angiotensin receptor blockers are more effective in reducing renal outcomes in patients with DM, independent of their BP-lowering effect. These agents are now used as first-line BP agents in patients with DM and proteinuria, with calcium-channel blockers as second line.

Preventing complications: multifactorial intervention

Steno 2: Intensified multifactorial intervention in patients with type 2 diabetes mellitus and microalbuminuria.

AUTHORS: Gaede P, Vedel P, Parving H *et al.*
REFERENCE: Lancet (1999) 353, 617–22.
STUDY DESIGN: RCT
EVIDENCE LEVEL: 1b

Key message

Addressing all diabetes-related co-morbidities using a multifactorial approach, and treating patients to targets is effective in reducing cardiovascular (CV) and microvascular complications.

Impact

Intensified multifactorial treatment has now become a cornerstone in the management of type 2 diabetes mellitus (DM) and associated co-morbidities. So-called treating-to-target is being recommended by UK national (National Institute of Health and Clinical Excellence, NICE) as well as various international guidelines.

Aims

Previous studies had shown the benefit of intensified control of modifiable risk factors (blood sugar, blood pressure, lipids, and smoking cessation) in reducing CV diseases, but none had addressed the effectiveness of such an intensified approach to target multiple risk factors at the same time. The Steno 2 study was conducted to assess the effectiveness of this multifactorial strategy in reducing complications in patients with type 2 DM.

Methods

Patients: 160 patients at 1 centre in Denmark.

Inclusion criteria: Type 2 DM:
- Age 40–65y;
- Persistent microalbuminuria (albumin excretion rate (AER) 30–300mg/24h).

Exclusion criteria:
- Serum C-peptide concentration <600pmol/L (6min post-injection of 1mg glucagon);
- Pancreatic insufficiency or DM secondary to pancreatitis;
- Alcohol abuse;
- Non-diabetic kidney disease;
- Malignancy;
- Life-threatening disease with death probable within 4y.

Groups:
- Intervention group: Specific dietary advice, smoking cessation, antihypertension treatment, vitamin supplements, 150mg aspirin, stepwise treatment of DM, treatment of raised cholesterol (n=80).
- Conventional group: routine care (n=80).

Primary endpoint (CV arm): Composite of death from CV causes, non-fatal myocardial infarction (MI), non-fatal stroke, revascularisation, and amputation from lower limb ischaemia.

Secondary endpoint (microvascular arm): Nephropathy (median albumin excretion rate >300mg/24h in ≥1 of the two-yearly examinations); neuropathy and retinopathy.

Follow-up: Every 3 months, for 8y.

Results

Primary endpoint:
- The unadjusted HR of the composite primary endpoint in the intensive group relative to the conventional group was 0.47 (95% CI: 0.24 to 0.73; p=0.008).
- After adjusting for diabetes control, age, sex, smoking, and baseline CV status, HR=0.47; 95% CI: 0.22 to 0.74; p=0.01).

Secondary endpoint	RR (intensive vs conventional)	95% CI	p
Nephropathy	0.39	0.17 to 0.87	0.003
Retinopathy	0.42	0.21 to 0.86	0.02
Autonomic neuropathy	0.37	0.18 to 0.79	0.002

Discussion

This study demonstrated that targeted, long-term, intensified intervention in people with type 2 DM and microalbuminuria reduced the rate of vascular events. The data suggest that the NNT over the 7.8y F/U period to prevent one CV event was 5. This study demonstrated the impact of targeted multifactorial therapy in the management of type 2 DM. Of particular note, almost every individual component assessed in the intervention group (BP, cholesterol, blood glucose, etc) has been shown in subsequent trials to be effective in reducing CV endpoints. Today, integrated multiple risk factor assessment and therapy has become the pinnacle of DM management.

Preventing complications: statins

> **CARDS (Collaborative AtoRvastatin Diabetes Study):** Primary prevention of cardiovascular disease with atorvastatin in type 2 diabetes.
>
> AUTHORS: Colhoun H, Betteridge J, Durrington P et al.
> REFERENCE: Lancet (2004) 364, 685–96.
> STUDY DESIGN: RCT
> EVIDENCE LEVEL: 1b

Key message

Atorvastatin 10mg daily is safe and effective in preventing the onset of first CV events in people with type 2 diabetes mellitus (DM) without high LDL cholesterol.

Impact

Statin therapy is now indicated for primary prevention in people with type 2 DM and one additional risk factor for CV disease, including those patients with 'normal' cholesterol levels.

Aims

Available evidence on statin use in primary prevention of CV disease in type 2 DM had been extrapolated from studies (e.g. Heart Protection Study) where DM was not the main focus, and this was reflected by the reluctance of those caring for people with DM to prescribe these agents. This trial sought to clarify whether atorvastatin 10mg was better than placebo in the primary prevention of CV diseases in patients with type 2 DM.

Methods

Patients: 2838 patients at 132 centres in the UK.

Inclusion criteria: Type 2 DM:
- Age 40–75y;
- No previous history of CV disease;
- LDL cholesterol ≤4.14mmol/L;
- Triglycerides ≤6.79mmol/L;
- One of: retinopathy/hypertension/albuminuria/current smoking.

Groups:
- Atorvastatin 10mg od (n=1428);
- Matching placebo od (n=1410).

Primary endpoint:
Time to first occurrence of any of:
- Acute coronary heart disease (CHD) events (myocardial infarction, unstable angina, CHD death, resuscitated cardiac arrest);
- Coronary revascularisation;
- Stroke.

Secondary endpoints:
- Total mortality;
- Hospital-verified CV endpoint.

Follow-up: Monthly for the first 3 months; then at 6 months; then every 6 months, for endpoints, BP measurement and weight.

Results

	Number of patients with an event			
	Placebo	Atorvastatin	HR	*p*
Primary endpoint	**127**	**83**	**0.63**	**0.001**
Acute coronary event	77	51	0.64	
Coronary revascularisation	34	24	0.69	
Stroke	39	21	0.52	
Secondary endpoint				
Death from any cause	82	61	0.73	0.06
Primary endpoint	189	134	0.68	0.001

Discussion

Diabetes management was initially focused on blood sugar control until the recognition that most deaths in these patients were due to CV disease. Since then, hypertension management has also been considered integral to diabetes care. Patients with DM present with dyslipidaemia where HDL cholesterol is low, triglycerides are raised. and the classical culprit, LDL cholesterol, may be normal—a different lipid profile from patients in whom statins were previously found to be beneficial. This study demonstrated, that in patients with at least one other risk factor for CV disease, statin therapy reduced death and CV endpoints. The NNT over 4y was 27 patients to prevent one major vascular event. The benefits of statin therapy were so significant that the study was terminated 2y prior to its expected end date. In a recent paper (*Diabetes Care* (2006) 29, 2378–84), Neil *et al.* demonstrated the safety and efficacy of a similar approach in elderly people aged 65–75y.

Nephropathy: ACE inhibitors

The effect of angiotensin-converting enzyme inhibition on diabetic nephropathy.

AUTHORS: Lewis E, Hunsicker L, Bain R et al.
REFERENCE: N Engl J Med (1993) 329, 1456–62.
STUDY DESIGN: RCT
EVIDENCE LEVEL: 1b

Key message

ACE inhibitors (ACE-Is) provide additional benefit beyond blood pressure (BP) control in slowing diabetic nephropathy.

Impact

ACE-Is are the first choice antihypertensive in patients with diabetes mellitus (DM), especially those with proteinuria.

Aims

The progression of diabetic nephropathy is due to haemodynamic rather than metabolic factors. Prior to this trial, it was known that strict BP control could slow the progression, but it remained unclear whether ACE-Is could have additional benefits, independent of their antihypertensive effect. This study aimed to resolve the issue.

Methods

Patients: 409 patients at 30 nephrology centres in the USA.

Inclusion criteria: Diabetic nephropathy:
- Age 18–49y;
- Type 1 DM for ≥7y with onset before age 30y;
- Diabetic retinopathy;
- Urinary protein excretion >0.5 g/d;
- Serum creatinine <221 µmol/L.

Groups: Both groups had target BP <140/90 mmHg:
- Captopril (n=207);
- Placebo (n=202).

Primary endpoint: Time to doubling of baseline serum creatinine.

Secondary endpoints:
- Time to death, dialysis, or transplantation;
- Hyperkalaemia.

Follow-up:
- At 2wk, 1 month, and then every 3 months until the patient died, started dialysis, or had renal transplant.
- Median F/U=3y.

Results

Primary endpoint	Captopril	Placebo	*p*
Doubling of baseline creatinine	25	43	0.007
Secondary endpoints			
Death	8	14	Not reported
Death, dialysis, or transplantation	23	42	0.006
Hyperkalaemia	3	0	Not reported

Discussion

This study confirmed the central role of ACE-Is in the treatment of diabetic nephropathy. It was the first study to clearly demonstrate that they had additional benefits beyond simple lowering of BP.

Problems

- In current practice, the BP control would no longer be considered optimal, so the additional benefits of ACE-Is if BP was already <130/80mmHg might not be as apparent.
- The rate of progression of renal disease in the control group was higher than expected from the contemporary literature. However, as this was an RCT, effects causing this accelerated decline should have impacted equally on both groups.
- The patients were quite highly selected, but are still probably representative of the general type 1 DM population.

Nephropathy: angiotensin II receptor antagonists

> **RENAAL (Reduction of Endpoints in NIDDM with the Angiotensin II Antagonist Losartan) study:** Effects of losartan on renal and cardiovascular outcomes in patients with type 2 diabetes and nephropathy.
>
> **AUTHORS:** Brenner B, Cooper ME, Zeeuw D et al.
> **REFERENCE:** N Engl J Med (2001) 345, 861–9.
> **STUDY DESIGN:** RCT
> **EVIDENCE LEVEL:** 1b

Key message

The angiotensin receptor blocker (ARB), losartan, reduces renal endpoints, independent of its blood pressure (BP)-lowering effect in patients with type 2 diabetes mellitus (DM) and advanced nephropathy.

Impact

ARBs have become the first-line agents in lowering BP in patients with type 2 DM and nephropathy. This has also made ARBs (together with angiotensin-converting enzyme inhibitors, ACE-Is), first-line agents in patients with DM and microalbuminuria or proteinuria, even in the absence of hypertension.

Aims

DM is the commonest cause of end-stage renal disease (ESRD). Interruption of the renin angiotensin system is known to slow the progression of renal disease in type 1 DM. However, type 2 DM is the most common form of diabetes. This trial was designed to assess the role of the ARB, losartan, in patients with type 2 DM and nephropathy. It specifically sought to determine whether there was any benefit independent of its BP-lowering effect.

Methods

Patients: 1513 patients at 250 centres in 28 countries.

Inclusion criteria:
- Age 31–70y;
- Type 2 DM;
- Nephropathy: ratio of urinary albumin to urinary creatinine ≥300 (or urinary protein excretion ≥0.5g/d) and serum creatinine values between 1.3–3.0mg/dL (115–265µmol/L).

Primary endpoint: Time to ESRD, death, or doubling of baseline serum creatinine.

Secondary endpoints:
- Composite of morbidity/mortality from cardiovascular (CV) causes;
- Changes in the level of proteinuria;
- Rate of progression of renal disease (inverse of serum creatinine).

Follow-up: At 1 month (titration of dose of losartan to 100mg), at 3 months (to titrate other antihypertensive medications to achieve BP ≤140/90), and subsequently every 3 months (to assess endpoints) up to a mean F/U of 3.4y.

Results

	Losartan (n=751)	Placebo (n=762)	*p*	RRR (95 % CI)
Composite primary endpoint	327	359	0.02	16 (2 to 28)
Doubling of serum creatinine	162	198	0.006	25 (8 to 39)
ESRD	147	194	0.002	28 (11 to 42)
Death	158	155	0.9	−2 (−27 to 19)

Discussion

Previous trials had shown that ARBs (irbesartan) reduced the progression from microalbuminuria to overt diabetic nephropathy in patients with DM and hypertension *(IRMA. N Engl J Med (2001) 345, 870–8)*. However, none had examined their effects on overt nephropathy. This study extended the scope of ARBs by demonstrating their usefulness in reducing renal endpoints in hypertensive patients with DM and nephropathy. It also confirmed previous suggestions that ARBs could reduce CV endpoints (data not shown) in these patients, although the study was not sufficiently powered to specifically examine this endpoint.

Problems

- This trial was terminated prematurely as concurrent evidence from the HOPE trial *(N Engl J Med. 2000; 342(3):145-53)* suggested that ACE-Is (closely related in mechanism of action) were effective at reducing CV endpoints in patients with renal impairment, including those with DM. ACE-I therapy was one of the exclusion criteria in the RENAAL study. Hence, the steering committee voted to discontinue the study. However, it is being argued that had the study continued to its intended 4.5y mean F/U period, this would only have increased the power and heightened the strength of an association that had already been proven to exist.
- Although analyses were done on an intention-to-treat basis, there still remained a worryingly high proportion of patients who discontinued the study from both the placebo (53.5%) and losartan (46.5%) groups.

Gestational diabetes: screening and treatment

ACHOIS (**A**ustralian **C**arbo**H**ydrate **I**ntolerance **S**tudy in pregnancy) trial: Effect of treatment of gestational diabetes mellitus on pregnancy outcomes.

AUTHORS: Crowther C, Hiller J, Moss J et al.
REFERENCE: N Engl J Med (2005) 352, 2477–86.
STUDY DESIGN: RCT
EVIDENCE LEVEL: 1b

Key message

Routine screening for and intensive treatment of gestational diabetes in women reduces the rates of serious perinatal complications.

Impact

Although uncertainty remains as to the cut-off levels for glucose intolerance in pregnancy (or gestational diabetes), it is now standard, internationally recommended practice to screen at-risk women, and intensively manage gestational diabetes with diet, glucose monitoring, and insulin, as needed: this is reflected in the current American Diabetes Association, American College of Obstetrics and Gynaecology, and National Institute of Health and Clinical Excellence (NICE) guidelines.

Aims

The risks associated with gestational diabetes are well known, but the benefits of screening and treatment of this condition were uncertain. The ACHOIS trial was designed to determine whether treatment of women with gestational diabetes reduced the risk of perinatal complications.

Methods

Patients: 1000 patients at 14 Australian and four UK centres.

Inclusion criteria: Women with singleton or twin pregnancy:
• Between 16–30wk gestation;
• ≥1 risk factors for gestational diabetes on selective screening *or* a positive 50g oral glucose challenge test (OGGT, glucose levels 1h after challenge ≥7.8mmol/L.);
• 75g OGGT at 24–34wk gestation with fasting venous plasma glucose (FPG) <7.8mmol/L and 2h value of 7.8–11.0mmol/L post-load.

Exclusion criteria: More severe glucose impairment.

Groups:
• Intervention group: Individualised dietary advice, monitoring of blood glucose, insulin therapy with dose readjustments (n=490).
• Routine-care group: Care left to the discretion of the attending clinician (n=510).

Primary endpoints:
- *Infants:* Composite measure of serious perinatal complications: death, shoulder dystocia, bone fracture, and nerve palsy; admission to neonatal nursery; jaundice requiring phototherapy.
- *Mothers:* Need for induction of labour and caesarean section.

Secondary endpoints:
- *Infants*: Gestational age at birth.
- *Mothers*: Number of prenatal visits, mode of birth, weight gain, number of antenatal admissions, presence or absence of pregnancy-induced hypertension.

Follow-up: Until birth.

Results

Primary endpoints	Intervention	Routine care	p
Any serious perinatal complications	7 (1%)	23 (4%)	0.01
Admission to neonatal nursery	357 (71%)	321 (61%)	0.01
Induction of labour	189 (39%)	150 (29%)	<0.001

Discussion

This RCT showed that treatment of women with gestational diabetes—including dietary advice, blood glucose monitoring, and insulin therapy—reduced the rate of serious perinatal outcomes. In addition, the infants born to mothers in the intervention group were less likely to be large for gestational age or macrosomic, and were not more likely to be small for gestational age. Earlier studies had shown that infants with macrosomia or large for gestational age were more likely to develop diabetes mellitus (DM) or glucose intolerance, and that female infants would go on to develop gestational diabetes. Therefore, it is tempting to speculate that intensive treatment of gestational diabetes could reduce the risk of infants developing DM in later life. The health gains demonstrated in this study were obtained without significant harm (such as hypoglycaemia).

Problem

- There is controversy as to which diagnostic test is best in screening for gestational diabetes, and whether screening should be routine or selective. However, in a recent paper, van Leeuwen et al (*Diabetes Care* 2007; 30:2779-84) showed that the 50g glucose challenge test performed better than conventional fasting blood glucose as a screening test. This makes it hard to translate the findings of this study into practical recommendations as the cost-effectiveness of intensive management would depend on proper identification of patients and targeted individualised therapy.

Chapter 6

Emergency medicine

Introduction

The specialty of emergency medicine was until recently 'Accident and Emergency Medicine' in the UK. It is often known as 'A&E' or even 'Casualty', a name last used officially in 1972 but perpetuated by a television series.

Most casualty departments were staffed by junior doctors with no supervision or training. A consultant orthopaedic surgeon was nominally in charge and visited regularly every Christmas. Sensible doctors followed advice from experienced casualty nurses who had seen it all before. Patients waited many hours to be seen. Research was unknown and evidence-based emergency medicine had not been invented.

In the 1970s, several A&E consultants were appointed and training schemes started to train more. Much has changed since then. There are now more staff but ever increasing numbers of patients, with all sorts of emergencies or other problems. A few patients have major trauma. Many have minor injuries, often treated by nurses rather than doctors. Emergency medicine has become more complicated, with political pressures and targets for waiting times, changes in other hospital specialties and general practice, and lack of beds to admit patients. Many emergency departments have short stay wards or Clinical Decisions Units with protocols for rapid diagnosis and treatment.

Most of current practice in emergency medicine is based on experience rather than research. But there is some good evidence from the UK, USA, Canada, and elsewhere, which has changed (or should change) what we do.

Much more research is needed in emergency medicine. Here is some of the key clinical evidence available now.

Cervical spine trauma imaging

The Canadian C-spine rule for radiography in alert and stable trauma patients.

AUTHORS: Stiell I, Wells G, Vandemheen K *et al.*
REFERENCE: JAMA (2001) 286, 1841–8.
STUDY DESIGN: Prospective cohort study
EVIDENCE LEVEL: 2b

Key message

The Canadian C-spine rule is a highly sensitive decision rule for the use of cervical spine radiographs in alert and stable trauma patients.

Impact

This decision rule is used in many Emergency Departments (EDs). It avoids unnecessary radiographs and allows some patients to be released more quickly from cervical spine immobilisation.

Aims

Cervical spine radiographs are taken in many trauma patients, but very few have a C-spine injury. This study aimed to produce a clinical decision rule that would be highly sensitive for detecting C-spine injury and allow selective use of radiography in alert and stable trauma patients.

Methods

Patients: 8924 patients at 10 EDs in Canada.

Inclusion criteria: Adult patients presenting with blunt trauma to head or neck, stable vital signs, and Glasgow Coma Score (GCS) of 15.

Study design:
- Doctors evaluated 20 standardised clinical findings before radiography;
- Some patients were assessed independently by a second doctor;
- Plain radiographs of cervical spine only if requested by treating doctor;
- Radiologists who reported films were blinded to clinical findings;
- Patients who did not have radiographs were followed up by telephone and recalled for review and radiographs if necessary.

Outcome measures:
- Clinically important cervical spine injuries (evaluated by plain radiographs, CT, and telephone F/U);
- All cervical spine injuries were considered important unless the patient was neurologically intact and had an isolated avulsion of an osteophyte, an isolated transverse process fracture not involving a facet joint, an isolated spinous process fracture not involving the lamina, or a simple compression fracture involving <25% of vertebral body height;
- Logistic regression analysis and recursive partitioning techniques were used to find the best combination of clinical variables which detected important injuries with the highest possible sensitivity and specificity.

Results
- 6,145 (68.9%) of the study patients had cervical spine radiographs.
- 151 (1.7%) patients had important cervical spine injuries.
- 28 (0.3%) had clinically unimportant cervical fractures.
- 11 (0.1%) developed neurological deficits.

Canadian cervical spine rule: This was derived from this study and comprises 3 main questions:
- Is there any high risk factor that mandates radiographs (age ≥65y, dangerous mechanism of injury, or limb paresthesiae)?
- Is there a low risk factor to allow assessment of range of motion (simple rear end motor vehicle collision, walking since injury, delayed onset of neck pain, or absence of midline cervical spine tenderness)? Radiographs are indicated if there is no low risk factor.
- Can the patient actively rotate the neck 45° to left and right despite pain? If this is possible, cervical spine radiographs are not needed. Radiographs are indicated if active movement is <45° to either side.
- Use of this rule would have identified all 151 patients with important cervical spine injuries (sensitivity 100%, specificity 42.5%).
- The rule would also have found 27 out of 28 patients with clinically unimportant fractures; the one not identified was aged 63y with a small C3 osteophyte avulsion and was treated in a cervical collar.
- If this rule had been used, radiographs would have been taken in 58.2% of the study cohort, a relative reduction of 15.5% from 68.9%.

Discussion
This study resulted in a simple clinical decision rule that can help ED staff to decide whether cervical spine radiographs are needed. This decision rule also allows patients who do not need radiographs to be released more quickly from cervical spine immobilisation. Another clinical decision rule for the use of cervical spine radiography in trauma is NEXUS, which was assessed in a study of 34,069 patients (*N Engl J Med* (2000) 343, 94–9). The Canadian C-spine rule appears to have better sensitivity and specificity than NEXUS, with less requirement for radiography.

Problems
- Cervical spine radiographs were only taken in 69% of patients studied, since it was thought unethical to X-ray all patients considered at low risk of injury. Telephone F/U was used to confirm recovery or to recall patients for review and radiography.
- Clinical decision rules such as this require validation in other cohorts of patients to confirm reliability and acceptability in widespread use.

Ankle injury imaging

Multicentre trial to introduce the Ottawa ankle rules for use of radiography in acute ankle injuries.

AUTHORS: Stiell I, Wells G, Laupacis A *et al.*
REFERENCE: BMJ (1995) 311, 594–7.
STUDY DESIGN: Controlled clinical trial
EVIDENCE LEVEL: 2a

Key message

Introduction of the Ottawa ankle rules reduces the number of ankle radiographs without increasing the risk of missing fractures.

Impact

The Ottawa ankle rules are widely used to determine which patients with ankle injuries require radiographs.

Aims

Ankle injury is a common presenting complaint to the Emergency Department (ED). During the acute phase, it can be difficult to determine whether radiography is necessary to exclude fracture. This study aimed to assess the feasibility and impact of introducing a set of clinical rules, the Ottawa ankle rules, to doctors in a wide range of hospitals.

Methods

Patients: 12,777 patients at 8 EDs in Canada.

Inclusion criteria: All adult patients presenting with ankle injury.

Groups: 'Before and after' design:
- Control group: patients seen in 1y period before intervention (n=6288);
- Intervention group: patients seen in 1y period after intervention (n=6489).

Intervention:
- A single 1h lecture on Ottawa ankle rules in each study hospital;
- Handouts, pocket cards, and posters (as in figure);
- Doctors asked to complete a data form about each patient;
- Decision on radiography made by the doctor treating each patient.

Follow-up and analysis:
- Telephone F/U at 10d for all intervention group patients without radiographs, and patients with radiographs seen in first 7d of each month: patients who had not improved were recalled;
- 6 months F/U of patients with fractures found after leaving ED;
- All included patients were analysed, whether or not the doctor had completed a data form or complied with the decision rules.

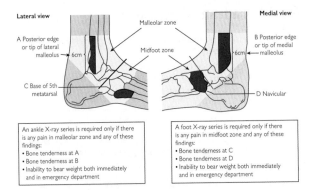

Lateral view

Malleolar zone

Midfoot zone

A Posterior edge or tip of lateral malleolus — 6cm

C Base of 5th metatarsal

Medial view

B Posterior edge or tip of medial malleolus — 6cm

D Navicular

An ankle X-ray series is required only if there is any pain in malleolar zone and any of these findings:
• Bone tenderness at A
• Bone tenderness at B
• Inability to bear weight both immediately and in emergency department

A foot X-ray series is required only if there is any pain in midfoot zone and any of these findings:
• Bone tenderness at C
• Bone tenderness at D
• Inability to bear weight both immediately and in emergency department

Main outcome measures:
• Numbers of patients referred for radiographs of ankle and/or foot;
• Fractures missed at the first visit to the ED.

Results

• Ankle radiographs were taken in 5207/6288 (83%) of control patients, but only in 3955/6489 (61%) of intervention patients (p<0.001).
• The number of foot radiographs was reduced in 3 hospitals, but unchanged in 5 hospitals after introduction of the Ottawa rules.
• Physicians accurately interpreted the rules in 97% and complied with them in 95% of patients. Radiographs were performed but judged unnecessary in 5% of patients.
• Important fractures were found in 1030/6288 (16%) of control patients and 1082/6489 (17%) of intervention group patients.
• In the intervention group, 6 (0.6%) important malleolar or midfoot fractures were diagnosed in the ED when the rules were interpreted as negative, but radiographs were taken because of gross swelling.
• 10 (0.5%) of 2,033 patients followed up by telephone had a fracture diagnosed after discharge from the ED. 3 (0.4%) of 732 had had radiographs in the ED. 7 (0.5%) of 1301 had not had radiographs, but in only 1 had the rules been applied correctly. All 10 fractures diagnosed after leaving the ED healed without long-term effects.

Discussion

This study showed that introduction of the Ottawa ankle rules reduced the number of ankle radiographs, saving time and cost in the ED, without increasing the risk of missing fractures. The rules may be unreliable when clinical assessment is difficult, or in a few patients in whom gross swelling makes it impossible to palpate the posterior edge of the malleoli. Radiographs may be needed in such cases. Whether or not radiographs are taken, patients should be advised to seek F/U if their pain and ability to bear weight do not improve.

Rapid trauma ultrasound

Prospective analysis of a rapid trauma ultrasound examination performed by emergency physicians.

AUTHORS: Ma O, Mateer J, Ogata M *et al.*
REFERENCE: J Trauma (1995) 38, 879–85.
STUDY DESIGN: Cohort study
EVIDENCE LEVEL: 2b

Key message
Ultrasound scanning by emergency physicians allows rapid detection of pericardial, pleural, and peritoneal bleeding in trauma patients.

Impact
Ultrasound is used increasingly often in emergency medicine.

Aims
Previous studies had shown ultrasound (US) scans detect peritoneal bleeding from blunt trauma. This study aimed to assess rapid US scans by emergency physicians for blunt and penetrating trauma of the chest and abdomen.

Methods
Patients: 245 patients at 1 Emergency Department (ED) (level 1 trauma centre) in the USA.

Inclusion criteria: Age ≥18y with major blunt or penetrating trauma to torso.

Exclusion criteria:
- US scans might delay emergency procedure or operation;
- Study physician not available immediately.

Training:
- 9 emergency physicians trained to perform rapid US scan (duration <5min) for free fluid in pericardial sac, pleural cavity, peritoneal cavity, and pararenal retroperitoneum;
- Training was >10h of lectures, videotape reviews, and supervised practice with >15 videotaped scans on normal or non-trauma patients.

Ultrasound examination technique:
- 6 areas were scanned, using a sweeping motion of the probe;
- Subxiphoid four-chamber view of heart for pericardial fluid;
- Right intercostal oblique and coronal views for right pleural effusion and fluid in Morison's pouch, paracolic gutter, and retroperitoneum;
- Left intercostal oblique and left coronal views for left pleural effusion and fluid in perisplenic area, left paracolic gutter, and retroperitoneum;
- Suprapubic views for free fluid in pelvis or pouch of Douglas;
- US scan was done with the patient supine, immediately after initial trauma team assessment and before other diagnostic studies;
- US scan results were not used in patient management decisions;
- Scans were videotaped and reviewed later by a surgical sonologist who was blinded to clinical details and emergency physician interpretations.

Results
- 245 patients: 165 blunt trauma, 37 gunshot wounds, 43 stab wounds.
- 60 patients had free peritoneal or pleural fluid (shown by CT scan, peritoneal lavage, laparotomy, thoracostomy, or echocardiography).
- 9 patients had free fluid in two different body cavities.
- Mean duration of US scans=4.0min (range 2–12min).
- US scan results were analysed as true/false and positive/negative, using CT scans, other test results, and operative findings as the 'gold standard'.

Location of free fluid	Total US scan examinations	True positive	True negative	False positive	False negative
Pericardial	245	6	238	1	0
Pleural	240	25	214	0	1
Intraperitoneal	245	32	207	1	5
Retroperitoneal	245	1	243	0	1
Total	975	64	902	2	7

- In 165 blunt trauma patients, US scan assessment for free fluid was 90% sensitive, 99% specific, and 99% accurate.
- In 80 penetrating trauma patients, US scan assessment for free fluid was 91% sensitive, 100% specific, and 99% accurate.
- A correct US scan result would have altered the patient's management in only 2 of 7 false negatives and none of 2 false positive scans.
- The sonologist reviewing the videotaped US scan examinations agreed with the emergency physician's interpretation in 95% of cases.

Discussion
This study showed that rapid trauma US scan was sensitive, specific, and accurate in detecting free peritoneal, pleural, and pericardial fluid. It showed that appropriately trained emergency physicians can perform and interpret trauma US scans rapidly and accurately. US scans detected traumatic haemothorax within seconds in supine and immobilised patients, allowing prompt treatment. US scans allowed rapid detection of pericardial fluid, which is particularly helpful in a hypotensive trauma patient. US scans also detected intraperitoneal fluid, showing the need for laparotomy or further imaging to assess organ damage.

Problems
- It is unclear how much training is necessary before trauma US scans can be performed and interpreted accurately. Some authors have suggested that experience of over 200 scans is needed.

Nasal diamorphine for analgesia in children

Multicentre randomised controlled trial of nasal diamorphine for analgesia in children and teenagers with clinical fractures

AUTHORS: Kendall J, Reeves B, Latter V.
REFERENCE: BMJ (2001) 322, 261–5.
STUDY DESIGN: RCT
EVIDENCE LEVEL: Ib

Key message

Nasal diamorphine provides effective and acceptable analgesia for children in acute pain from fractures.

Impact

Nasal diamorphine is now used in many Emergency Departments (EDs) as the preferred choice of analgesia for children with severe pain who do not need immediate intravenous access.

Aims

To compare the effectiveness and acceptability of nasal diamorphine spray and intramuscular morphine for analgesia in children with pain from a suspected fracture, and to assess the safety of nasal diamorphine.

Methods

Patients: 404 children (EDs in 8 UK hospitals).

Inclusion criteria:
- Children aged 3–16 years;
- Clinical fracture of upper or lower limb.

Main exclusion criteria:
- Staff not available for prompt recruitment to trial;
- Child not accompanied by parent or guardian;
- Need for immediate intravenous access;
- Head injury;
- Upper respiratory tract infection or blocked nose.

Groups:
- Nasal diamorphine 0.1mg/kg: 204 patients. A nasal spray device gave 0.1mL of solution prepared by dissolving freeze dried diamorphine in a volume of diluent appropriate for the child's weight.
- Intramuscular (IM) morphine 0.2mg/kg: 200 patients.

Rescue analgesia with intramuscular morphine 0.2mg/kg was given if the child was still in extreme pain 20–30min after treatment.

Outcome measures:
- Pain assessment by patients, parents, and staff using Wong Baker face pain scale (1–6) before treatment and after 5,10, 20, and 30min.

- Nurses noted the child's reaction to drug administration.
- Nurses' and parents' assessment of acceptability of treatment.
- Adverse events observed within 30min of treatment.

Results

Effectiveness

- Nasal diamorphine relieved pain faster than IM morphine, with lower pain scores at 5, 10, and 20min but no difference at 30min (χ^2 test for trend of distribution of patients' Wong Baker pain scores: p value 0.04 at 5min, 0.003 at 10min, 0.002 at 20min, 0.20 at 30min).
- No difference between nasal diamorphine and IM morphine in the adequacy of analgesia, assessed by the use of rescue analgesia.

Acceptability

- Nasal diamorphine was much more acceptable than IM morphine, as assessed by patients, parents and staff (χ^2 tests for trends $p<0.0001$).

Safety

- No unexpected adverse effects were seen. 24% of nasal diamorphine group and 19% of IM morphine group had adverse events, which were almost all mild, mostly irritation at the site where the drug was given.
- One child given nasal diamorphine had abdominal pain and vomiting; one given IM morphine had nausea and vomiting.
- 8% of nasal diamorphine group and 11% of IM morphine group had $SaO_2 < 95\%$ at any time in the 30min observation period.

Discussion

Patients in acute pain need prompt and effective analgesia. Injections may be painful and distressing, especially in children, but oral analgesia may be inadequate. Rectal administration has limited acceptability and slow and variable onset of analgesia.

Some drugs are absorbed rapidly by the nasal route. This trial showed that nasal diamorphine gives effective and acceptable analgesia in children with limb fractures, avoiding painful injections in patients who do not need immediate intravenous access.

Problems

- The trial was not blinded, because it was thought unethical to give dummy IM injections in the nasal diamorphine group.
- IM injections are painful, with variable drug absorption, so opioids are rarely given intramuscularly in emergency departments. A trial comparing nasal diamorphine with intravenous or oral morphine would have been more useful. However, IM analgesia was still standard practice in some hospitals when this study was approved in 1996–97.
- Few EDs have the nasal spray devices used in this trial, so nasal diamorphine is usually given dissolved in 0.2mL of saline and dripped into the nose from a syringe.
- Since this trial, medicinal diamorphine has been in short supply in the UK, and it is not available in all countries. Further studies have been done of the nasal administration of other opioids, such as alfentanyl.

Corticosteroids after head injury

CRASH (Corticosteroid **R**andomisation **A**fter **S**ignificant **H**ead injury) trial: Effect of intravenous corticosteroids on death within 14 days in 10,008 adults with clinically significant head injury.

AUTHORS: CRASH trial collaborators.
REFERENCE: Lancet (2004) 364, 1321–8, Lancet (2005) 365, 1957–9.
STUDY DESIGN: RCT
EVIDENCE LEVEL: 1b

Key message

Routine corticosteroid use following head injury increases risk of death.

Impact

Before this trial, corticosteroids were often used to treat head injuries and a systematic review had suggested that these drugs reduced mortality by 1–2%. As a result of CRASH, corticosteroids are no longer used in the treatment of head injuries.

Aims

Corticosteroids were a common treatment after head injury; this practice was supported by a systematic review in 1997, which suggested that they reduced the risk of death from head injury by 1–2%. This international, multicentre RCT aimed to confirm or refute these findings.

Methods

Patients: 10,008 patients at 239 hospitals in 49 countries.

Inclusion criteria:

- Adults of age ≥16y, presenting within 8h of head injury;
- Glasgow coma score (GCS) in hospital ≤14.

Groups:

- Corticosteroids: Methylprednisolone (2g over 1h in 100mL 0.9% saline; then 0.4g/h for 48h in 20mL/h infusion) (n=5007);
- Placebo (n=5001).

Primary outcome measures:

- Death from any cause within 2wk of injury;
- Death or disability at 6 months from injury;
- Prespecified subgroup analyses for time since injury and severity of head injury (based on GCS at randomisation).

Data recorded included:

- Results of first CT head scan;
- Number of days in intensive care, seizures, haematemesis or melaena requiring transfusion, wound infection with pus, pneumonia treated with antibiotics, antibiotics for other reasons, whether patient had a neurosurgical operation, presence of major extracranial injury.

Results

Primary endpoint	Steroid	Placebo	p
Death within 2wk	21% (n=1052)	18% (n=803)	0.0001
Death within 6 months	25.7%	22.3%	0.0001
Death/severe disability at 6 months	38.1%	36.3%	0.08

- Subgroup analysis: Relative increase in deaths in the corticosteroid group did not differ by time since injury ($p=0.05$), injury severity ($p=0.22$) nor between 8 CT scan diagnosis subgroups (in 7,812 patients (78%) who had a CT scan) nor with the presence or absence of major extracranial injury.

Discussion

This was a major international, double-blinded trial, with strong methodology. The trial groups were well balanced for all variables and 99.6% of both groups had complete data at 2wk. Analysis was on an intention-to-treat basis. There were significantly more deaths in the corticosteroid group compared with placebo, so enrollment was stopped after 10,008 patients had been recruited. The final report of this trial (*Lancet* (2005) 365, 1957–9) showed similar results, with significantly more deaths at 6 months in the corticosteroid group (1,248 deaths, 26%) than the placebo group (1075, 22%), relative risk 1.15 (95% CI 1.07 to 1.24), $p=0.0001$. There was no significant increase in the risk of infection or gastrointestinal bleeding with corticosteroids. This trial refuted previous evidence supporting the routine use of corticosteroids in the management of head injury.

These results could also have implications for treating spinal cord injury, in which corticosteroid use is controversial. The NASCIS-2 study (*N Engl J Med* (1990) 322, 1405–11) showed some evidence of neurological benefit in a subgroup of patients treated within 8h of spinal cord injury. However, trials of corticosteroids in spinal cord patients have been small, and subgroup analyses may cause confusing results, so larger studies of spinal cord injuries are needed.

Problems

- The mechanism of increased mortality in the corticosteroid group was unclear. However, clinicians' opinions of the cause of each death were not recorded, and establishing the main cause of death is often difficult if there are multiple factors related to trauma.
- Concurrent treatments may have varied between countries/units (and were not recorded); however, this should not have affected outcomes since similar numbers were allocated to either group in every hospital.

Tubigrip® bandage for ankle sprain

A randomised controlled trial to determine the effectiveness of double Tubigrip® in grade 1 and 2 (mild to moderate) ankle sprains.

AUTHORS: Watts B, Armstrong B.
REFERENCE: Emergency Med J (2001) 18, 46–50.
STUDY DESIGN: RCT
EVIDENCE LEVEL: 1b

Key message
Tubigrip® increases pain without speeding recovery from ankle sprains.

Impact
This study suggested that Tubigrip® may be harmful rather than helpful. More research is needed to assess treatments for ankle sprains.

Aims

Ankle sprains are common and often treated with Tubigrip®, a tubular elastic bandage. This study aimed to assess whether a double Tubigrip® bandage affected patients' functional recovery from ankle sprains.

Methods

Patients: 400 patients from the Emergency Departments (EDs) of 2 UK hospitals.

Inclusion criteria: Grade 1 (mild) or grade 2 (moderate) lateral ankle sprains.

Main exclusion criteria:
- Patients expressing a treatment preference;
- Age <16y. Time since injury >24h;
- Non-English speaking; no telephone; intoxicated.

Groups:
- Tubigrip®: Double Tubigrip® bandage (DTG) on injured ankle (n=200);
- No Tubigrip®: no bandage (n=200);
- Block randomisation using sealed opaque envelopes;
- Both groups received the same advice sheet describing ankle exercises and advising simple analgesia, if necessary;
- Telephone F/U after 1wk by ED reception staff, asking standardised questions.

Outcome measures:
- Pain (sleep disturbance, need for analgesia);
- Mobility (days until walking unaided);
- Number of days off work.

Results

- Many patients (51%) were lost to F/U because data sheets were incomplete or lost, or telephone F/U was unsuccessful.
- 105 Tubigrip® and 92 'no Tubigrip®' patients completed the trial.
- Treatment groups were well matched for age, sex, and occupation. Patients completing the trial were well matched with those who did not.

Outcome measure	Tubigrip® (n=105)	No Tubigrip® (n=92)	p
Did the injury keep you awake at night?	54 (51.4 %)	44 (47.8 %)	0.7
Did you take pain killers?	81 (77.9 %)	50 (54.3 %)	0.001
Did you take days off work?	54 (51.4 %)	48 (52.2 %)	0.07
How many days off work? (mean±SD)	3.37±2.33	3.21±2.02	0.9
How many d until walking unaided? (mean±SD)	2.65±1.86	2.32±1.99	0.2

- There was no significant difference between the treatment groups in the number of days off work or the time before walking unaided.
- There was no significant difference for whether the injury kept the patient awake at night ($p=0.7$), but significantly more of the Tubigrip® patients took analgesia ($p=0.001$).

Discussion

Ankle sprains are common. Initial treatment is often based on 'RICE' (Rest, Ice, Compression, Elevation), but the evidence for this is poor. There are very few RCTs of treatments for sprains in typical ED patients (rather than athletes or military recruits). Tubigrip® bandage is widely used for ankle sprains in the hope of reducing ankle swelling and providing some support. This study showed no benefit from Tubigrip® in the time taken for the patient to walk unaided or return to work. Tubigrip® appears to increase the need for analgesia, perhaps because the tubular bandage forms a tight band across the front of the ankle, especially if applied or reapplied incorrectly. This study suggests that Tubigrip® may be harmful rather than helpful for ankle sprains.

Problems

- This study shows the difficulties of research on a common injury, which often resolves without needing F/U.
- The authors recruited 400 patients, as required by their power calculation, but the high dropout rate could have affected the findings.
- F/U was only for 1wk. Patient satisfaction was not measured.
- Telephone F/U might have been better with a research assistant.
- Further studies are needed to assess treatments for ankle sprains.

Penetrating trauma: timing of fluid resuscitation

Immediate vs delayed fluid resuscitation for hypotensive patients with penetrating torso injuries.

AUTHORS: Bickell W, Wall M, Pepe P, *et al.*
REFERENCE: N Engl J Med (1994) 331, 1105–9.
STUDY DESIGN: Controlled trial
EVIDENCE LEVEL: 2a

Key message
Intravenous fluid resuscitation should be delayed until the time of surgery in hypotensive patients with penetrating torso injuries.

Impact
This study emphasised the need for prompt surgery to stop bleeding, rather than giving large amounts of fluid to replace lost blood.

Aims
Traditional resuscitation for trauma patients with hypotension had involved giving large amounts of fluid pre-operatively. This study aimed to assess whether delaying fluids to the time of surgery would improve survival.

Methods
Patients: 598 patients from 1 trauma service in the USA.

Inclusion criteria:
- Adults (age ≥16y) with penetrating torso injuries;
- Pre-hospital systolic blood pressure ≤90mmHg.

Exclusion criteria: Included:
- Revised Trauma Score zero at scene of injury;
- Fatal gunshot wound of head (as well as torso injury).

Groups:
- Immediate resuscitation group (on even numbered days of month): intravenous fluid resuscitation (rapid infusion of crystalloid solution) given pre-hospital and in trauma centre before operation, with packed red cells following standard criteria of American College of Surgeons (n=309);
- Delayed resuscitation group (on odd numbered days of month): intravenous fluid resuscitation was delayed until operation (n=289).
- Once in theatre and anaesthetised, both groups received IV crystalloid (Ringer's acetate) and packed red cells to keep systolic BP ≥100mmHg, haematocrit ≥25% and urine ouput ≥50mL/h. Treatment protocols were identical, except for pre-operative fluids. Operative treatment included thoracotomy (at trauma centre and in operating theatre), laparotomy, neck, and groin exploration.

Outcome measures:
- Survival until discharge from hospital;
- Postoperative complications: wound infection, respiratory distress syndrome, sepsis syndrome, renal failure, coagulopathy, pneumonia;
- Analyses were by intention-to-treat.

Results

- The groups were well matched, with 309 patients in the immediate resuscitation group and 289 in the delayed resuscitation group.
- About 70% of patients had gunshot wounds and 30% stab wounds.
- 22 delayed resuscitation patients were inadvertently given rapid intravenous fluids transiently before operation.

Variable (mean±SD)	Immediate resuscitation (n=309)	Delayed resuscitation (n=289)	p
Ringer's acetate given pre-hospital	870 ± 667mL	92±309mL	< 0.001
Ringer's acetate given in trauma centre	1608±1201mL	283±722mL	< 0.001
Survival to discharge from hospital	193/309 patients (62%)	203/289 patients (70%)	0.04
Length of hospital stay	14±24d	11±19d	0.006
Length of intensive care unit stay	8±16 d	7±11d	0.3

- Survival rate was significantly higher in the delayed resuscitation group.
- Immediate resuscitation group had significantly longer hospital stays.
- Intensive care unit stay did not differ significantly between groups.
- There was a trend towards more complications in the immediate resuscitation group (*p*=0.08, ns).

Discussion

This study showed that fluid resuscitation should be delayed until operation in hypotensive patients with penetrating torso injuries. The findings were consistent with animal studies that had showed that fluids given before surgical control of bleeding accentuated ongoing haemorrhage, disrupting effective thrombus and diluting coagulation factors. The results of this study challenged the traditional practice of giving large amounts of intravenous fluids to injured patients with hypotension, which is presumed to result from blood loss.

Problems

- Randomisation was not feasible because it would have caused delays in care, so treatment groups were allocated by the date of injury.
- This study involved only penetrating trauma and so is not directly relevant to other patients with blunt trauma.

Cardiac arrest: defibrillation

Multicentre RCT of 150-J biphasic shocks compared with 200- to 360-J monophasic shocks in the resuscitation of out-of-hospital cardiac arrest victims.

AUTHORS: Schneider T, Martens P, Paschen H *et al.*
REFERENCE: Circulation (2000) 102, 1780–7.
STUDY DESIGN: RCT
EVIDENCE LEVEL: 1b

Key message

Biphasic shocks are much more effective than monophasic shocks in treating ventricular fibrillation and restoring spontaneous circulation. Survivors of cardiac arrest have better neurological recovery after biphasic shocks than after monophasic shocks.

Impact

This paper and other studies have resulted in biphasic automatic external defibrillators (AEDs) replacing monophasic AEDs.

Aims

Rapid response programmes have improved survival after cardiac arrest. Laboratory and hospital studies showed higher defibrillation rates with biphasic AEDs than with traditional monophasic defibrillators. This study aimed to compare monophasic and biphasic AEDs in out-of-hospital arrest.

Methods

Patients: 115 patients from 4 emergency services in Germany, Belgium, and Finland.

Inclusion criteria:
- Patients weighing ≥36kg in out-of-hospital cardiac arrest attended by emergency medical services (EMS) systems and treated with AEDs;
- Initial cardiac rhythm ventricular fibrillation (VF).

Main exclusion criteria:
- Cardiac arrest witnessed by EMS personnel;
- Cardiac arrest from non-cardiac causes, such as trauma or drowning.

Groups: Randomisation by day for use of monophasic or biphasic AEDs.
- Monophasic: up to 3 shocks (200, 200, 360J) from monophasic AED (n=61);
- Biphasic: up to 3 defibrillation shocks (all 150J) from biphasic AED (n=54).

Primary endpoint:
- Percentage of patients initially in VF defibrillated in ≤3 shocks.

Secondary endpoints:
- Defibrillation with first shock or second shock;
- Return of spontaneous circulation (ROSC);
- Survival to hospital admission and discharge;
- Neurological status at discharge from hospital.

Results

- Monophasic and biphasic AED groups were well matched.
- Comparisons were made by treatment group and by intention-to-treat.

Endpoint	Monophasic (n=61)	Biphasic (n=54)	p
Defibrillation on first shock	36 (59 %)	52 (96 %)	<0.0001
Defibrillation in ≤2 shocks	39 (64 %)	52 (96 %)	<0.0001
Defibrillation in ≤3 shocks	42 (69 %)	53 (98 %)	<0.0001
ROSC	33 (54 %)	41 (76 %)	0.01
Survival to hospital admission	31 (51 %)	33 (61 %)	0.3
Survival to hospital discharge	19 (31 %)	15 (28 %)	0.7

- Biphasic shocks were much more effective than monophasic shocks in defibrillating patients in VF.
- Rates of survival to hospital admission and discharge were similar.
- Cerebral status of survivors discharged from hospital was better in biphasic shock patients than monophasic: 13/15 (87%) biphasic and 10/19 (53%) monophasic had 'good' neurological status (p=0.04).

Discussion

Biphasic shocks were much more effective than monophasic shocks in treating VF and restoring spontaneous circulation in patients with out-of-hospital cardiac arrest. Neurological recovery was better after biphasic than monophasic shocks, perhaps because of shorter time to ROSC and better cardiac output after defibrillation with lower energy shocks. Less energy is needed for biphasic shocks, so biphasic AEDs can be smaller, lighter, and cheaper than monophasic AEDs.

Problems

- Randomisation was by date rather than by patient.
- Responders were not blinded to the type of AED used.
- Other biphasic AEDs may use different wave forms and energy levels from those used in this study. It is unclear which parameters of a biphasic wave form influence the effectiveness of defibrillation, and so different models of biphasic AEDs might not be equally effective.

Septic shock: early goal-directed therapy

Early goal-directed therapy in the treatment of severe sepsis and septic shock.

AUTHORS: Rivers E, Nguyen B, Havstad S *et al.*
REFERENCE: N Engl J Med (2001) 345, 1368–77.
STUDY DESIGN: RCT
EVIDENCE LEVEL: 1b

Key message
Early goal-directed therapy reduces the high mortality of severe sepsis and septic shock.

Impact
This work has stimulated many other studies and an international campaign to reduce the number of deaths from sepsis.

Aims
Goal-directed therapy for septic shock involves adjusting cardiac preload, afterload, and contractility to improve oxygen delivery and correct tissue hypoxia. This study aimed to assess the value of early goal-directed therapy.

Methods
Patients: 263 patients at 1 Emergency Department in a tertiary care hospital in the USA.

Inclusion criteria:
- Adults age ≥18y;
- 2 of 4 criteria for systemic inflammatory response syndrome (SIRS): T <36 or ≥38°C; pulse >90/min; resp rate >20/min or P_aCO_2 <32mmHg; WBC >12,000 or <4,000/mm^3 or >10% immature band forms;
- Systolic BP ≤90mmHg after fluid challenge (crystalloid 20–30mL/kg over 30min), or blood lactate ≥4mmol/L.

Groups: Random allocation to early goal-directed therapy (EGDT) or standard therapy. Critical care physicians took over care of all patients after admission from the ED and were unaware of patients' group allocations:
- EGDT (n=130):
  - Crystalloid bolus (500mL every 30min until central venous pressure (CVP) 8–12mmHg);
  - Vasoactive drugs if MAP <65mmHg *or* >90mmHg;
  - Continuous $S_{CV}O_2$ monitoring: if $S_{CV}O_2$ <70% red cell transfusion to haematocrit ≥30%, then IV dobutamine 2.5–20mcg/kg/min;
  - Treatment in ED for ≥6h, then admission to first available bed.
- Standard therapy (n=133):
  - Haemodynamic support to keep CVP 8–12mmHg, MAP ≥65mmHg, and urine output ≥0.5mL/kg/h;
  - Critical care consultation, with inpatient care as soon as possible.

Primary outcome: In-hospital mortality.

Secondary outcome measures: Resuscitation endpoints, organ dysfunction scores, coagulation-related variables, administered treatments, use of health care resources.

Results

Therapy	Standard (n=133)	Early goal-directed (n=130)	p
In-hospital mortality	59 (46.5 %)	38 (30.5 %)	0.009

Percentages calculated by the Kaplan–Meier product-limit method.

- Standard therapy group had a higher mortality rate than EGDT group, with more deaths from sudden cardiovascular collapse ($p=0.02$), but similar numbers of deaths from multi-organ failure ($p=0.27$, ns).
- In the first 6h, the EGDT group received more fluids, red cell transfusions, and inotropic support than the standard therapy group ($p<0.001$), but similar numbers had vasopressors ($p=0.62$, ns) and mechanical ventilation ($p=0.90$, ns).
- At 7–72h the standard therapy group had lower mean arterial pressure ($p<0.001$), lower $S_{CV}O_2$ ($p<0.001$), lower pH ($p<0.001$), and higher lactate ($p=0.02$) than the EGDT group.
- Organ dysfunction scores from 7–72h after start of treatment were worse with standard therapy than with EGDT ($p<0.001$).

Discussion

Severe sepsis and septic shock are common and have a high mortality, with many deaths associated with sudden cardiovascular collapse. This study showed the benefits of EGDT with rapid correction of fluid deficit and tissue hypoxia. Measurement of central venous oxygen saturation was particularly helpful to identify patients with insidious illness, with global tissue hypoxia but stable vital signs, who were liable to deteriorate suddenly. Prompt correction of global tissue hypoxia prevented sudden cardiovascular collapse and the resulting complex problems. EGDT clearly reduced mortality from sepsis.

Problems

- This study showed what can be achieved by prompt and expert intensive care in an ED, but this standard of care would be beyond the capabilities and resources of most centres.

Deep vein thrombosis: type of heparin

Subcutaneous low molecular weight heparin compared with continuous intravenous heparin in the treatment of proximal vein thrombosis.

AUTHORS: Hull R, Raskob G, Pineo F et al.
REFERENCE: N Engl J Med (1992) 326, 975–82.
STUDY DESIGN: RCT
EVIDENCE LEVEL: 1b

Key message

Weight adjusted low molecular weight heparin (LMWH) given subcutaneously (once a day, with no monitoring) is at least as effective as intravenous unfractionated heparin (UFH) adjusted according to the activated partial thromboplastin time (APTT).

Impact

These findings revolutionised the treatment of deep vein thrombosis (DVT), moving its management to outpatient care.

Aims

Prior to this study, the conventional initial treatment for DVT had been initial continuous IV UFH. LMWH has a high bioavailability when administered subcutaneously, with a longer half-life than UFH. Furthermore, unlike UFH, LMWH does not require regular monitoring of APTT. This study aimed to compare fixed dose subcutaneous LMWH (given once daily) with adjusted dose intravenous UFH (given by continuous IV infusion) for the initial treatment of patients with proximal vein thrombosis, using objective documentation of clinical outcomes.

Methods

Patients: 432 patients at 15 centres in the USA and Canada.

Inclusion criteria: Consecutive patients:
• Age ≥18y;
• Proximal DVT of lower limb on venography (popliteal or more proximal veins);
• Previous venous thromboembolism.

Exclusion criteria:
• Current active bleeding or history of protein C deficiency;
• Disorder contraindicating anticoagulant therapy (including allergy to heparin, bisulphites, or fish; or heparin-induced thrombocytopaenia);
• Preganancy;
• ≥2 previously documented episodes of DVT or pulmonary embolism;
• Severe malignant hypertension (systolic BP ≥250mmHg, diastolic ≥350mmHg);
• Severe hepatic failure (encephalopathy) or renal failure (necessitating dialysis).

Groups: Patients stratified according to study centre. All patients received warfarin for 3 months.

- UFH: 5000U bolus followed by continuous IV infusion, started at 1680U/h or 1240U/h depending on bleeding risk) and adjusted according to APTT (target=1.5–2.5x mean normal) (n=219);
- LMWH: 175U/kg od SC (n=213).

Primary endpoint: Recurrent venous thromboembolism, major and minor bleeding.

Follow-up: All patients followed for 3 months.

Results

	LMWH (n=213)	UFH (n=219)	p
Recurrence	6 (2.8%)	15 (6.9%)	0.07
Major bleeding	1 (0.5%)	11 (5.0%)	0.006
Minor bleeding	7 (3.3%)	7 (3.2%)	ns
Deaths	10 (4.7%)	21 (9.6%)	0.05

Discussion

This study showed that subcutaneous LMWH given without any monitoring was at least as effective and as safe as intravenous UFH monitored carefully using the APTT. The LMWH also resulted in significantly fewer major bleeds. The intravenous heparin group also had a higher mortality ($p=0.062$). LMWH was much more convenient to administer, and the authors correctly predicted that, with no need for laboratory monitoring, it would allow patients with uncomplicated proximal DVT to be cared for in an outpatient setting, a finding confirmed by other studies *(Lancet (2006) 339, 441–5; N Engl J Med (1996) 334, 677–81)*.

Problems

- Only 51% of eligible patients were randomised; it is unclear why. This may have introduced an element of selection bias.

Pulmonary embolism: D-dimer testing

D-dimer testing for suspected pulmonary embolism in outpatients.

AUTHORS: Perrier A, Desmarais S, Goehring C et al.
REFERENCE: Am J Respir Crit Care Med (1997) 156, 492–6.
STUDY DESIGN: Cohort Study
EVIDENCE LEVEL: 2a

Key message

A negative D-dimer (<500mcg/L by ELISA) reliably excludes pulmonary embolism (PE) in outpatients suspected of having PE.

Impact

D-dimer measurement is an important tool in the assessment of patients who attend the emergency room with low or intermediate clinical probability of PE. In the appropriate clinical context, a negative D-dimer may assist the clinician in early and safe hospital discharge.

Aims

The plasma level of D-dimer, a degradation product of crosslinked fibrin, is increased in the presence of venous thromboembolism. A cutoff of >500mcg/L has high sensitivity (97%), but low specificity (20–50%). The British Thoracic Society recommends the use of D-dimer testing in patients with low or intermediate clinical probability of PE, with further investigation if the test is positive. This study extended previous observations aiming to determine the safety of withholding anticoagulation from prospective patients suspected of having a PE who had a negative D-dimer over a 3 months F/U, and to evaluate the sensitivity and specificity of D-dimer testing.

Methods

Patients: 671 outpatients at 1 emergency centre in Geneva.

Inclusion criteria:
• Age >16y;
• PE suspected by primary care or emergency ward physician.

Exclusion criteria:
• Suspected PE during hospital stay;
• Symptoms of DVT as principal presenting complaint;
• Occurrence of DVT <3 months before inclusion.

Preparation: All patients underwent clinical evaluation, and clinical probability of PE was rated between 0 and 100%. Within 24h, all patients underwent a ventilation/perfusion (V/Q) scan, D-dimer assay, and lower limb venous compression ultrasonography (US). Pulmonary angiography was done in patients with inconclusive initial results.

Groups:
- No PE: as judged by a negative D-dimer, normal V/Q scan, or normal angiogram; or, in patients with low clinical probability, a non-diagnostic V/Q scan. Median age=67y. Not anticoagulated (n=475).
- PE: high probability V/Q scan, DVT on US, and non-diagnostic V/Q scan, or positive pulmonary angiogram. 15 patients adjudged to have PE were too unwell to undergo angiography. Median age=70y. Anticoagulated (n=196).

Endpoint: Sensitivity and specificity of D-dimer.

Follow-up: 3 months during which all adverse events were recorded: venous thromboembolism, deaths, or severe haemorrhage.

Results

	PE (n=196)	No PE (n=475)
D-dimer ≥500mcg/L	195	278
D-dimer <500mcg/L	1	197
95% CI	Sensitivity=99.5% 97.2 to 100.0	Specificity=41.4% 37.0 to 45.9

Discussion

The prevalence of PE in the population was 29%, and the study demonstrated that a cutoff D-dimer level of 500mcg/L was associated with a sensitivity of 99.5% and a specificity of 41.4% (lower in older patients). Of the 198 patients with a negative D-dimer, 197 were considered free of PE and not anticoagulated. At 3 months F/U, none of these patients had adverse events. The study validated the use of a D-dimer level below 500mcg/L alone to exclude PE. Withholding anticoagulation had a risk of <1% venous thromboembolic events at 3 months.

Problems

- The study highlighted the poor specificity of a positive D-dimer level in predicting PE. 473 patients in total had a D-dimer ≥500mcg/L, while only 195 had a PE. The specificity of D-dimer concentration was greatly influenced by age, with a maximum value of 72% in the 30–39y age group, but a value as low as 9% in patients over the age of 80y.
- The findings rely on an enzyme-linked immunosorbant assay (ELISA) test, which comes as batch kits and is labour-intensive in determining D-dimer concentration. The results cannot be extrapolated to bedside latex red cell agglutination tests for measuring D-dimer concentration, commonly used in clinical practice, but associated with different sensitivity and specificity.
- In this study, a negative D-dimer excluded PE in 2 of 3 patients under the age of 60, but in only 1 in 5 patients older than 60y. A cost analysis would be useful to further justify D-dimer measurement in older patients.
- Pulmonary angiography was not performed in all patients, so the gold standard of PE diagnosis was taken as positive V/Q scan or non-diagnostic scan + DVT; however, all patients were followed up for 3 months.

Paracetamol poisoning: intravenous acetylcysteine

Intravenous N-acetylcysteine: the treatment of choice for paracetamol poisoning.

AUTHORS: Prescott LF, Illingworth RN, Critchley JA, *et al.*
REFERENCE: BMJ (1979) 2, 1097–100.
STUDY DESIGN: Cohort study
EVIDENCE LEVEL: 3

Key message

Intravenous acetylcysteine provides virtually complete protection if started within 8h of paracetamol overdose. Later treatment is less effective. Acetylcysteine has minimal side effects and is more effective than cysteamine or methionine.

Impact

Since this study, intravenous acetylcysteine has been the standard treatment for paracetamol poisoning.

Aims

Paracetamol overdose can cause fatal liver failure and renal damage. This study aimed to assess the efficacy of intravenous (IV) acetylcysteine in preventing liver damage, renal impairment, and death from paracetamol poisoning, compared to historical control groups given only supportive treatment (before specific treatment was available), IV cysteamine, or IV methionine.

Methods

Patients: 100 overdoses in 87 patients treated with IV acetylcysteine at 1 centre in the UK. Historical control groups=57 patients with supportive treatment only; 40 patients given IV cysteamine; 20 given IV methionine.

Inclusion criteria:
- Paracetamol overdose within 24h;
- Plasma paracetamol above treatment line (straight line on semilog graph from 200mg/L at 4h to 30mg/L at 15h, extrapolated to 24h).

Treatment with IV acetylcysteine (in 5% dextrose):
- Acetylcysteine 150mg/kg in 200mL dextrose over 15min, 50mg/kg in 500mL dextrose over 4h, then 100mg/kg in 1L dextrose over 16h;
- About half the patients were given IV acetylcysteine as Airbron® (a 20% sterile aqueous solution manufactured for intrabronchial use) and half had a similar solution specially prepared for IV use.

Outcome measures:
- Severe liver damage (defined as serum AST or ALT >1000iu/L);
- Renal impairment (plasma creatinine increased from normal to >300micromol/L);

- Death;
- 'High risk' patients (plasma paracetamol above line 300mg/L at 4h to 45mg/L at 15h) were analysed with other patients and also separately.

Results
- Patients given acetylcysteine were comparable to the historical control groups, except that more of the acetylcysteine group had taken alcohol or other drugs (especially Distalgesic®) in addition to paracetamol.
- Severe liver damage occurred in one of 62 patients given acetylcysteine at <10h, compared to 33 of 57 patients with supportive treatment.
- Acetylcysteine given at <8h gave almost complete protection against liver damage and was more effective than cysteamine or methionine.
- Acetylcysteine was less effective at >8h and ineffective at >15h.

Treatment	Patients (n)	No (%) high risk	Severe liver damage (%)	Renal damage (%)	Deaths from liver failure (%)
Acetylcysteine <10h	62	33 (53)	1 (2)	0	0
Acetylcysteine 10–24h	38	27 (71)	20 (53)	5 (13)	2 (5)
Cysteamine or methionine <10h	42	24 (57)	3 (7)	0	0
Cysteamine or methionine 10–24 h	18	14 (78)	8 (44)	1 (6)	1 (6)
Supportive	57	28 (49)	33 (58)	6 (11)	3 (5)

Discussion
It would have been unethical to withhold active treatment in a clinical trial, so this study used a historical control group of 57 patients treated before any specific therapy for paracetamol poisoning was available. IV acetylcysteine was more effective than IV cysteamine, IV or oral methionine, and oral acetylcysteine in preventing liver damage. Vomiting is common in severe paracetamol poisoning, so IV treatment is more reliable than oral treatment.

Problems
- The treatment line was based on a limited number of historical cases and liver damage may occur with levels below this line, so the authors suggested lowering the line to 150mg/L at 4h and 25mg/L at 15h.
- Current protocols still use the original treatment line, with a lower line (100mg/L at 4h) for patients at high risk of paracetamol liver damage because of enzyme-inducing drugs, alcoholism, or malnourishment.
- Occasional dose-related anaphylactoid reactions to acetylcysteine (rashes, asthma, hypotension) have been noted since this study.

Endocrinology

Introduction

One of the first properly described endocrine diseases arose in 1855 when Thomas Addison, a British scientist, reported a patient with Addison's disease. However, the modern concept of endocrinology, whereby a chemical messenger is secreted into the circulation to cause systemic effects, was born on June 1st 1889. On this date, Professor Charles-Edouard Brown-Sequard reported to a meeting in Paris that self-administration of guinea pig and dog testes aqueous extracts improved physical strength, mental capacity, and sexual potency. In 1891, George Murray first treated a myxoedematous female patient with thyroid extract, and in 1894, Oliver and Schafer reported on epinephrine in the adrenal medulla. At the start of the 20th century, endocrinology was still in its infancy. The medical term 'hormone', (derived from the Greek 'hormoa' (to excite)), was only introduced by Ernest Starling in 1905 to describe chemical secretion from an endocrine gland. Since then, there has been tremendous progress in the field of endocrinology as a result of advances in biochemistry, physiology, genetics, and molecular biology.

In 1909, Harvey Cushing successfully carried out the first modern-day endocrine surgery entailing removal of a portion of the anterior pituitary gland in an acromegalic patient. Otto Loewi first identified neurohormones with the discovery of acetylcholine, for which he was subsequently awarded the Nobel Prize with Henry Dale in 1936. In 1971, Earl Sutherland was awarded the Nobel Prize for developing the concept of second messenger pathways following work involving norepinephrine and cyclic AMP. Recently, advances in molecular biology, particularly sequencing of the human genome, have led to unravelling of hormone receptor–post-receptor mechanisms. These discoveries have uncovered novel therapeutic targets for endocrine disease.

Hyperthyroidism: radioiodine

Long-term follow-up study of radioiodine treatment for hyperthyroidism.

AUTHORS: Metso S, Jaatinen P, Huhtala H *et al.*
REFERENCE: Clin Endocrinol (2004) 61, 641–8.
STUDY DESIGN: Cohort
EVIDENCE LEVEL: 2a

Key message
The majority of patients with Graves' disease are rendered hypothyroid with radioiodine treatment.

Impact
Radioiodine therapy is an effective treatment for Graves' disease.

Aims
Hyperthyroidism is common, affecting approximately 2% of women and 0.2% of men. Untreated thyrotoxicosis can lead to cardiovascular (CV) and metabolic complications, which can be fatal. Radioactive iodine (RAI) has long been used to treat this condition, and has been found to be safe and effective. The dose administered to give prompt control generally induces hypothyroidism, which can be treated with thyroxine to make the patient euthyroid. This study aimed to determine the long-term incidence of hypothyroidism after a fixed dose (259 MBq) of RAI therapy and to evaluate whether clinical factors could predict the likelihood of hypothyroidism.

Methods
Patients: 2043 patients at 1 University hospital in Finland.

Inclusion criteria:
- All patients with biochemical evidence of hyperthyroidism;
- Classified into Graves' disease, toxic multinodular goitre (MNG), or toxic adenoma.

Endpoints:
- Incidence of hypothyroidism;
- Number of radioiodine treatments needed to control hyperthyroidism;
- Clinical factors predicting the likelihood of hypothyroidism.

Follow-up: Started at the time of first RAI treatment. Study ran from 1965–2002 (study end) *or* patient moved out of the area *or* death. Median F/U=9.8y.

Results

Endpoint	Graves' disease	Toxic MNG or adenoma
1y incidence of hypothyroidism	24%	4%
10y incidence of hypothyroidism	59%	15%
25y incidence of hypothyroidism	82%	32%

- Median time to development of hypothyroidism was 2y (minimum 1 month, maximum 25·4y).

Clinical factors	Relative risk			
	Graves' disease (n=1086)	p	Toxic MNG or adenoma (MNG n=749) (adenoma n=208)	p
Female	1.53	<0.01	0.65	0.1
Age at first RAI (RR per y)	0.97	<0.01	0.95	<0.01
Antithyroid drugs	0.47	<0.01	1.43	0.4
Previous partial thyroidectomy	1.63	<0.01	1.59	0.03
Remission after first radioiodine dose	0.99	0.97	1.00	0.99

Discussion

The majority of patients with Graves' disease became hypothyroid by 25y following radioiodine therapy. However, this only happened in 32% of patients with MNG. Previous partial thyroidectomy and age at first RAI treatment were significantly associated with an increased risk of hypothyroidism. Graves' patients, unlike MNG patients, showed a decreased risk of hypothyroidism with previous antithyroid medication use, and an increased risk of hypothyroidism with female gender. A total of 75% of patients were hypothyroid after a single dose of radioiodine, whereas 25% needed two to six doses, with no significant differences between the different aetiologies of the hyperthyroidism.

Problems

- The majority of patients who participated had Graves' disease (53%) compared with toxic MNG (37%) and toxic adenoma (10%).
- The long-term CV and metabolic safety of radioiodine therapy was not investigated.

Hyperthyroidism: methimazole

Effect of long-term continuous methimazole treatment of hyperthyroidism: comparison with radioiodine.

AUTHORS: Azizi F, Ataie L, Hedayati M *et al.*
REFERENCE: Eur J Endocrinol (2005) 152, 695–701.
STUDY DESIGN: RCT
EVIDENCE LEVEL: 1b

Key message

Hyperthyroidism is treated safely with long-term antithyroid medication.

Impact

Prolonged treatment with antithyroid medication is an alternative, safe option to radioiodine therapy in patients with relapsed toxic goitre.

Aims

Patients with relapsed hyperthyroidism are usually treated with radioiodine therapy. This study aimed to investigate whether long-term antithyroid medication was a suitable alternative option to radioiodine therapy.

Methods

Patients: 67 patients at 1 centre in Iran.

Inclusion criteria:
- Age >40y;
- Hyperthyroidism due to diffuse toxic goitre;
- Recurrence of hyperthyroidism after initial treatment with antithyroid drugs for 1½y.

Groups:
- Methimazole (n = 26);
- Radioiodine (n = 41).

Endpoints:
- Thyroid function tests;
- Antithyroperoxidase antibodies;
- Cholesterol;
- Goitre rate;
- Bone mineral density;
- Serious adverse events;
- Cost of treatment.

Follow-up: Median F/U=10.2y.

Results

Endpoint	Methimazole	Radioiodine	p
Free T_4 (ng/dL)	1.55±0.50	1.63±0.44	ns
Free T_3 (pg/mL)	3.66±0.72	3.44±0.77	ns
TSH (mU/L)	1.7±1.7	4.3±6.4	ns
Antithyroperoxidase antibody (IU/mL)	244±277	45±81	<0.05
Cholesterol (mg/dL)	190±47	224±46	<0.01
LDL cholesterol (mg/dL)	99±41	132±46	<0.01
Total goitre rate (%)	50	25	<0.05
Total bone mineral density at the hip (Z score)	−0.31±0.84	−0.54±0.94	ns
Total bone mineral density at the radius (Z score)	−1.41±1.20	−1.70±1.11	ns
Serious adverse events	0	0	ns
Cost of management (US$)	631±32	691±36	<0.001

LDL=low-density lipoprotein; TSH=thyroid stimulating hormone.

Discussion

This study demonstrated that in patients with diffuse toxic goitre, long-term methimazole was a safe and cost-effective alternative to radioiodine. Compared with radioiodine, 10y of methimazole treatment resulted in no significant difference in thyroid function tests or bone mineral density, a higher goitre rate and level of antithyroperoxidase antibodies, but a reduction in total and LDL cholesterol. In the UK, the treatment of choice for patients with relapsed hyperthyroidism remains radioiodine therapy, but long-term antithyroid medication may be considered a safe and cost-effective alternative.

Problems

- The study was limited to patients >40y of age with diffuse toxic goitre, and did not include the more prevalent Graves' patients who make up an important group of thyroid patients seen in the endocrine clinic.
- There was a high dropout rate of 8% which may have biased the results, and the numbers in each group were small, thus limiting the power of the study.
- The cost comparison was based on each group being followed up on a six monthly basis, but in clinical practice, the methimazole group may have to be followed up more frequently to alter the dose of treatment. This may also be a significant factor in adverse compliance outside the setting of a controlled study.

Hypothyroidism: levothyroxine

The starting dose of levothyroxine in primary hypothyroidism treatment.

AUTHORS: Roos A, Linn-Rasker S, van Domburg R et al.
REFERENCE: Arch Intern Med (2005) 165, 1714–20.
STUDY DESIGN: RCT
EVIDENCE LEVEL: 1b

Key message

A full starting replacement dose of levothyroxine in patients with primary hypothyroidism (without known cardiac disease) is a safe treatment option.

Impact

This was the first prospective study to investigate the safety and efficacy of initial levothyroxine starting doses in patients with primary hypothyroidism.

Aims

Hypothyroidism is common, particularly in women. It is most often due to autoimmune thyroiditis. Suggested starting doses for replacement therapy vary considerably. This study aimed to investigate the safety of higher initial replacement doses of levothyroxine.

Methods

Patients: 50 patients at 1 centre in the Netherlands.

Inclusion criteria:
- Untreated primary autoimmune hypothyroidism;
- Serum thyrotropin >4.2mIU/L, free T4 <10pmol/L.

Exclusion criteria:
- History of cardiac disease;
- Patients on cardiac medications.

Groups:
- Full starting dose: levothyroxine (1.6mcg/kg) (n=25);
- Low starting dose: levothyroxine (25mcg, dose increased every 4wk) (n=25).

Endpoints:
- Cardiac adverse events;
- Thyroid function tests;
- Lipids;
- Exercise performance (bicycle ergometer);
- Quality of life (QoL) scores.

Follow-up: Up to 48wk. Review every 4wk (first 24wk of treatment), then every 12wk. Included clinical symptom score, cardiac assessment, and patient questionnaires.

Results

Endpoint	(Full dose) Levothyroxine 1.6 mcg/kg	(Low dose) Levothyroxine 25 mcg	p
Time to normalisation of thyrotropin levels	4wk	16wk	–
4wk median thyrotropin levels (mIU/L)	4.2	26.7	0.005
4wk median free T4 levels (pmol/L)	19	12	<0.01
Significant change in cholesterol levels (number of patients)	0	0	Not reported
Cardiac symptoms/events (number of patients)	0	0	Not reported
Change in exercise performance (%)	10	0	<0.001
Change in QoL score (%)	+19	+26	Not reported

Discussion

This study demonstrated that a 1.6mcg/kg dose of levothyroxine was safe in patients without known cardiac disease. Greater increases were observed in 4wk free T4 levels and exercise performance in the higher dose levothyroxine group, compared with the group starting on the lower dose of 25mcg. There were no significant changes in QoL scores or cholesterol levels. The authors postulated that the high dose regime might be more cost-effective and convenient, thus improving compliance. However, this conclusion was not formally evaluated in this study.

Problems

- Levothyroxine was given in a liquid formulation rather than the more widely used tablet preparation.
- Only 25 patients in each group were studied, which may make the study insufficiently powered to arrive at meaningful conclusions.
- The mean patient age was 47y. Even though some elderly patients were included, the application of these results to older populations needs to be done with caution.
- This study did not address the safe starting dose of levothyroxine in patients with cardiac disease.

Primary hyperparathyroidism: medical treatment

Cinacalcet hydrochloride maintains long-term normocalcaemia in patients with primary hyperparathyroidism.

AUTHORS: Peacock M, Bilezikian J, Klassen P et al.
REFERENCE: J Clin Endocrinol Metab (2005) 90, 135–41.
STUDY DESIGN: RCT
EVIDENCE LEVEL: 1b

Key message
Calcium and parathyroid hormone (PTH) levels are rapidly and effectively reduced with cinacalcet therapy.

Impact
Medical treatment with cinacalcet can be considered as a non-surgical option for the maintenance of normocalcaemia in patients with mild to moderate primary hyperparathyroidism.

Aims
There are limited therapeutic alternatives for patients who are either not cured by, or have contraindications to, parathyroidectomy. This trial was designed to see whether the calcimimetic, cinacalcet, could safely reduce calcium and PTH levels in this group. Additionally, it aimed to explore the metabolic effects of therapy on bone structure.

Methods
Patients: 78 patients from 18 centres in the USA.

Inclusion criteria:
- Serum calcium level >2.57mmol/L and <3.12mmol/L;
- PTH level >4.73pmol/L.

Exclusion criteria:
- Creatinine clearance <50mL/min;
- Treatment with bisphosphonates or fluoride;
- Familial hypocalciuric hypercalcemia;
- Patients who required drugs that are metabolised by cytochrome P450.

Groups:
- Cinacalcet (30mg bd, increased up to 50mg bd, if needed) (n=40);
- Placebo (n=38).

Primary endpoint: Serum calcium ≤2.57mmol/L and a reduction from baseline of ≥0.12mmol/L.

Secondary endpoints:
- Plasma PTH, serum and urine biochemistry, biochemical measures of bone turnover (bone-specific alkaline phosphatase (BALP), N-telopeptide (NTx));
- Adverse events.

Follow-up: Total F/U=52wk. Included clinical/biochemical measurement and modification of dosage, if required.

Results

Primary endpoint	Cinacalcet	Placebo	*p*
Calcium ≤ 2.57mmol/L	73%	5%	<0.001
Secondary endpoint			
PTH change	−7.6%	+7.7%	<0.01
Serum phosphorus	+18.5%	−3.6%	<0.001
Calcium/creatinine	−38.5%	+12.0%	<0.001
Serum BALP	+35.3%	+4.4%	<0.05
Serum NTx	+27.8%	No change	<0.05
Urine NTx/creatinine	+60.4%	−4.7%	<0.001
Tubular reabsorption of calcium	+5.7%	No change	<0.001
Tubular reabsorption of phosphorus	+29.6%	No change	<0.001
BMD (Z score) change	Lumbar: 0.00 Femur: −0.01 Radius: −0.05	Lumbar: 0.03 Femur: −0.02 Radius: −0.01	ns

Discussion

This trial demonstrated the effectiveness of cinacalcet in reducing serum calcium levels, reducing PTH levels, and increasing bone resorption and formation markers. In 90% of patients, the dose needed to maintain normocalcaemia was 30mg bd. Importantly, the trial found cinacalcet to be well tolerated with non-significant adverse effects. Two thirds of patients not previously cured by parathyroidectomy reached the primary endpoint with cinacalcet.

Problems

- The trial was of only 52wk duration, so the long-term complications of primary hyperparathyroidism were not analysed. No data were collected on hard endpoints such as mortality, skeletal fractures, renal stones, cardiovascular disease, or gastrointestinal manifestations.
- The trial was limited to patients with mild to moderate hyperparathyroidism, so patients with severe hypercalcaemia or asymptomatic hyperparathyroidism were not analysed.
- The trial was not designed to look at the cost benefit of cinacalcet vs parathyroidectomy.

Primary hyperparathyroidism: surgical treatment

Randomised controlled clinical trial of surgery vs no surgery in patients with mild asymptomatic primary hyperparathyroidism.

AUTHORS: Rao DS, Phillips E, Divine G *et al.*
REFERENCE: J Clin Endocrinol Metab (2004) 89, 5415–22.
STUDY DESIGN: RCT
EVIDENCE LEVEL: 1b

Key message

Parathyroidectomy in patients with mild asymptomatic hyperparathyroidism is beneficial in improving bone mineral density (BMD), quality of life (QoL), and psychological function, compared with no surgery.

Impact

This was the first RCT to have been conducted to investigate the benefits of surgery vs no surgery in asymptomatic patients with primary hyperparathyroidism.

Aims

Parathyroidectomy is well recognised as the most appropriate treatment of symptomatic hyperparathyroidism. However, surgery in the absence of symptoms remains controversial. This trial aimed to evaluate the benefits of parathyroidectomy vs no surgery in patients with mild asymptomatic hyperparathyroidism.

Methods

Patients: 53 patients at 1 centre in the USA.

Inclusion criteria:
- Age 50–75y;
- Corrected calcium levels 10.1–11.5mg/dL (2.52–2.87mmol/L);
- Parathyroid hormone (PTH) >20pg/mL (20 ng/L);
- Creatinine <1.5mg/dL (133micromol/L);
- Forearm BMD within 2SD adjusted for age, sex, and race (Z scores);
- Absence of symptoms and complications due to hypercalcaemia or excess PTH levels.

Exclusion criteria:
- Familial hyperparathyroidism;
- Previous neck surgery;
- Active thyroid disease requiring surgical intervention;
- Non-traumatic vertebral or hip fractures;
- Nephrolithiasis within the past 2y;
- Women within 5y of the menopause;
- Medications known to affect bone and mineral metabolism;
- Adverse echocardiogram findings (that would preclude surgery).

Groups:
- Parathyroidectomy (n=25);
- No surgery (n=28).

Endpoints:
- BMD and bone biochemistry;
- QoL.

Follow-up: Included clinical/biochemical assessment, and QoL/psychosocial well-being questionnaires. Median F/U=42 months.

Results

% change in BMD per y	Surgery	No Surgery	p
Spine	1.2	0.5	Not reported
Femoral neck	0.4	-0.4	0.01
Total hip	0.3	-0.6	0.001
Forearm	0.4	0.2	Not reported

	Before surgery	After surgery	p
Calcium (mg/dL)	10.41±0.51	9.22±0.42	<0.001
PTH (pg/mL)	87±27	39±28	<0.001
Urine calcium (mg/d)	252±135	147±86	<0.001
Urine calcium/creatinine (mg/mg)	0.15±0.08	0.11±0.14	Not reported

- Biochemical parameters were unchanged in patients without surgery.
- Social (p=0.007) and emotional function (p=0.012) was better in the parathyroidectomy group compared with the non-surgery group.
- Anxiety (p=0.003) and phobia (p=0.024) declined in the parathyroidectomy group compared with the non-surgery group.

Discussion

The ideal treatment of asymptomatic hyperparathyroid patients has been controversial. This was the first RCT to evaluate this question. There were benefits seen in BMD (only at the femoral neck and total hip), QoL, and psychological function in the parathyroidectomy group. However, these slight benefits need to be weighed up against the complications of parathyroid surgery.

Problems

- The surgical group had a higher mean age.
- Patients aged <50y, in whom there is a high prevalence of hypercalcaemic complications, were not included.
- The numbers in this study were small, and the F/U period was too short to assess morbidity and mortality data.

Postmenopausal osteoporosis: bisphosphonates

FIT (Fracture Intervention Trial): Randomised trial of effect of alendronate on risk of fracture in women with existing vertebral fractures.

AUTHORS: Black D, Cummings S, Karpf D *et al.*
REFERENCE: Lancet (1996) 348, 1535–41.
STUDY DESIGN: RCT
EVIDENCE LEVEL: 1b

Key message

Post-menopausal women with low bone mass and a previous history of vertebral fractures have a lower incidence of fractures with alendronate therapy.

Impact

Alendronate is the most commonly used therapy in postmenopausal osteoporosis.

Aims

In women, the risk of osteoporosis increases after the menopause. Several treatments have been shown to have efficacy in increasing bone mass, including bisphosphonates. This trial aimed to evaluate the effect of the bisphosphonate, alendronate, on the clinical and radiological incidence of vertebral and non-vertebral fractures, in postmenopausal women with a previous history of vertebral fractures.

Methods

Patients: 2027 women from 11 centres in the USA.

Inclusion criteria:
- ≥2y postmenopause;
- Femoral neck bone mineral density (BMD) of ≤0.68g/cm^2;
- At least one previous vertebral fracture at recruitment.

Exclusion criteria:
- Peptic ulcer disease or dyspepsia requiring treatment;
- Abnormal renal function;
- Major medical problems likely to stop participation for 3y.
- Severe malabsorption syndrome;
- Uncontrolled hypertension (BP systolic >210, diastolic >105);
- Myocardial infarction during previous 6 months or unstable angina;
- Abnormal thyroid or parathyroid function;
- Previous bisphosphonates or sodium fluoride use.

Groups:
- Alendronate (n=1022);
- Placebo (n=1005).

Primary endpoints: New morphometric vertebral fractures.

Secondary endpoints:
• Any clinical fracture;
• Bone mass;
• Adverse effects, in particular gastrointestinal (GI).

Follow-up: Mean F/U=2.9y. Included BMD (at 1, 2, and 3y) and radiographs (at 2 and 3y).

Results

Endpoint	Alendronate	Placebo	HR (95% CI)
≥1 morphometric vertebral fractures	78 (8.0%)	145 (15.0%)	RR=0.53 (0.41 to 0.68)
Clinical vertebral fractures	23 (2.3%)	50 (5.0%)	0.45 (0.27 to 0.72)
Any clinical fracture	139 (13.6%)	182 (18.2%)	0.72 (0.58 to 0.90)
Any non-vertebral fracture	122 (11.9%)	148 (14.7%)	0.80 (0.63 to 1.01)
Hip fracture	11 (1.1%)	22 (2.2%)	0.49 (0.23 to 0.99)
Wrist fracture	22 (2.2%)	41 (4.1%)	0.52 (0.31 to 0.87)
Upper GI disturbance	422 (41.3%)	402 (40.0%)	p=0.67

Endpoint	Alendronate vs placebo	p
Femoral bone mass	4.1%	<0.001
Total hip bone mass	4.7%	<0.001
Lumbar spine bone mass	6.2%	<0.001

Discussion

Postmenopausal women with low bone mass and previous vertebral fractures had a lower incidence of clinical and radiological fractures. The alendronate group had 47% fewer radiographic vertebral fractures and 55% fewer clinical vertebral fractures. No significant differences in adverse GI events were seen.

Problems

• This arm of the FIT trial did not study fracture risk in women without a pre-existing history of vertebral fractures. Additionally, only women with low BMD were included.
• The ethnic diversity was limited, 97% of patients being Caucasian.
• There were no long-term data, the trial being limited to 3y.
• The cost–benefit ratio of alendronate treatment was not assessed.

Paget's disease: bisphosphonates

Comparison of a single infusion of zoledronic acid with risedronate for Paget's disease.

AUTHORS: Reid I, Miller P, Lyles K *et al.*
REFERENCE: N Engl J Med (2005) 353, 898–908.
STUDY DESIGN: RCT
EVIDENCE LEVEL: 1b

Key message

A single infusion of zoledronic acid is a rapid and effective treatment regime for patients with Paget's disease.

Impact

Bisphosphonate therapy is the first-line treatment for patients with Paget's disease and, as a result of this study, zoledronic acid is considered the most effective way to achieve sustained remission.

Aims

Paget's disease is characterised by increased bone turnover, often resulting in bone pain. Bisphosphonates can suppress this process. This study aimed to compare the effects of two different bisphosphonates, IV zoledronic acid and oral risedronate, on biochemical markers of Paget's disease activity and quality of life (QoL) measures.

Methods

Patients: 357 patients from 76 centres in ten countries.

Inclusion criteria:
- Age >30y;
- Radiological evidence of Paget's disease.

Exclusion criteria:
- Serum vitamin D <37nmol/L;
- Primary hyperparathyroidism, hepatic; or renal disease;
- History of uveitis, iritis, upper gastrointestinal disorders, diabetic nephropathy, or retinopathy;
- Paget's disease therapy in preceding 180d.

Groups:
- Zoledronic acid 5mg IV (n=182);
- Risedronate 30mg PO (n=175).

Primary endpoints: Alkaline phosphatase (ALP) normalisation or reduction of ≥75% of ALP excess (from midpoint of reference range).

Secondary endpoints:
- Biochemical markers of bone resorption and formation;
- QoL (Medical Outcomes Study 36-item Short-Form General Health Survey (SF36));

- Adverse events;
- Loss of primary endpoint at median 190d after study.

Follow-up: 6 months.

Results

Endpoint	Zoledronic acid	Risedronate	*p*
Primary endpoint	96%	74.3%	<0.001
Mean time to primary endpoint	64d	89d	<0.001
ALP normalisation	88.6%	57.9%	<0.001
Loss of primary endpoint at median 190d after study	0.9%	25.6%	<0.001
Adverse events (1–3d)	53.7%	25%	<0.01
Adverse events (after 3d)	66.1%	73.3%	0.2

Secondary endpoints:

- Bone formation marker: N-terminal propeptide of type 1 collagen showed significant decrease in both groups from baseline, with the response being greater in the zoledronic acid group.
- Bone resorption markers: Beta C-telopeptide of type 1 collagen and ratio of urinary alpha C-telopeptide of type 1 collagen to creatinine showed greater reductions in the zoledronic acid group.
- SF36 (QoL): The zoledronic acid group showed a significant increase from baseline at 3 and 6 months, and was significantly greater than the risedronate group at 3 months.

Discussion

Treatment with zoledronic acid resulted in a greater significant effect in suppressing Paget's disease activity, which was more rapid, sustained, and associated with improvements in QoL. In the zoledronic acid group, there were twice the number of adverse events in the first 3d, mostly due to influenza-like symptoms (which mainly resolved after 4d). After 3d, the rate of adverse events was similar in the two groups.

Problems

- The study was only for 6 months, so longer-term data are needed to evaluate treatment response and adverse events.
- The majority of patients were male (68%).

Male hypogonadism: testosterone replacement

A novel testosterone gel formulation normalises androgen levels in hypogonadal men with improvements in body composition and sexual function.

AUTHORS: McNicholas T, Dean J, Mulder H *et al.*
REFERENCE: Br J Urol (2003) 91, 69–74.
STUDY DESIGN: RCT
EVIDENCE LEVEL: 1b

Key message
Testosterone gel preparation is an effective alternative route for testosterone replacement in hypogonadal males.

Impact
With the recent availability of testosterone gel preparations, patients have been offered an alternative choice for testosterone replacement, which is more tolerable than traditional transdermal testosterone patches.

Aims
Declining testosterone levels in men can lead to altered mood and sexual function. Testosterone replacement through transdermal patches, oral formulations, or intramuscular injections were all previously used. However, all had associated problems (e.g. pain, inconvenience). Although patches were the most convenient for patients, a gel preparation had been proposed to provide more consistent therapeutic levels of testosterone. This study aimed to compare the effects of testosterone gel (Testim™) with the more established transdermal testosterone patch (Andropatch®) as a way of administering testosterone replacement in hypogonadal patients.

Methods
Patients: 208 patients from 29 European centres.

Inclusion criteria:
- Hypogonadal men (morning testosterone <10.4nmol/L);
- ≥1 symptom of hypogonadism.

Groups:
- Testim 50 (containing 5mg testosterone) (n=68);
- Testim 100 (containing 10mg testosterone) (n=72);
- Testosterone patch (containing 5mg testosterone) (n=68).

Measurements:
- Androgen levels;
- Body composition (i.e. lean body mass, fat mass, % of body fat and bone mineral density (BMD) of L1–L4 section of lumbar spine by dual-energy X-ray absorptiometry, DEXA);
- Sexual function and mood;
- Adverse events.

Follow-up: Clinical assessment (including sexual function and mood questionnaires) at 30, 60, and 90d.

Results

Measurement change	Testim 50	Testim 100	Andropatch
Testosterone (nmol/L)	6.54	12.41	3.82
DHT (nmol/L)	0.91	1.39	0.03
Free testosterone (pmol/L)	22.07	47.83	15.74
Spontaneous erections (mean/wk)	0.6	0.5	0.3
Motivation (mean/wk)	0.4	0.4	0.5
Desire (mean/d)	0.8	0.7	0.5
Performance (mean/wk)	0.3	0.4	0.3
Lean body mass	0.9	1.5	1.0
Fat mass	−0.1	−0.2	−0.1
% fat	−0.4	−0.7	−0.3
Adverse events	35%	29%	63%

DHT=dihydrotestosterone

Discussion

Compared with the transdermal patch, testosterone delivered in a gel preparation was more effective at normalising androgen levels in a dose-dependent manner. Additionally, there was a significant improvement in sexual function, mood, and body composition. The transdermal patch had more adverse effects, mainly due to skin irritation, which resulted in a greater discontinuation rate. This is an important factor as testosterone replacement in hypogonadal patients is a long-term therapy.

Problems

- No comparison was made between other testosterone replacement therapies, in particular the more common testosterone injections.
- The majority of patients had secondary rather than primary hypogonadism.

Acromegaly: octreotide

Primary treatment of acromegaly with LAR octreotide: prospective study of its efficacy in the control of disease activity and tumour shrinkage.

AUTHORS: Cozzi R, Montini M, Attanasio R et al.
REFERENCE: J Clin Endocrinol Metab (2006) 91, 1397–403.
STUDY DESIGN: Cohort study
EVIDENCE LEVEL: 2b

Key message
Long-acting repeatable (LAR) octreotide is an effective primary therapy in acromegalic patients with large or invasive adenomas and high growth hormone levels.

Impact
LAR octreotide is considered the first treatment option for acromegalic patients with large invasive adenomas who are poor surgical candidates.

Aims
Whilst surgical management is the treatment of choice for acromegaly, in some patients, this is not an option and so medical therapy is required. This trial aimed to study the effect of the somatostatin analogue, LAR octreotide, as primary treatment for patients with acromegaly.

Methods
Patients: 67 patients (72% macroadenomas) at one centre in Italy.

Inclusion criteria:
- Clinical symptoms and signs of acromegaly;
- Elevated growth hormone (GH) not suppressed after an oral glucose tolerance test;
- High age-adjusted insulin-like growth factor-1 (IGF-1) levels;
- MRI showing macroadenoma or invasive microadenoma;
- No previous neurosurgery or radiotherapy.

Exclusion criteria:
- Intrasellar microadenoma (except patients refusing or unable to have neurosurgery);
- Ophthalmological or neurological involvement;
- Hepatic or renal disease.

Endpoints:
- GH level <2.5mcg/L;
- Normal age-matched IGF-1 level;
- Tumour shrinkage on MRI.

Follow-up: Up to 48 months. Assessment at 3–6 monthly intervals during first year, then annually thereafter. MRI before start of treatment, and at 6 and 12 months.

Results

GH level <2.5 mcg/L (% of patients)	68.7%
Percentage decrease in GH	81.5±21.7%
Normal age-matched IGF-1 level (% of patients)	70.1%
Percentage decrease in IGF-1	59±27%
Tumour decreased in size (% of patients)	82.1%
Amount of tumour decrease from baseline	62±31%
Tumour shrinkage >75% (% of patients)	44%

Discussion

LAR octreotide therapy in treatment-naive patients with acromegaly resulted in a normalisation of GH and IGF-1 levels in over two thirds of patients. This occurred regardless of the baseline levels of GH or IGF-1, although the greatest normalisation occurred in those patients with higher baseline values. Tumour shrinkage occurred more frequently with macroadenomas compared with microadenomas.

Problems

- A total of 49% of patients initially having LAR octreotide decided to change to alternative treatment for their acromegaly (surgery or addition of lanreotide or cabergoline).
- The majority of patients had macroadenomas, and the study did not include acromegalic patients with only intrasellar adenomas.
- There was no control group in the trial.

Acromegaly: pegvisomant

Long-term treatment of acromegaly with pegvisomant, a growth hormone receptor antagonist.

AUTHORS: van der Lely A, Hutson R, Trainer P *et al.*
REFERENCE: Lancet (2001) 358, 1754–9.
STUDY DESIGN: Cohort study
EVIDENCE LEVEL: 2b

Key message
Pegvisomant reduces insulin-like growth factor-1 (IGF-1), fasting insulin, and fasting glucose levels in patients with acromegaly.

Impact
Pegvisomant is the first highly selective growth hormone receptor antagonist that has been shown to be an effective medical treatment option for acromegalic patients.

Aims
Traditional management of acromegaly involves either surgery or medication (dopamine agonists/somatostatin analogues). This trial aimed to assess the efficacy of a novel drug, subcutaneous pegvisomant (a growth hormone receptor agonist) in patients with acromegaly.

Methods
Patients: 160 patients at multiple international centres.

Inclusion criteria:
• Age >18y;
• IGF-1 levels ≥1.3 times the upper end of age-adjusted normal range;
• Somatostatin analogues discontinued for ≥2wk;
• Dopamine agonists discontinued for ≥5wk.

Endpoints:
• Pituitary tumour volume change assessed by MRI;
• GH levels;
• IGF-1 levels;
• Fasting insulin levels;
• Fasting glucose levels.

Follow-up: 425d.

Results

Endpoint	6 months cohort (n=131)	12 months cohort (n=90)	18 months cohort (n=39)	p
Decrease in IGF-1 (mcg/L)	467	526	523	<0.001
Increase in GH (mcg/L)	12.5	12.5	14.2	<0.001
Decrease in fasting insulin (mU/L)	7.2	10.6	10.9	0.039
Fasting glucose (mg/L)	191	147	80	0.013

- A total of 97% of patients treated for >52wk had a normal IGF-1 level.
- A total of 16.9% developed antibodies to GH (but no tachyphylaxis occurred).
- Mean tumour volume decreased by 0.033cm^3 at 11.46 months ($p=0.353$, ns).

Discussion

This study demonstrated a significant reduction in IGF-1, insulin, and glucose levels with pegvisomant therapy. GH levels rose in the first 6 months and remained stable thereafter. The mechanism by which this happened was unclear. Serum GH is not a good marker of acromegalic activity in patients treated with pegvisomant. Mean tumour volume did not decrease significantly.

Problems

- A total of 18.8% of patients withdrew from the study.
- The effect of pegvisomant on symptoms and quality of life (QoL) were not assessed.
- Long-term F/U is needed to exclude an increase in tumour volume (Nelson's syndrome-like effect—rapid pituitary tumour enlargement occurring post-bilateral adrenalectomy).
- The trial did not study the efficacy of pegvisomant compared with other forms of medical therapy for acromegaly, including dopamine agonists and somatostatin analogues.

Hyperprolactinaemia: dopamine agonists

A comparison of cabergoline and bromocriptine in the treatment of hyperprolactinaemic amenorrhoea.

AUTHORS: Webster J, Piscitelli G, Polli A *et al.*
REFERENCE: N Engl J Med (1994) 331, 904–9.
STUDY DESIGN: RCT
EVIDENCE LEVEL: 1b

Key message

In patients with hyperprolactinaemic amenorrhoea, cabergoline therapy is more efficacious and tolerable than bromocriptine.

Impact

The dopamine agonist, cabergoline, is considered first-line treatment for patients with hyperprolactinaemia.

Aims

Dopamine agonists are the treatment of choice for hyperprolactinaemia. This trial aimed to compare cabergoline, a newer long-acting dopamine agonist, with the former gold standard, bromocriptine.

Methods

Patients: 459 patients, from multiple international centres (279 microprolactinomas, 3 macroprolactinomas, 1 craniopharyngioma, 167 idiopathic hyperprolactinaemia, 9 empty sella).

Inclusion criteria:
- Females with amenorrhoea >3 months;
- Serum prolactin level at least twice the upper limit of normal;
- ≥4wk discontinuation of previous prolactin therapy.

Exclusion criteria:
- Any previous side effects to either one of the dopamine agonists;
- Any disorder preventing normal menstruation after normalisation of prolactin;
- Hyperprolactinaemia due to polycystic ovary syndrome, thyroid or adrenal disorders, renal or hepatic disease.

Groups:
- Cabergoline (0.5–1.0mg twice weekly) (n = 223);
- Bromocriptine (2.5–5.0mg twice weekly) (n = 236).

Endpoints:
- Occurrence of menses and ovulation;
- Serum prolactin levels;
- Adverse events.

Follow-up: Clinical assessment (including checking side-effects) and serum prolactin measurements at baseline, and at 2, 4, 6, 8, 12, 14, 16, 20, and 24wk after initiation of therapy.

Results

Endpoint	Cabergoline	Bromocriptine	*p*
Normoprolactinaemia	83%	59%	<0.001
Ovulatory cycles or pregnancy	72%	52%	<0.001
Persistence of amenorrhoea	7%	16%	ns
Adverse events	68%	78%	0.03
Drug intolerance	3%	12%	<0.001

Discussion

This study demonstrated cabergoline to be more effective at normalising prolactin levels and restoring normal menstruation and ovulation compared with bromocriptine. Adverse events were significantly fewer and tolerability significantly better in the cabergoline group.

Problems

- Treatment was only double-blinded for the first 8wk, then continued open-labelled. The authors state that most side effects occurred within the first few weeks, though continuing the double-blind design would have been a better study design.
- Only 72% in the bromocriptine group and 83% in the cabergoline group completed the 24wk study.

Gastroenterology

Introduction

'One good set of bowels is more important than any amount of brain' were the wise words that inspired gastroenterologists for centuries. Fittingly, an earnest gastroenterologist spent good time on ward rounds stool gazing. Arrival of flexible endoscopy brought glamour to the specialty which had long been monopolised by cardiology. Despite being sneered upon by intellectuals as 'just a tool', endoscopy continues to challenge surgery and radiology, driving both of these specialties to advances in laparoscopic techniques and newer sophisticated imaging modalities. The discovery of *Helicobacter pylori* has made surgery for 'peptic ulcers' history. Refinements in endoscopic haemostatic techniques are even raising concerns that surgical trainees may not get sufficient experience in dealing with acute gastrointestinal bleeding.

Over the last two decades, there has been a marked improvement in the quality of study design and statistical rigour. However, the complexity of gastroenterological problems has limited the size of the studies which still do not compare with those performed in cardiology. Biological therapy in inflammatory bowel disease has been a therapeutic landmark in therapeutics in gastroenterology, not only for increasing the sophistication in study design, but also for stimulating debate on fundamental goals of therapy. In hepatology, antiviral therapy has established large and robust multi-national randomised controlled trials. Interventions in hepatology are now judged by their effect on hard clinical endpoints, including long-term survival.

Clinical gastroenterology has matured into a specialty that challenges both the intellect and dexterity.

Gastric cancer: *Helicobacter pylori* eradication

Helicobacter pylori eradication to prevent gastric cancer in a high-risk region of China.

AUTHORS: Wong B, Lam S, Wong W *et al.*
REFERENCE: JAMA (2004) 291, 187–94.
STUDY DESIGN: RCT
EVIDENCE LEVEL: 1b

Key message

In *Helicobacter* (*H.*) *pylori* carriers without precancerous lesions on presentation, eradication therapy decreases the development of gastric cancer.

Impact

Despite persuasive evidence implicating *H. pylori* as the main cause of gastric cancer, clinical benefits of eradication therapy in asymptomatic *H. pylori* carriers without peptic ulcer is not well established. This was the first population-based study to demonstrate that eradication therapy reduced the risk of gastric cancer in subjects without precancerous lesions already. However, the role of *H. pylori* eradication in preventing gastric cancer continues to be debated.

Aims

H. pylori infection is an established risk factor for the development of gastric cancer. This study aimed to determine whether treating *H. pylori* infection reduces the incidence of gastric cancer.

Methods

Subjects: 1630 healthy carriers of *H. pylori* infection, from centres in Fujinan Province, China. A total of 988 patients were without precancerous lesions (gastric atrophy, intestinal metaplasia, or gastric dysplasia).

Inclusion criteria: Healthy subjects with normal endoscopy and confirmed *H. pylori* infection:
- Endoscopic gastric antral biopsy positive for rapid urease test;
- *H. pylori* confirmed on histology of gastric antral biopsy.

Exclusion criteria:
- History of *H. pylori* eradication therapy;
- Ulcer on endoscopy;
- Equivocal or negative rapid urease test or histology;
- Age <35y and >65y;
- Severe comorbidity.

Groups:
- Treatment: received triple therapy followed by carbon-13 urea breath test (^{13}C-UBT). Those with unsuccessful eradication received quadruple therapy followed by repeat ^{13}C-UBT in 6wk (n=817).
- Placebo (n=813).

Primary endpoint: Incidence of gastric cancer during F/U.

Secondary endpoints: Incidence of gastric cancer in subjects with or without precancerous lesions.

Follow-up: Six monthly review, biannual ^{13}C-UBT for *H. pylori* status. Repeat endoscopy at 5y or when upper gastrointestinal symptoms appeared. Total F/U=7.5y.

Results

Primary endpoint	Placebo (n=813)	*H. pylori* eradication (n=817)	*p*
New cases of gastric cancer	11	7	0.33
Secondary endpoint	**Placebo (n=503)**	***H. pylori* eradication (n=485)**	
New cases of gastric cancer	6	0	0.02

Discussion

After 7.5y of F/U, gastric cancer developed in seven subjects who received *H. pylori* eradication and 11 in the placebo group. Among 18 new cases of gastric cancer, six developed in subjects without precancerous lesions, whereas 12 developed in those with such lesions. None in the *H. pylori*-treated group without pre-malignant lesions developed gastric cancer during the study period, suggesting that eradication therapy was beneficial in this group. However, *H. pylori* treatment had no benefit in subjects with precancerous lesions. It could be argued that during the development of precancerous lesions, the benefit of *H. pylori* eradication diminishes and a 'point of no return' may be reached. Other studies have demonstrated that *H. pylori* eradication results in regression of gastric atrophy and intestinal metaplasia in 15–30% of cases. Therefore, larger sample size and longer F/U are required to investigate whether *H. pylori* eradication is beneficial in this subgroup.

Problems

- A small number of cancers were detected and the duration of F/U was too short for this study to be conclusive. Longer F/U would have been particularly useful in investigating the effect of eradication therapy in those with precancerous lesions at the time of initial endoscopy.
- The study was based in a high-risk population. It is unclear whether these results are applicable to low-risk areas in Western countries.

Peptic ulcer disease: *Helicobacter pylori* eradication

Eradication therapy for peptic ulcer disease in *Helicobacter pylori*-positive patients (Cochrane review).

AUTHORS: Ford A, Delaney B, Forman D *et al.*
REFERENCE: Cochrane Database of Systematic Reviews (2006) Issue 2.
STUDY DESIGN: Systematic review
EVIDENCE LEVEL: 1a

Key message
All *Helicobacter* (*H.*) *pylori*-positive peptic ulcer disease patients should receive eradication therapy.

Impact
The seminal discovery that *H. pylori* infection is the cause of 95% of duodenal and 70% of gastric ulcers radically changed the management of dyspepsia. The majority of peptic ulcers can now be cured by *H. pylori* eradication therapy and surgical interventions are rarely indicated.

Aims
RCTs of short- and long-term treatment of peptic ulcer disease in *H. pylori*-positive adults were analysed to assess the proportion of patients with peptic ulcers, and the proportion of patients who remained free from relapse after eradication therapy.

Methods
Trials included: 56 of 63 eligible trials.

Inclusion criteria: RCTs of short- and long-term treatment of peptic ulcer disease in *H. pylori*-positive adults:
- ≥1wk of *H. pylori* eradication;
- Comparison with ulcer healing drug, placebo, or no treatment;
- Patients assessed at 2wk or after eradication therapy.

Exclusion criteria: Trials from which data extraction was not possible.

Types of interventions included:
- Proton pump inhibitor (PPI) dual or triple therapy (one or two antibiotics);
- H_2 receptor antagonist triple therapy;
- Bismuth triple or quadruple therapy;
- PPI, H_2 receptor antagonists, bismuth salts, sucralfate, antacids as monotherapy;
- Placebo;
- No treatment.

Primary endpoints:
- Proportion of ulcers healed initially;
- Proportion of patients free from recurrence following successful healing.

Results

Primary endpoints	Eradication therapy vs ulcer healing drugs	Eradication therapy vs no treatment
Duodenal ulcer persisting with therapy	RR: 0.66 95% CI: 0.58 to 0.76	RR: 0.37 95% CI: 0.26 to 0.53
Duodenal ulcer recurring with therapy	RR: 0.73 95% CI: 0.42 to 1.25	RR: 0.20 95% CI: 0.15 to 0.26
Gastric ulcer persisting with therapy	RR: 1.25 95% CI: 0.88 to 1.76	—
Gastric ulcer recurring with therapy	—	RR: 0.29 95% CI: 0.20 to 0.42

Discussion

About 10% of the Western population develops a gastric or duodenal ulcer during their lifetime. The cost to health care runs into billions of pounds. In the 1970s and 80s, therapy for peptic ulcer disease was mainly aimed at reducing acid secretion using H_2 receptor antagonists and PPIs. Recognition of the role of *H. pylori* in the development and recurrence of peptic ulcers and confirmation that this could be prevented by eradication of the organism has transformed the management of peptic ulcer disease. This review concluded that eradication therapy was clearly indicated in *H. pylori*-positive peptic ulcer disease, as there were definite benefits in terms of ulcer healing and prevention of recurrence. Benefits were more marked in duodenal ulcers. This was consistent with international guidelines. Use of *H. pylori* eradication therapy reduced the use of health care resources during F/U compared with conventional ulcer healing drugs, and therefore, should be the preferred approach from a health economic perspective.

Problems

- This review reported ulcer healing rates of 75–85% and ulcer recurrence rates of 12–14%. These figures are much lower than previous systematic reviews, which report healing rates of 90–95% and recurrence rates <10%. This was due to the analysis used, where all patients lost to F/U in the trials were assumed to be treatment failures.
- The review found no significant benefit in symptom relief with *H. pylori* eradication therapy over other regimens. The number of trials included reporting this outcome was small and none of the trials evaluated symptoms beyond 6wk, thereby potentially overlooking the long-term effects of *H pylori* eradication.

Peptic ulcer disease: managing antiplatelet bleeding risk

> Clopidogrel vs aspirin and esomeprazole to prevent recurrent ulcer bleeding.
>
> **AUTHORS:** Chan F, Ching J, Hung L *et al.*
> **REFERENCE:** N Engl J Med (2005) 352, 238–44.
> **STUDY DESIGN:** RCT
> **EVIDENCE LEVEL:** 1b

Key message

In patients taking aspirin with bleeding peptic ulcers, once the ulcer has healed, restarting aspirin in combination with a proton pump inhibitor (PPI) is better than introducing clopidogrel in preventing recurrent bleeding.

Impact

In the past two decades, many millions have started taking aspirin to prevent myocardial infarction (MI) and stroke. Aspirin, even at low doses, doubles the risk of upper gastrointestinal (GI) bleeding. Two strategies that allow maintenance of cardiovascular (CV) protection and minimise GI adverse events were compared in this study. Based on the firm evidence provided, combination of aspirin with a PPI should be the standard management in this situation. The results raise doubt about the GI safety of clopidogrel.

Aims

PPI therapy heals ulcers and reduces the risk of bleeding. Clopidogrel, an effective antiplatelet agent, does not induce ulcers. Therefore, patients who have had one episode of GI bleeding from ulcers whilst on aspirin can either receive the combination of aspirin and PPI, or clopidogrel (instead of aspirin). This study aimed to compare the effectiveness of these two strategies in the prevention of recurrent bleeding in high-risk patients.

Methods

Patients: 320 patients at one centre in Hong Kong.

Inclusion criteria: Consecutive users of low-dose aspirin (≤325mg/d) with upper GI bleeding due to peptic ulcer (confirmed on index endoscopy):
• Triple therapy if *H. pylori*-positive;
• Withdrawal of aspirin and PPI therapy to heal the ulcer;
• Healed ulcer plus successful *H. pylori* eradication on repeat endoscopy at 8wk.

Exclusion criteria: Concomitant use of NSAIDs, cyclooxygenase-2 inhibitors, and anticoagulants.

Groups:
• Clopidogrel (75mg) plus placebo bd (n=161);
• Aspirin (80mg) plus esomeprazole (20mg) bd (n=159).

Primary endpoint: Recurrent ulcer bleeding with endoscopically documented ulcers or erosions.

Secondary endpoints: Lower GI bleeding.

Follow-up: 12 months.

Results

Primary endpoint	Clopidogrel+ placebo	Aspirin+ esomeprazole	p
Cumulative incidence of recurrent ulcer bleeding	8.6% (95% CI 4.1 to 13.1%)	0.7% (95% CI 0 to 2.0%)	0.001
Secondary endpoint			
Cumulative incidence of lower GI bleeding	4.6% (95% CI 1.3 to 7.9%)	4.6% (95% CI 1.3 to 8.0%)	0.98

Discussion

A previous study reported about 15% of patients with a history of ulcer bleeding to develop recurrent bleeding within 1y of aspirin therapy. Current opinions regarding GI safety of clopidogrel have been based on secondary analysis of studies that did not use prespecified criteria to report GI complications. This study's findings challenge the American College of Cardiology/American Heart Association guidelines, which recommend the use of clopidogrel in patients with major GI side effects from aspirin. The majority (71%) of rebleeding episodes were from recurrent ulcers at the same location as seen during the initial endoscopy. The mechanisms leading to recurrent bleeding among patients receiving clopidogrel are unknown. Clopidogrel inhibits platelet-derived growth factors, which may impair ulcer healing and induce recurrent bleeding from the previously damaged mucosa. Alternatively, comorbidity may predispose patients to the development of ulcers in the absence of *H. pylori* or NSAIDs.

Problems

- The study did not include a group of patients who were restarted on aspirin without PPI, as this was considered unethical. Therefore, it was not possible to assess whether clopidogrel was safer than aspirin.
- The efficacy of PPI is known to vary among ethnic groups and this may have influenced the significance of the results.
- Study drugs were repackaged from the commercially available form; this may have influenced their therapeutic effects.

Peptic ulcer disease: endoscopic control of bleeding

Dual therapy vs monotherapy in the endoscopic treatment of high-risk bleeding ulcers.

AUTHORS: Marmo R, Rotondano G, Piscopo R et al.
REFERENCE: Am J Gastroenterol (2007) 102, 279–89.
STUDY DESIGN: Meta-analysis
EVIDENCE LEVEL: 1a

Key message

Treatment using thermal probe/haemoclip as monotherapy is as effective as dual modality therapy. Therefore, routine combined endoscopic therapy is not recommended. In patients with active arterial bleeding, dual therapy assures a higher rate of initial haemostasis.

Impact

Combined therapy using adrenaline injection plus thermal coagulation is increasingly being offered as the gold standard management for bleeding peptic ulcers. However, adrenaline injection is still the most widely used treatment. While this meta-analysis supports dual therapy, it also suggests that if a single modality of endoscopic intervention is to be delivered, it should be thermal coagulation. Therefore, every endoscopist should become proficient with thermal coagulation treatment.

Aims

Endoscopic techniques of haemostasis such as injection, thermal, and mechanical methods are complementary in the management of bleeding peptic ulcers. This study aimed to assess the efficacy of dual vs single endoscopic intervention in improving clinical outcomes.

Methods

Studies: 20 studies.

Inclusion criteria: Studies comparing efficacy of dual endoscopic therapy vs any other form of endoscopic monotherapy:
- Patients with bleeding from peptic ulcer;
- Stigmata of bleeding at the ulcer base (active bleeding, visible vessel, or adherent clot).

Exclusion criteria: Studies without detail on safety of techniques used.

Groups: Injection of two agents vs injection of single agents. Four groups: Dual therapy vs controls, dual therapy vs injection therapy, dual therapy vs thermal coagulation, dual therapy vs mechanical treatment.

Primary endpoint: Control of bleeding:
- Risk of rebleeding;
- Risk of emergency surgery;
- Risk of death.

Secondary endpoints: Procedure-related complications.

Results

Primary endpoints	Dual vs controls OR (95% CI)	Dual vs injection OR (95% CI)	Dual vs thermal OR (95% CI)	Dual vs mechanical OR (95% CI)
Rebleeding	0.59 (0.44 to 0.80)	0.36 (0.18 to 0.73)	0.67 (0.40 to 1.20)	1.04 (0.45 to 2.45)
Emergency surgery	0.66 (0.49 to 0.89)	0.40 (0.19 to 0.83)	0.89 (0.45 to 1.76)	0.49 (0.50 to 4.87)
Death risk	0.68 (0.46 to 1.02)	0.88 (0.35 to 2.22)	0.51 (0.24 to 1.10)	1.28 (0.34 to 4.86)
Secondary endpoints	Dual therapy	Monotherapy	p	
Procedure-induced bleeding	18/1069	18/1068	>0.05	
Perforation	7/1069	0/1068	0.03	

Discussion

Evolution of endoscopic techniques has allowed primary haemostasis to be achieved in up to 95% of bleeding peptic ulcers. Adrenaline injection is simple, cheap, and safe. However, thermal coagulation and haemoclip were more effective. As different interventions may be complementary, combination of adrenaline injection and thermal coagulation is increasingly offered as the gold standard. In high-risk peptic ulcer bleeding, this study confirmed that dual endoscopic therapy (additional thermal probe or haemoclip application) was superior to adrenaline injection alone. However, when bleeding had first been controlled using thermal or mechanical treatment, further injection therapy had no additional benefit. Therefore, the logical approach should be to use thermal probes first; if this achieves haemostasis, no further treatment is necessary. In ongoing bleeds during endoscopy, initial adrenaline injection followed by thermal coagulation achieves better control of bleeding. Routine application of combined endoscopic therapy in all patients is not warranted.

Problems

- The number of studies and patients was not large enough to have sufficient power to detect small (but potentially significant) differences between dual therapy and thermal coagulation.
- Dual therapy is associated with an increased risk of perforation.
- Expertise and sound judgement are of paramount importance when treating high-risk bleeding peptic ulcer patients. Haemoclips are effective but also require technical expertise, limiting their applicability.

Upper GI bleeding: intravenous proton pump inhibitor

APPE study: **A**dministration of intravenous **P**roton **P**ump Inhibitor prior to **E**ndoscopy in patients with upper gastrointestinal bleeding.

AUTHORS: Lau J, Leung W, Wu J *et al.*
REFERENCE: N Engl J Med (2007) 356, 1631-40.
STUDY DESIGN: RCT
EVIDENCE LEVEL: 1b

Key message
Infusion of a proton pump inhibitor (PPI) before endoscopy leads to early resolution of upper gastrointestinal (GI) bleeding, also reducing the need for endoscopic therapy and duration of hospital stay.

Impact
Endoscopic therapy is the key step in the management of suspected upper GI bleeding and has an established role in the care of these patients. However, out-of-hours endoscopy is not uniformly available in hospitals in the UK. Early presumptive infusion of PPI may become a common practice in patients with suspected upper GI bleeding.

Aims
A neutral gastric pH is critical for the stability of clot over bleeding arteries. Therefore, it has been proposed that earlier acid suppression with PPI therapy for any GI bleeds (before the cause is known) may lead to better outcomes. This study aimed to investigate the effect of presumptive infusion of omeprazole (before endoscopy) on the need for endoscopic therapy.

Methods
Patients: 638 patients at one centre in Hong Kong.

Inclusion criteria: Consecutive patients with overt signs of upper GI bleeding:
- Age >16y;
- Fresh haematemesis and/or melaena;
- Haemodynamically stable (after volume resuscitation, if and as required).

Exclusion criteria: Chronic low dose aspirin use.

Groups: Both groups received 80mg IV bolus followed by 8mg/h infusion for 72h:
- Omeprazole (n=319);
- Placebo (n=319).

Primary endpoint: Control of bleeding at the time of endoscopy.

Secondary endpoints:
- Transfusion requirement;
- Rate of rebleeding;
- Need for emergency surgery;
- 30d mortality;
- Duration of hospital stay.

Follow-up: 30d from the time of admission or until the time of discharge (if >30d), or death.

Results

Primary endpoints	Placebo	Omeprazole	p
Need of endoscopic therapy	28.4%	19.1%	0.007
Active bleeding on endoscopy	14.7%	6.4%	0.01
Clean base ulcer on endoscopy	47.4%	64.2%	0.001
Secondary endpoints			
Mean units of blood transfusion	1.88	1.54	0.1
Rebleeding	2.5%	3.5%	0.5
Need of emergency surgery	1.26%	0.95%	1.0
30d mortality	2.52%	2.22%	0.8
<3d hospital stay	60.5%	49.2%	0.005

Discussion

A systematic review had suggested that PPI therapy reduced the risk of rebleeding and surgery in patients with bleeding peptic ulcer. It is now standard practice to perform an early endoscopy in patients with upper GI bleeding, with an intention to establish the underlying aetiology and to treat (endoscopic haemostatic methods) as well as to assess the risk of rebleeding (active bleeding, visible vessel at endoscopy) and mortality (using Rockall score). Patients confirmed to have peptic ulcer and estimated to be at high risk of rebleeding were treated with IV PPI for 72h. This study suggested that it was beneficial to treat all cases of upper GI bleeding with IV PPI, even pre-endoscopy. Early PPI treatment may assist endoscopic diagnosis and may reduce the need for endoscopic therapy.

Problems

- There were no significant differences in clinically important secondary endpoints such as rebleeding, need for surgery, and death.
- The proportion of patients with bleeding due to peptic ulcer was much higher than that seen in many Western countries. So the impact of PPI therapy will vary depending on the case mix of patients with differing aetiologies of upper GI bleeding.
- Previous studies had suggested that PPIs perform better for peptic ulcer bleeds in Asian patients compared with other ethnic groups. Therefore, the findings cannot be extrapolated to all patient groups.
- The cost-effectiveness of early IV PPI was not assessed.

Variceal bleeding: somatostatin analogues

Early administration of vapreotide for variceal bleeding in patients with cirrhosis.

AUTHORS: Cales P, Masliah C, Bernard B *et al.*
REFERENCE: N Engl J Med (2001) 344, 23–8.
STUDY DESIGN: RCT
EVIDENCE LEVEL: 1b

Key message

In patients with cirrhosis and variceal bleeding, the combination of vaso-active drug and endoscopic therapy is more effective than endoscopy alone. Prompt administration of vasoactive drug prior to endoscopy achieves early haemostasis, hence potentially facilitating endoscopic intervention.

Impact

The combination of vasoactive drug (somatostatin or vasopressin analogues) and endoscopic intervention is now the standard care for patients with variceal bleeding. In cases where there is a high index of clinical suspicion that upper gastrointestinal (GI) bleeding is related to portal hypertension, early administration of vasoactive drugs before endoscopy is justified.

Aims

Variceal bleeding can be controlled in a proportion of patients by either vasoactive drugs or endoscopic therapy. The aim of this trial was to eval-uate the effects of early administration of a somatostatin analogue (vapre-otide) followed by endoscopic treatment in patients with bleeding varices.

Methods

Patients: 227 patients at 22 centres in France.

Inclusion criteria: Consecutive patients with cirrhosis and upper GI bleeding:
- Fresh haematemesis and/or melaena;
- Initial episode of bleeding <24h at enrolment;
- <6h from the time of hospital admission;
- Age between 18–75y.

Exclusion criteria:
- Variceal bleeding within last 6wk;
- Previous shunt procedure;
- Child-Pugh score >13;
- Hepatocellular carcinoma, non-cirrhotic portal hypertension, or com-plete portal vein thrombosis.

Groups: 31 patients whose bleeding was not caused by portal hypertension were excluded:
- Vapreotide: 50mcg IV bolus, then 50mcg/h infusion, for 5d (n=98);
- Placebo (n=98).

Primary endpoint:
- Control of bleeding and survival for 5d.

Secondary endpoints:
- Absence of active bleeding at the time of initial endoscopy;
- Transfusion requirement during 5d;
- Incidence of late rebleeding (d6–42);
- 42d survival.

Follow-up: 42d or death.

Results

Primary endpoint	Placebo (n=98)	Vapreotide (n=98)	*p*
Control of bleeding and survival for 5d	50%	66%	0.02
Secondary endpoints			
Absence of active bleeding on endoscopy	54%	69%	0.03
Mean units of blood transfusion in 5d	2.8	2.0	0.04
Late rebleeding (d6–42)	11%	16%	0.4
42d survival	79%	86%	0.2

Discussion

The results emphasised the importance of the timing of vasoactive drug administration. Two other studies using somatostatin and terlipressin early after the onset of upper GI bleeding have also shown significant improvement in the initial control of bleeding. Furthermore, the study in which the first dose of terlipressin was given before hospitalisation also showed significant reduction in mortality. Therefore, it is reasonable to recommend that patients with upper GI bleeding with clear clinical evidence of portal hypertension should receive vasoactive drug therapy as soon as possible. Vasoactive drugs may ensure haemodynamic stability and haemostasis at the time of initial endoscopy which contributes to overall success of the procedure.

Problems

- One third of patients screened were excluded due to stringent entry criteria. So one cannot be certain as to whether the benefits of early vasoactive drugs will be better or worse when used in routine practice.
- Overall, 42d mortality was similar in both groups. On multivariate analysis, higher Child-Pugh score, age, and source of bleeding other than oesophageal varices predicted worse outcome. Treatment with vapreotide was not a significant factor (*p*=0.07), confirming a well recognised fact that overall mortality in these patients is dependent on factors other than control of bleeding.

Variceal bleeding: primary prevention

Comparison of endoscopic ligation and propranolol for the primary prevention of variceal bleeding.

AUTHORS: Sarin S, Lamba G, Kumar M *et al.*
REFERENCE: N Engl J Med (1999) 340, 988–93.
STUDY DESIGN: RCT
EVIDENCE LEVEL: 1b

Key message
In patients with high-risk oesophageal varices, endoscopic ligation of the varices is safe and effective for the primary prevention of variceal bleeding.

Impact
This study highlighted the superiority of variceal banding. As beta (β)-blockers are inexpensive and generalists are able to prescribe them, some guidelines still recommend non-selective β-blockers as the first-line treatment for primary prevention of variceal bleeding. In subjects who are intolerant to or non-compliant with β-blocker therapy, prophylactic variceal banding is now an established intervention.

Aims
β-blockers and endoscopic variceal ligation have independently been shown to decrease the risk of first-episode variceal bleeding. This study compared propranolol therapy with banding for the primary prevention of variceal bleeding.

Methods
Patients: 89 patients at one centre in India.

Inclusion criteria: Patients with large varices that were at high risk of bleeding:
- Varices >5mm diameter;
- At least one 'red sign' (cherry-red spot, red wale, haematocystic spot).
- No history of haematemesis or melaena.

Exclusion criteria:
- Concomitant hepatoma;
- On antiviral therapy;
- Contraindications to β-blockers.

Groups:
- Propranolol group: 40mg/d, to increase daily until resting heart rate decreases by 25% of the baseline (or systolic BP <80mmHg, HR <55) (n=44);
- Band ligation group: 3–9 bands placed in the lower 5–7cm of variceal columns. Procedure was repeated weekly to obliterate varices (n=45).

Primary endpoint: Variceal bleeding.

Secondary endpoints:
- Transfusion requirement;
- Death.

Follow-up: 18 months.

Results

Primary endpoints	Propranolol (n=44)	Banding (n=45)	*p*
Cumulative probability of variceal bleeding in 18 months	43%	15%	0.04
Secondary endpoints			
No. of patients needing blood transfusion	1	7	0.03
Mean no. of transfusions per patient	0.1	0.4	0.03
Proportion of patients hospitalised	27%	11%	0.09
Deaths	11%	11%	0.8

Discussion

Although β-blockers have proven efficacy in preventing bleeding from varices, they have a variable and unpredictable effect on hepatic venous pressure gradient (HVPG), and hence the portal pressure. β-blocker therapy needs to be given for prolonged periods, and long-term non-compliance raises the risk of bleeding to pre-treatment levels. In addition, contraindications and intolerance limit the use of propranolol. This study showed endoscopic variceal ligation to be more effective and safer than sclerotherapy. Varices could be obliterated within about a month. Therefore, ligation offered a distinct advantage over lifelong β-blocker therapy. In this study, risk of bleeding was lower with ligation than with propranolol. No serious complication occurred due to banding, but two patients in the propranolol group stopped treatment due to side effects.

Problems

- The efficacy of β-blockers in patients without cirrhosis is less established. When patients without cirrhosis were excluded (leaving 41 patients in each group), actuarial probability of bleeding was 43% in propranolol group and 17% in banding group (not significant; *p*=0.08).
- There may be ethnic variations in the metabolism of propranolol which, in turn, may influence its efficacy. Therefore, the findings of this study may not be entirely applicable to a Caucasian population.
- The costs of each strategy were not compared.

GI bleeding with cirrhosis: antibiotic prophylaxis

Antibiotic prophylaxis for the prevention of bacterial infections in cirrhotic patients with gastrointestinal bleeding: a meta-analysis.

AUTHORS: Bernard B, Grange J, Khac E *et al.*
REFERENCE: Hepatology (1999) 29, 1655–61.
STUDY DESIGN: Meta-analysis
EVIDENCE LEVEL: 1a

Key message

In patients with cirrhosis and upper gastrointestinal (GI) bleeding, antibiotic prophylaxis for 7d significantly increases short-term survival.

Impact

This meta-analysis showed, for the first time, that systemic antibiotic prophylaxis improved survival in patients with cirrhosis and GI haemorrhage. Benefits gained by this simple and inexpensive measure are comparable to endoscopic interventions in their importance. Current guidelines recommend antibiotic prophylaxis in these patients.

Aims

Bacterial infections complicate 35–66% of GI bleeding episodes in patients with cirrhosis, and these predict rebleeding and poor outcome. The aim of this meta-analysis was to assess the efficacy of antibiotic prophylaxis in the prevention of infections and its effect on survival rates in patients with cirrhosis and upper GI bleeding.

Methods

Trials: Five trials (534 patients).

Inclusion criteria: Prospective randomised trials:
- Patients with cirrhosis and GI bleeding.

Exclusion criteria:
- Trials comparing two different treatments;
- Trials including patients without GI bleeding.

Groups:
- Antibiotic group: treatment for 4–10d (n=264);
- No antibiotic group (n=270).

Follow-up: Mean of 12d.

Primary endpoints:
- Proportion of patients free of infection;
- Proportion of patients free of spontaneous bacterial peritonitis;
- Proportion of patients surviving.

Results

Primary endpoints	No antibiotic prophylaxis	Antibiotic prophylaxis	p
Proportion free of infection	55%	86%	<0.001
Proportion free of spontaneous bacterial peritonitis	87%	95%	0.006
Proportion of patients surviving	76%	85%	0.004

Discussion

Although the incidence of infections, including spontaneous bacterial peritonitis, varied between trials, the efficacy of antibiotic prophylaxis was clearly established. Benefits were more marked in patients with more severe liver disease. Sensitivity analysis suggested that absorbable antibiotics were superior. Antibiotic prophylaxis also increased the mean survival rate by 9% (95% CI 2.9 to 15.3%). Considering the fact that overall mortality in cirrhosis with upper GI bleeding can be up to 30%, the benefits of antibiotic prophylaxis were highly significant. The risk of short duration of treatment (4–10d) seems to be very low. Development of resistant strains in those receiving antibiotics was not observed. Moreover, one study demonstrated that the cost of antibiotic prophylaxis was lower than the cost of treatment of infection.

Problems

- There was significant heterogeneity between the control groups for the proportion of individuals free of infection or spontaneous bacterial peritonitis. This was due to variations in the severity of underlying liver disease included in the different trials.
- Data on adverse events of treatment were not consistently recorded in the trials.

Alcoholic hepatitis: pentoxifylline

Pentoxifylline improves short-term survival in severe acute alcoholic hepatitis: a double-blind, placebo-controlled trial.

AUTHORS: Akriviadis E, Botla R, Briggs W et al.
REFERENCE: Gastroenterology (2000) 119, 1637–48.
STUDY DESIGN: RCT
EVIDENCE LEVEL: 1b

Key message

Treatment with pentoxifylline decreases the development of hepatorenal syndrome and improves short-term survival in patients with severe acute alcoholic hepatitis.

Impact

This study has raised awareness among non-specialist clinicians regarding the distinction between acute alcoholic hepatitis and decompensated cirrhosis. It has provided an incentive for accurate diagnosis and active management of these patients.

Aims

About 40–50% of patients with severe alcoholic hepatitis die within 3 months, a prognosis worse than breast, colon, prostate, or lung cancer. Tumour necrosis factor (TNF) is an important mediator of inflammation in alcoholic hepatitis. Pentoxifylline, an inhibitor of TNF synthesis, is a relatively inexpensive and safe drug that has been shown to improve short-term outcome in these patients. This study aimed to investigate whether pentoxifylline could improve outcomes in this condition.

Methods

Patients: 101 patients at one centre in the USA.

Inclusion criteria: Patients admitted with the diagnosis of alcoholic hepatitis:
• Jaundice;
• Maddrey discriminant factor (DF) ≥32 (DF=bilirubin in mg/dL+prothrombin time above control in seconds x 4.6);
• ≥1 of the following: tender hepatomegaly, fever, leucocytosis, hepatic encephalopathy, hepatic bruit.

Exclusion criteria:
• Chronic low dose aspirin use;
• Bacterial infection;
• Active gastrointestinal bleeding;
• Severe cardiac or respiratory disease.

Groups: Both groups received 400mg drug or placebo tds:
• Pentoxifylline group (n=49);
• Placebo group (n=52).

Primary endpoints:
- Short-term survival;
- Progression to hepatorenal syndrome.

Follow-up: 4wk treatment and review at 5wk from entry into the trial.

Results

Primary endpoints	Placebo	Pentoxifylline	p
In-hospital (28d) deaths	46.1%	24.5%	0.04
Development of hepatorenal syndrome	34.6%	8.2%	0.002

Discussion

Alcoholic hepatitis has a dismal short-term prognosis. If these patients survive complications in the short term, then abstinence from alcohol consumption allows remarkable recovery in a proportion of patients with good long-term survival. Therefore, improving short-term survival is important. Hepatorenal syndrome is a common complication of alcoholic hepatitis leading to death. It is plausible that TNF is a key contributor to the development of this complication. Although pentoxifylline is a weak inhibitor of TNF, its efficacy in preventing hepatorenal syndrome demonstrated in this study was impressive. If these results were reproduced in a larger, better characterised cohort of patients, then pentoxifylline would be a very useful and feasible intervention in alcoholic hepatitis.

Problems

- Liver biopsies were not performed. Reliability of clinical criteria for the diagnosis of alcoholic hepatitis is debatable.
- There was no significant difference in the course of TNF levels between the two groups, which does not support the initial hypothesis. However, survivors had a lower rise in TNF levels compared with non-survivors.
- Significantly more patients withdrew from the pentoxifylline group due to adverse effects (14% vs 2%; $p=0.028$). However, patients generally tolerate pentoxifylline well in routine clinical practice.

Alcoholic hepatitis: corticosteroids

Corticosteroids improve short-term survival in patients with severe alcoholic hepatitis: individual data analysis of the last three randomised, placebo-controlled, double-blind trials of corticosteroids in severe alcoholic hepatitis.

AUTHORS: Mathurin P, Mendenhall L, Carithers RJ *et al.*
REFERENCE: J Hepatol (2002) 36, 480–7.
STUDY DESIGN: Meta-analysis
EVIDENCE LEVEL: 1a

Key message

In patients with severe alcoholic hepatitis (AH), corticosteroid therapy improves short-term survival. For every five patients treated, corticosteroids prevents one death.

Impact

This study argues that if patients are chosen for corticosteroid therapy using Maddrey discriminant factor (DF), then therapy proves to be effective. It is still unclear whether histological or clinical criteria should be used to diagnose AH. Use of Maddrey DF in clinical practice as well as corticosteroid therapy in this condition is increasing. However, debate regarding the role of corticosteroid continues to polarise opinions and clinicians.

Aims

RCTs that evaluated corticosteroids in AH had used a variety of definitions, inclusions, and exclusions. This study analysed individual data of patients with severe AH with Maddrey DF ≥32 from the last three trials to investigate the effect of corticosteroid treatment on short-term survival.

Methods

Trials: Three RCTs (215 patients).

Inclusion criteria:
- Severe AH with Maddrey DF ≥32 (DF=bilirubin in mg/dL + prothrombin time above control in seconds x 4.6);
- Diagnosis of AH based on clinical criteria or liver biopsy.

Exclusion criteria:
- Active peptic ulcer;
- Active infection.

Groups: Corticosteroid regime in three studies included prednisolone 60mg/d to taper 4wk or 40mg/d for 28d, and methylprednisolone 32mg/d for 28d:
- Corticosteroid group (n=113);
- Placebo group (n=102).

Primary endpoint: Survival at 28d.

Follow-up: 28d from the onset of treatment or death.

Results

Primary endpoint	Placebo	Corticosteroid	p
Proportion who survived at 28d	65.1%	84.6%	0.001
Secondary endpoint			
Median difference in Maddrey DF between d28 and d0	−16	−25	0.002

Discussion

Two meta-analyses evaluating the role of steroid therapy in AH had included trials that were too heterogenous and drew contradictory conclusions. This study highlighted factors regarding the case definition, assessment of severity, and exclusions that may explain these inconsistencies. Maddrey DF is a well validated measure of severity while hepatic encephalopathy correlates poorly with clinical outcome. Studies that included patients with encephalopathy failed to demonstrate benefits of steroid therapy. Similarly, the protective effect of steroids depends upon exclusion of patients with gastrointestinal bleeding. Using data from patients with Maddrey DF ≥32, the authors demonstrated that corticosteroid-treated patients had a higher survival in each individual trial included in the analysis. Benefit of treatment was highly significant overall. Multivariate analysis identified corticosteroid treatment ($p<0.01$) as an independent predictor of favourable outcome in these patients.

Problems

- Data from only three trials were suitable for analysis in contrast with 11 and 13 trials included in two previous meta-analyses.
- The definition of AH was based on histology in one trial while liver biopsy was not required in the other two. This adds significant heterogeneity to the study population.
- Protective effects of corticosteroid depend on exclusion of patients with gastrointestinal bleeding. One of the trials did not exclude these patients.

Ascites: fluid replacement following paracentesis

Randomised trial comparing albumin, dextran 70, and polygeline in cirrhotic patients with ascites treated by paracentesis.

AUTHORS: Gines A, Fernandez-Esparrach G, Monescillo A *et al.*
REFERENCE: Gastroenterology (1996) 111, 1002–10.
STUDY DESIGN: RCT
EVIDENCE LEVEL: 1b

Key message

In patients undergoing large volume therapeutic paracentesis, 20% albumin solution is the best plasma expander to prevent post-paracentesis circulatory dysfunction and associated complications.

Impact

This was one of the first studies to highlight the role of 20% albumin in the management of ascites and related complications. Albumin is now accepted as the best plasma expander in cirrhosis although there is incomplete agreement regarding the threshold for its use and the magnitude of its impact.

Aims

Large volume paracentesis with plasma volume expansion is an effective and safe therapy for tense ascites in cirrhosis. This study aimed to compare the efficacy of albumin, dextran 70, and polygeline in preventing post-paracentesis circulatory dysfunction and its consequences.

Methods

Patients: 289 patients at 12 hospitals in Spain, Italy, and Argentina.

Inclusion criteria: Patients with cirrhosis and tense ascites.

Exclusion criteria:
- Bilirubin >170micromol/L; prothrombin time <40%, platelets <40,000/mm^3, serum creatinine >280micromol/L;
- Gastrointestinal bleeding within the preceding month;
- Hepatocellular carcinoma;
- Respiratory, cardiac, or renal disease.

Groups: All groups had 8g/L of ascitic fluid drained. 50% of the dose was given within the first 2h and the rest 6–8h after paracentesis;
- Albumin group: 20% albumin solution (n=97);
- Dextran 70 group: 6g dextran 70 per 100mL dextrose solution (n=93);
- Polygeline group: 3.5% saline solution of polygeline (n=99).

Primary endpoint: Post-paracentesis circulatory dysfunction:
- Increase in plasma renin activity (PRA) of >50% of the pre-treatment value to a level of >4ng/mL/h.

Secondary endpoints: Clinical outcome in those with and without post-paracentesis circulatory dysfunction:

- Time to first readmission;
- Survival.

Follow-up: Up to 6 months.

Results

Primary endpoint	Albumin group	Dextran 70 group	Polygeline group	*p*
Proportion developing post-paracentesis circulatory dysfunction	18.5%	34.4%	37.8%	<0.02

Secondary endpoints	With post-paracentesis circulatory dysfunction	Without post-paracentesis circulatory dysfunction	*p*
Time for first readmission (mean in months)	1.3	3.5	0.03
Survival (mean in months)	9.3	16.9	0.01

Discussion

The study demonstrated that post-paracentesis circulatory dysfunction did not resolve spontaneously, but persisted during F/U. Amongst the three plasma expanders investigated, 20% albumin was least frequently associated with circulatory dysfunction. Although the number of patients studied was inadequate to detect significant differences in clinical endpoints between the groups, subgroup analysis confirmed that circulatory dysfunction was associated with poor clinical outcome during F/U. Circulatory dysfunction is characterised by marked activation of natriuretic systems and accentuated renal sodium retention, leading to rapid reaccumulation of ascites. Post-paracentesis circulatory dysfunction was also an independent predictor of survival.

Problems

- The majority of guidelines recommend therapeutic paracentesis in patients with refractory (diuretic-resistant or diuretic-intolerant) ascites. In this study, patients with tense ascites were recruited, irrespective of response to diuretic therapy.
- There were no significant differences in clinically important endpoints between the treatment groups. The study was powered to detect differences in post-paracentesis circulatory dysfunction between the treatment groups.

Coeliac disease: serological testing

Pre-endoscopy serological testing for coeliac disease: evaluation of a clinical decision tool.

AUTHORS: Hopper A, Cross S, Hurlstone D *et al.*
REFERENCE: BMJ (2007) 334, 729–32.
STUDY DESIGN: Cohort study
EVIDENCE LEVEL: 2a

Key message
Pre-endoscopy serology for tissue transglutaminase antibody (TTGA) followed by duodenal biopsy for those who are positive and those identified as 'high risk' (with weight loss, diarrhoea, or anaemia) with negative serology detects all cases of coeliac disease.

Impact
A decision tool that achieves 100% sensitivity in disease detection is a rare accomplishment. If validated in different cohorts, this algorithm will become standard practice.

Aims
Serological markers are cheap, non-invasive, and are suitable for use in primary care. The study aimed to develop an effective diagnostic method of detecting all cases of coeliac disease without using a combination of serological test and duodenal biopsy.

Methods
Patients: 1464 patients from one centre in the UK.

Inclusion criteria: Had both gastroscopy and duodenal biopsy.

Retrospective analysis and clinical decision tool developed:

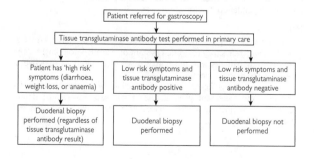

Results

Prospective evaluation of clinical decision tool:

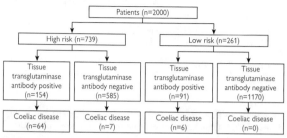

Hopper, A. D et al. BMJ 2007;334:729.

Discussion

Positive IgA antibody to tissue transglutaminase on its own was highly sensitive and specific for the diagnosis of coeliac disease. However, demonstration of villous atrophy on duodenal biopsy is the internationally accepted 'gold standard' diagnostic test. Because of antibody-negative coeliac disease, many centres recommend routine duodenal biopsy. The clinical decision tool evaluated in this study used a combination of pre-endoscopy serology and assessment of symptoms to improve the detection of coeliac disease without the need for routine endoscopic duodenal biopsy. The decision tool was derived using a large database of 1464 patients and validated in a prospective cohort of 2000 patients. Pre-endoscopy serology for TTGA followed by duodenal biopsy for those who were positive and those identified as 'high risk' (with weight loss, diarrhoea, or anaemia), irrespective of serology, detected all cases of coeliac disease in a cohort of 2000 patients. In 1170 low-risk patients with negative serology, none was found to have coeliac disease on duodenal biopsy. The strategy recommended by this study would significantly reduce the workload associated with processing and reporting duodenal biopsies. However, 60% of high-risk patients with positive serology did not have coeliac disease on duodenal biopsy, so it is essential that biopsy is performed in these patients. Alternatively, it could be argued that serology should only be performed in low-risk subjects and duodenal biopsy in those at high risk.

Problems

- Implementation of the decision tool has not been tested in primary care where prevalence of the disease will be lower.
- Inter-individual variability in assigning patients to the 'high risk' group was not considered in the study. This may reduce the performance of the decision tool.
- This is a single centre study. In a multicentre setting, variability of serological tests and reporting of duodenal biopsies may alter the performance of the decision tool.

Ulcerative colitis: ciclosporin

Randomised, double-blind comparison of 4mg/kg vs 2mg/kg intravenous ciclosporin in severe ulcerative colitis.

AUTHORS: Van Assche G, D'Haens G, Noman M *et al.*
REFERENCE: Gastroenterology (2003) 125, 1025–31.
STUDY DESIGN: RCT
EVIDENCE LEVEL: 1b

Key message
Intravenous (IV) low dose (2mg/kg) ciclosporin is as effective as high dose (4mg/kg) in the treatment of acute severe ulcerative colitis (UC).

Impact
Since the first report of its efficacy in 1990, ciclosporin therapy has remained the only alternative to colectomy in patients with acute severe colitis who fail to respond to IV corticosteroids. Lower dose therapy has the potential to reduce adverse effects and widen the use of ciclosporin therapy in these patients.

Aims
Intravenous corticosteroids remain the mainstay of treatment for acute severe flares of UC. However, in non-responders, IV ciclosporin had been demonstrated to be an alternative to colectomy. The first placebo-controlled trial of IV ciclosporin in acute severe colitis as well as several uncontrolled trials had used a starting dose of 4mg/kg over the first 24h. A lower dose of ciclosporin had also previously been used successfully in solid organ transplantation. This trial aimed to evaluate the additional clinical benefit of 4mg/kg over 2mg/kg IV ciclosporin dose in the treatment of acute severe UC.

Methods
Patients: 73 patients at a single centre in Belgium.

Inclusion criteria: Consecutive patients admitted for acute severe UC:
- Age 18–70y;
- Lichtiger clinical activity index ≥10.

Exclusion criteria:
- Serum creatinine >2mg/dL;
- Serum cholesterol <150mg/dL;
- Uncontrolled hypertension;
- Positive stool culture or *Clostridium difficile* toxin.

Groups: Both groups received continuous IV infusion of ciclosporin, and blood ciclosporin levels were maintained at 250–350ng/mL in the '4mg/kg' group and 150–250ng/mL in the '2mg/kg' group:
- 4mg/kg group (n=38);
- 2mg/kg group (n=35).

Primary endpoint: Proportion of patients with a clinical response.

Secondary endpoints:
- Time to response;
- Colectomy rates;
- Adverse effects.

Follow-up: Response assessed on d8 and colectomy rates on d14.

Results

Primary endpoint	4mg/kg	2mg/kg	*p*
Response rate	84.2%	85.7%	ns
Secondary endpoints			
Median time to response	4 (1–7)d	4 (1–8)d	ns
Colectomy rate within 14d	13.1%	8.6%	ns
New diastolic hypertension	23.7%	8.6%	<0.08
10% increase in serum creatinine	18.4%	17.1%	ns
Neurotoxicity	7.9%	5.7%	ns

Discussion

The value of ciclosporin therapy in acute severe UC is widely accepted, but concerns regarding toxicity have limited its use. Because most of the adverse effects of ciclosporin are dose-dependent, it is logical to recommend the lowest effective dose for treatment. This study showed that a higher dose of ciclosporin did not add any clinical benefit. Although no statistically significant difference in the frequency of adverse events was seen between the groups, this was likely to be due to a type 2 error. A trend towards the development of diastolic hypertension was seen in the high dose group. The blood levels of the drug were significantly different between the two groups, so it is logical to presume that if the sample size were bigger, a lower dose would have been shown to be less toxic.

Problems

- Only half of the patients in both groups were on concomitant corticosteroid therapy. Despite the evidence for the efficacy of ciclosporin as monotherapy, it is still reserved for steroid non-responsive patients in most centres.
- The sample size was too small to demonstrate the difference in adverse events between the two groups.

Crohn's disease: infliximab

Infliximab for the treatment of fistulas in patients with Crohn's disease.

AUTHORS: Present D, Rutgeerts P, Targan S et al.
REFERENCE: N Engl J Med (1999) 340, 1398–405.
STUDY DESIGN: RCT
EVIDENCE LEVEL: 1b

Key message
Infliximab is effective for the treatment of fistulae in patients with severe Crohn's disease (CD).

Impact
Infliximab and other biological agents are increasingly used in the management of patients with severe active CD, particularly when disease has proven refractory to treatment with corticosteroids and other immuno-modulating drugs. Infliximab maintenance therapy is now an established treatment for fistulising CD and selected patients without fistulae.

Aims
Enterocutaneous and perianal fistulae are common complications of CD and are difficult to treat. Medical treatments had otherwise proven ineffective, whereas surgery usually involved the formation of stomas—undesirable to most patients. Following reports that infliximab, a genetically constructed IgG1 murine-human chimeric monoclonal antibody against tumour necrosis factor-α (TNF-α), was safe and effective in the treatment of refractory CD, this double-blind, placebo-controlled trial was specifically designed to evaluate the efficacy of infliximab in healing established, enterocutaneous fistulae.

Methods
Patients: 94 patients from multiple centres in the USA and Europe.

Inclusion criteria
- Age 18–65y;
- Single or multiple abdominal or perianal fistulae of ≥3 months duration, as a complication of CD.

Exclusion criteria:
- Concurrent treatment with ciclosporin;
- Other complications of CD (e.g. current strictures or abscesses);
- No recent surgery or stoma formation (within previous 6 months);
- Previous treatment with infliximab *or* known allergy to murine proteins.

Groups
- IV infliximab (5mg/kg at wk 0, 2, and 6) (n=31);
- IV infliximab (10mg/kg at wk 0, 2, and 6) (n=32);
- Placebo (n=31).

Primary endpoint: Reduction of ≥50% in the number of draining fistulae at two consecutive visits.

Secondary endpoints:
- Complete response (absence of any draining fistulae);
- Duration of response;
- Measures of disease activity;
- Incidence of adverse events.

Follow-up: Clinical and laboratory assessments at wk 2, 4, 10, 14, and 18.

Results

Primary endpoint	5mg/kg	10mg/kg	Placebo
At least 50% response	68%*	56%*	26%
Secondary endpoints			
Complete response	55%*	38%*	13%
Duration of response (median)	84d	99d	86d
Disease activity (median score)	108%	111	171
Adverse events (any)	65%	84%	65%

* Statistically significant difference from placebo (p<0.05).

Discussion

Infliximab is a monoclonal antibody against TNF-α, a cytokine implicated in the pathogenesis of various chronic inflammatory conditions, including CD and rheumatoid arthritis. These data suggested, for the first time, that infliximab was effective not only in achieving remission in patients with severe, refractory CD (as shown in previous studies), but also in healing CD-related enterocutaneous and perianal fistulae. The larger (306 patients across 45 centres) ACCENT II trial *(N Engl J Med* (2004) 350, 876–85) confirmed these findings, and demonstrated that infliximab infusion every 8wk was effective in keeping CD fistulae dry over a period of 1y, leading to an improved quality of life. Those who lose response during maintenance therapy with 5mg/kg of infliximab may respond to 10mg/kg.

Problems

- The median duration of response after three doses of infliximab was approximately 3 months. Subsequent trials have shown that repeated doses can maintain fistula healing for longer periods of time.
- Although no serious adverse events were reported, concerns have been raised about the possibility of serious infection, autoimmune reaction, and even carcinogenesis associated with infliximab. Careful monitoring of patients and auditing of adverse reactions is essential.
- Infliximab is expensive; this study was not designed to evaluate its cost-effectiveness. Future studies should also include economic analyses.
- Only patients with CD were recruited. However, subsequent studies have demonstrated the efficacy of infliximab in the management of ulcerative colitis.

Hepatitis B: lamivudine

CALM (**C**irrhosis **A**sian **L**amivudine **M**ulticentre) study: Lamivudine for patients with chronic hepatitis B and advanced liver disease.

AUTHORS: Liaw Y, Sung J, Chow W *et al.*
REFERENCE: N Engl J Med (2004) 351, 1521–31.
STUDY DESIGN: RCT
EVIDENCE LEVEL: 1b

Key message
In patients with chronic hepatitis B, treatment with lamivudine delays the development of hepatic decompensation and hepatocellular carcinoma.

Impact
The current study offers great promise because of the large benefit observed after treatment with lamivudine, although the development of the genotypic resistance tyrosine, methionine, aspartate, aspartate (YMDD) mutation reduced overall benefit. Hence, strategies to counter the development of mutations are necessary to realise the maximum benefits of antiviral therapy in chronic hepatitis B.

Aims
Worldwide, there are about 450 million chronic carriers of hepatitis B virus (HBV). About 1.2 million die annually from HBV-related liver disease. Lamivudine suppresses HBV, reduces hepatic necro-inflammation, and improves liver function. This trial aimed to assess the efficacy of lamivudine in reducing the clinical progression of chronic hepatitis B.

Methods
Patients: 651 patients at 41 sites across Australia, China, Hong Kong, Malaysia, New Zealand, Philippines, Singapore, Taiwan, and Thailand.

Inclusion criteria: Chronic hepatitis B with advanced fibrosis on liver biopsy (Ishak score ≥4):
- Age >16y;
- Positive hepatitis B surface antigen;
- Positive HBeAg or detectable HBV DNA.

Exclusion criteria: Complications of cirrhosis at study entry:
- Hepatocellular carcinoma;
- Renal insufficiency;
- Bleeding varices;
- Spontaneous bacterial peritonitis.

Groups: Both groups received 100mg/d of the drug or placebo:
- Lamivudine (n=436);
- Placebo (n=215).

Primary endpoint: First occurrence of any of the following:
- An increase of ≥2 points in Child-Pugh score;
- Spontaneous bacterial peritonitis;
- Renal insufficiency;

- Variceal bleeding;
- Hepatocellular carcinoma;
- Death related to liver disease.

Follow-up: The study was terminated after a median duration of treatment of 32.4 months (0–42 months).

Results

Primary endpoints	Placebo	Lamivudine	*p*
Overall disease progression	17.7%	7.8%	0.001
Increase in Child-Pugh score	8.8%	3.4%	0.02
Hepatocellular carcinoma	7.4%	3.9%	0.05

- No significant difference between the two groups for other endpoints.

Discussion

The study was stopped early because of large differences between the two groups with respect to primary endpoints. However, the number of endpoints observed in this study was inadequate to demonstrate potential improvements in survival. In 49% of patients in the lamivudine group and 5% in the placebo group, YMDD mutation emerged during the study period. Once this occurred, patients with YMDD mutations were more likely to develop complications of cirrhosis compared with those unaffected. However, patients with YMDD mutations still had fewer complications compared with the placebo group (11% vs 18%; $p>0.05$). So the authors concluded that YMDD mutations reduced the benefits of lamivudine without negating them altogether.

Problems

- Five cases of hepatocellular carcinoma were diagnosed during the first year, suggesting that these may have been missed at the time of entry into the study. When these cases were excluded, the HR was 0.47 (95% CI 0.22 to 1.00; $p=0.052$).
- The study was terminated, based on interim analysis. There were insufficient numbers of patients who reached important endpoints such as renal insufficiency or variceal bleeding. There were no liver-related deaths in either group.
- The emergence of YMDD mutation, an inevitable outcome with lamivudine monotherapy, significantly reduced the benefits of treatment. It is likely that lamivudine could only delay the complications of cirrhosis in the long term.
- The high cost of long-term treatment.

Hepatitis C: peginterferon and ribavirin

Peginterferon α-2b plus ribavirin compared with interferon α-2b plus ribavirin for initial treatment of chronic hepatitis C.

AUTHORS: Manns M, McHutchison J, Gordon S *et al.*
REFERENCE: Lancet (2001) 358, 958–65.
STUDY DESIGN: RCT
EVIDENCE LEVEL: 1b

Key message

The combination of peginterferon and ribavirin is the most effective therapy for chronic hepatitis C. The benefit of this combination is most significant in patients with genotype 1 infections.

Impact

The addition of the polyethyleneglycol molecule to interferon allowed more convenient once-weekly dosing, making treatment more acceptable to patients. Peginterferon also contributed to a significant increase in sustained virological response (SVR) rates, in particular for genotype 1 infection, otherwise the least responsive genotype. Combination of peginterferon and ribavirin has replaced the conventional interferon-based treatment for chronic hepatitis C.

Aims

The most effective initial therapy for patients with chronic hepatitis C virus (HCV) infection had been demonstrated to be a combination of interferon A-2b plus ribavarin. Pegylation produces a biologically active molecule with a longer half-life and more favourable pharmacokinetics. This study aimed to assess the safety and efficacy of two different regimens of peginterferon A-2b plus ribavirin vs conventional interferon A-2b plus ribavirin.

Methods

Patients: 1530 patients at 62 centres in Europe, Canada, Argentina, and the USA.

Inclusion criteria: Previously untreated chronic hepatitis C:
- HCV RNA detectable in serum by PCR;
- Liver biopsy within 1y consistent with chronic hepatitis;
- Elevated alanine aminotransferase.

Exclusion criteria:
- Low haemoglobin, white blood cell count, platelet count;
- Decompensated cirrhosis, raised α-fetoprotein, previous transplantation;
- HIV infection;
- Pre-existing psychiatric disease, seizure disorders.

Groups:
- High-dose peginterferon group: Peginterferon α-2b 1.5mcg/kg/wk plus ribavirin 800mg/d (n=511);

- Low-dose peginterferon group: Peginterferon α-2b 1.5mcg/kg/wk for 4wk followed by 0.5mcg/kg/wk plus ribavirin 1000–1200mg/d (n=514);
- Interferon group: Interferon α-2b 3MU three times per wk plus ribavirin 1000–1200mg/d (n=505).

Primary endpoint: SVR defined as detectable HCV RNA in serum at the end of F/U.

Follow-up: Treatment was for 48wk, and patients were followed up for 24wk after the end of therapy.

Results

Primary endpoints	High-dose peginterferon	Low-dose peginterferon	Interferon	p
SVR at the end of treatment (all patients)	65%	56%	54%	<0.001
SVR at the end of F/U (all patients)	54%	47%	47%	0.01
Genotype 1	42%	34%	33%	0.02
Genotype 2/3	82%	80%	79%	0.5
Genotype 4/5/6	50%	33%	38%	0.7

Discussion

This large RCT demonstrated that combination of high-dose peginterferon and ribavirin treatment significantly increased the SVR rates compared with a conventional interferon-based regime. In this study, SVR reported with the conventional interferon group was higher than expected. Despite this, peginterferon-based treatment was clearly superior. In addition, SVR was associated with a decrease in hepatic inflammation on liver biopsy. The benefit of high-dose peginterferon was most apparent in those with genotype 1 infection, which generally responds poorly to antiviral therapy. The side effect profiles were similar between groups. As compliance is a major factor in determining SVR rates in these patients, ease of once-weekly injection of peginterferon is a distinct advantage.

Problems

- All patients were treated for 48wk, so the efficacy of a shorter duration of treatment in genotype 2 and 3 patients could not be evaluated.
- Peginterferon α-2b-based treatment did not lower the frequency of adverse reactions.

Genitourinary medicine

Introduction

The name 'genitourinary medicine' replaced venereology in the UK 32 years ago. What used to be called venereal disease (VD) in the 19th and 20th centuries referred to syphilis, gonorrhoea, and chancroid—still the legally defined VD. The devastating effect of syphilis on the British army (33% of sick cases) prompted government legislation (the Contagious Diseases Act 1864) to force prostitutes to be examined for VD and admitted to Lock hospitals for treatment. Meanwhile, 'normal' hospitals shunned VD. After widespread protests against its iniquity, the Act was repealed in 1886. Lobbying by various interested medical, social, and feminist campaigners produced a Royal Commission enquiry from 1913 to 1916, followed in 1917 by the development of public services which were free, confidential, and open to anyone.

Despite the success of the VD service and subsequent incorporation into the UK's National Health Service, sexually transmitted disease (STD) clinics, venereologists, and those affected by STD continued to be stigmatised. The name 'genitourinary medicine' was chosen to minimise the stigma and to reflect changing epidemiology as STDs with genitourinary manifestations overshadowed the legally defined VDs. Elsewhere, the specialty is part of dermato-venereology or other disciplines such as infectious diseases.

Since the advent of HIV infection, many genitourinary medicine specialists have also undertaken the management of HIV and AIDS. There is also a move towards closer links or integration with contraception/family planning under the umbrella of sexual health. Advances in diagnostic technology and treatment continue to make this specialty as fascinating and satisfying as ever, combining the science of medicine with the art of clinical practice.

Syphilis: antibiotic treatment

Doxycycline compared with benzathine penicillin for the treatment of
early syphilis.

AUTHORS: Ghanem K, Eberlding E, Cheng W *et al.*
REFERENCE: Clin Infect Dis (2006) 42, 45–9.
STUDY DESIGN: Case-control study
EVIDENCE LEVEL: 3

Key message
Doxycycline (100mg bd for 14d) is an effective treatment for early syphilis.

Impact
The results of this study support the use of an oral regimen for treatment of early syphilis as an alternative to parenteral penicillin.

Aims
Although doxycycline was considered the preferred second-line treatment of syphilis, there had been no controlled trial data of its efficacy.
Previous observational studies on small numbers of patients had shown
>90% response to doxycycline treatment, and data published in the 1950s
had demonstrated the efficacy of chlortetracycline and oxytetracycline.
This study aimed to provide more substantial evidence for the use of a
2wk oral doxycycline (100mg bd) regime.

Methods
Patients: Retrospective study of patients treated for primary, secondary,
or early latent syphilis between October 1993 and June 2000 at two public
sexually transmitted disease clinics in the USA. Study patients drawn from
a total of 1558 patients treated with either doxycycline (100mg bd PO for
14d) or a single dose of benzathine penicillin (BPG, 2.4MU IM).

Inclusion criteria:
- Diagnosed using the Centre for Disease Control (USA) criteria;
- Age ≥18y;
- Reactive rapid plasma reagin (RPR) test (a serological, non-treponemal
  test to look for antibodies) confirmed by reactive fluorescent trepo-
  nemal antibody absorption test before treatment;
- Clear documentation of complete treatment;
- Documented treponemal serology results at the time of treatment and
  ≥1 F/U serology titre 270–400d after treatment.

Groups:
- Doxycycline (n=34);
- Benzathine penicillin (n=73).
- Demographic/clinical features evenly distributed: 56% female; 98% black;
  45% symptomatic; 28% contacts of syphilis; 32% (group 1) and 19%
  (group 2) early latent; 6% (group 1) and 13% (group 2) HIV positive;
  85% with rapid plasma reagin (RPR)>1:16.

Primary outcome: Serological response (failure defined as the lack of 4-fold drop in RPR titre 270–400d after treatment *or* a 4-fold increase in RPR titre 30–400d after treatment, without evidence of re-infection on the basis of health adviser records).

Secondary outcome: Time to 4-fold drop in RPR titre.

Follow-up: Until a serology titre was recorded 270–400d after treatment. Median number of serology titres recorded=3 (doxycycline group) and 2.8 (BPG group).

Results

	Doxycycline (n=34)	BPG (n=73)
Serological failure (%, 95% CI)	0 (0%, 0 to 10.3%)	4 (5.5%, 1.6% to 13.8%)
Median time to serological response (95% CI)	106d (75 to 149d)	137d (111 to 172d)

- No significant differences between groups in serological failure (after excluding re-infection) or time to serological response in responders;
- Two of the four failures were HIV-positive. There were no relapses.

Discussion

This study provided reassuring data on the efficacy of doxycycline in comparison with BPG in the treatment of early syphilis. These findings were consistent with previous reports from uncontrolled studies. The failure in the BPG group was consistent with the range reported in previous studies. Re-infection in these cases was not categorically excluded despite careful study of the records.

Problems

- The 107 patients evaluated were only about 40% of all those screened to be eligible; therefore, the results may not represent the population at large. The loss to F/U is unlikely to have biased the results as it was equal in both groups.
- Only 40% of patients treated with doxycycline and 37% of randomly selected penicillin-treated controls had F/U serological tests to enable evaluation of treatment efficacy.
- While a larger controlled trial is necessary for head-to-head comparison of doxycycline with parenteral penicillin, such a study is not feasible because of the strong evidence available for the efficacy of parenteral penicillin regimens.

Gonorrhoea: antibiotic resistance

GRASP (<u>G</u>onococcal <u>R</u>esistance to <u>A</u>ntimicrobial <u>S</u>urveillance <u>P</u>rogramme).

AUTHORS: Fenton K, Herring A, Ison C *et al.*
REFERENCE: GRASP Annual Report, Year 2000 collection; 1–30.
STUDY DESIGN: Systematic Review
EVIDENCE LEVEL: 1a

Key message

National monitoring of patterns of antibiotic resistance in *Neisseria gonorrhoea* (gonococcus, GC) ensures that there is still effective treatment for this disease in the UK.

Impact

Intense monitoring of GC antibiotic resistance since 2000 detected an increasing resistance to fluroquinolones which had previously been extensively used to treat GC. In 2005, treatment was switched to cephalosporins, and so far, GC remains susceptible to these antibiotics. An annual update on GC antibiotic resistance is now produced.

Aims

GC antibiotic resistance first appeared in the UK in the early 1990s. However, until the first GRASP study, reports of resistance had been *ad hoc* and provided limited data. By centralising the collection of GC isolates, it became possible to determine a national demographic pattern of antibiotic resistance, and thus provide appropriate information about which antibiotic to use. This review presented the results of this data collection.

Methods

GC isolates: 2987 collected over 3 months.

Inclusion criteria:
- Genitourinary medicine (GUM) clinics with close working relationships with local microbiology laboratories;
- Any patient diagnosed with GC during the 3 months collection period (June–August 2000);
- Two monitoring laboratories: Genitourinary Infections Reference Laboratory (GUIRL), Bristol; Imperial College, London.

Groups:
- GUM clinics in London (13);
- GUM clinics outside London (17).

Primary endpoint: Resistant antibiotic and type of resistance (i.e. plasmid or chromosomally acquired).

Secondary endpoints: Clinical characteristics of patients infected with GC (e.g. age, sexual behaviour).

Results

Primary endpoints	London	Non-London	p
Total number of isolates	1988	999	–
Penicillin resistance	168 (8.5%)	110 (11.0%)	0.004
Ciprofloxacin resistance	18 (0.81%)	37 (3.70)	0.0005
Ceftriaxone resistance	0 (0%)	0 (0%)	–
Secondary endpoints			
Gay/bisexual men	25% of GC	19% of GC	Not reported

Discussion

Unlike previous investigations, the GRASP study provided data for England and Wales about both GC antibiotic resistance and the epidemiology of the disease. The advantage of this methodology was that it made information available about disease transmission and high-risk groups, and therefore, could be used in health promotion. This study also showed the advantages of collaboration between the clinician, laboratory scientist, and epidemiologist.

Problems

- As this was an annual study, it could have missed a rapidly emerging antibiotic-resistant isolate.
- This study required good collaboration between GUM clinics and microbiology laboratories. Therefore, data collection was limited to London teaching hospitals and large metropolitan areas elsewhere. This may have led to sample bias.
- Seasonal bias may have stemmed from the time period during which samples were acquired (June to August 2000). It is possible that characteristics of these patients are different from those who become infected at other times of the year.

Chlamydia: antibiotic treatment

A controlled trial of a single dose of azithromycin for the treatment of chlamydial urethritis and cervicitis.

AUTHORS: Martin DH, Mroczkowski TF, Dalu Z *et al.*
REFERENCE: N Engl J Med (1992) 327, 921–5.
STUDY DESIGN: RCT
EVIDENCE LEVEL: 1b

Key message

A single 1g dose of oral azithromycin is as effective as a 7d course of doxycycline in the treatment of uncomplicated genital chlamydia infection.

Impact

Single dose oral azithromycin should be considered as first-line therapy to reduce rates of treatment failure as a result of non-compliance with multi-dose regimens.

Aims

Traditional treatment of genital chlamydia infection with 7d multi-dose regimens of doxycycline or erythromycin is associated with high rates of non-compliance, especially among asymptomatic patients. Azithromycin, an azalide antibiotic, has good *in vitro* activity against *Chlamydia (C.) trachomatis,* with substantial bioavailability and a long tissue half-life. This trial evaluated the efficacy and safety of a single 1g dose of oral azithromycin compared to the standard 7d course of doxycycline (100mg bd) for the treatment of uncomplicated genital tract chlamydia infection.

Methods

Patients: 457 patients from 12 centres in the USA.

Inclusion criteria: Attendees at sexual health, college student and adolescent health, and family planning clinics:
- Age >16y;
- Positive *C. trachomatis* antigen test;
- No evidence of complicated infection (epididymitis, salpingitis);
- No systemic antibiotic therapy within 72h of enrolment.

Groups: Open-labelled, no placebo group. Antibiotics commenced 48h after examination and culture specimens for chlamydia (men—urethra, women—urethra and endocervix):
- Azithromycin (1g on d1) (n=237: 85 male, 152 female);
- Doxycycline (100mg bd for 7d) (n=220: 73 male, 147 female).

Primary endpoint: Bacteriological cure (negative *C. trachomatis* culture result at F/U).

Secondary endpoints:
- Complete resolution of signs and symptoms (clinical cure);
- No significant adverse effects with azithromycin.

Follow-up: At 5–11d, then at 12–20d, and finally at 31–35d.

Results

- Patients with negative culture at initial visit were excluded from analysis of biological and clinical outcomes (hence, only 141 (azithromycin) and 125 (doxycycline) patients included).

Primary endpoint	Azithromycin (n=141)	Doxycycline (n=125)
Bacteriological cure	136 (96%)	122 (98%)
Secondary endpoints		
Clinical cure—Male	97%	91%
Female	98%	95%
Adverse side effects	41/237 (17%)	43/220 (20%)

Discussion

A previous study had demonstrated 98% efficacy for azithromycin given as a single 1g dose against uncomplicated genital chlamydia infection. This trial, comparing that same dose to the standard doxycycline treatment, showed similar efficacy. Azithromycin was as effective as doxycycline, and its use as a first-line agent overcame the problems of non-compliance associated with multi-dose regimens. Azithromycin was well tolerated with only occasional gastrointestinal side effects (similar to doxycycline).

Problems

- Clinical cure is very subjective, and the higher rates in the azithromycin group may be related to its efficacy against organisms other than chlamydia which also cause urethritis.
- Not all patients attended the three F/U sessions. Some were only assessed at the first F/U (d5–11 after treatment) when the majority of patients that failed treatment were detected. Could this have been too soon to assess?

Cervical cancer: human papillomavirus vaccine

> **FUTURE II** (**F**emales **U**nited **T**o **U**nilaterally **R**educe **E**ndo/
> **E**ctocervical disease) **study:** Quadrivalent vaccine against human pap-
> illomavirus to prevent high-grade cervical lesions.
>
> **AUTHORS:** The FUTURE II Study Group.
> **REFERENCE:** N Engl J Med (2007) 356, 1915–27.
> **STUDY DESIGN:** RCT
> **EVIDENCE LEVEL:** 1b

Key message

High-grade cervical lesions associated with human papillomavirus (HPV)
16 and 18, such as cervical intraepithelial neoplasia (CIN) (grade 2 and
3) and adenocarcinoma *in situ*, could be prevented by the use of a quadrivalent HPV 6/11/16/18 vaccine.

Impact

Mass vaccination of female children and adolescents who have yet to be
infected with HPV 16 and 18 is likely to reduce related cervical disease,
including cervical carcinoma. Vaccination programmes have already been
approved and are being rolled out in several countries.

Aims

Cervical cancer is the second most common malignancy in women worldwide. It accounts for large numbers of deaths each year, particularly in
developing countries that have not yet been able to effectively implement
the Papanicolaou (Pap) smear screening programme (often due to its cost).
Up to 70% of cervical cancers are caused by infection with human papillomavirus (HPV) 16 and 18. Prophylactic vaccines had been developed using
virus-like particles (VLPs). However, their efficacy had not been evaluated
in RCTs. The aim of this trial was to demonstrate the efficacy of one such
vaccine against high-grade cervical lesions attributed to HPV 16 and 18.

Methods

Patients: 12,167 women at 90 study sites in 13 countries.

Inclusion criteria:
- Women aged 15–26y;
- Not pregnant at enrolment;
- No abnormal results on Pap smear;
- Lifetime number of no more than four sexual partners.

Groups: Double-blinded study. Both groups received injections at d1,
month 2, and month 6:
- Quadrivalent vaccine to HPV 6/11/16/18 (with aluminium adjuvant)
  (n=6087);
- Placebo (containing aluminium) (n=6080).

Primary endpoint: CIN grade 2 or 3; adenocarcinoma *in situ*; or invasive carcinoma of the cervix, with the detection of DNA from HPV 16, HPV 18, or both, in ≥1 of three adjacent biopsy specimens of the same abnormal cervical lesion sampled at colposcopy.

Analysis: Case ascertainment 1 month after the third dose of vaccine or placebo:
- Subjects with negative results on DNA and serological testing for HPV 16 and 18 at enrolment and remained DNA negative 1 month after the third dose;
- Received all doses within 1y;
- No protocol violations (e.g. pregnancy).

Follow-up: Medical history/gynaecological examination, cervical samples for Pap testing and ano-genital swabs at six sites for HPV DNA testing at first-day visit. F/U at 1 and 6 months after third injection; then at months 24, 36, and 48. Abnormal cervical lesions referred for colposcopy.

Results

HPV 16/18 associated lesions (populations)	Vaccine group	Placebo group	Vaccine efficacy
Subjects in per protocol	1/5305	42/5260	98%
Subjects in unrestricted	3/5865	62/5863	95%
Subjects in intention-to-treat	83/6087	148/6080	44%

Discussion

This trial demonstrated 98% vaccine efficacy in preventing HPV 16 and 18 related high-grade cervical lesions over a 3y period. However, this was only the case in those patients who had not been previously exposed to those virus subtypes. The efficacy decreased to just 44% when those previously exposed were included. Therefore, it is only useful as a prophylactic vaccine and the target population should be those who have yet to become sexually active. In the short term, the vaccination appeared safe with very few initial side effects.

Problems

- Only effective against HPV 16 and 18; no effect against other HPV types that can cause neoplasia (will not completely eradicate cervical carcinoma and may open a niche for other subtypes).
- Does immunity wane and will a booster dose be required? A 15y F/U study is underway.

Genital warts: immunomodulator cream

Topical imiquimod 5% cream in external anogenital genital warts.

AUTHORS: Arican O, Guneri F, Bilgic K et al.
REFERENCE: J Dermatol (2004) 31, 627–31.
STUDY DESIGN: RCT
EVIDENCE LEVEL: 1b

Key message

Imiquimod, a novel immunomodulator, is an effective and reliable treatment for external genital warts.

Impact

Imiquimod will result in complete clearance of external genital warts in over two thirds of patients, if used for up to 12wk. It has minimal side effects with low recurrence rates. It is an ideal treatment in patients who have had recurrent episodes of warts and are looking for a treatment they can use safely at home.

Aims

Standard treatments for warts, including ablative methods such as cryotherapy, electrosurgery, and chemical destruction with trichloracetic acid and podophyllin, have little impact on viral clearance and infectivity, with limited success and high recurrence rates. This study aimed to assess the effects of a novel immunomodulator, imiquimod.

Methods

Patients: 45 patients (each with ≥5 external genital warts) from three centres in Turkey.

Inclusion criteria:
• Age >18y;
• No wart treatment in the last 3 months (local or systemic);
• No serious systemic/immunosuppressive disorder, drug and alcohol dependence, or frequently occurring genital herpes.

Groups: Double-blind trial. Both groups applied medicament three times a week, every other day for 12wk:
• Imiquimod 5% cream (n=23 male, 11 female);
• Placebo (vaseline cream) (n=9 male, 2 female).

Primary endpoint: Clearance rates greater than placebo.

Follow-up: Full blood count, biochemistry, HIV, syphilis serology, and pregnancy test at first visit. Lesions mapped, location and duration of warts recorded. F/U monthly for 6 months, and then at the end of therapy (either at 12wk or earlier, if clearance had occurred) for re-mapping of lesions and side effect assessment.

Results

Clearance		0–10%	11–50%	51–99%	Complete
Imiquimod	Male	–	4.5%	40.9%	54.5%
	Female	–	–	–	100%
Placebo	Male	87.5%	–	–	12.5%
	Female	50%	–	50%	–

- Differences between placebo and treatment group statistically significant ($p<0.001$);
- Resolution of warts most common wk 6–12 in the treatment group, female patients demonstrating an earlier improvement;
- Imiquimod was more effective at clearing warts in the perianal region than at other genital sites;
- Side effects occurred in 55% of the treatment group (mainly erythema due to immune response associated with lesion resolution).

Discussion

Imiquimod 5% cream was more effective than placebo, with complete clearance rates of 69.7% vs 12.5%. However, success rates were lower than with ablative techniques. Advantages of imiquimod include a low reccurrence rate (18.2%) with tolerable side effects, resulting in no patients prematurely terminating treatment—cryotherapy and surgery can be painful and leave scarring. This trial demonstrated imiquimod to be a safe and effective alternative that patients could use as a home treatment.

Problems

- Although the two groups were matched for age and duration of warts, there were low numbers of patients in the placebo group and the ratio of females to males were considerably different. A higher, more equitable ratio in the placebo group may have influenced the results.
- Cost-effectiveness was not discussed within this study. At present, imiquimod cream is much more expensive than the other treatment options, and is hence often only prescribed in patients with frequent recurrences.

Genital herpes simplex: antiviral therapy

Valaciclovir vs acyclovir in the treatment of first-episode genital herpes infection.

AUTHORS: Fife K, Barbarash R, Rudolph T *et al. (*Valaciclovir International Herpes Simplex Virus Study Group).
REFERENCE: Sexually Transmitted Diseases (1997) 24, 481–6.
STUDY DESIGN: RCT
EVIDENCE LEVEL: 1b

Key message
A twice-daily dose of valaciclovir (VACV), a pro-drug of acyclovir (ACV), is as effective and well tolerated as the latter, given five times daily in the treatment of the first episode of genital herpes.

Impact
The results of this study have led to the introduction of a twice-daily regimen—more convenient than the five times daily dosing of ACV.

Aims

ACV had been in use for a decade as an effective and well tolerated drug for the treatment of the first episode of genital herpes, after early RCTs had shown evidence of its efficacy. VACV, the L-valine ester pro-drug of ACV, had been demonstrated to be better absorbed than ACV, with more rapid and complete metabolism to ACV. This study aimed to determine whether twice-daily VACV was more efficacious than the standard five times daily regimen of ACV in treating patients with first presentations of genital herpes simplex virus (HSV).

Methods
Patients: 643 patients from 54 sites (mostly student sexually transmitted disease or family planning clinics) in the USA, UK, and Australia.

Inclusion criteria:
- Age >18y;
- First clinical episode of genital herpes;
- Presenting within 72h of lesion onset.

Exclusion criteria:
- Pregnant or breastfeeding;
- HIV antibody-positive.

Groups: Double-blinded study.
- VACV (1g: 2 tablets bd) and placebo (1 capsule 5x/d), for 10d (n=323);
- ACV (200mg: 1 capsule 5x/day) and placebo (2 tablets bd) for 10d (n=320).

Primary endpoints: Time to healing of all lesions and duration of viral shedding.

Secondary endpoints: (see table below). Intention-to-treat (ITT) analysis of all 643 patients for primary endpoints and adverse events, and subset analysis of 605 HSV-confirmed patients for all endpoints.

Follow-up: Lesions staged as macule/papule, vesicle, ulcer, or healed. Lesion swabs for culture taken on d1, 2, 3, 5, 7, 10, and 14, and thereafter 2x weekly (if needed) until full healing. HSV 1 and 2 antibody test on d1 and 14. Clinical laboratory studies at baseline, d1 and d7 (haemoglobin, white and platelet cell counts, creatinine and liver enzymes).

Results

Efficacy Endpoints		Median (mean)		HR (95% CI)	p
		VACV	ACV		
Days to healing	ITT	9 (9.2)	9 (9.5)	1.08 (0.92 to 1.27)	0.4
	HSV+	9 (9.3)	9 (9.5)	1.08 (0.91 to 1.27)	0.4
Duration of viral shedding, d	ITT	3 (3.7)	3 (4.1)	1 (0.84 to 1.18)	1.0
	HSV+	3 (3.9)	3 (4.3)	1.01 (0.85 to 1.2)	0.9
Duration of pain, d	HSV+	5 (5.3)	5 (5.3)	1 (0.85 to 1.18)	1.0
Days to resolution of symptoms	HSV+	9 (10.9)	9 (10.6)	1.02 (0.85 to 1.22)	0.9
Proportion with new lesions at 48h	HSV+	0.217	0.241	–	Not reported
Maximum no. of lesions	HSV+	8 (10.5)	8 (12.1)	–	Not reported

- **Side effects:** no difference between groups—headache in 41 (VACV) and 33 (ACV); nausea in 18 (VACV) and 20 (ACV);
- **Lab tests:** no adverse changes in either group.

Discussion

Despite previous pharmacokinetic data showing VACV (1g bd) to produce three times as much ACV exposure as ACV (200mg 5x daily), the clinical efficacy of the two agents in this study did not differ significantly. There was also no difference in the type, incidence, and severity of adverse events. This study, with the largest number of patients evaluated, added further evidence for the use of thymidine kinase inhibitors in the treatment of first episode genital herpes.

Problems

- No placebo control. However, previous placebo-controlled trials had already established the efficacy of ACV.
- Study was not powered to detect <10% difference, but such a difference would be clinically insignificant.

Genital herpes: prevention of outbreaks

A meta-analysis to assess the efficacy of oral antiviral treatment to prevent genital herpes outbreaks.

AUTHORS: Lebrun-Vignes B, Bouzamondo A, Dupuy A et al.
REFERENCE: J Am Acad Dermatol Med (2007) 57, 238–46.
STUDY DESIGN: Meta-analysis
EVIDENCE LEVEL: 1a

Key message

Oral acyclovir (ACV), famciclovir (FCV) and valaciclovir (VACV) for prophylaxis against recurrent episodes of genital herpes of high clinical efficacy.

Impact

As the first meta-analysis on the topic, this study strengthens the evidence base for continuous suppressive regimens of the three antiviral agents for the prevention of genital herpes outbreaks. Implications include a positive impact on individual health-related quality of life, economic benefit, and reduced transmission at community level.

Aims

This meta-analysis aimed to compare the clinical efficacies of three oral antiviral drugs (oral ACV, FCV, and VACV), already established as suitable for prophylaxis against recurrent episodes of genital herpes.

Methods

Databases searched: Medline, EMBASE, and Cochrane controlled trials register.

Inclusion criteria:
- Placebo-controlled RCT;
- Study patients not immunocompromised or pregnant;
- No reviews or cross-over trials;
- Oral prophylactic treatment;
- Study endpoint to include the number of patients developing ≥1 episode of disease recurrence during the trial;
- Article in English.

Data extraction: The following items were extracted from each RCT:
- Number and characteristics (sex, mean age) of patients included;
- Frequency of recurrences chosen for inclusion;
- Treatment duration;
- Antiviral drug used and evaluated total daily dose and regimen;
- Number of recurrence-free patients.

Statistics: The pooled estimate of the global RR of recurrence during the trials was calculated for each study using the inversed variance-weighted RR in a fixed model. This yielded bilateral 95% CI for trials and for the meta-analysis.

Results
- **Baseline:**
  - 14 trials evaluated: 10 ACV, 2 FCV, 3 VACV (1 both ACV and VACV);
  - 6,158 patients evaluated.
- **RR:**
  - Significant benefit of oral ACV, FCV, or VACV (RR ranging from 0.16 to 0.73);
  - RR of developing recurrence reduced by 47% (95% CI=45 to 49%).
- **NNT**=2.15 (95% CI=2.06 to 2.25).
- **Regimens:** The following regimens showed efficacy:
  - ACV: 200mg 2–5x/day, 400mg bd, or 800mg od;
  - VACV: 250mg od or bd, 500 or 1,000mg od;
  - FCV: 125 or 250mg, bd or tds;
  - Higher doses of VACV and FCV were more effective;
  - The best regimens were ACV 200mg qds or 400mg bd, VACV 250mg bd or 500mg od, and FCV 250mg bd;
  - VACV 500mg od appeared to be better than FCV 250mg bd in suppression of recurrent episodes and associated viral shedding;
  - ACV 400mg bd and VACV 500mg bd were equally efficacious.
- One of the RCTs was continued as open study for 5y after the controlled phase and reported sustained efficacy.
- **Side effects:**
  - Minor/transient adverse effects such as nausea, diarrhoea, and headache were not significantly associated with any of the three antivirals vs placebo.
  - No serious adverse effects were attributable to these oral regimens in a long-term F/U study (up to 9y).

Discussion
This evidence, along with other studies showing improvement in genital herpes-associated psychosocial morbidity and the possible reduction in infection transmission to an uninfected partner, supports the use of prophylactic suppressive antiviral treatment against recurrent genital herpes. Long-term studies showing good tolerance are also encouraging.

Problems
- Only English language articles were included in the analysis. However, the only non-English article excluded also showed efficacy for a bd ACV regimen.
- Duration of F/U in most studies was relatively short, except for one that provided long-term open-label F/U data on efficacy and tolerance.
- Data on interruption of transmission to uninfected sexual partners remain scarce.

Pelvic inflammatory disease: inpatient vs outpatient treatment

PEACH (Pelvic Inflammatory Disease Evaluation and Clinical Health) study: Effectiveness of inpatient and outpatient treatment strategies for women with pelvic inflammatory disease.

AUTHORS: Ness R, Soper D, Holley R *et al.*
REFERENCE: Am J Obstet Gynecol (2002) 186, 929–37.
STUDY DESIGN: RCT
EVIDENCE LEVEL: 1b

Key message

The first RCT to show similar rates of pregnancy and complications among women with mild to moderate pelvic inflammatory disease (PID) treated with a cephalosporin and doxycycline, in either the outpatient or inpatient setting.

Impact

Women presenting with mild to moderate PID can be treated as outpatients rather than being admitted to a gynaecology ward.

Aims

A cephalosporin and doxycycline combination is effective treatment for women with mild to moderate PID. However, these women have previously been treated in hospital despite the potential to give these two antibiotics orally in an outpatient setting. This study was designed to compare the effectiveness of outpatient and inpatient treatments in both short- and long-term management.

Methods

Patients: 831 women at 13 sites (including emergency departments, clinics, and sexually transmitted disease units) throughout Eastern, Southern, and Central USA.

Inclusion criteria: Clinically suspected PID:
- Age 14–37y and able to attend F/U (homeless patients excluded);
- A history of pelvic discomfort for a period of ≤30d;
- Pelvic organ (uterine or adnexal) tenderness on vaginal examination;
- Leucorrhoea and/or mucopurulent cervicitis and/or untreated known positive gonococcal or chlamydial cervicitis.

Exclusion criteria:
- Pregnant or foetal termination/delivery in previous 14d;
- Gynaecological surgery in previous 14d or previous hysterectomy/bilateral salpingectomy;
- Antimicrobial agent use within previous 7d;
- Allergy to study medications or vomited after anti-emetic treatment;
- Suspected tubo-ovarian abscess/other condition requiring surgery.

Groups:
- Inpatient treatment: cefoxitin (second generation cephalosporin, 2g qds IV), doxycycline (100mg bd IV for minimum 48h), then doxycycline (100mg bd PO for 14d) (n=409);
- Outpatient treatment: single dose of cefoxitin (2g IM), plus probenecid (1g PO), then doxycycline (100mg bd PO for 14d) (n=422).

Primary endpoints: Frequency of (and time to) documented pregnancy (i.e. positive urine/blood test (β-HCG), doctor's diagnosis, or live birth).

Secondary endpoints: <u>Short-term:</u> Change in treatment; tubo-ovarian abscess; adverse reaction; phlebitis; tender on examination at 30d; gonorrhoea, chlamydia, or endometritis at 30d. <u>Long-term:</u> Involuntary infertility (1y of unprotected intercourse without conception); self-reported repeat PID; hysterectomy; ectopic pregnancy; chronic pelvic pain; evidence of tubal obstruction by HSG (hysterosalpingogram).

Follow-up: At d5 and 30; then at 3 monthly intervals in the first year; thereafter every 4 months, until study end. Gynaecological examination, and cervical and endometrial specimens performed at the 30d visit. Subsequent F/U generally conducted by telephone.

Results

Primary endpoint	Inpatient	Outpatient	p
Pregnancy	41.7%	42%	1.0
Secondary endpoints			
Neisseria gonorrhoea	2.4%	2.7%	0.4
Chlamydia trachomatis	3.6%	2.7%	0.5
Ectopic pregnancies	0.3%	1.0%	0.4
Tubal obstruction	33.3%	41.2%	0.7
Chronic pelvic pain	29.8%	33.7%	0.3
Involuntary infertility	17.9	18.4%	0.9

Discussion

Previous studies which only evaluated short-term outcomes of treating women with mild to moderate PID in an outpatient setting had shown excellent rates of microbiological cure, but varying rates of clinical cure (72% to 97%). This larger and longer study, which compared the short- and long-term outcomes of women treated either as inpatients or outpatients, demonstrated no significant difference between the groups.

Problems

- Participants were primarily recruited from inner city medical centres and therefore, were mainly low-income African-American women—not representative of all women who develop mild to moderate PID.
- PID is a difficult clinical diagnosis with definitive confirmation only possible in less than two thirds of cases. Gonorrhoea and chlamydia were excluded in the majority of women in this study (66% of outpatients and 60% of inpatients), suggesting either that their symptoms were not due to PID or were due to mild PID most likely to respond to outpatient therapy.

Bacterial vaginosis: antibiotic treatment

Vaginal clindamycin and oral metronidazole for bacterial vaginosis.

AUTHORS: Paavonen J, Mangioni C, Martin M *et al.*
REFERENCE: Obstet Gynecol (2000) 96, 256–60.
STUDY DESIGN: RCT
EVIDENCE LEVEL: 1b

Key message
Clindamycin is an effective and better tolerated alternative to metronidazole in the treatment of bacterial vaginosis (BV) with similar cure rates.

Impact
Clindamycin is used in women with metronidazole allergy and in cases of metronidazole-resistant BV. An oral preparation has been used to try to prevent preterm labour in pregnancy.

Aims
BV is a vaginal infection that may cause an offensive vaginal discharge. It is linked with pelvic infections following abortions, normal deliveries, and transvaginal hysterectomies. In pregnancy, it is associated with late miscarriages and preterm labour. Metronidazole is the standard treatment for BV. However, it has unpleasant side effects, including a disulfiram-like adverse reaction when taken with alcohol. This trial aimed to compare the effectiveness and safety of clindamycin (vaginal ovules containing 100mg clindamycin) with standard therapy (oral metroniadazole) in women suffering from BV.

Methods
Patients: 233 women from 23 centres in Europe.

Inclusion criteria: Laboratory criteria of BV:
- Vaginal discharge of pH >4.5;
- Presence of clue cells on wet mount slide;
- Fishy amine odour from vaginal discharge after adding 10% potassium hydroxide (positive amine test).

Groups:
- Clindamycin (100mg ovules intravaginally for three consecutive days) plus placebo (capsules bd PO for 7d) (n=113);
- Metronidazole (500mg bd PO for 7d) plus placebo (ovules intravaginally for 3d) (n=120).

Primary endpoint: Overall clinical outcome: cure (resolution of amine odour and clue cells at F/U visit), failure, adverse effect failure (i.e. stopped treatment due to side effects), and non-assessable (i.e. insufficient data to categorise as cure or failure).

Secondary endpoints: Side effects and patient evaluation.

Follow-up: At 12–16d and 28–42d after the start of treatment. A vulvovaginal examination was performed, with vaginal discharge described. Diagnostic tests for positive amine and clue cells were repeated.

Results

Primary endpoint	Clinical status	Clindamycin (n=113)	Metronidazole (n=120)	*p*
1st and 2nd F/U visit	Cured	77 (68.1%)	80 (66.7%)	0.8
1st F/U visit	Cured	98 (86.7%)	102 (85.7%)	1.0
	Clinical failure	13 (11.5%)	15 (12.6%)	–
	Adverse effect failure	2 (1.8%)	2 (1.7%)	–
	Non-assessable	0	1	–
2nd F/U visit	Cured	85 (78.7%)	87 (76.3%)	0.7
	Clinical failure	23 (21.3%)	27 (23.7%)	–
	Non-assessable	5	6	–
Secondary endpoints				
Side effects		21 (10.3%)	32 (16.3%)	0.1
Patient evaluation	Cured	83/106 (78.3%)	90/103 (79.6%)	–

Discussion

Other trials had also shown 3d regimens of intravaginal clindamycin to be as effective as oral metronidazole for treating BV with better tolerance. This study also showed that overall cure rates remained acceptable for both agents up to 6wk after the start of treatment. This finding is based on the number of women who were defined as cured at both F/U visits. In other studies, cure rates were calculated from the number of participants at each visit. Both agents have also been shown to be efficacious for treating BV in pregnancy, with treatment before 20wk gestation reducing the incidence of preterm birth—a complication associated with infection (*Cochrane Database of Systemic Reviews 2007, Issue 1*).

Problems

- 399 women were originally enrolled, but only 233 (58%) were found to be eligible after proper assessment. However, the authors claimed there were enough participants to make the study statistically viable.
- The study involved the use of ovules, a clinical preparation of clindamycin not in common use.
- Each participating centre determined instances of BV themselves rather than using a central assessor(s). However, because some of the criteria used to diagnose BV are subjective, it is possible that some women were misdiagnosed and wrongly included (and vice versa).

Geriatric medicine

Introduction

The medicine of older people is plagued with manifestations of the Inverse Care Law—that those in most need of medical care are least likely to receive it. There is a prejudice that Geriatric Medicine is simple. Yet the reality is of routine complexity—a result not least of multiple causation, chronic fluctuating course, and attendant functional and social factors. Such complex aetiology mandates multifactorial assessments and multi-factorial interventions.

Complexity sits disguised beneath a simple veneer—the predominant geriatric presentations of immobility, instability, incontinence, and cognitive impairment invite a hasty, restricted response. But outcomes are optimised only when the covert issues beneath the wrapper are considered, sought, and treated. And what outcomes! There is nothing more important to the patient or rewarding to the doctor than enhancing functional independence or enabling a return home.

Therapeutic responses are often dominated by apathy (non-engagement, for example catheterising an undiagnosed incontinent patient), sympathy (platitudes, but feeble medicine) or antipathy (overt or covert criticism). The missing factor is empathy: in this context, the empathetic response is of diagnostic and therapeutic action. Worryingly, the former ineffectual responses are now codified in a health and social care system that emphasises care rather than diagnosis and cure. The epidemics of frailty and other geriatric syndromes demand the highest levels of diagnostic and therapeutic precision; yet contemporary management dogma is to keep older people out of hospital and expedite their discharge home if that threshold is crossed.

The naïve view of disease in older people leads to the notion—often implemented—that 'anyone can do it'. But experience—and increasingly evidence—shows that many cannot. Not all older people need the skills of a geriatrician or specialist geriatric team, but appropriate skills must either be embedded within systems managing older people, or else effective screening tools developed that enable non-specialists to recognise patients who benefit from more specialist assessment.

A further paradox is that older people as a group face the greatest burden of disease, and stand to benefit most from quality research—yet there is less of it. Determining the effect of complex interventions on heterogeneous populations afflicted by complex disease is inherently difficult, and is made more so by high fatality, difficult follow-up, and cognitive impairment. Such 'difficult' patients are routinely excluded from trials that seek answers to simpler—but less common and less important—clinical questions.

Atrial fibrillation: warfarin therapy

BAFTA (**B**irmingham **A**trial **F**ibrillation **T**reatment of the **A**ged) **study:** Warfarin vs aspirin in an elderly community population with atrial fibrillation.

AUTHORS: Mant J, Hobbs F, Fletcher K *et al.*
REFERENCE: Lancet (2007) 370, 493–503.
STUDY DESIGN: RCT
EVIDENCE LEVEL: 1b

Key message
Compared with aspirin, warfarin is as safe and more effective in preventing stroke in elderly people with atrial fibrillation (AF).

Impact
This widely applicable trial should lead to an increased uptake of warfarin, an effective stroke prevention treatment, in a population in which it has previously been underutilised.

Aims
AF is a common arrhythmia in older people and a strong risk factor for stroke. Warfarin is effective in reducing this risk, but the perceived risk of bleeding in older people had limited its use. This large study aimed to assess the efficacy of warfarin compared with aspirin in a primary care population of elderly patients with AF.

Methods
Patients: 973 patients from 234 general practices in England and Wales.

Inclusion criteria:
- Age >75y;
- AF or atrial flutter on ECG within the previous 2y.

Exclusion criteria:
- Rheumatic heart disease;
- Major non-traumatic haemorrhage in the previous 5y;
- Intracranial haemorrhage;
- Oesophageal varices or recent proven peptic ulcer disease;
- Terminal illness;
- Surgery in past 3 months;
- Blood pressure >180/110mmHg.

Primary endpoint: Composite of first occurrence of fatal or non-fatal disabling stroke (ischaemic or haemorrhagic), any other intracranial haemorrhage, or clinically significant arterial embolism.

Secondary endpoints:
- Major extracranial haemorrhage;
- Other admissions to hospital with haemorrhage;
- All-cause mortality.

Follow-up: Mean F/U=2.7y.

Results

Primary endpoint	Warfarin (annualised no. of events)	Aspirin (annualised no. of events)	RR (95% CI) Warfarin vs aspirin
Stroke, other intracranial haemorrhage, or systemic embolism	24 (1.8%)	48 (3.8%)	0.48 (0.28 to 0.80)
Secondary endpoints			
Major extracranial haemorrhage	18 (1.4%)	20 (1.6%)	0.87 (0.43 to 1.73)
Other admissions to hospital with haemorrhage	24 (1.8%)	19 (1.5%)	1.22 (0.64 to 2.36)
All-cause mortality	107 (8.0%)	108 (8.4%)	0.95 (0.72 to 1.26)

Discussion

Given its setting (in primary care) and its pragmatic approach to monitoring control (patients had their international normalised ratio measured and controlled according to local protocols), this trial reflects widespread primary care practice and addressed a gap in the evidence for treatment. Physicians should now be more willing to prescribe warfarin to older people as the benefits are clear and the risks of treatment low. Although the trial was not powered to show a difference, the low rates of haemorrhage were also reassuring.

Problems

Assessment of risk vs benefit in the individual patient remains difficult. Older people with AF vary enormously in their risk of ischaemic stroke (e.g. higher in those with structural heart disease or previous embolism) and their risk of haemorrhage (e.g. higher in those who fall). Although this trial saw an overall advantage of treatment, subgroups may have gained no benefit or else been harmed by warfarin.

Falls: multifactorial intervention

PROFET (**PR**evention **O**f **F**alls in the **E**lderly **T**rial)

AUTHORS: Close J, Ellis M, Hooper R et al.
REFERENCE: Lancet (1999) 353, 93–7.
STUDY DESIGN: RCT
EVIDENCE LEVEL: 1b

Key message
Multidisciplinary assessment and intervention reduce disability and the risk of further trauma in older people presenting with a fall.

Impact
As a result of this study (and others that developed its findings), the UK National Institute for Health and Clinical Excellence (NICE) recommends that all older people at risk of falls should undergo an individualised multifactorial intervention, including strength and balance training, home hazard reduction, optimisation of vision, and review of medication. Specialist falls services for older people are now widely developed.

Aims
The cost of falls is high: to the individual, they represent physical and psychological trauma, loss of independence, and even death; to the health service, they include a high cost and bed occupancy. Previous management of falls had commonly focused on dealing with the injury itself. However, this approach fails to address the root of the problem. This study aimed to examine whether patients would benefit from a systematic assessment of the underlying causes and functional consequences of falls.

Methods
Patients: 397 patients at the Emergency Department (ED) of one UK teaching hospital.

Inclusion criteria:
- Patients presenting with a fall to the ED;
- Aged ≥65y.

Exclusion criteria:
- Significant cognitive impairment: abbreviated mental test score (AMTS) <7;
- No regular carer or not local, thereby hampering postal F/U.

Groups:
- Control: standard management (ED letter to GP who assessed or referred for specialist assessment, if considered appropriate) (n=213);
- Intervention (n=184);
  - Medical assessment (vision, cardiovascular and neurological status, balance, cognition);
  - Occupational therapy: home assessment and intervention visit (removal or modification of hazards, provision of equipment).

Primary endpoint: Total reported number of falls.

Secondary endpoints:
- Proportion of patients unable to go out alone;
- Serious injury from falls.

Follow-up: By postal questionnaire at 4, 8, and 12 months.

Results

Primary endpoint	Control (n=163)	Intervention (n=141)	p
Total reported falls	510	183	0.0002
Secondary endpoints			
Able to go outside alone	106 (65%)	108 (77%)	0.04
Serious injury	16 (8%)	8 (4%)	0.05

- Bidisciplinary assessment resulted in many referrals to outpatients, geriatric day hospital, optician, or general practitioner (e.g. for drug modification). In only 16% of assessments was no further action required.

Discussion
There are myriad causes of falls in older people; each fall is usually the result of the interplay between several factors—both patient-centred ('intrinsic' factors, e.g. drugs, impaired vision, poor footwear) and environmental ('extrinsic' factors, e.g. poor lighting, trip hazards). Therefore, the most effective interventions are likely to be those that screen for multiple causes and intervene on an individual basis, depending on the relevant risk factors for each individual. Such 'individualised multifactorial intervention' is at the heart of most contemporary falls prevention programmes. Unlike this study, most protocols include a programme of muscle strengthening and balance retraining delivered by a nurse specialist, occupational therapist, or physiotherapist.

Problems
- Although such interventions reduce falls, much less is known about their effects on fall-related injuries.
- Those with significant cognitive impairment were excluded from this study, as consent would be more difficult and recall of falls impaired. This exclusion is unfortunate as many older people who fall have a dementia syndrome, and the combination of falls and dementia is a frequent reason for long-term institutional care. Although interventions are more challenging in people with dementia, comorbidities which impact on falls risk are more frequent, and these individuals are likely to benefit from environmental interventions.

Falls: vitamin D

Effect of vitamin D on falls.

AUTHORS: Bischoff-Ferrari H, Dawson-Hughes B, Willett W *et al.*
REFERENCE: JAMA (2004) 291, 1999–2006.
STUDY DESIGN: Meta-analysis
EVIDENCE LEVEL: 1a

Key message
Vitamin D supplements significantly reduce falls in elderly people living at home or in care homes, in addition to their known beneficial effect on bone mineral density.

Impact
Administration of vitamin D (with calcium) to elderly people at high risk of falls is now standard practice in most specialist clinical settings, although this treatment is not prescribed routinely to all elderly people. The UK's National Institute for Health and Clinical Excellence (NICE) falls prevention guidance was unfortunately published too early to consider this meta-analysis.

Aims
Falls are common in older people and lead to injury, institutional care, and sometimes death. There are theoretical benefits of vitamin D on both bone density and muscle strength, but studies of vitamin D to prevent falls have given inconsistent results. This analysis sought to synthesise all published evidence of high quality and arrive at a conclusion of greater confidence than any single trial could achieve.

Methods
Search strategy: Systematic review of all English and non-English articles using Medline, EMBASE, and the Cochrane Controlled Trials Register. Additional contact with experts, and searches of reference lists and abstracts.

Eligible studies:
- **Design:** Double-blind RCTs;
- **Intervention:** Any type of vitamin D compared with matching placebo;
- **Population:** Elderly people living in the community or institutional care;
- Must include a definition of a fall and how falls were ascertained.

Ineligible studies:
- Uncontrolled or observational studies;
- Studies focusing on those with alcoholism or unstable health, e.g. following acute hospitalisation;
- Unacceptable methodological quality.

Primary outcome:
- Relative risk of having ≥1 fall.

Results

Systematic review identified 38 potentially relevant trials. These were screened independently by three investigators. A total of 33 were excluded according to the criteria above, leaving five studies involving 1,237 participants suitable for the primary outcome analysis. Outcomes were analysed on an intention-to-treat basis.

Data synthesis:
- Corrected pooled odds ratio (OR) for vitamin D supplementation preventing a person from falling was 0.78 (95% CI 0.64 to 0.92).
- Pooled risk difference was 7% (95% CI 2 to 12%), giving an NNT of 15.
- The inclusion of a further five trials (trials that failed to define a fall or those in unstable patients) in the meta-analysis did not alter the study conclusions.
- Subgroup analysis demonstrated that effect size was independent of:
  - Type of vitamin D;
  - Calcium supplementation;
  - Duration of therapy or F/U.

Discussion

Falls were remarkably common, affecting 16–63% of participants in the included trials. Older people are at risk of vitamin D deficiency due to nutritional issues and lack of exposure to sunlight. The mechanism of action of vitamin D on muscle is uncertain, but other studies have detected prompt improvements in body sway and strength. This study did not detect an effect of including calcium with vitamin D. However, other studies suggest that the beneficial effect of vitamin D is lost in those with poor dietary calcium intake. Therefore, recommended preparations include Adcal-D$_3$® or Calcichew D$_3$ Forte®; two tablets each day provide calcium 1g and cholecalciferol 800 units.

Problems

- The most clinically effective dose and formulation is uncertain, as is the cost-effectiveness of targeting supplementation based on pre-treatment vitamin D levels.
- Calcium preparations are often poorly tolerated. Explaining the rationale for treatment and exploring alternatives such as dispersible tablets may improve compliance.

Delirium in hospital

Reducing delirium after hip fracture.

AUTHORS: Marcantonio E, Flacker J, Wright R et al.
REFERENCE: J Am Geriatr Soc (2001) 49, 516–22.
STUDY DESIGN: RCT
EVIDENCE LEVEL: 1b

Key message
Proactive patient assessment by specialists in elderly care reduces delirium ('acute brain failure').

Impact
This is one component of a broad spectrum of evidence which supports a geriatric approach to the acutely unwell older person, including those with hip fracture. The UK National Services Framework (NSF) for Older People states 'at least one general ward in an acute hospital should be developed as a centre of excellence for orthogeriatric practice'. Several trials have described and compared different models of orthogeriatric care. There is no single effective model, but all seek to place appropriately skilled specialists (geriatricians, surgeons, anaesthetists, nurses, and therapists) close to the patient at critical points in the care pathway. Nevertheless, implementation of this guidance is incomplete; in many UK hospitals, patients only receive reactive specialist medical care.

Aims
Delirium (often referred to as 'acute confusional state' or 'acute brain failure') is a transient global disorder of cognition, and is common after hip fracture, affecting up to 50% of patients. It results from the interplay of a brain with limited cognitive reserve (or one manifesting overt dementia) and extra-cerebral factors such as drug administration, fluid depletion, pain, and an unfamiliar environment. Delirium is often severe and associated with adverse long-term cognitive and physical outcomes. This trial aimed to determine whether proactive involvement of elderly care specialists would reduce incidence of acute brain failure.

Methods
Patients: 126 patients at the orthopaedic unit of a large tertiary US hospital.

Inclusion criteria:
● Admitted emergently for surgical repair of hip fracture;
● Age >65y.

Exclusion criteria:
● Metastatic cancer;
● Life expectancy <6 months secondary to comorbid condition(s).

Groups:
● Reactive: Management by orthopaedic team, with reactive involvement of medical or geriatric specialists, if requested by orthopaedic team (n=64);

- Proactive: Daily assessment by geriatrician (beginning preoperatively, where possible) with targeted recommendations based on structured protocol (n=62). The most commonly applied interventions were:
  - Optimisation of O_2 delivery, fluid/electrolyte balance, nutrition;
  - Treatment of pain;
  - Reduction in unnecessary medications;
  - Early mobilisation;
  - Early prevention, identification, and treatment of complications.

Primary endpoint: Cumulative incidence of delirium.

Secondary endpoints:
- Cumulative incidence of severe delirium;
- Length of stay.

Follow-up: Daily assessment until discharge. No longer term F/U. Assessor blinded to treatment allocation.

Results

Endpoint	Reactive	Proactive	p
Delirium (cumulative)	50%	32%	0.04
Severe delirium (cumulative)	29%	5	12%
Length of stay (days)	5	0.02	0.4

Discussion

This study showed that multifactorial intervention, addressing basic but important aspects of care, results in a reduced incidence of brain failure in an at-risk population. This result has been replicated in studies from other settings. The nature of the intervention suggests that it might be delivered effectively, at least in part, by other suitably trained doctors (including surgeons) or by specialist nurses.

Problems

- The proactive consultation service provided advice only. Adherence to that advice by the orthopaedic team was highly variable—ranging from 32–100% for common interventions. Improved adherence may increase the power of the intervention.
- F/U was short-term. Impact on longer term outcomes (including cognition, residency status, and physical dependency) is unknown. There was no financial evaluation.
- Future studies should test the application of these results to other clinical settings, and the extent to which the interventions can be optimised and delivered by other health professionals.

Mild cognitive impairment: preventing progression

Vitamin E and donepezil for the treatment of mild cognitive impairment.

AUTHORS: Petersen R, Thomas R, Grundman M *et al.*
REFERENCE: N Engl J Med (2005) 352, 2379–88.
STUDY DESIGN: RCT
EVIDENCE LEVEL: 1b

Key message

Donepezil and vitamin E are not effective in preventing progression from mild cognitive impairment (MCI) to Alzheimer's disease (AD).

Impact

The prospect of dementia terrifies patients and carers, who often take empiric over-the-counter medication (e.g. vitamin E) in an attempt to prevent its onset. This trial highlighted the difficulties in design of clinical trials in the prevention of AD, and the limitations of treatment. It gave clinicians and patients strong evidence that drugs currently offer no useful effect on progression.

Aims

MCI is an acquired cognitive impairment that does not interfere significantly with daily activities, and therefore, does not meet the diagnostic criteria for a dementia syndrome. People with MCI progress to AD at a rate of 10–15% per year, although such progression is not inevitable. This study aimed to determine if treatment with vitamin E or donepezil could delay the diagnosis of AD in subjects with the amnestic form of MCI.

Methods

Patients: 769 patients from 69 centres across the USA.

Inclusion criteria: Age 55–90 with:
• Amnestic form of MCI, with significantly impaired memory;
• Clinical Dementia Rating 0.5 (i.e. very mild dementia symptoms);
• Mini-Mental State Examination (MMSE) score 24–30.

Exclusion criteria:
• Significant cerebrovascular disease (modified Hachinski score >4);
• Depression (Hamilton Depression Rating Scale >12);
• Central nervous system infarct or infection, or focal lesions on brain scan;
• Medical or psychiatric disease that could interfere with participation;
• Restrictions on concomitant use of medication with potential adverse cognitive effects.

Primary endpoint: Development of possible or probable AD.

Secondary endpoints:
• MMSE;
• AD assessment scale (cognitive subscale);
• Global Clinical Dementia Rating;

- Mild Cognitive Impairment Activities of Daily Living Scale;
- Global Deterioration Score;
- Neuropsychological battery of tests.

Follow-up: 36 months.

Results

Primary endpoint		HR	95% CI	p
Donepezil vs placebo	12 months	0.42	0.24 to 0.76	0.004
	36 months	0.80	0.57 to 1.13	0.2
Vitamin E vs placebo	12 months	0.83	0.52 to 1.32	0.4
	36 months	1.02	0.47 to 1.41	0.9

- There were no sustained differences at 3y between donepezil and placebo or vitamin E and placebo in any of the secondary outcomes.

Discussion

The trial showed the neccesity of adequate F/U in this type of prevention trial. There were apparent benefits at 12 months that were not seen in longer term F/U; a shorter study would have given a misleading impression of treatment efficacy. This study is best viewed as a secondary preventon trial as substantial degenerative change is already present at the stage of MCI. Determining whether planned trials are either primary or secondary preventative in nature will have an important effect on trial design, impacting on estimates of treatment effect, sample size, and required duration of F/U. Best evidence at present suggests that maintaining a healthy lifestyle, control of vascular risk factors, and maintaining cognitive activity (e.g. social interaction) are more important than drug treatment.

Problems

For some patients, MCI is an interim phase on the path to dementia, but this is not true for all. Until a more robust way of distinguishing between these two groups is found (perhaps through the use of biomarkers), it will be difficult to demonstrate treatment effects in prevention trials.

Alzheimer's disease: donepezil

AD2000 study: Long-term donepezil treatment in 565 patients with Alzheimer's disease.

AUTHORS: AD2000 Collaborative Group.
REFERENCE: Lancet (2004) 363, 2105–15.
STUDY DESIGN: RCT
EVIDENCE LEVEL: 1b

Key message
Donepezil has modest clinical effectiveness and may not be cost-effective.

Impact
This was one of several trials that cast doubt on the clinical benefit and cost-effectiveness of cholinesterase inhibitors (CHEIs), thereby influencing the 2007 decision of the UK National Institute for Health and Clinical Excellence (NICE) to restrict the use of these agents to patients with moderate disease (at its simplest, MMSE score of 10–20). This decision has been very controversial, but was supported by judicial review.

Aims
Alzheimer's dementia is a common, irreversible brain disease, which causes progressive patient disability and carer stress, and has major economic implications for health and social services. The advent of the CHEIs, including donepezil, has offered hope that an effective treatment is finally available. This trial aimed to answer several important, yet unanswered, questions: what is the extent of improvement in non-cognitive symptoms of dementia; what is the optimal dose; for how long do any benefits persist; and is this medicine cost-effective?

Methods
Patients: 486 patients from 22 centres in the UK.

Inclusion criteria: Community-resident patients with mild to moderate Alzheimer's disease who completed a 12wk run-in period:
- Clinical diagnosis of Alzheimer's disease±vascular dementia;
- Attending UK memory clinic;
- Living in the community with regular carer.

Groups:
- Donepezil, sub-randomised to either 5mg or 10mg (n=242);
- Placebo (n=244).

Primary endpoints:
- Entry to institutional care;
- Progression of disability, defined as loss of either 2/4 basic, or 6/11 instrumental activities on the Bristol Activities of Daily Living Scale.

Follow-up: At 12wk intervals until 60wk, and then annually.

Results

Entry to institutional care	Donepezil	Placebo	*p*
1 y	9%	14%	0.2
3 y	42%	44%	0.4
Progression of disability			
1 y	13%	19%	0.3
3 y	55%	53%	0.9

Discussion

There remains considerable uncertainty regarding the role of CHEIs in the management of dementia. For the foreseeable future, this issue will remain unresolved.

Problems

- Sample size: Recruitment to this trial was hugely under target, largely due to the issue of NICE guidance regarding the use of CHEIs in this patient group.
- Cost-effectiveness data: There is intense debate and controversy over interpretations of cost-effectiveness data, both for this trial and for the recent NICE review. These are highly sensitive to changes in basic assumptions, including purchase price of CHEIs and costs of social care.
- Co-prescription: AD2000 sub-randomised participants to low dose aspirin or aspirin avoidance, complicating the evaluation of outcomes.
- Diagnostic uncertainty: There is no diagnostic test for what is essentially a pathologically-defined disease, and AD2000 recruited a sample in which many may have had vascular dementia.

Alzheimer's disease: memantine

Reisberg's study: Memantine in moderate to severe Alzheimer's disease.

AUTHORS: Reisberg B, Doody R, Stöffler A *et al.* (for the Memantine Study Group).
REFERENCE: N Engl J Med (2003) 348, 1333–41.
STUDY DESIGN: RCT
EVIDENCE LEVEL: 1b

Key message
Memantine may reduce rate of decline in patients with moderate to severe Alzheimer's disease (AD).

Impact
Memantine remains one of the few treatment options for patients with advanced AD. However, after appraisal of this trial and two others, the UK National Institute for Health and Clinical Excellence (NICE) concluded that the evidence base was limited, that treatment benefits appeared to be modest, and that treatment with memantine was not cost-effective.

Aims
Glutamate neurons are implicated in the cognitive and functional decline seen in AD. Memantine may protect neurons from glutamate-mediated excitotoxicity. This study aimed to determine whether memantine reduces the rate of cognitive and functional decline in the later (moderate and severe) stages of AD.

Methods
Patients: 252 community-dwelling patients referred to 32 treatment centres in the USA.

Inclusion criteria: Probable AD (by clinical diagnosis):
• Mini-Mental State Examination (MMSE) score of 3–14 (i.e. moderate to severe impairment);
• Age >50y;
• Reliable caregivers;
• No clinically significant medical conditions or laboratory abnormalities.

Groups:
• Memantine: 20mg/d (n=126);
• Placebo (n=126).

Primary endpoints:
• Clinician's Interview-Based Impression of Change plus Caregiver Input (CIBIC-Plus) score at 28wk;
• Change from baseline to 28wk in Alzheimer's Disease Cooperative Study Activities of Daily Living Inventory (ADCS-ADL).

Secondary endpoints: Other scales, including the Severe Impairment Battery (SIB), Mini-Mental State Examination (MMSE), Global Deterioration

Scale (GDS), Functional Assessment Staging scale (FAST), NeuroPsychiatric Inventory (NPI), and Resource Utilisation in Dementia (RUD).

Follow-up: At randomisation, and at 12 and 28wk.

Results

Primary endpoints (at 28wk)	Memantine	Placebo	*p*
Change in CIBIC-Plus	4.591.1	4.891.1	0.06
Change in ADCS-ADL	−3.196.8	−5.296.3	0.02
Secondary endpoints (at 28wk)			
Change in SIB	−4.0±11.3	−10.1±13.5	<0.001
Change in MMSE	−0.5±2.4	−1.2±3.0	0.2
Change in GDS	0.1±0.5	0.2±0.5	0.1
Change in NPI	0.5±15.8	3.8±16.1	0.3
Change in FAST	0.2±1.2	0.6±1.4	0.02

- Care required, measured by RUD score, was significantly less in memantine group (difference=45.8h/month; 95% CI 10 to 81).

Discussion

There is a lack of effective treatments for the common, irreversible, neuro-degenerative diseases (like AD), that place a major burden on formal and informal carers. This study provided evidence that memantine reduces the rate of cognitive and functional decline with clinically meaningful effects. The same research group has also published encouraging cost-effectiveness data, but these are complex and difficult to interpret. In the UK, there has been intense scrutiny of the limited available evidence for the effectiveness and cost-effectiveness of memantine for Alzheimer's dementia: a stormy debate continues.

Problems

- Possibility of bias: The withdrawal rate was higher in the placebo group with an overall dropout rate of almost 30%, probably due to the late stage of disease studied. However, sensitivity analysis for managing missing data demonstrated that the main result was robust.

Alzheimer's disease: antipsychotics and cognitive decline

> **Ballard's study:** Quetiapine and rivastigmine and cognitive decline in Alzheimer's disease.
>
> **AUTHORS:** Ballard C, Margallo-Lana M, Juszczak E *et al.*
> **REFERENCE:** BMJ (2005) 330, 874–7.
> **STUDY DESIGN:** RCT
> **EVIDENCE LEVEL:** 1b

Key message
Quetiapine (and therefore, possibly other antipsychotics) is associated with accelerated cognitive decline in Alzheimer's disease (AD).

Impact
Antipsychotics, both typical and atypical, have been commonly used in the management of the non-cognitive/behavioural symptoms of dementia. This trial was one of several which shifted practice away from pharmacological treatment and towards behavioural interventions, and when antipsychotics have to be used, towards their short-term use alone.

Aims
Dementia can be associated with intrusive neuropsychiatric symptoms. Treatment strategies often include an antipsychotic agent. However, these have substantial adverse effects, including parkinsonism and tardive dyskinesia. This study aimed to compare the effects of quetiapine (an atypical antipsychotic) and rivastigmine (a cholinesterase inhibitor, CHEI) on agitation and cognition in people with AD living in institutional care.

Methods
Patients: 93 patients from residential care settings in the UK.

Inclusion criteria:
- Age >60y;
- Probable or possible AD;
- Clinically significant agitation for ≥6wk;
- Scores ≥4 on the aberrant motor behaviour or irritability scales of the neuropsychiatric inventory;
- No use of antipsychotics or CHEIs for 4wk before study entry.

Groups:
- Quetiapine (n=31, of which 26 started treatment);
- Rivastigmine (n=31, of which 25 started treatment);
- Placebo (n=31, of which 29 started treatment).

Primary endpoint: Agitation (at 6wk).

Secondary endpoints: Cognitive function at 6 and 26wk; agitation at 26wk.

Follow-up: At 0, 6, 12, and 26wk, with Cohen-Mansfield agitation inventory (CMAI) and severe impairment battery (SIB).

Results

	Mean difference in change from baseline (95% CI)		
	Rivastigmine vs placebo	Quetiapine vs placebo	Rivastigmine vs quetiapine
To 6wk			
In CMAI	4.1 (−4.2 to 12.3) $p=0.3$	3.5 (−3.7 to10.8) $p=0.3$	0.3 (−8.0 to 8.6) $p=0.9$
In SIB	−3.5 (−13.1 to 6.2) $p=0.5$	−14.6 (−25.3 to −4.0) $p=0.009$	12.0 (0.8 to 23.2) $p=0.04$
To 26wk			
In CMAI	2.2 (−5.3 to 9.7) $p=0.6$	2.0 (−4.2 to 8.3) $p=0.5$	−0.5 (−8.0 to 6.9) $p=0.9$
In SIB	−7.5 (−21.0 to 6.0) $p=0.3$	−15.4 (−27 to −3.8) $p=0.01$	8.3 (−5.6 to 22.3) $p=0.2$

Discussion

Concerns have arisen regarding use of the atypical antipsychotics, risperidone and olanzapine, in people with dementia due to increased rates of cerebrovascular death (*JAMA* (2005) 294, 1934–43), culminating in a Committee on Safety of Medicines (CSM) warning in early 2004. Quetiapine was an attractive alternative. However, this study supported the use of neither CHEIs nor atypical antipsychotics in the management of Alzheimer's related agitation. Indeed, it provided evidence of accelerated cognitive decline with quetiapine. If antipsychotics are to be used in the management of behavioural symptoms, they should be used cautiously and for short periods. There are limited therapeutic options available for the management of dementia-related agitation. Behavioural interventions are an important approach, but rely heavily on the availability of staff with time, skill, and motivation. Medical and nursing assessment to rule out simple causes of agitation (such as untreated pain, constipation, and urinary retention) is crucial.

Problems

- Placebo response: In the participants receiving placebo, both agitation and cognition improved a little between baseline and 6wk. This may well be due to the influence of the research project itself.
- Sample size: The study was small, raising the possibility of a type 2 error, i.e. lack of evidence of an effect when one actually exists.

New onset epilepsy

New onset geriatric epilepsy: a study of gabapentin, lamotrigine, and carbamazepine.

AUTHORS: Rowan A, Ramsay R, Collins J et al.
REFERENCE: Neurology (2005) 64, 1868–73.
STUDY DESIGN: RCT
EVIDENCE LEVEL: 1b

Key message

Newer antiepileptic drugs (AEDs)—lamotrigine (LTG) and gabapentin (GBP)—are better tolerated than carbamazepine (CBZ) in older people with new onset epilepsy.

Impact

Guidelines continue to reflect traditional prescribing practice, favouring the older AEDs, e.g. CBZ, phenytoin, and valproate. However, prescribing practice is shifting away from the older AEDs, supported by studies such as this, and as familiarity with newer drugs increases.

Aims

In older people, the incidence of epilepsy is much higher, but antiepileptic drugs (AEDs) are less well tolerated. Treatment is complicated by comorbidity, polypharmacy, and altered pharmacokinetics and pharmacodynamics. This study was the first to compare two newer AEDs (LTG and GBP) with a well established drug (CBZ) that is often the drug of choice, but frequently causes serious treatment-limiting side effects.

Methods

Patients: 593 patients presenting to 18 Veteran Affairs centres in the USA.

Inclusion criteria:
- Age >60y with newly diagnosed seizures (≥1 in last 3 months) of any type;
- Either untreated, treated short-term (<4wk), or treated longer term but at sub-therapeutic levels.

Exclusion criteria:
- Taking long-term AEDs;
- Terminal illness or progressive neurological disease;
- Illicit drug use, alcoholism, severe psychiatric disease.

Groups: Dosing above (if poor seizure control) or below (if toxicity) target was permitted. Patients were withdrawn from the study if side effects co-existed with poor control:
- CBZ: target dose 600mg/d (n=198);
- GBP: target dose 1500mg/d (n=195);
- LTG: target dose 150mg/d (n=200).

Primary endpoint: Retention in trial for 12 months, as an indicator of efficacy and tolerability.

Secondary endpoints:
• Seizure-free retention rate (SFRR) at 1y. SFRR is an intention-to-treat measure of the proportion of patients who remain seizure-free and who were not withdrawn from the study;
• Drug toxicity.

Follow-up: Double-blind, double-dummy. At least bimonthly clinical evaluation until 12 months.

Results

Primary endpoint	CBZ	GBP	LTG	*p*
Early termination	64.5%	51%	44.2%	0.0002
Secondary endpoints				
SFRR (1y)	22.8%	23.2%	28.6	0.33
Terminated drug due to toxicity	31%	21.6%	12.1%	0.001

Discussion

This study of seizures in older people is the largest to date. It reflects real clinical practice, in that patients with concurrent disease were included, and both target doses and pace of dose titration were lower than is standard for younger patients. The study provides convincing evidence of improved tolerability and similar efficacy of the newer AEDs.

Problems

• The low SFRR indicates that the ideal AED has yet to be identified. At 1y, 56% of patients randomised to the LTG arm remained in the trial, but only 51% of these were seizure-free. There were no significant differences in seizure-free rates between drugs.
• Subjects were enrolled after only one seizure. In older people, this may be reasonable clinical practice: adverse consequences of seizures are more common as are risk factors (e.g. cerebrovascular disease) and recurrence rates are higher (66–90%).
• Although generally well tolerated, LTG has some side effects which are serious but rare (e.g. skin and haematological reactions).

Assessment before care home placement

Specialist clinical assessment of older people prior to care home entry.

AUTHORS: Challis D, Clarkson P, Williamson J *et al.*
REFERENCE: Age Ageing (2004) 33, 25–34.
STUDY DESIGN: RCT
EVIDENCE LEVEL: 1b

Key message

Specialist medical (geriatric) assessment before care home placement identifies covert morbidity and reduces dependency, carer distress, and emergency service contacts.

Impact

The UK National Service Framework (NSF) for Older People advises full multidisciplinary assessment for older people at risk of long-term care, accessed via a 'Single Assessment Process'. This should facilitate comprehensive geriatric assessment that includes a medical evaluation. In practice, implementation of guidance is patchy; multidisciplinary teams often have no specialist geriatric medical component, and many assessors are untrained in identification of the need for specialist medical assessment. Therefore, specialist clinical assessment before care home admission is far from universal.

Aims

Accurate needs assessment is essential prior to consideration of care home placement, in order to ensure that those with the greatest need are awarded places. However, disagreement had existed as to the precise criteria required of such an assessment process, leading to multiple and varied assessments by different members of the multidisciplinary team. This study aimed to evaluate the effect of additional specialist (geriatric) medical assessment at the time of consideration of care home placement.

Methods

Patients: 256 patients from two social services areas in the UK.

Inclusion criteria:
- Older people with mental or physical deterioration being considered for care home placement;
- Living at home.

Exclusion criteria:
- Emergency care home admissions; team unable to assess prior to admission;
- Terminal illness;
- Recent specialist (geriatric) medical assessment.

Groups:
- Control: Usual assessment by care manager (n=127);
- Clinical: Additional domiciliary clinical assessment by experienced geriatrician or psychogeriatrician. Assessment of cognitive function, affect and activities of daily living, with brief clinical examination. Report to care managers, including diagnoses, prognosis, care needs, and treatment options (n=129).

Primary endpoint: Admission to care home.

Secondary endpoints:
- Service use and costs;
- Dependency and behaviour;
- Carer stress and burden.

Follow-up: Unblinded. Interview at 6 months, including assessment of cognition, mood, physical dependency, and quality of life.

Results

	Control	Clinical	*p*
Admission to care home, 6 months (%)	47%	42%	ns
Total NHS costs (including trial assessment, £)	10,592	9461	0.03
Total social services costs (£)	24,138	22,619	ns
Change in dependency, 0 to 6 months (Barthel index, (mean, SD))	−6.4 (14)	−2.5 (13)	0.04

Discussion

Although there was no significant reduction in overall care home admissions (both residential and nursing), there were reductions in time spent in nursing homes, contact with emergency medical services, physical functional decline, and carer stress. There was a high rate of detection of potentially treatable conditions. The intervention was valued by care managers who often lacked the detailed diagnostic and prognostic information required to assist decision-making. It is possible that the limited overall effect on care home admission concealed a greater number of occasions where clinical assessment affected decision-making—in some cases accelerating admission (e.g. untreatable progressive disease) whilst in others, delaying or averting it (e.g. treatable behavioural problems).

Problems

- The study was small and had limited power to detect meaningful effect. Multiple outcome measurements increase the risk of type 1 errors.
- Effective cross-professional collaborative working is essential, but may be difficult to deliver where there is a culture of separate practice.
- Issues for future research include whether a similar, more structured intervention may be delivered more cost-effectively by specialist nurses, and whether there are subgroups that benefit most from specialist assessments.

Haematology

Introduction

One of the great British contributions to medicine has been the development of the prospective randomised clinical trial (RCT) as a method of assessing whether novel treatments demonstrate superiority over established therapy. This replacement of hunch, clinical impression, and anecdote by the design and rigorous evaluation of the results of well-designed studies has been enthusiastically embraced by practising haematologists the world over.

Enthusiastic adoption of RCTs is probably the consequence of a number of factors. First, the training of haematologists has always involved an understanding of the pathological and scientific processes that underlie blood disorders, engendering a rational clinical approach. Secondly, the treatments used in the management of haematological disorders (especially leukaemias and lymphomas) are toxic and difficult to use, involving considerable clinical expertise and expense; there is little justification here for individual clinicians dabbling with such agents. Thirdly, the prognosis of untreated patients is poor with often only one chance of success.

Haematologists, then, need no reminding of the importance of clinical trials. The infrastructure originally established by the Medical Research Council to perform clinical studies in acute leukaemia has been widely replicated.

The studies summarised here are an excellent example of how well-designed RCTs have influenced day to day clinical practice with immense and progressive benefit to patients. One can only hope that the increased regulation surrounding clinical trial design and execution, and the delays in incorporating their results into clinical practice now experienced by UK clinicians will not reverse this process.

Packed red cell transfusion threshold

> **TRICC (**T̲ransfusion R̲equirements I̲n C̲ritical C̲are**) study:** A multi-centre RCT trial of transfusion requirements in critical care
>
> **AUTHORS:** Hebert P, Wells G, Blajchman M *et al.*
> **REFERENCE:** N Engl J Med (1999) 340, 409–17.
> **STUDY DESIGN:** RCT
> **EVIDENCE LEVEL:** 1b

Key message

A restrictive transfusion strategy (haemoglobin (Hb) threshold 7g/dL) is as effective, and possibly superior to, a liberal transfusion strategy (Hb threshold 10g/dL) in adult critical care patients without ischaemic heart disease. The restrictive strategy is associated with a reduction in the overall use of red cell transfusions.

Impact

This has perhaps been one of the most widely applied intensive care papers ever written. A threshold Hb concentration of 7g/dL has since become standard practice for adult critical care patients without significant comorbidity, and is widely used in other clinical settings.

Aims

Critical care patients frequently require red cell transfusions. However, whilst conferring benefits, transfusions themselves are associated with risks *(N Engl J Med (2001) 354, 1230–6)*. For this reason, optimal transfusion practice for this group of patients had yet to be established. This study was designed to determine whether a restrictive approach to red cell transfusion was equivalent to a more liberal strategy.

Methods

Patients: 838 patients at 22 intensive care units (ICUs) in Canada.

Inclusion criteria: ICU patients of age >16y, with:
- Expected stay in ICU >24h;
- Hb concentration <9.0g/dL within 72h of admission;
- Euvolaemic, with no active blood loss.

Exclusion criteria:
- Unable to receive blood, active blood loss, *or* chronic anaemia;
- Brain death or imminent death;
- Routine cardiac surgery.

Groups:
- Liberal: Hb concentration maintained between 10–12g/dL with a threshold of 10g/dL for red cell transfusion (n=420);
- Restrictive: Hb concentration maintained in the range 7–9g/dL with a threshold of 7g/dL for red cell transfusion (n=418).

Primary endpoint: All-cause mortality in the 30d after randomisation.

Secondary endpoints:
- Mortality: 60d; during hospital stay; during ICU stay;
- Length of hospital and ICU stay;
- Multiple organ dysfunction (MOD) score.

Follow-up: To 60d or death.

Results

	Restrictive (n=418)	Liberal (n=420)	*p*
Primary endpoint			
30d mortality	n=78 (18.7%)	n=98 (23.3%)	0.1
Secondary endpoints			
60d mortality	n=95 (22.7%)	n=111 (26.5%)	0.2
Intensive care unit mortality	n=56 (13.6%)	n=68 (16.2%)	0.3
Hospital mortality	n=93 (22.2%)	n=118 (28.1%)	0.05
MOD score	10.7±7.5	11.8±7.7	0.03
Length of ICU stay (d)	11±10.7	11.5±11.3	0.5
Length of hospital stay (d)	34.8±19.5	35.5±19.4	0.6

- Overall survival curves similar between groups, but significantly different in the subgroup with APACHE (<u>a</u>cute <u>p</u>hysiology <u>a</u>nd <u>c</u>hronic <u>h</u>ealth <u>e</u>valuation) score ≤20 (*p*=0.02) and those <55y old (*p*=0.02).

Discussion

Although this was largely a negative trial, its findings were nonetheless extremely important. Publication came at a time when worldwide awareness of the hazards of transfusion was rising. It reassured clinicians that withholding red cell transfusion was, at the very least, not harmful, and possibly also of benefit in critically ill patients. The results indicated that a transfusion threshold of 7g/dL, combined with maintenance of Hb in the range 7–9g/dL, was as effective (and possibly superior) to a liberal transfusion strategy. Patients in the restrictive transfusion group also had a 54% reduction in the average number of red cell units transfused.

Problems

- Potential selection bias: 3206 patients were eligible, but only 838/2039 (41%) of those screened for consent agreed to participate in the study.
- This trial only considered adult patients. However, similar results have been found in critically ill neonates and children.
- Debate continues about the optimal transfusion strategy in those with significant comorbidity, e.g. severe ischaemic heart disease, although there is general acceptance that a higher threshold is appropriate.
- Barely 50% of the numbers required by the power calculation were enrolled.
- Patients received non-leucodepleted RBCs. Results might be different with current RBC products, because the infusion of donor leucocytes with the red cells, or the infusion of RBCs modified by storage in the presence of leucocytes, may have adverse effects on outcome.

Platelet transfusion threshold

The threshold for prophylactic platelet transfusions in adults with acute myeloid leukemia.

AUTHORS: Rebulla P, Finazzi G, Marangoni F *et al.*
REFERENCE: N Engl J Med (1997) 337, 1870–5.
STUDY DESIGN: RCT
EVIDENCE LEVEL: 1b

Key message

There is no increased risk of major bleeding between a prophylactic platelet transfusion threshold of 10 and 20×10^9/L in patients undergoing remission induction therapy for acute myeloblastic leukaemia (AML). The lower threshold is associated with a 21.5% reduction in the number of platelet transfusions.

Impact

Other trials have confirmed these findings and a threshold platelet count of 10×10^9/L is now the standard of care for prophylactic platelet transfusions in patients with haematological malignancies.

Aims

The ready availability of platelet concentrates has undoubtedly made a major contribution to the development and safety of intensive treatment for haematological and other malignancies. However, platelet transfusions are associated with a number of complications and are costly. This study aimed to investigate the frequency and severity of haemorrhage in patients with AML receiving prophylactic platelet transfusions at two different thresholds of platelet counts: 10 and 20×10^9/L.

Methods

Patients: 255 patients at 21 centres in Italy.

Inclusion criteria:
- Patients with newly diagnosed AML;
- Age >16y;
- Receiving platelet transfusions during first course of remission induction therapy.

Exclusion criteria:
- Acute promyelocytic leukaemia;
- Secondary AML;
- Blood transfusion before diagnosis of leukaemia.

Groups:
- Control: prophylactic platelet transfusions when platelet count <20×10^9/L (n=120).
- Restrictive: prophylactic platelets transfusions when platelet count <10×10^9/L, or between 10–20×10^9/L when temperature >38°C in the

presence of fresh minor or major bleeding or if invasive procedures necessary (n=135).

Primary endpoint: Frequency and severity of haemorrhage.

Secondary endpoints:
- Number of platelet and red cell transfusions;
- Number of patients achieving complete remission;
- Mortality.

Results

	Restrictive	Control	p
Primary endpoint			
Patients with major bleeding episodes	n=29 (21.5%)	n=24 (20.0%)	ns
Days with major bleeding episodes	n=123 (3.1%)	n=65 (2.0%)	ns
Secondary endpoints			
Number of platelet transfusions (median/range)	6 (1–22)	8 (2–27)	0.001
Complete remission	n=76 (56.3%)	n=76 (63.3%)	ns
Death	n=18 (13.3%)	n=9 (7.5%)	ns

Discussion

A threshold platelet count of 20×10^9/L for prophylactic platelet transfusions in patients with bone marrow failure became accepted in the 1960s, although no clinical studies directly supported this practice. The data from this study suggested that it was safe to lower the threshold to 10×10^9/L. In doing so, the use of platelet transfusions was significantly reduced. Other trials have since confirmed these findings.

Problems

- In the restrictive group, 22.6% of platelet transfusions were given when the platelet count was $>10 \times 10^9$/L due to the presence of concomitant risk factors e.g. fever, bleeding, or invasive procedure.
- There was one fatal cerebral haemorrhage in the restrictive group, although the platelet count was 32×10^9/L when the haemorrhage began.
- 21 patients did not complete F/U and were excluded in the analysis.

Sickle cell anaemia: hydroxyurea

HUSOFT (<u>H</u>ydroxy<u>U</u>rea <u>S</u>afety and <u>O</u>rgan <u>T</u>oxicity) extension study: Long-term hydroxyurea therapy for infants with sickle cell anaemia.

AUTHORS: Hankins J, Ware R, Rogers Z et al.
REFERENCE: Blood (2005) 106, 2269–75.
STUDY DESIGN: Cohort Study
EVIDENCE LEVEL: 2a

Key message
The first study to demonstrate the long-term efficacy and safety of hydroxyurea (HU) therapy in very young children with sickle cell anaemia (SCA).

Impact
When used in this age group, HU is able to significantly reduce or prevent chronic organ damage associated with this disease. HU is increasingly used in SCA and a large RCT is currently underway.

Aims
SCA results in chronic haemolysis and end-organ damage, secondary to repeated intravascular sickling and vaso-occlusion. Almost every organ system can be involved and damage starts very early in life. Indeed, many children lose splenic reticuloendothial function by 2 years of age, and are at risk of renal, cerebral, and pulmonary disease. Lower levels of foetal haemoglobin (HbF) and a higher white blood cell (WBC) count are associated with higher incidence of SCA-related events. HU is an antimetabolite which increases production of HbF, lowers WBC and platelet counts, and reduces the adhesion of red cells to vascular endothelium. In this study, the investigators sought to determine the feasibility, toxicity, and efficacy of HU treatment in infants, focusing on its effects on splenic function and HbF levels.

Methods
Patients: 28 patients at 4 paediatric centres in the USA.

Inclusion criteria: Unselected for disease severity:
- Infants aged 6-24 months;
- Homozygous SCA (HbSS) or HbS beta-thalassaemia.

Therapy: HU 20mg/kg/d for first 2y, then gradually increased to a target dose of 30mg/kg/d.

Primary endpoint: Haematological efficacy: Hb, mean cell volume (MCV), HbF, F cells, reticulocyte, WBC and platelet count.

Secondary endpoints:
- Clinical events: pain and acute chest syndrome;
- Organ function and growth rates;
- Treatment-related toxicity.

Follow-up: Nov 1996–June 1997. Bi-weekly physical examination. Regular blood counts. HbF levels every 6 months. Splenic filtrative function measured by technetium 99m (Tc99m) sulphur-colloid uptake measurement at baseline, and 2 and 4y of therapy. MRI/MRA of brain at 2y intervals.

Results

	Baseline (n=28)	Y2 (n=21)	Y4 (n=17)	CSSCD age 4–5	p	Y6 (n=11)
Hb (g/dlL)	8.5	8.8	9.1	8.1	<0.001	9.0
MCV (fL)	81.7	90.0	95.1	88.0	<0.001	96.0
HbF (%)	21.8	20.3	23.7	9.0	<0.001	23.3
Retic count (%)	9.2	8.6	8.2	12.4	<0.001	5.5
WBC x10⁹/L	12.6	10.1	10.1	14.3	<0.001	8.9

CSSCD: Cooperative Study of Sickle Cell Disease— a prospective, multicentre study of the natural history of SCD, provided age-matched figures for comparison with HU treatment group.

Discussion

Assessment of haematological efficacy showed a significant benefit in the HU-treated group vs age-matched controls from the CSSCD trial. HbF values were significantly higher after dose escalation to 30mg/kg/d, and this response was sustained in contrast with declining levels seen in untreated children. There were also fewer episodes of acute chest syndrome in the HU-treated group (7.5 vs 24.5 events per 100 person years, $p=0.001$). Of 14 children with splenic function assessment, 6 (43%) were functionally asplenic at the end of F/U (vs 94% expected in untreated group, $p<0.001$), and 2 children were found to have regained normal splenic uptake after 4y of HU therapy. Growth rates were better in the HU-treated group and similar to those of healthy controls. Toxicity was minor and transient, and dose escalation tolerated in 95% of children.

Problems

- Longer F/U needed to assess HbF and address ongoing concerns about myelodysplasia and malignancy secondary to HU.
- Small number of patients.
- Improved splenic function may increase risk of acute sequestration.
- 12 of 28 excluded due to poor compliance or parental withdrawal.

Acute lymphoblastic leukaemia: bone marrow transplant

> **Medical research council (MRC) UKALL XII/ECOG E2993:** In adults with standard-risk acute lymphoblastic leukemia, the greatest benefit is achieved from a matched sibling allogeneic transplant in first complete remission, and an autologous transplant is less effective than conventional consolidation/maintenance chemotherapy in all patients: final results of the international ALL trial.
>
> **AUTHORS:** Rowe J, Buck G, Fielding A *et al.*
> **REFERSENCE:** Blood (2008) 111, 1827–33.
> **STUDY DESIGN:** RCT
> **EVIDENCE LEVEL:** 1b

Key message

Sibling allogeneic bone marrow transplant (BMT) is indicated for standard-risk patients with acute lymphoblastic leukaemia (ALL) during first complete remission. All other Philadelphia-chromosome negative patients should receive chemotherapy based consolidation and maintenance, rather than autologous BMT.

Impact

This is now the standard for treating ALL in adults.

Aims

Treatment of ALL in children had improved considerably, with long-term survival rates of 80% being achieved. In adults, survival was considerably poorer, with survival rates of (at most) 40% for those <60y old, and <10% for those >60y old. Furthermore, the low incidence of ALL in adults had made obtaining sufficient numbers for study difficult. With the graft vs leukaemia effect having been described for adult patients, the aim of this study was to prospectively define optimal therapy for ALL in adults up to the age of 60, particularly with regards to the role of allogeneic BMT in first complete remission (CR1). In addition, although protracted consolidation/maintenance chemotherapy had been the mainstay of treatment (largely based upon paediatric studies), this study aimed to assess the benefits of a single autologous transplant.

Methods

Patients: 1980 patients from multiple centres in the UK and USA.

Inclusion criteria: All patients aged 15 to 60y (extended to 65y from 2004), with newly diagnosed ALL.

Groups: All patients received 8wk of identical induction therapy with response evaluated at wk4 and 8. All in CR1 went on to treatment allocation/randomisation. Intensification phase prior to transplant/consolidation:
- Philadelphia +ve: matched unrelated donor search, if no sibling donor;
- Philadelphia –ve: with HLA-matched sibling donor, assigned to allogeneic BMT;
- Other patients: randomised to autologous BMT or standard consolidation/maintenance chemotherapy.

Primary endpoint: Overall survival (OS) at 5y after enrolment.

Secondary endpoints: Event-free survival (EFS) and relapse risk.

Follow-up: Median F/U=4y, 11 months (range 1 month to 13y and 11 months).

Results

5y data: Philadelphia –ve group	Number	OS (%)	EFS (%)	Relapse (%)
Donor vs no donor	388 vs 527	53 vs 45	50 vs 41	29 vs 54
High risk	170 vs 230	39 vs 36	38 vs 32	36 vs 63
Standard risk	218 vs 286	63 vs 51	59 vs 48	25 vs 48
Auto. vs chemo.	220 vs 215	37 vs 46	33 vs 42	61 vs 54
Sibling allo. vs chemo.	384 vs 418	54 vs 44	50 vs 40	29 vs 55
High risk	168 vs 190	41 vs 35	38 vs 31	36 vs 63
Standard risk	216 vs 223	64 vs 51	59 vs 47	24 vs 48

High risk=age >35y; high WCC (>30,000x10^9/L for B-lineage or >100,000x10^9/L for T lineage) at presentation. Philadelphia +ve patients not included in analysis.

Discussion

Philadelphia –ve patients with sibling donors who received allogeneic transplants in CR1 had improved OS, EFS, and relapse rates, in comparison with other treatment arms ($p<0.05$). However, high treatment-related mortality in the high-risk group meant that benefit from allogeneic BMT was restricted to the standard-risk group. In those with no sibling donor, autologous transplantation offered no benefit over chemotherapy and was associated with a higher relapse rate ($p<0.05$). In addition, it was found that disease monitoring after induction therapy and intensification was highly predictive of outcome in non-allograft patients (OS 70% vs 22%, $p=0.001$).

Problems

- It is becoming increasingly evident that cytogenetic abnormalities other than t(9;22) (e.g. t(4;11) and t(8;14)) are important for risk stratification in ALL. Their role in guiding therapy should be the subject of future trials.

Acute promyelocytic leukaemia: transretinoic acid

Effect of all transretinoic acid in newly diagnosed acute promyelocytic leukaemia. Results of a multicentre randomised trial. European APL 91 Group.

AUTHORS: Fenaux P, Le Deley M, Castaigne S et al.
REFERENCE: Blood (1993) 82, 3241–9.
STUDY DESIGN: RCT
EVIDENCE LEVEL: 1b

Key message
This study demonstrates the efficacy of all transretinoic acid (ATRA) in (1) reducing the incidence of induction deaths and potentially fatal disseminated intravascular coagulation (DIC); (2) reducing relapse rate; and (3) improving event-free and overall survival, when combined with standard chemotherapy in the treatment of acute promyelocytic leukaemia (APL).

Impact
ATRA combined with chemotherapy has now become standard therapy in the management of APL. The current trial question is whether there is a role for conventional chemotherapy.

Aims
Coagulopathy, comprising disseminated intravascular coagulation (DIC), fibrinolysis, and proteolysis, is an often fatal complication of APL. Patients with APL have a unique form of acute myeloid leukaemia characterised by t(15;17) translocation and high incidence of severe coagulopathy. Although conventional chemotherapeutic agents such as anthracycline and cytosine-based agents achieved remission rates of 90%, patients would often relapse within 24 months of completion, unsuccessful treatments often also resulting in fatal haemorrhage. ATRA, a vitamin A analogue, had been previously shown to induce differentiation and improve coagulopathy in APL. This study aimed to compare intensive chemotherapy alone vs intensive chemotherapy with ATRA in order to determine whether there was an improvement in remission rates, deaths at induction, and overall survival.

Methods
Patients: 101 patients at 46 centres in France.

Inclusion criteria:
• New morphological diagnosis of APL (French-American-British criteria), subsequently confirmed by presence of t(15;17) translocation;
• Age ≤65y.

Groups: Non-blinded. Each group received 3 courses of chemotherapy:
- Chemotherapy: Course 1=daunorubicin (60mg/m^2/d, for 3d) and cytarabine (200mg/m^2/d, for 1wk). Repeated for course 2. Course 3=daunorubicin (60mg/m^2/d, for 3d) and cytarabine (1g/m^2/12 hourly, for 4d) (n=47);
- ATRA: 45mg/m^2/d to complete remission (CR), followed by 3 courses of chemotherapy, as above (n=54).

Primary endpoint: (EFS) (events=failure to achieve CR, relapse, and death in CR).

Secondary endpoints: CR rate, relapse-free survival, overall survival (OS).

Follow-up: Median F/U=11 months (chemotherapy) and 11.5 months (ATRA).

Results
- Median age=40y (range 6–67y)

	Chemotherapy (n=47)	ATRA (n=54)	p
Primary endpoint			
EFS (at 1y)	50% (±9%)	79% (±6%)	0.001
*EFS (at 4y)	17%	63%	0.001
Secondary endpoints			
Complete response	n=38 (81%)	n=49 (91%)	0.3
Early (induction) deaths	n=4 (8%)	n=5 (9%)	0.9
OS(1y)	80% (±7%)	91% (±4%)	0.3
*OS (4y)	49%	76%	0.02

* Follow-up report: Fenaux *et al.* Leukemia (2000) **14**, 1371–7.

Discussion
This was the first study in which a differentiating agent demonstrated clear efficacy over cytotoxic chemotherapy. The trial was stopped early after the first interim analysis clearly demonstrated improvement in EFS with ATRA. The ATRA group showed faster resolution of significant coagulopathy (3 vs 6d, $p<0.001$). Subsequent studies have also reported a reduction in early deaths. These data have been confirmed by a larger subsequent USA-based intergroup study.

Problems
- The study was underpowered to demonstrate improvement in response rates or induction deaths. Furthermore, the initial report did not show a survival benefit. However, the 73 months data did show an improvement in overall survival.
- Not all patients had molecular or cytogenetic confirmation of APL.
- The value of concurrent ATRA and chemotherapy was not addressed, although a benefit has subsequently been demonstrated. Concurrent ATRA and chemotherapy is now standard therapy.

Chronic myeloid leukaemia: imatinib

IRIS (**I**nternational **R**andomised study of **I**nterferon and **STI**571): Imatinib compared with interferon and low-dose cytarabine for newly diagnosed chronic-phase chronic myeloid leukaemia.

AUTHORS: O'Brien S, Guilhot F, Larson R et al.
REFERENCE: N Engl J Med (2003) 348, 994–1004.
STUDY DESIGN: RCT
EVIDENCE LEVEL: 1b

Key message

This study demonstrates unequivocal superiority of the novel BCR-ABL tyrosine kinase inhibitor, imatinib mesylate, over the best previous standard medical therapy for chronic myeloid leukaemia (CML).

Impact

Imatinib is now the treatment of choice for CML. Previous standard treatment with interferon is largely redundant and the indications for allogeneic transplant are now restricted to imatinib resistance.

Aims

The Philadelphia chromosome (t(9;22) reciprocal translocation) is present in 90% of patients with CML and results in juxtaposition of DNA sequences from BCR and Abl genes. Imatinib (Gleevec®) is an oral, selective inhibitor of BCR-Abl tyrosine kinase, and has been demonstrated to be highly effective in patients with CML resistant to interferon (IFN) and those with advanced disease. This study aimed to compare imatinib with the then best available medical therapy of IFN and cytarabine.

Methods

Patients: 1106 patients at 177 centres worldwide (mainly Europe and USA).

Inclusion criteria: Patients aged 18–70y with chronic phase CML:
• Within 6 months of diagnosis;
• Previously untreated (except hydroxycarbamide);
• Creatinine <1.5x upper limit of normal;
• Eastern Cooperative Oncology Group (ECOG) performance status <3.

Exclusion criteria:
• Pregnant or breastfeeding;
• Serious medical comorbidities;
• Prior haematopoietic stem cell transplantation.

Groups: Non-blinded. Groups well balanced except for more cytogenetic abnormalities in addition to t(9;22) in the imatinib arm (12.1 vs 7.6%). Crossover allowed for non-responders, loss of response, or intolerance (National Cancer Institute Common Toxicity Criteria for non-haematological toxicity ≥ grade 3 despite dose reductions).
• IFN (escalating dose to a target of 5MU/m²/d subcutaneous) and cytarabine (20mg/m²/d subcutaneous for 10d per month) (n=553);
• Imatinib mesylate (400mg od) (n=553).

Primary endpoint: Progression-free survival.

Secondary endpoints: Haematological and cytogenetic response (complete [0% Ph positive cells] vs partial [<35% Ph positive cells]), safety, and tolerability.

Follow-up: Median F/U=19 months. Updated to 54 months (abstract form).

Results
- Median age=50.5y (range 18–70).

	IFN and cytarabine	Imatinib	*p*
Primary endpoint			
Progression free survival (1y)	79.9%	96.6%	<0.001
Secondary endpoints			
Complete cytogenetic response	14.5% (10.5–18.5)	76.2% (72.5–79.9)	<0.001
Major cytogenetic response (<35%)	34.7% (29.3–40.0)	87.1% (84.1–90.0)	<0.001
Complete haematological response	55.5% (51.3–59.7)	95.3% (93.2–96.9)	<0.001
Crossover (n)	318	11	–

Discussion
Imatinib was a more effective and better tolerated drug. The 60 months F/U data (published in abstract form, *N Engl J Med* (2006) 355, 2408–17) confirmed complete and major cytogenetic response rates of 92% and 87%, respectively, with overall and progression free survivals of 89% and 83%, respectively. Outcomes were better in patients experiencing a complete cytogenetic response or major molecular response (>3 log reduction in BCR-ABL transcripts). More recent studies have considered the issue of imatinib resistance, which can develop in a significant proportion of patients due to mechanisms including BCR-ABL mutations and activation of alternate oncogenic pathways *(N Engl J Med* (2006) 354, 2531–41 and 2542–51).

Problems
- There were very high rates of crossover and treatment discontinuation in the IFN arm with only 3% of patients remaining on IFN at 5y. A survival advantage for the imatinib arm is unlikely to be demonstrated.
- The high crossover rate for IFN intolerance may underestimate the response rate in the IFN arm. However, an analysis with patients censored at crossover for intolerance did not alter the results.
- This study did not address the question of duration of therapy.
- Longer F/U will be required to determine the rate of resistance and impact upon life expectancy.

Non-Hodgkin's lymphoma: chemotherapy

> Comparison of a standard regimen (CHOP) with three intensive chemotherapy regimens for advanced non-Hodgkin's lymphoma.
>
> **AUTHORS:** Fisher R, Gaynor E, Dahlberg S *et al.*
> **REFERENCE:** N Engl J Med (1993) 328, 1002–6.
> **STUDY DESIGN:** RCT
> **EVIDENCE LEVEL:** 1b

Key message

CHOP (cyclophosphamide, doxorubicin, vincristine and prednisolone) chemotherapy is as effective as newer, more intensive regimens and associated with fewer adverse reactions in the treatment of high-grade non-Hodgkin's lymphoma (NHL).

Impact

There has been much interest in the use of more intensive and toxic regimens in the treatment of high-grade NHL. This trial elegantly demonstrated that each combination must be tested against existing standards in a phase III clinical trial, prior to being introduced into routine clinical practice. CHOP is now the standard chemotherapy regimen for high-grade lymphomas.

Aims

High-grade, aggressive lymphomas had been treated with intravenous, combination chemotherapy since the 1960s, with initial cure rates of up to 40%. Arguing that more chemotherapy would mean higher response rates, newer regimens were developed and initial phase II studies suggested improved rates of cure. However, supportive care (such as antibiotic therapy and growth factor therapy) was also developing over this time period and it was unclear whether improved outcomes were due to the chemotherapy regimens alone. This study aimed to compare the standard treatment at the time (CHOP) with more intensive regimens.

Methods

Patients: 899 patients at multiple centres in the USA.

Inclusion criteria: Biopsy-confirmed non-Hodgkin's lymphoma:
- Bulky stage II, stage III, or stage IV disease;
- Histology suggesting intermediate or high-grade disease.

Exclusion criteria:
- Lymphoblastic lymphoma or overt CNS lymphoma;
- Previous malignancy or treatment with chemotherapy/radiotherapy;
- HIV/AIDS or significant cardiac/renal dysfunction.

Groups:
- CHOP chemotherapy: 8 courses (n=225);
- ProMACE-CytaBOM (prednisolone, doxorubicin, cyclophosphamide, and etoposide, followed by cytarabine, bleomycin, vincristine, and methotrexate) (n=233);
- MACOP-B (methotrexate, doxorubicin, cyclophosphamide, vincristine, prednisolone, and bleomycin) (n=218);
- m-BACOD (methotrexate, bleomycin, doxorubicin, cyclophosphamide, vincristine, dexamethasone) (n=223).

Primary endpoints: Response to treatment and time to failure.

Secondary endpoint: Overall survival and toxicity.

Follow-up: Repeated staging by CT scanning. Median F/U=35 months. Maximum F/U=6y.

Results

	Response to treatment		Alive at 3y with no disease‡	Overall survival*
	Partial	Complete		
CHOP	36%	44%	41%	54%
ProMACE-CytaBOM	31%	56%	46%	50%
MACOP-B	32%	51%	41%	50%
m-BACOD	34%	48%	46%	52%

Response to treatment between groups=ns / ‡ $p=0.4$ / * $p=0.9$

- **Toxicity:** CHOP and ProMACE-CytaBOM associated with significantly fewer serious toxic side effects (fatal/life-threatening) than MACOP-B or m-BACOD ($p=0.001$).

Discussion

This study highlighted an important principle: for a chemotherapy regimen to be deemed superior to current treatment, it must be evaluated in a large, phase III RCT. Previous phase II studies had shown significantly improved survival figures than for CHOP chemotherapy. This may have been due to a) phase II studies having used historical controls for comparison (not taking into account improvements in supportive care), and b) inadequate F/U (indeed, prolonged F/U of some of the phase II trials observed a dramatic fall in predicted 5y survival). After the negative outcome of this study, there was a feeling that lymphoma treatment had been set back several years. However, it was truly an advance to define the optimal treatment regimen for a given patient population, particularly with the regimen in question being easy to administer and associated with relatively mild toxicity.

Diffuse large B-cell lymphoma: rituximab

> CHOP chemotherapy plus rituximab compared with CHOP alone in elderly patients with diffuse large B-cell lymphoma.
>
> **AUTHORS:** Coiffier B, Lepage E, Brière J et al.
> **REFERENCE:** N Engl J Med (2002) 346, 235–42.
> **STUDY DESIGN:** RCT
> **EVIDENCE LEVEL:** 1b

Key message

Addition of rituximab to CHOP (cyclophosphamide, doxorubicin, vincristine, and prednisolone) chemotherapy (R-CHOP) improves response rates and prolongs event-free survival in elderly patients with diffuse large B-cell lymphoma (DLBCL) without significant extra toxicity.

Impact

This was the first therapeutic use of a monoclonal antibody for a haematological malignancy. R-CHOP regime is now standard first-line chemotherapy for advanced-stage DLBCL (i.e. bulky stage II or stage III, IV disease).

Aims

DLBCL is the most frequent histological subtype of non-Hodgkin's lymphoma (NHL), accounting for 40% of new lymphoma cases. Standard CHOP chemotherapy induces complete response in only 40–50% of elderly patients, with only 35–40% overall survival. Attempts to improve this using more intensive regimens had been unsuccessful, instead leading to increased toxicity and no survival benefit. Rituximab, a chimeric IgG monoclonal antibody, targets CD20 (a surface protein occurring almost exclusively on mature B cells) leading to lysis of malignant B cells. Phase II trials had previously demonstrated efficacy and good safety profile when used in combination with CHOP. This study aimed to be the first RCT to compare CHOP plus rituximab with CHOP alone.

Methods

Patients: 399 patients at 86 centres in France, Belgium, and Switzerland.

Inclusion criteria: Untreated DLBCL (REAL/WHO classification):
- Age 60–80y;
- Stage II, III, or IV disease, with ECOG (Eastern Cooperative Oncology Group) performance status 0–2 (i.e. good-fair).

Exclusion criteria:
- History of indolent lymphoma/T-cell lymphoma/concurrent malignancy;
- Central nervous system (CNS) involvement or peripheral neuropathy;
- Active medical condition preventing completion of therapy;
- Cardiac contraindications to doxorubicin;
- HIV/Hepatitis B virus (HBV) positive status.

Groups: Randomised and stratified according to age-adjusted International Prognostic Index (IPI) score. Granulocyte-colony stimulating factor (G-CSF) added following an episode of Grade 4 or febrile neutropaenia:
- CHOP (every 21d for 8 cycles) (n=197);
- R-CHOP (CHOP plus rituximab on d1 of each cycle, every 21d for 8 cycles) (n=202).

Primary endpoint: Response to chemotherapy (CR=complete response, CRu=unconfirmed CR, PR=partial response, SD=stable disease, PD= progressive disease).

Secondary endpoints: Overall survival (OS) and event-free survival (EFS) at 2y, and treatment-related toxicity.

Follow-up: Median F/U=24 months. CT scan to assess response.

Results

	CR/CR$_U$	PD	EFS	OS
CHOP	63%	22%	38%	57%
R-CHOP	76%	9%	57%	70%
p	0.003	Not reported	<0.001	0.007

- Rituximab addition reduced risk of events by 42% (vs CHOP alone).

Discussion
R-CHOP treated patients had significantly better response rates, EFS, and OS than those treated with CHOP alone. This benefit was seen in patients with both low- and high-risk disease and was independent of adverse risk factors. Treatment-related toxicity was similar in both groups. Grade 3/4 infusion-related reactions (chills, fever, decresed BP, bronchospasm) were seen in 9% receiving rituximab, but all disappeared after stopping/slowing the infusion. There were no associated deaths. Mean nadir neutrophil counts were slightly lower in the R-CHOP group, but this did not translate to an increase in febrile episodes or the use of more granulocyte-colony stimulating factor (G-CSF).

Problems
- Subsequent analyses suggest the survival benefit of R-CHOP is restricted to DLBCL with BCL-2 expression, an immunohistochemical marker associated with poor prognosis and chemotherapy resistance.
- This trial considered a limited patient group (elderly with advanced disease). However, subsequent studies have confirmed the efficacy of rituximab in younger patients and in those with limited staging.

Hodgkin's disease: chemotherapy

Chemotherapy of advanced Hodgkin's disease with MOPP, ABVD, or MOPP alternating with ABVD.

AUTHORS: Cannellos G, Anderson J, Propert K *et al.*
REFERENCE: N Engl J Med (1992) 327, 1478–84.
STUDY DESIGN: RCT
EVIDENCE LEVEL: 1b

Key message

The ABVD (adriamycin, bleomycin, vinblastine, dacarbazine) regime has higher efficacy with less toxicity than the former standard MOPP regime (mechlorethamine, vincristine, procarbazine, prednisolone) in patients with Hodgkin's disease.

Impact

ABVD has now replaced MOPP as standard first-line chemotherapy in Hodgkin's disease, regardless of the clinical stage at presentation.

Aims

Combination chemotherapy has significantly improved survival in advanced Hodgkin's disease over the last 30y. In 1992, MOPP was considered standard therapy, but was associated with considerable toxicity, including sterilisation, severe myelosuppression, and secondary acute myeloid leukaemia. This trial aimed to show that ABVD was an effective and less toxic first-line therapy in patients with advanced Hodgkin's disease.

Methods

Patients: 361 patients at 13 centres in the USA.

Inclusion criteria:
- Age ≥16y;
- Biopsy proven Hodgkin's disease;
- Untreated patients with stage IIIA2, IIIB, IVA, or IVB disease;
- Recurrence at least 3 months after primary radiotherapy (RT) for localised Hodgkin's disease;
- ≥1 tumour mass on physical/radiological examination;
- Adequate renal and hepatic function;
- Normal bone marrow reserve (unless impairment secondary to marrow involvement with Hodgkin's disease).

Groups: Patients risk stratified, then randomised into 3 well-matched groups:
- MOPP alone (n=123);
- ABVD alone (n=115);
- MOPP-ABVD (n=123).

Primary endpoint: Response to chemotherapy: complete remission (CR), partial remission (PR) or no response/progressive disease.

Secondary endpoints:
- Failure-free survival (FFS);
- Overall survival (OS);
- Treatment-related toxicity.

Follow-up: Median 6y (minimum 4y).
- Every 2 cycles of treatment;
- Every 3 months for the first 2y after treatment, then every 6 months;
- CXR every 2 cycles, plus any radiological assessment that was abnormal at presentation.

Results

	MOPP	ABVD	MOPP-ABVD	*p*
CR (%)	67	82	83	0.006
No response (%)	4	2	0	Not reported
FFS (%)	50	61	65	0.02
OS (%)	66	73	75	0.3

p value refers to comparison of MOPP with the other regimen.

Discussion

Response rates and FFS with regimens containing ABVD were significantly better than with MOPP alone, particularly for patients with adverse prognostic factors. One possible explanation is that patients treated with MOPP alone required more dose reductions due to the greater myelosuppression and higher incidence of infective complications associated with this regimen. Secondary acute leukaemia was limited to MOPP containing regimens, but there were three fatalities from pulmonary toxicity in the ABVD only group. There was no significant difference in overall survival.

Problems

- Some concerns over bleomycin-related pulmonary toxicity.
- No significant difference in overall long-term survival.
- Had G-CSF (granulocyte-colony stimulating factor) been available at the time of this trial, there *may* have been improved response rates with MOPP as a result of reduced neutropaenia, infective complications, and dose reductions.

Myeloma: melphalan

Medical Research Council (MRC) Myeloma VII Trial: High-dose chemotherapy with haematopoietic stem-cell rescue for multiple myeloma.

AUTHORS: Child J, Morgan G, Davies F et al. (MRC Adult Leukaemia Working Party).
REFERENCE: N Engl J Med (2003) 348, 1875–83.
STUDY DESIGN: RCT
EVIDENCE LEVEL: 1b

Key message
The largest study to demonstrate progression-free and overall survival benefit for high-dose melphalan in newly diagnosed myeloma.

Impact
High-dose melphalan is currently considered the standard of care for patients under the age of 65 with myeloma in first remission.

Aims
Conventional dose chemotherapy followed by dose escalated melphalan supported with autologous stem cell rescue results in improved response rates in myeloma. However, the survival benefits were inconclusive in previous non-randomised and randomised studies. This trial aimed to compare standard doxroubicin, carmustine, cyclophosphamide, and melphalan (ACBM) with cyclophosphamide, vincristine, doxorubicin, and methylprednisolone (C-VAMP), followed by high-dose melphalan with autologous stem cell rescue.

Methods
Patients: 401 patients at 83 centres in the UK and New Zealand.

Inclusion criteria: Patients with previously untreated myeloma:
- <65y old;
- Fulfilling MRC criteria for initiation of treatment;
- Suitable candidates for high-dose therapy.

Groups: Both groups received maintenance interferon α-2a:
- Standard: ABCM (to maximum response, median 6 cycles, range 1–13) (n=196; 30 patients also received high-dose melphalan off-protocol);
- Intensive: C-VAMP (to maximal response, median 5 cycles, range 1–9; followed by melphalan 200mg/m^2 with autologous stem cell rescue) (n=197; 150 received high-dose melphalan).

Primary endpoints: Overall survival (OS) and progression-free survival (PFS).

Secondary endpoints: Complete and partial response rates (European Group for Blood and Marrow Transplantation: International Bone Marrow Transplant Registry criteria).

Follow-up: Median F/U of survivors=42 months.

Results
- Median age 55y (33–66); 56%=male.

	Standard	Intensive	p
Primary endpoints			
OS (median)	42 months (33–52)	54 months (45–65)	0.04
PFS	20 months (16–22)	32 months (27–38)	<0.001
Secondary endpoints			
Complete response	8%	44%	<0.001
Partial response	40%	42%	0.7
No change/minimal response	33%	5%	<0.001
Progression	10%	1%	Not reported

Discussion
The intention-to-treat analysis demonstrated an improvement in remission rates and a survival advantage of 1y for patients receiving intensive treatment with high-dose melphalan. Previous studies had compared early vs late transplantation, single vs double transplantation, high vs intermediate dose melphalan, or had only randomised those patients who responded to treatment. However, combined analysis with this study confirmed a progression-free and overall survival advantage. It is important to note that this therapy is not curative, and that the survival benefits demonstrated were only modest.

Problems
- Quality of life was not studied. However, the IFM study of early vs late transplantation showed no survival benefits, but did show an improvement in quality of life in patients receiving immediate vs delayed high-dose melphalan.
- Improved outcomes in myeloma with newer agents such as thalidomide, lenolidamide, and bortezomib used alone or in combination have again questioned the value of autologous transplantation, particularly in those patients achieving a complete or near complete remission prior to transplantation.

Myeloma: thalidomide

Oral melphalan and prednisolone chemotherapy plus thalidomide compared with melphalan and prednisolone alone in elderly patients with multiple myeloma.

AUTHORS: Palumbo A, Bringhen S, Caravita T *et al.* (GIMEMA trials group)
REFERENCE: Lancet (2006) 367, 825–31.
STUDY DESIGN: RCT
EVIDENCE LEVEL: 1b

Key message

The first RCT of thalidomide in previously untreated patents with myeloma. It was the first study to show an improvement over melphalan and prednisolone (which have been standard therapy for elderly patients with myeloma since the 1960s).

Impact

The use of novel agents such as thalidomide in combination with steroid with or without alkylating agents is now acknowledged as the preferred standard of care.

Aims

Thalidomide had been demonstrated to be effective as a single agent in relapsed myeloma with response rates of 25–35%, increased to 50% in combination with steroid, and to 70% with the further addition of alkylating agents. This study aimed to assess the benefits of the addition of thalidomide to the previously accepted standard of melphalan and prednisolone.

Methods

Patients: 331 patients at 54 centres in Italy.

Inclusion criteria: Patients with previously untreated myeloma:
• Age >65y (or younger but unsuitable for high-dose chemotherapy);
• Salmon and Durie stage II–III;
• Measurable disease;
• Suitable candidates for high-dose therapy.

Exclusion criteria: Peripheral neuropathy.

Groups: Non-blinded:
• **MP:** melphalan and prednisolone (n: randomised=164, F/U to >6 months=126);
• **MPT:** melphalan, prednisolone and thalidomide (n: randomised=167, F/U to >6 months=129);

Primary endpoints: Response rates (complete response, CR; partial response, PR; minimal response, MR) and event-free survival (EFS).

Secondary endpoints: Overall survival (OS), time to response and adverse events.

Follow-up: Median F/U of survivors=15.2 and 17.6 months in the MP and MPT groups, respectively.

Results

- Median age=72y (60–85).

	MP	MPT	Difference	p / 95% CI
Primary endpoints				
CR	2.4%	15.5%	13%	16.5 to 39.1%
PR	45.2%	60.4%	15.2%	3.0 to 26.9%
No change / MR	31.8%	10.8%	−21%	Not reported
Progression	16.7%	7.8%	−8.9	−17.2 to −0.8
EFS (at 2y)	27% (16–22)	54% (27–38)	27%	0.0006
Secondary endpoints				
OS (at 3y)	80%	64%	−16%	0.2
Time to PR	3.1 months (25–210d)	1.4 months (22–200d)	−1.7 months	Not reported

Discussion

This study demonstrated clear superiority of the addition of thalidomide to melphalan and prednisolone, with similar results in age groups greater and less than 70y of age. This benefit was achieved at the expense of greater toxicity, although the risk of thromboembolism was effectively reduced by low molecular weight heparin.

Problems

- The median duration of thalidomide therapy was short (8 months).
- Thalidomide was associated with increased grade 3–4 toxicity (particularly neuropathy, infection, and venous thromboembolism). The latter complication was significantly reduced by the introduction of prophylactic enoxaparin half way through the study.
- The F/U of this study was short. No survival benefit has been demonstrated as yet.
- The MPT group received thalidomide as maintenance as well as initial therapy. The duration of therapy was therefore longer in the MPT arm, and the relative merits of thalidomide as induction therapy vs thalidomide as maintenance therapy remain unknown.
- It is possible, even likely, that thalidomide will be superseded by agents such as lenalidamide or bortezomib either alone, or in combination, in the near future.

HIV/AIDS

Introduction

HIV/AIDS is a dynamic and fast-moving specialty. It is not yet 30 years since the recognition of the acquired immune deficiency syndrome in 1981, when first reports described homosexual men in the USA presenting with unusual infections (e.g. *Pneumocystis* pneumonia) and malignancies (e.g. Kaposi's sarcoma). The cause of this syndrome, a virus related to simian retroviruses, was established in 1983.

Retrospectively, it now seems likely that cases had occurred since at least the 1930s in parts of Africa, and phylogenetic study of human and simian retroviruses has established the zoonotic origins of HIV-1 from chimpanzees and HIV-2 from sooty mangabeys.

Initially, mortality was high, and treatment limited to management and prevention of opportunistic infections. For those living in developed countries, treatment improvements have meant that HIV has been transformed from a fatal condition to a chronic infection with dramatic improvements in life expectancy. This change was heralded by the development of protease inhibitors and the strategy of using three drugs in combination—so called 'highly active antiretroviral therapy' (HAART)—in 1996.

Therefore, the outlook for people living with HIV in developed countries is cause for optimism. However, this is not yet the case for the majority of the 33 million people living with HIV across the world, particularly in sub-Saharan Africa where the prevalence of HIV infection is highest. Access to medication and health professionals trained in managing HIV greatly determines the improvement in life expectancy, so that the prognosis for an HIV-infected individual in a developing country does not nearly resemble that found in the Western world. Between 2001 and 2007 the steepest increases in prevalence have been seen in regions of Asia and Europe.

Here, we present some of the evidence which guides current practice, much of it recent, and some of it likely to be superseded by newer trials in the months and years to come. This evidence largely refers to treatment of HIV-1 infection; HIV-2 is much less prevalent and requires an adjusted therapeutic approach.

See also:
For up-to-date UK treatment guidelines, visit the British HIV Association website at:
www.bhiva.org

Boosted vs unboosted protease inhibitors

> Lopinavir-ritonavir vs nelfinavir for the initial treatment of HIV infection.
>
> **AUTHORS:** Walmsley S, Bernstein B, King M *et al.*
> **REFERENCE:** N Engl J Med (2002) 346; 2039–46.
> **STUDY DESIGN:** RCT
> **EVIDENCE LEVEL:** 1b

Key message

Combination antiretroviral therapy (ART) containing a protease inhibitor (PI) given with low dose ritonavir ('boosted' regime) is more effective in suppressing HIV replication than an 'unboosted' regime.

Impact

Ritonavir-boosted PIs are now used in preference to unboosted PIs in combination ART, with lopinavir-ritonavir recommended as one of the first-line alternatives to efavirenz for patients naïve to treatment. Boosted PIs are also used as second-line therapy for patients failing treatment with non-nucleoside reverse transcriptase inhibitors (this is also the World Health Organisation recommendation for use in resource-poor settings).

Aims

PIs are effective at suppressing HIV replication. The cytochrome p450 enzyme-inhibiting properties of the PI, ritonavir, were exploited in formulating the then new ART agent, lopinavir, with a low-dose of ritonavir to increase its serum levels and half-life. This allows levels >75% higher than that needed to inhibit HIV replication, leaving more flexibility in the dosing schedule. With their combined activity having been demonstrated in small studies, this RCT aimed to compare lopinavir-ritonavir with the standard of care unboosted PI nelfinavir in terms of virological suppression and tolerability.

Methods

Patients: 653 patients from 93 centres in 13 countries (in North and South America, Europe, Africa, and Australia).

Inclusion criteria:
- Age >12y, confirmed HIV infection, viral load >400 copies/mL;
- Treatment naïve.

Groups: All given open-label stavudine and lamivudine as backbone:
- Boosted: Lopinavir-ritonavir (400/100mg bd) and nelfinavir placebo (tds) (n=326);
- Unboosted: Nelfinavir (750mg tds) and lopinavir-ritonavir placebo (bd) (n=327). NB. Nelfinavir license changed during study and 30 patients switched to 1250mg bd.

Primary endpoint: Undetectable (<400 copies/mL) viral load at 24wk and time to loss of virological response (up to 48wk). Longer-term response measured with <50 copies/mL at 48wk (a more relevant result as the aim of ART is maintenance of an undetectable viral load at <50 copies/mL).

Secondary endpoints:
- Laboratory abnormalities including lipid levels;
- Resistance mutations in HIV protease;
- Side effects including diarrhoea.

Follow-up: Every 4wk for the first 24wk; then every 8wk for following 24wk.

Results

Primary endpoint	Lopinavir-ritonavir	Nelfinavir	*p*
<400 copies/mL at wk24	79%	71%	<0.05
<50 copies/mL at wk48	67%	52%	<0.001
Secondary endpoints			
Total cholesterol >7.76mmol/L*	9.0%	4.9%	ns
Triglycerides >8.47mmol/L*	9.3%	1.3%	<0.001
Protease mutations	0/37‡	25/76‡	<0.001

* Conversion from mg/dL ‡tested where VL >400 copies/mL.

Discussion

This RCT showed improved efficacy durability of a boosted PI vs unboosted nelfinavir. The sustained virological response at 48wk and lack of evidence for resistance to PIs in those failing the boosted regime were encouraging, as most patients need several regimens in their lifetime, possibly using PIs again in other combinations. The significant differences in triglyceride levels may increase cardiovascular risk, but must be seen in the context of overall health improvement with effective ART. Newer data with other boosted PIs have demonstrated similar virological efficacy and protection against primary PI resistance. However, the dosing regimen of boosted-lopinavir required twice daily administration and was associated with generic side effects of boosted PIs (dyslipidaemia, central obesity, and diarrhoea).

Problems

- As in many HIV trials, F/U of trial participants vs duration of treatment required was very short; many years of F/U are required to truly test ART regimens. However, data have been presented since showing virological suppression is still better with lopinavir-ritonavir than nelfinavir at 96wk.

Initial treatment: number of nucleoside agents

Triple nucleoside regimens vs efavirenz-containing regimens for the initial treatment of HIV-1 infection.

AUTHORS: Gulick R, Ribaudo H, Shikuma C et al. (Aids Clinical Trials Group, ACTG 5095 team).
REFERENCE: N Engl J Med (2004) 350, 1850–61.
STUDY DESIGN: RCT
EVIDENCE LEVEL: 1b

Key message

Triple nucleoside combination regimens are inferior to regimens containing efavirenz plus nucleosides in providing virological control of HIV infection. A companion article from the group demonstrated that there is no advantage in adding a fourth nucleoside, abacavir, to an efavirenz/ZDV/3TC combination.

Impact

Nucleoside-only regimens are no longer recommended for treatment of HIV and two-class, three-drug combinations remain the optimal treatment for HIV.

Aims

The triple nucleoside regimen of abacavir/ZDV/3TC has been used in HIV treatment because of improved patient adherence, lack of interactions, and the strategic sense of sparing the two other major classes of antiretrovirals (ARV) for the later development of virological failure. This double-blind, placebo-controlled RCT aimed to investigate the efficacy of nucleoside reverse transcriptase inhibitor (NRTI) regimens only or with non-NRTIs, and to compare whether additional benefit is derived from the use of abacavir, a further nucleoside in efavirenz-containing dual NRTI regimens.

Methods

Patients: 1147 patients at multiple centres in the USA.

Inclusion criteria: HIV-1 infected adults:
- Antiretroviral naïve;
- Viral load (VL) >400 copies/mL.

Groups:
- Zidovudine-lamivudine-abacavir (n=382);
- Zidovudine-lamivudine-efavirenz and zidovudine-lamivudine-abacavir-efavirenz (combined n=765).

Design and analysis: Non-inferiority design; intention-to-treat analysis; stratified by initial VL above or below 100,000 copies/mL.

Primary endpoint: Virological failure (defined by 2 successive HIV-1 RNA values ≥200 copies/mL, at least 16wk after randomisation).

Follow-up: Every 4wk to 24wk; every 8wk thereafter, with adherence questionnaires at 4, 12, 24, 48wk.

Results

	Virological failure during study time	Viral load <50 copies/mL at 48wk	CD4 change at wk48 (cells/mm^3)
ZDV & 3TC & ABC	82/382 (21%)	61% (50–72)	+174 (151–197)
ZDV & 3TC & EFV*	85/765 (11%)	83% (78–88)	+173 (152–194)
ZDV & 3TC & ABC & EFV*			*p*=0.58

Results did not differ between strata based on initial VL. * These results were consistent at 156wk F/U, published in a separate paper.

Discussion

The results of the first analysis of this study substantiated earlier evidence that triple nucleoside regimens were inferior to a two-class combination. It also demonstrated the excellent virological efficacy of efavirenz-containing regimens. This triple NRTI arm of the trial was stopped early (with pre-specified stopping rules), and the results were presented for the combined efavirenz-containing groups vs the triple nucleoside group. In the comparison of the two efavirenz-based arms, there were no differences in any of the endpoints evaluated. Subsequent analysis demonstrated that the speed of viral load fall was identical in both efavirenz arms; this argues against initial induction with more drugs. The findings of this study were published in two papers.*

Problems

- A double-blind study design using placebo does not assess the role of convenience of a regimen in its success. However, adherence to the study regimens was excellent, and there was still a difference in rate of virological failure.

* See also Gulick *et al.* JAMA (2006) 296, 769–81.

Nucleoside reverse transcriptase inhibitor: optimal agents

Tenofovir DF, emtricitabine, and efavirenz vs zidovudine, lamivudine, and efavirenz for HIV.

AUTHORS: Gallant J, DeJesus E, Arribas J et al.
REFERENCE: N Engl J Med (2006) 354, 251–60.
STUDY DESIGN: RCT
EVIDENCE LEVEL: 1b

Key message
When combined with efavirenz, the nucleotide/nucleoside backbone of tenofovir and emtricitabine (TDF/FTC) provides superior virological control and improved tolerability to fixed dose combination zidovudine and lamivudine.

Impact
TDF/FTC, available as a fixed dose combination, is now a recommended first-line nucleoside reverse transcriptase inhibitor (NRTI) backbone.

Aims
Long-term treatment of HIV infection depends on the availability of durable, tolerable, non-toxic, antiretroviral regimens which can be adhered to over many years. All recommended initial regimens include two nucleoside/nucleotide reverse transcriptase inhibitors. Zidovudine/lamivudine (ZDV/3TC) was previously the standard backbone to antiretroviral therapy, but is associated with suboptimal tolerability and long-term extremity fat loss. Many other combinations have also been evaluated. This non-inferiority trial aimed to compare ZDV/3TC with TDF/FTC. A subgroup analysis examining fat loss was also included.

Methods
Patients: 487 patients at 67 centres in 5 European countries and the USA.

Inclusion criteria:
- Age >18y, HIV-1 infection with viral load (VL) >10,000 copies/mL;
- Antiretroviral naïve.

Groups: Both open-label:
- Efavirenz plus tenofovir and emtricitabine (n=244);
- Efavirenz plus zidovudine and lamivudine (n=243).

Primary endpoint: Non-inferiority of TDF/FTC to ZDV/3TC by HIV viral load <400 copies/mL at 48wk and 96wk.

Secondary endpoints:
- Non-inferiority by HIV VL <50 copies/mL and changes in CD4$^+$ count;
- Resistance mutations in those with virological failure.

Subgroup analysis: Limb fat loss by DEXA scan.

Follow-up: At wk2, 4, and 8; then every 8wk to wk48; then every 12wk thereafter to wk96. Data to 3y F/U reported.

Results

Primary endpoint	TDF/FTC	ZDV/3TC	*p*
VL<400 copies/mL at 48wk	84%	73%	0.002
Secondary endpoints			
VL <50 copies/mL at 48wk	80%	70%	0.02
Change in limb fat 48–96wk by DEXA*	+0.3kg (*p*=0.01)	−0.7kg (*p*=0.001)	–

* These results were published in a F/U paper.

- **Resistance:**
  - No significant difference in development of resistance to efavirenz between groups.
  - M184V (resistance to 3TC and FTC) occurred more frequently in ZDV/3TC group.

Discussion

This study indicated that TDF/FTC was significantly more active in achieving viral suppression with less likelihood of adverse effects than ZDV/3TC. With the published extended data to 96wk, the durability and safety of this combination was confirmed. The lower frequency of resistance mutations seen in the TDF/FTC group may be due to the longer half-lives of TDF and FTC. Subgroup analysis of those who had DEXA scans revealed significantly less limb fat loss in those in the TDF/FTC arm.

Problems

- The tenofovir/emtricitabine combination was non-inferior to zidovudine/lamivudine, but superior in terms of virological undetectability at 400 copies/mL. However, when judged by usual clinical criteria for undetectable VL (<50 copies/mL), the difference between the groups did not reach statistical significance at 96wk. This does demonstrate non-inferiority, but not superiority.
- The open-label design was a potential source of bias and more patients discontinued treatment on ZDV/3TC than TDF/FTC. This may have been due to anaemia attributed to ZDV. The open-label design allowed the effect of pill burden and dosing frequency to be included in overall efficacy.
- There were many exclusion criteria (largely biochemical), which may limit the extent to which these results can be extrapolated to a routine clinic population.

* See also Pozniak *et al.* J Acquired Immune Deficiency Syndrome (2006) 43, 535–40.

Continuous vs intermittent antiretrovirals

SMART (Strategies for Management of AntiRetroviral Therapy) study: CD4$^+$ count-guided interruption of antiretroviral treatment.

AUTHORS: El-Sadr W, Lundgren J, Neaton J et al (SMART Study Group).
REFERENCE: N Engl J Med (2006) 355, 2283–96.
STUDY DESIGN: RCT
EVIDENCE LEVEL: 1b

Key message
CD4$^+$ count-guided interruption of highly active antiretroviral therapy (HAART) is inferior to continuous HAART, with significantly higher rates of death, opportunistic disease, and renal, hepatic, and cardiovascular events in the drug conservation arm.

Impact
Whereas before this study, patient groups and physicians were considering interrupting therapy for patients with higher CD4$^+$ counts in the interests of reduced cost and side effects, all now recommend continuous therapy outside of clinical trials.

Aims
Long-term antiretroviral therapy is associated with side effects, a high financial cost, and risk of developing resistance to antiretroviral drugs. Prior to this publication, several smaller studies had investigated treatment strategies to potentially allow intermittent therapy, thus reducing these risks and costs. These demonstrated 'safe' interruption of HAART, even in individuals with previous AIDS-defining conditions. This study aimed to conclusively compare the safety and efficacy of two treatment strategies: continuous treatment (virological suppression) with CD4-guided interrupted treatment (drug conservation).

Methods
Patients: 5472 patients at 318 centres in 33 countries.

Inclusion criteria: HIV infection, plus:
- Age >13y and not pregnant or breastfeeding;
- CD4 count >350 cells/mm^3;
- Consent to start, stop, or change HAART according to protocol.

Groups:
- Viral suppression (VS): received uninterrupted HAART, aiming for continuous suppression of viral replication (n=2752);
- Drug conservation (DC): HAART given if CD4 <250 cells/mm^3 and discontinued if >350 cells/mm^3 (n=2720).

Primary endpoint: New/recurrent opportunistic disease/death (any cause).

Secondary endpoints:
- Serious opportunistic disease;
- Major cardiovascular, hepatic, or renal disease;

- Grade 4 toxicity: potentially life-threatening events requiring medical intervention (as per toxicity tables of the National Institute of Allergy and Infectious Diseases).

Follow-up: At 1 and 2 months; then every 2 months thereafter in the first year; then every 4 months in each following year. Included history, examination, ECG, HIV viral load (VL), and CD4 count. Patients also seen and assessed as per clinical need.

Results

	Event rate per 100 person y		
Primary endpoint	**VS**	**DC**	***p***
Death from any cause	1.3	3.3	<0.001
Serious opportunistic disease	0.1	0.4	0.01
Secondary endpoints			
Major cardiovascular, renal, or hepatic disease	1.1	1.8	0.009
Grade 4 event or death from any cause	4.7	5.9	0.03

Discussion

There were relatively few deaths due to opportunistic infection and, unexpectedly, the DC group did not have fewer grade 4 events than the VS group. The higher rate of cardiovascular disease in the DC group challenges the belief that cardiovascular toxicity in HIV is entirely related to medication, and raises questions about the pro-inflammatory effects of untreated HIV infection. Those stopping treatment had a rapid fall in CD4 count and rise in viral load: HAART was taken 94% of the F/U time in the VS group vs 33% in the DC group. The study was stopped early, with an average of 16 months F/U (rather than the planned 6y) due to the high rate of disease progression and death in the DC group.

Problems

- Early interruption of study recruitment and F/U: data were not as long-term as intended.
- No data from SMART on the development of drug resistance with each treatment strategy; this was examined in previous small studies.
- Further evidence is needed to assess whether interrupting treatment at higher CD4 counts may be of benefit.

HIV and hepatitis C co-infection

> **APRICOT** (**A**IDS **P**egasys **R**ibavirin **I**nternational **C**oinfection **T**rial) **study group:** Pegylated α-2a plus ribavirin for chronic hepatitis C virus infection in HIV-infected patients.
>
> **AUTHORS:** Torriani F, Rodriguez-Torres M, Rockstroh J *et al.*
> **REFERENCE:** N Engl J Med (2004) 351, 438–50.
> **STUDY DESIGN:** RCT
> **EVIDENCE LEVEL:** 1b

Key message

In HIV co-infected patients, combined weekly pegylated interferon α-2a and ribavirin is more effective in producing a sustained virological response (SVR) to hepatitis C virus (HCV) than three times weekly pegylated interferon α-2a alone or standard interferon-α plus twice daily ribavirin. However, the rate of SVR is less than that achieved in HIV-negative HCV-infected (monoinfected) patients.

Impact

This trial demonstrated that HCV in HIV co-infected patients could be effectively treated with 1y of pegylated interferon α and ribavirin. It also confirmed that the absence of an early virological response (>2 log fall in viral load by 12wk) was highly predictive of treatment failure, and further informed guideline recommendations that treatment be stopped at 12wk in these patients.

Aims

Co-infection with HIV has a deleterious effect on HCV due to the accelerated development of hepatic fibrosis. With improved antiretroviral therapy and fewer opportunistic infections, HCV infection is now a major cause of morbidity and mortality among HIV-positive individuals. Therefore, its treatment has the potential to increase longevity. The established treatment for HCV monoinfection is pegylated interferon α plus weight-based ribavirin. This trial aimed to assess its efficacy in HIV co-infection, where HCV treatment had previously been less successful.

Methods

Patients: 868 patients at 95 centres in 19 countries in Europe, Australia, North and South America.

Inclusion criteria: HIV and HCV, plus:
- Age >18y;
- Detectable serum HCV RNA levels;
- Elevated alanine aminotransferase and compensated liver disease;
- Evidence of chronic HCV infection on liver biopsy.

Groups:
- Interferon α-2a and ribavirin (n=289);
- Pegylated interferon α-2a and placebo (n=289);
- Pegylated interferon α-2a and ribavirin (n=290).

Primary endpoint: SVR: serum HCV RNA below limit of detection of assay at 50iu/mL.

Secondary endpoints: Factors independently associated with SVR and predictive value of early virological response.

Follow-up: 48wk treatment period followed by 24wk F/U.

Results

Intention-to-treat analysis — percentage of patients in each group with SVR at 72wk.

Genotype	pegIFN and rib (n=285)	pegIFN (n=286)	IFN and rib (n=289)
1	29	14	7
2/3	62	36	20
All patients	40	20	12

Secondary endpoints
Non-genotype 1 and lower baseline HCV RNA load associated with SVR

p<0.001 for comparisons of pegIFN and ribavirin with other treatments in all patients.

Discussion

This trial confirmed that successful treatment of HCV is possible despite the presence of HIV. For co-infected patients, SVR was less likely in patients with non-2/3 genotypes, high baseline HCV VL, and cirrhosis. Adverse event rates were comparable to those seen in monoinfection. In addition to the clear benefit of dual therapy with pegylated interferon α-2a and ribavirin, pegylated interferon α alone could be considered for those with contraindications to ribavirin, as a better SVR rate was seen than with standard interferon α and ribavirin.

Problems

- Extensive exclusions may mean that response rates can be extrapolated only to similarly straightforward patients. The majority of patients had CD4 counts >500 cells/mL and were on HAART; in practice, one often has more advanced patients to manage.
- Subsequent studies have demonstrated that improved responses are achieved with weight-based ribavirin.

Antiretroviral therapy and cardiovascular risk

> **D:A:D study (Data collection on Adverse events of anti-HIV Drugs):**
> Class of antiretroviral drugs and the risk of myocardial infarction.
>
> **AUTHORS:** Friis-Møller N, Reiss P, Sabin C *et al.* (D:A:D study group)
> **REFERENCE:** N Engl J Med (2007) 356, 1723–35.
> **STUDY DESIGN:** Cohort study
> **EVIDENCE LEVEL:** 3

Key message
Use of highly active antiretroviral therapy (HAART) is associated with increased risk of myocardial infarction (MI). This risk increases with longer duration of treatment, is primarily associated with protease inhibitor (PI) use and may be partially explained by dyslipidaemia.

Impact
Strong evidence now underlines the importance of assessing and reducing modifiable cardiovascular risk factors and, where possible, choosing components of HAART which do not aggravate dyslipidaemia.

Aims
Although combination antiretroviral therapy (ART) can significantly reduce morbidity and mortality in HIV-1, concerns have been raised about the risk of associated coronary heart disease. This prospective, observational cohort study aimed to detect the incidence of cardiovascular and cerebrovascular events, and to assess the association between these events and treatment with antiretroviral agents. Specifically, it examined risk profiles for MI, and their association with PIs and non-nucleoside reverse transcriptase inhibitors (nNRTIs). Further analysis of this dataset has shown a significant association between certain NRTIs (abacavir and didanosine) and coronary heart disease.

Methods
Patients: 23,437 patients from 19 European countries, USA, and Australia.

Inclusion criteria: HIV-1 infected adults.

Groups:
- Cohort data analysed by class of ART:
  - PI-containing regimens;
  - NNRTI-containing regimens.

Primary endpoint: MI: definite, possible, or unclassifiable; recorded as fatal or non-fatal.

Follow-up: Every 8 months through period of study by patient interview, physical examination, and case note review for status of HIV infection, cardiovascular risk, and events. Mean F/U=4.5y per patient; total 94,469 person-y.

Results

Primary endpoint	nNRTI relative risk	PI
MI (adjusted relative rate/y of exposure to ART)	1.05 (0.98–1.13)	1.16 (1.1–1.23)
	$p = 0.17$	$p = <0.001$
Adjusted for serum lipid levels	1.00 (0.93–1.09)	1.10 (1.04–1.18)

Discussion

Previous studies had demonstrated an association between the use of ART and MI. However, this analysis from the D:A:D cohorts (with longer F/U) showed a clear association limited to PI use only that accumulated with each year on therapy, to a doubling of risk over 5y. Much of this risk clearly depended on underlying known risk factors for coronary disease, and the risk attributable to PIs was unchanged with age. There was no effect of viral load or CD4+ count. Although an observational study, thorough adjustment models for possible confounders gave consistent results. The effect of PIs on (increasing) lipid levels did not seem to completely explain the increased cardiovascular risk. Many patients in the cohort were young (median age 39y) and many were smokers (60.8%); the benefits of PI therapy still outweighed the additional risks in most cases.

Problems

- This was an observational study. A causal relationship between drug exposure and outcomes cannot conclusively be established.
- Awareness of a possible link between PIs and MI could mean that cohort patients deemed to be at high risk were prescribed other therapies. However, this would have only weakened the observed association.

Infectious diseases and tropical medicine

Introduction

Some of the earliest clinical trials were conducted in infectious diseases. In the 1940s the development of the first antibiotics for treating tuberculosis coincided with the recognition that rigorous clinical trials were required to determine optimum drug combinations and duration of treatment. Key early trials funded by the MRC included a study comparing streptomycin with the then standard treatment for pulmonary tuberculosis – bed rest.[1] The joint efforts of bacteriologists, clinicians, and statisticians promoted the development of clinical trials acknowledging that clinically valid end-points and careful statistical analysis are vital for trials to provide evidence of sufficient quality to guide clinical practice.

Infectious diseases was then dominated by antibiotic trials, often funded by drug companies with their own agendas. However, the last decade has seen the publication of a range of important trials, many conducted in resource poor settings and addressing important clincial questions.

For this chapter, we chose key questions in our field that had been addressed by good quality trials. We wanted our chapter to be useful for both clinicians in the UK and overseas. We then used a democratic process to evaluate the evidence whereby key papers were allocated to clinicians at the Hospital for Tropical Diseases, London and our Evidence Based Medicine sessions were used to evaluate the trials following a structure very similar to that used in the *Oxford Handbook of Key Clinical Evidence*.[2] All the medical staff contributed to these sessions which generated intense discussions resulting in the rejection of a number of trials judged to be of inferior quality, not representative, or not relevant. It was sometimes difficult to select a single trial in any one area since clinical practice often evolves based on the collated evidence of multiple trials, each with their own strengths and weaknesses.

We chose trials that generated key data such as the study in Vietnam which examined the effect of adding corticosteroids to the treatment regime for tuberculous meningitis; based on this study, adjunct steroids have now become part of routine practice. Another key trial is the comparison of quinine vs artesunate for the treatment of falciparum malaria which shows that in Asia, treatment with artesunate results in reduced mortality. Other trials address clinical problems that are important worldwide and less commonly seen in the UK, such as the management of cerebral cysticercosis where critical evaluation of current trials might be difficult.

Despite the early studies on tuberculosis, this disease is again becoming a major clinical problem worldwide. Amongst other appropriately designed trials we hope that in future editions we shall be reporting trials looking at novel anti-tuberculous drugs.

References

1. Streptomycin treatment of pulmonary tuberculosis. BMJ 1948 (2):769–82.
2. Integrating evidence based medicine into routine clinical practice: seven years' experience at the Hospital for Tropical Diseases, London. Lockwood DNJ, Armstrong M and Grant A. BMJ, Oct 2004; 329: 1020–23.

Bacterial meningitis: steroids

Dexamethasone in adults with bacterial meningitis.

AUTHORS: de Gans J, van de Beek D.
REFERENCE: N Engl J Med (2002) 347, 1549–56.
STUDY DESIGN: RCT
EVIDENCE LEVEL: 1b

Key message
The first double-blind RCT to show a reduction in morbidity and mortality in adults with bacterial meningitis, treated early with adjuvant corticosteroids. Subgroup analysis shows particular benefit of corticosteroids in meningitis caused by *Streptococcus pneumoniae*.

Impact
Steroids are now recommended for administration with the first dose of empiric antibiotics (and for 4d thereafter) in adults with bacterial meningitis, particularly if pneumococcal meningitis is likely.

Aims
A number of trials assessing children with acute bacterial meningitis had suggested benefit from early corticosteroid use in pneumococcal meningitis and reduced auditory complications in *Haemophilus influenzae* type B meningitis. However, a large placebo-controlled double-blind study in adults was lacking. This trial aimed to examine neurological outcome and mortality in adults with bacterial meningitis treated with conventional antibiotics, with and without adjuvant corticosteroids. All patients underwent cerebrospinal fluid (CSF) sampling, enabling subgroup analysis of outcome on the basis of causative organism.

Methods
Patients: 301 patients from multiple centres in the Netherlands, Belgium, Germany, Austria, and Denmark.

Inclusion criteria:
- Age >17y, with suspected meningitis and ≥1 of the following:
- Bacteria seen in CSF on Gram stain (n=215);
- CSF white cell count >1000/mm^3 (n=80);
- Cloudy CSF (n=6).

Groups:
- Dexamethasone (10mg IV) given with OP 15–20min before first dose of antibiotics, then every 6h, for a total of 4d (n=157);
- Placebo (administered identically) (n=144).

Primary endpoint: Score on Glasgow Outcome Scale: 1=death, 2=vegetative state, 3=severe disability, 4=moderate disability, 5=mild or no disability. Favourable outcome=score of 5. Unfavourable outcome=score of 1–4.

Secondary endpoints:
- Death;
- Focal neurological abnormalities (including aphasia, cranial nerve palsy, severe ataxia, monoparesis, and hemiparesis);

- Hearing loss;
- Gastrointestinal haemorrhage (clinically significant, with a drop in serum haemoglobin);
- Others (fungal infection, herpes zoster, hyperglycaemia >8mmol/L).

Follow-up: Neurological examination 8wk after admission (262 of 301 patients). Last observation 'carried forward' in remaining 39 patients, so all 301 patients were included in endpoint analyses.

Results

Primary endpoint	Dexamethasone (n=157)	Placebo (n=144)	p
Unfavourable outcome (all patients)	15%	25%	0.03
Streptococcus pneumoniae	26% (15/58)	52% (26/50)	0.006
Secondary endpoints			
Death (all patients)	7%	15%	0.04
Streptococcus pneumoniae	14% (8/58)	34% (17/50)	0.02

Discussion

These data provided the first unequivocal demonstration of benefit from adjuvant corticosteroids started early (before or with the first dose of antibiotic) in adults with acute bacterial meningitis. The overall reduced risk of neurological deficit and death was primarily a result of significant benefit for patients with pneumococcal meningitis. There was no demonstrable effect on outcome in cases of meningococcal or other non-pneumococcal meningitis. Rates of focal neurological abnormalities and hearing loss were not improved by dexamethasone therapy, and this may be partly explained by the greater proportion of severely ill patients surviving to 8wk in the dexamethasone vs placebo group. However, there was no overall increase in severe neurological sequelae in the dexamethasone group.

Problems

- Although study inclusion criteria were reliant on CSF findings, a delay in administering antibiotics and corticosteroids whilst a lumbar puncture is performed (with preceding cerebral imaging in a proportion of cases) is not recommended.
- The majority (77%) of patients in this study were initially prescribed amoxicillin and penicillin (appropriate microbiological coverage in >97% of CSF culture positive cases). UK guidelines recommend a third generation cephalosporin (usually ceftriaxone) as initial empiric therapy for acute bacterial meningitis because of the small risk of penicillin resistance.
- The failure to demonstrate improved outcome in non-pneumococcal meningitis has led some to advocate restriction of steroid use to situations where pneumococcal meningitis is strongly suspected; this approach is likely to lessen the overall beneficial impact of early adjuvant steroids in adult bacterial meningitis.

Tuberculous meningitis: steroids

Dexamethasone for the treatment of tuberculous meningitis in adolescents and adults.

AUTHORS: Thwaites G, Bang N, Dung N *et al.*
REFERENCE: N Engl J Med (2004) 351, 1741–51.
STUDY DESIGN: RCT
EVIDENCE LEVEL: 1b

Key message

In tuberculous meningitis 6–8wk dexamethasone, administered with initial anti-tuberculous chemotherapy, reduces overall mortality compared with placebo. In patients presenting with mild (Grade I) disease, dexamethasone also reduces the combined risk of death or severe disability.

Impact

Corticosteroids are considered safe in the management of tuberculous meningitis and are routinely administered as part of its management.

Aims

Tuberculous meningitis (TBM) is one of the most severe forms of *Mycobacterium tuberculosis* infection. Although initial small studies had suggested a reduction in severity, and subsequently improved outcomes following steroid use to diminish the inflammatory response, these results had not been substantiated by RCTs. This trial was designed to examine the effect of dexamethasone on mortality and neurological outcome in the treatment of TBM in adolescents and adults.

Methods

Patients: 545 patients at 2 centres in Ho Chi Minh City, Vietnam.

Inclusion criteria:
- Age >14y;
- Meningism and cerebrospinal (CSF) abnormalities;
- Acid-fast bacilli seen in CSF ('definite' TBM); *or* seen in any other specimen/evidence of active pulmonary/extrapulmonary tuberculosis ('probable' TBM); *or* ≥4 of tuberculosis (TB) history, CSF lymphocytosis, CSF:plasma glucose <0.5, yellow CSF, altered consciousness, focal neurology, illness duration >5d ('possible' TBM).

Groups: All patients received streptomycin IM (3 months) and oral rifampicin, isoniazid, pyrazinamide (6 months). Ethambutol replaced streptomycin if HIV-infected; added for 3 months if previous TB treatment.
- Dexamethasone (n=274; including 44 with HIV infection);
- Placebo (n=271; including 54 with HIV infection).

Dosage: Dexamethasone group with Grade I disease (Glasgow Coma Scale (GCS) 15, no focal neurology) received 2wk dexamethasone IV (0.3mg/kg/d wk1; 0.2mg/kg/d wk2); then 4wk oral therapy (0.1mg/kg/d wk3; 3mg/kg/d wk4; reduced by 1mg each wk). Those with Grades II (GCS 11–14) and III (GCS ≤10) disease received 4wk dexamethasone IV (0.4mg/kg/d wk1; reduced by 0.1mg/kg/d each wk); then 4wk oral therapy (4mg total/d; decreased by 1mg each wk).

Primary endpoint: Death or severe disability at 9 months.

Secondary endpoints:
- Fever and coma-clearance time, time to discharge from hospital;
- Time to relapse (new focal neurology or decreased GCS);
- Adverse events inc. hepatitis, gastrointestinal bleeding, bacterial sepsis.

Follow-up: At 1, 2, 6, and 9 months. The latest assessment time point was carried forward in 10 patients lost to F/U at 9 months.

Results

Primary endpoint	Dexamethasone	Placebo	p
Death (all patients)	87 (31.8%)	112 (41.3%)	0.01
Death/severe disability (Grade I disease)	19/90 (21.1%)	30/86 (34.9%)	0.04
Secondary endpoints			
Fever clearance	Median 9d	Median 11d	0.03
Severe adverse events	26 (9.5%)	45 (16.6%)	0.02
Severe clinical hepatitis	0 (0.0%)	8 (3.0%)	0.004

Discussion

Although overall mortality was reduced, there was no reduction in the combined outcome of death or severe disability in the dexamethasone group. This may, in part, be due to the greater proportion of survivors in the dexamethasone group who presented with moderate or severe (Grade II or III) disease. In patients with mild (Grade I) disease, there was a small but significant reduction in the combined primary endpoint in the dexamethasone group. There was no significant difference in coma-clearance time, time to discharge, or relapse rates between the groups, but there were significantly fewer adverse events with dexamethasone.

Problems

- Dexamethasone regimes differed in patients with Grade I vs II/III disease, and although anti-tuberculous drugs were administered via nasogastric tube in those unable to swallow, dexamethasone was always administered IV for the first 2 or 4wk. As bioavailability of oral steroids is usually good, some advocate equivalent dose oral protocols rather than the dexamethasone regimes used here.
- 20% of TBM subjects had co-existent HIV infection (median CD4 count 66/mm^3). None were receiving antiretroviral therapy (ART). Overall mortality in these patients was higher (65%) than in HIV-negative subjects (28%) and occurred at a steady rate throughout F/U. The study was not sufficiently powered to assess the impact of corticosteroids in this population, although most clinicians would recommend their use in these situations.

Cerebral cysticercosis: anti-parasitic therapy

A trial of anti-parasitic treatment to reduce the rate of seizures due to cerebral cysticercosis.

AUTHORS: Garcia H, Pretell E, Gilman R *et al.*
REFERENCE: N Engl J Med (2004) 350, 249–58.
STUDY DESIGN: RCT
EVIDENCE LEVEL: 1b

Key message
In patients with cerebral cysticercosis and viable parenchymal cysts, a short course of albendazole and dexamethasone reduces the long-term rate of generalised seizures.

Impact
Anti-parasitic therapy with adjuvant corticosteroids is routinely considered in neurocysticercosis with viable cysts.

Aims
Neurocysticercosis (NCC), an infection of the central nervous system with *Taenia solium* larvae, is a common cause of acquired epilepsy in the developing world. Although albendazole is effective in killing cerebral cysts, its impact on seizure control had not been clearly established. This trial aimed to examine the effect of albendazole and dexamethasone vs placebo on the rate of seizures.

Methods
Patients: 120 adult patients at 1 centre in Lima, Peru.

Inclusion criteria: Parenchymal NCC, with:
- ≥1 viable cyst on cerebral CT (hypodense vesicle), including cysts with oedema or contrast enhancement (signs of inflammation), only if CT and MRI confirmed liquid contents (analysed separately);
- Serological confirmation of *Taenia solium*;
- ≥1 seizure in previous 6 months (but total seizure history <10y).

Exclusion criteria: Included: >20 cysts on cerebral CT or history of anti-parasitic treament or intracranial hypertension.

Groups: Both groups received a standard first-line anti-convulsant (phenytoin if not already on an anti-epileptic), and after one seizure-free year, anti-convulsants were tapered and stopped over 2 months:
- Albendazole (400mg bd) and dexamethasone (2mg tds) for 10d (n=57);
- Placebo (one of two forms) of similar appearance (n=59).

Primary endpoint: Number of seizures with generalisation (generalised and complex partial seizures; and partial with secondary generalisation).

Secondary endpoints:
- Resolution of parenchymal cysts (on MRI 6 months post-treatment);
- Side effects and adverse events.

Follow-up: At 1, 2, and 3 months; then every 3 months until 30 months post-treatment. F/U ended 6 seizure-free months after stopping treatment.

Results

- Over the 2–30 months F/U, the albendazole group had a non-significant reduction in all seizures vs placebo (46%, $p=0.30$, ns), and a significant reduction in seizures with generalisation (67%, $p=0.01$), persisting when the first month post-treatment was included in analysis (59%, $p=0.03$).
- No significant differences in side effects, except abdominal pain (8/57 treatment arm vs 0/59 placebo, $p=0.006$), likely due to dexamethasone. Three adverse events with placebo not directly related to NCC.

Primary endpoint (over 2–30 months)	Albendazole and dexamethasone (n=57)	Placebo (n=59)	p
Seizures with generalisation	22	68	0.01
Secondary endpoints (number of resolved cysts at 6 months)			
Non-inflamed	113/192 (59%)	36/279 (13%)	<0.001
Inflamed	38/48 (79%)	30/59 (51%)	0.01

Discussion

Despite an initial increase in seizure rate during the first month of anti-parasitic treatment (presumably due to immune-mediated pericyst oedema), the incidence of seizures with generalisation was reduced over 2½y F/U. There were no adverse effects related to treatment. Six months after treatment 59% of non-inflamed cerebral cysts had resolved in the albendazole group, whereas only 13% of untreated cysts resolved spontaneously.

Problems

- Although unlikely, a 10d course of dexamethasone in itself could have modified the host immune response to viable cerebral cysts, and thus affected long-term seizure control; a third 'dexamethasone alone' group would have addressed this possibility.
- The dose of dexamethasone to accompany albendazole anti-parasitic treatment advocated by most authorities is 4mg tds—double that employed in this trial. This may account for the negative impact on seizure control in the first month of treatment in this study.
- Judging by interquartile ranges, at least 25% of patients had a single viable cyst, suggesting albendazole and dexamethasone were appropriate for this group. However, the study was not powered to assess this and did not comment on outcome stratified according to the number of cysts.
- F/U duration was variable (only 18 months in many), as subjects left the trial if seizure-free 6 months after stopping the anti-convulsant. The actual number benefiting from the overall reduction in seizure number was relatively small; 44/57 in the albendazole and 37/59 in the placebo group experienced no seizures throughout F/U.

Treatment of falciparum malaria

SEAQUAMAT (South East Asian Quinine Artesunate MAlaria Trial): artesunate vs quinine for treatment of severe falciparum malaria.

AUTHORS: SEAQUAMAT group.
REFERENCE: Lancet (2005) 366, 717–25.
STUDY DESIGN: RCT
EVIDENCE LEVEL: 1b

Key message

In the treatment of severe falciparum malaria, artesunate reduces mortality by around one third vs standard treatment with quinine. Artesunate also results in reduced incidence of hypoglycaemia and is easier to administer than quinine.

Impact

Where quality assured supply is available, artesunate should replace quinine as the treatment of choice for severe falciparum malaria.

Aims

The artemisinin derivatives, artemether and artesunate, rapidly kill *Plasmodium (P.) falciparum* parasites and, in contrast to quinine, kill both circulating ring-form trophozoites and cytoadhering schizont stages. Unlike artemether, artesunate is water-soluble and can be administered IV. This trial was designed to establish whether artesunate IV could reduce mortality in the treatment of severe malaria, compared with established therapy using quinine IV.

Methods

Patients: 1461 patients (577 Myanmar, 453 Bangladesh, 289 Indonesia, 142 India).

Inclusion criteria: Clinical diagnosis of severe malaria, and:
- Age >2y;
- Positive blood antigen stick test for *P. falciparum* (95% subjects were peripheral blood film positive);
- Patients were excluded if treated with either quinine or artemisinin derivative for >24h prior to admission.

Groups: Both groups received doxycycline (100mg bd PO for 7d) if oral medication was tolerated (unless <8y or pregnant), and full supportive measures according to World Health Organization guidelines:
- Artesunate (2.4mg/kg IV as a bolus at 0, 12, and 24h, then daily); switched to PO when tolerated (2mg salt/kg/d); to complete a total course of 7d (n=730; 633 adults, 97 children [<15y]; 509 (70%) with severe malaria);
- Quinine dihydrochloride (20mg/kg IV loading dose over 4h); then 10mg/kg over 2–8h (tds); switched to PO (10mg/kg tds) when tolerated, to complete a total course of 7d (n=731; 626 adults, 105 children [<15y]; 541 (74%) with severe malaria).

Primary endpoint: Death from severe malaria (in-hospital mortality). Severe malaria: defined as a positive blood film and any one of the following: GCS <11/15 (adults), Blantyre coma scale <3 (children), shock, respiratory rate >32/min, plasma glucose <2.2mmol/L, blood bicarbonate <15mmol/L, haematocrit <20%, or jaundice and parasitaemia >100,000/microL, blood urea >17mmol/L, parasitaemia >10%.

Secondary endpoints:
- Incidence of neurological sequelae;
- Recovery times (times to eat, speak, sit) and time to hospital discharge;
- Development of severe complications.

Results

Primary endpoint	Artesunate	Quinine	p
Death	107/730 (15%)	64/731 (22%)	0.0002
Secondary endpoints			
Neurological sequelae	7/730 (1%)	3/731 (<1%)	0.2
Hypoglycaemia	6/730 (<1%)	19/731 (3%)	0.009

- No significant differences between the groups in recovery times and time to discharge.

Discussion

Overall mortality in this trial was 19% (24% in patients with severe malaria), ranging from 9.3% in Indonesia to 28% in Bangladesh. The superior efficacy of artesunate was consistent across high and low mortality centres. Most of the reduction in mortality attributable to artesunate occurred 24–48h after entry to the study (23 and 29 patients died on the day of admission in artesunate and quinine groups, respectively, *p*=0.4). Reduction in mortality was particularly marked in patients with parasitaemia >10% (mortality 23% artesunate group vs 53% quinine group) implying *in vivo* confirmation of artesunate's superior parasiticidal activity. Just as oral artemesinin derivatives are beginning to replace quinine as the treatment of choice for uncomplicated falciparum malaria, artesunate is now indicated as the optimum treatment for severe cases.

Problems

- The overall mortality in the 202 children <15y was only 8%, 5% in the artesunate group and 11% in the quinine group (*p*=0.2). Thus, although the treatment effect of artesunate mirrored that seen in adults, this study was not sufficiently powered to demonstrate an unequivocal benefit of artesunate vs quinine in children.
- Parenteral artesunate manufactured to appropriate standards is not routinely available in many parts of the world, compromising implementation of this trial's primary recommendation.

Enteric fever: antibiotic therapy

Randomised-controlled comparison of ofloxacin, azithromycin, and an ofloxacin-azithromycin combination for treatment of multidrug-resistant and nalidixic acid-resistant typhoid fever.

AUTHORS: Parry C, Anh Ho V, Thi Phuong L *et al.*
REFERENCE: Antimicrobial Agents Chemotherapy (2007) 51, 819–25.
STUDY DESIGN: RCT
EVIDENCE LEVEL: 1b

Key message

In the treatment of multidrug-resistant (MDR) *Salmonella (S.) enterica* serovar Typhi with reduced fluoroquinolone susceptibility, one week oral azithromycin is superior to ofloxacin and an ofloxacin-azithromycin combination, in terms of fever clearance times and faecal carriage rates immediately post-therapy.

Impact

Azithromycin may be considered in preference to fluoroquinolones in the treatment of uncomplicated typhoid fever acquired in settings where reduced fluoroquinolone susceptibility is common.

Aims

MDR typhoid is an increasing problem, particularly in Asian countries where disease is endemic. This study was designed to compare 7d oral azithromycin with ofloxacin or combined therapy in the treatment of uncomplicated typhoid fever due to MDR *S. enterica* serovar Typhi (resistant to ampicillin, chloramphenicol, and trimethoprim-sulphamethoxazole) and with reduced fluoroquinolone susceptibility (nalidixic acid-resistant).

Methods

Patients: 199 culture-positive patients at 1 infection ward in Vietnam.

Inclusion criteria: Fever ≥38°C for ≥4d and ≥1 of following: abdominal pain, diarrhoea/constipation, hepato- or splenomegaly, rose spots.

Exclusion criteria:
- Severe/complicated disease (intestinal bleeding/perforation, jaundice, myocarditis, pneumonia, renal failure, shock, or altered conscious level);
- Inability to swallow oral medication, drug hypersensitivity, pregnancy;
- Treatment with fluoroquinolone, extended-spectrum cephalosporin, or macrolide within 1wk of admission.

Groups:
- Ofloxacin (20mg/kg/d PO, max 400mg bd, for 7d) (n=63);
- Azithromycin (10mg/kg/d PO, max 500mg od, for 7d) (n=62);
- Ofloxacin (15mg/kg/d PO, max 300mg bd, for 7d) and azithromycin (10mg/kg/d PO, max 500mg od, for the first 3d) (n=62).

Primary endpoints: Clinical treatment failure (fever persistence and ≥1 typhoid-related symptom >7d after treatment start, or development of severe complication) and *microbiological treatment failure* (*S. enterica* serovar Typhi isolation from blood/other sterile site post-treatment).

Secondary endpoints:
- Faecal carriage immediately after treatment;
- Mean fever clearance time (time from treatment start to temperature ≤37.5°C and remaining ≤37.5°C for 48h);
- Relapse rates (recurrence of symptoms/signs and blood cultures positive for *S. enterica* serovar Typhi).

Follow-up: At 4wk, 3 months, and 6 months.

Results
- Of 187 eligible patients: 163 (87%)=age <15y; 165 (88%)=infected with MDR isolate; 173 (93%)=nalidixic acid-resistant isolate. All isolates susceptible to ofloxacin by disk test (majority had minimal inhibitory concentration (MIC) 0.5–1.0mcg/mL).

Primary endpoints	Ofloxacin	Ofloxacin and azithromycin	Azithromycin	*p*
Clinical failure	23 (36.5%)	15 (24.2%)	11(17.8%)	0.05
Microbiological failure	2 (3.2)	1 (1.6%)	2 (3.2%)	0.8
Secondary endpoints				
Fever clearance time	8.2d	7.1d	5.8d	<0.001
Faecal carriage	12 (19.4%)	4 (6.5%)	1 (1.6%)	0.006

Discussion
Clinical failure was more common with ofloxacin alone than with azithromycin and ofloxacin-azithromycin, and there was a significant difference in fever clearance times. Ofloxacin-treated patients were more likely to be faecal culture positive immediately post-treatment. There were no other outcome differences between the groups, including proportion with blood culture positivity after treatment, length of hospital stay, and faecal carriage rates at any time during 6 months F/U. There were no relapses and no treatment-limiting adverse effects of therapy.

Problems
- Despite evidence for first-line azithromycin in areas where nalidixic acid-resistant MDR strains are common, more evidence is required to change practice in settings where azithromycin's higher cost is an issue and when applying the results to adults (87% patients <15y old).
- Ceftriaxone remains the gold standard for MDR nalidixic acid-resistant typhoid fever. This study was unblinded and re-treatment after initial therapeutic failure was at the physician's discretion; all those re-treated responded to 7–10d ceftriaxone.

Brucellosis: antibiotic therapy

Doxycycline-rifampicin vs doxycycline-streptomycin in treatment of human brucellosis due to *Brucella melitensis*.

AUTHORS: Solera J, Rodriguez-Zapata M, Geijo P *et al.*
REFERENCE: Antimicrobial Agents Chemotherapy (1995) 39, 2061–7.
STUDY DESIGN: RCT
EVIDENCE LEVEL: 1b

Key message
Doxycycline-streptomycin is superior to doxycycline-rifampicin in the treatment of acute brucellosis, resulting in fewer early therapeutic failures and relapses 12 months after treatment. Both regimens are well tolerated with <5% patients experiencing treatment-limiting adverse effects.

Impact
Doxycycline-streptomycin should be considered for first-line treatment of acute brucellosis.

Aims
Brucellosis, although predominantly a disease of the Mediterranean, Middle East, and Latin America, can be acquired through contaminated dairy products and occupational exposure in other parts of the world. The optimum antimicrobial regimen for its acute treatment is not clearly established. Tetracycline-streptomycin combinations were considered standard therapy until the World Health Organization changed its recommendation to a 6wk doxycycline-rifampicin combination in 1986. This trial was designed to compare the efficacy and safety of doxycycline-streptomycin and doxycycline-rifampicin for the treatment of acute brucellosis due to *Brucella (B.) melitensis*.

Methods
Patients: 194 patients presenting to 5 hospitals in Spain.

Inclusion criteria:
- Age >7y;
- *Brucella* species isolated from blood or other fluid or tissue (n=120) *or* positive *Brucella* serology—agglutination titre for anti-*Brucella* antibodies >1:160 and compatible clinical findings (n=74).

Exclusion criteria: Including:
- Endocarditis or neurobrucellosis;
- Pregnancy, breastfeeding, or allergy to study antimicrobials;
- Antibiotic therapy for brucellosis within 7d of study entry.

Groups:
- Doxycycline (100mg bd PO) plus rifampicin (900mg od PO), for 45d (n=100);
- Doxycycline (100mg bd PO for 45d) plus streptomycin (1g od IM, for 14d) (n=94).

Primary endpoint: Absence of relapse (symptoms, signs, or new positive blood cultures 12 months after therapy completion).

Secondary endpoints:
- Early therapeutic failure (symptoms or signs persisting after 4wk of therapy);
- Time to defervescence.

Follow-up: Initial assessments at d0, 7–14, and 45; then at 1, 3, 6, and 12 months following completion of therapy.

Results

Primary endpoint	Doxycycline + rifampicin	Doxycycline + streptomycin	*p*
Relapses	16/100 (16%)	5/94 (5.3%)	0.02
Secondary endpoints			
Early therapeutic failure	8/100 (8%)	2/94 (2%)	0.1
Mean time to defervescence	4.6d	4.3d	ns

Discussion

Earlier trials for the treatment of brucellosis had shown relapse rates of 30–40% with doxycycline plus rifampicin given for <6wk, but rates of only 0–8% with >30d addition of tetracycline plus ≥14d streptomycin. Furthermore, previous small studies had failed to show significant differences between outcomes with doxycycline plus rifampicin (45d) and doxycycline (45d) plus streptomycin (14–21d). However, this larger trial, which combined relapses with early therapeutic failure, found 24% failed to respond to doxycycline-rifampicin vs only 7% failing to respond to doxycycline-streptomycin (*p*=0.002). Both regimens were well tolerated, with only 4 patients in the doxycycline-rifampicin and 2 in the doxycycline-streptomycin group experiencing treatment-limiting adverse effects.

Problems

- Clinical endpoints are difficult to define in human brucellosis. The study was not blinded as it was deemed unethical to include a 14d IM placebo group.
- The superior outcome with doxycycline-streptomycin must be weighed against the inconvenience, increased cost, and potential toxicity of IM streptomycin compared with oral rifampicin.
- Relapses (in which 13 out of 21 subjects had *Brucella* bacteraemias) could not be distinguished from re-infection with *B. melitensis*. Twenty of these 21 subjects responded to a second, alternative course of antibiotics (15 received doxycycline-streptomycin). One patient required a third antibiotic course after a second relapse.

Lyme disease: antibiotic therapy

Duration of antibiotic therapy for early Lyme disease.

AUTHORS: Wormser G, Ramanthan R, Nowakowski J et al.
REFERENCE: Ann Intern Med (2003) 138, 697–704.
STUDY DESIGN: RCT
EVIDENCE LEVEL: 1b

Key message
Clinical response rates do not differ significantly in patients treated for early Lyme disease with either 10 or 20d of doxycycline, and are not enhanced by the addition of a single initial dose of IV ceftriaxone.

Impact
Ten days doxycycline is regarded by some as sufficient treatment for early Lyme disease presenting as erythema migrans.

Aims
Erythema migrans is the most common manifestation of Lyme disease. The optimum duration of antibiotic therapy for an uncomplicated presentation had not been established, and it was also unclear whether outcomes were improved by routine use of a CSF-penetrating antibiotic. The aim of this trial was to evaluate prolonged vs short course oral doxycycline therapy for uncomplicated early Lyme disease, and to determine whether outcomes were improved by an initial bolus dose of IV ceftriaxone.

Methods
Patients: 180 outpatients at 1 centre in New York, USA.

Inclusion criteria:
- Age >16y, with diagnosis of uncomplicated early Lyme disease;
- Erythema migrans (annular skin lesion >5cm diameter).

Exclusion criteria:
- Received >48h antibiotic therapy for Lyme disease;
- Lyme meningitis or heart block;
- 'Any underlying condition' that might compromise assessment or F/U.

Groups:
- Single dose ceftriaxone (2g IV); then 10d doxycycline (100mg bd PO); then 10d placebo (PO) (n=60; 54 evaluable);
- Placebo (IV); then 10d doxycycline (100mg bd PO); then 10d placebo (PO) (n=61; 50 evaluable);
- Placebo (IV); then 20d doxycycline (100mg bd PO) (n=59; 45 evaluable).

Primary endpoints: Early response at 20d: Complete response (no recurrence of erythema migrans, no other objective manifestations of Lyme disease, return to pre-disease health); *partial response* (no recurrence of erythema migrans, but subjective symptoms); *failure* (any of: no clinical improvement by d10; recurrence of erythema migrans or fever attributable

to Lyme disease; objective cardiac, neurological, or rheumatological manifestations of disease not present in first 10d).
Late response at 3, 12, and 30 months: *Complete response* (as above); *partial
response* (as above, no objective manifestations but subjective symptoms
of uncertain aetiology); *failure* (objective manifestations of Lyme disease).

Secondary endpoints:
• Neurocognitive evaluation scores (baseline, 12, and 30 months);
• Drug-induced adverse events.

Follow-up: At 10 and 20d; then at 3, 6, 12, 24, and 30 months; included neurological examination and neurocognitive testing.

Results

Primary endpoints	10d doxycycline and ceftriaxone	10d doxycycline	20d doxycycline
Complete response (20d)	43/52 (65.4%)	34/48 (70.8%)	29/45 (64.4%)
Complete response (30 months)	32/37 (86.5%)	28/31 (90.3%)	26/31 (83.9%)
Partial response (30 months)	5/37 (13.5%)	2/31 (6.5%)	5/31 (31.0%)
Secondary endpoints			
Diarrhoea	21/60 (35.0%)	4/61 (6.6%)	5/59 (8.5%)

Discussion

There were no significant differences in complete response, partial
response, and failure rates between the three groups at all F/U time points.
Treatment failure occurred in only 1 patient (10d doxycycline group) who
developed Lyme meningitis at 18d and recovered fully after a 2wk course
of IV ceftriaxone. There were no significant differences between the three
groups in the results of neurocognitive testing. Significantly more patients
in the ceftriaxone-doxycycline group (35%) developed diarrhoea than in
the doxycycline alone groups ($p<0.001$).

Problems

• Uncertain impact of the broad exclusion criteria of 'any underlying
  condition'.
• Rates of post-Lyme disease syndrome were lower than expected, with
  >83% demonstrating a complete response at 30 months; the relatively
  small number of evaluable patients per group meant that the study was
  probably insufficiently powered to detect small differences in outcome.
• During 30 month F/U, a large proportion (range 48–65% for the
  3 groups) took additional antibiotics for intercurrent infections.
• In those deemed to have a partial response, there was no evaluation of
  the subjective symptoms to exclude causes other than Lyme disease.
• The *Borrelia burgdorferi* genospecies and clinical manifestations of
  disease differ between North America and Europe; conclusions drawn
  from this study are not necessarily applicable to European practice.

Neurology

Introduction

'[The neurologist is]......a brilliant and forgetful man with a bulging cranium, a loud bow tie, who reads Cicero in Latin for pleasure, hums Haydn sonatas, talks with ease about bits of the brain you'd forgotten existed, and—most importantly—never bothers about treatment.'

Richard Smith (BMJ Editor) 1999

Smith's stereotypical description is no longer recognisable to the 21st century neurologist. Neurologists are pragmatic, evidence-based wherever possible, and—most importantly—very bothered about treatment. Indeed, neurologists have been instrumental in designing and running RCTs of many therapies, including surgical treatments such as carotid endarterectomy. Neurological diseases present particular challenges for trialists. Many are uncommon or rare, making recruitment difficult. The more common ones such as epilepsy are very heterogeneous, and thus may not be suited to trials of 'one size fits all' treatments. Many neurological disorders (e.g. multiple sclerosis (MS), Parkinson's disease) cause increasing disability over many years, such that meaningful trials take time (and money). This approach does not suit the powerful pharmaceutical industry well, which, simply put, needs to recoup its investment in the expensive business of developing new drugs as soon as possible. Thus, controversies abound about how truly effective some currently licensed treatments are (e.g. β-interferon for MS, or anti-cholinesterase inhibitors for Alzheimer's disease). Finally, agreeing upon easily measured and useful outcome measures is always a challenge—counting dead bodies is rarely relevant in neurological disorders, and measuring disability is fraught with difficulty.

Despite these problems, neurologists have met the challenge, as the trials in this chapter (and others) show. It is no longer appropriate to suggest that neurologists are only useful as diagnosticians, and have nothing else to offer their patients. The last ten years in particular have seen an explosion of new therapies (and investigative techniques) for neurological disorders, and we now need to learn how best to use them.

Ischaemic stroke: aspirin and dipyridamole

> **ESPS-2 (European Stroke Prevention Study 2):** Dipyridamole and acetylsalicylic acid in the secondary prevention of stroke.
>
> **AUTHORS:** Diener H, Cunha L, Forbes C.
> **REFERENCE:** J Neurol Sci (1996) 143, 1–13.
> **STUDY DESIGN:** RCT
> **EVIDENCE LEVEL:** 1b

Key message

The first and only large-scale RCT to demonstrate efficacy of aspirin over placebo in long-term secondary stroke prevention. The trial results suggest equivalent efficacy for dipyridamole and a summative efficacy for the combination of the two agents.

Impact

Confirms the widely held, but poorly evidenced, assumption that anti-platelet agents are effective in preventing recurrent stroke.

Aims

An earlier study by the same group (ESPS-1) had found dipyridamole and aspirin combination produced a 38% reduction in secondary stroke. However, other studies had produced conflicting results, particularly with regard to the benefit of combination treatment, and due to a higher incidence of adverse events. This study aimed to assess the efficacy and safety of low-dose aspirin and modified-release dipyridamole, both individually and in combination, in the prevention of recurrent ischaemic stroke following first stroke or transient ischaemic attack (TIA).

Methods

Patients: 6602 patients from 13 European countries.

Inclusion criteria:
- Age >18y;
- Ischaemic stroke or TIA within preceding 3 months.

Groups:
- Acetylsalicylic acid (ASA) (aspirin) 25mg bd (n=1649);
- Modified-release dipyridamole (DP) 200mg bd (n=1654);
- Combined aspirin + dipyridamole (ASA + DP) (n=1650);
- Placebo (n=1649).

Primary endpoints: Stroke, death, or stroke and/or death.

Secondary endpoints:
- TIA;
- Myocardial infarction (MI);
- All ischaemic events (stroke, MI, sudden death);
- Other vascular events.

Follow-up: At 1 month after randomisation, thereafter every 3 months for 2y.

Results

	Stroke	RRR (%)	*p*	Stroke and/or death	RRR (%)	*p*	Death	RRR (%)	*p*
ASA (n=1649)	206	18.1	0.01	330	13.2	0.02	182	10.9	0.2
DP (n=1654)	211	16.3	0.04	321	15.4	0.02	188	7.3	0.5
ASA+ DP (n=1650)	157	37	<0.001	286	24.4	<0.001	185	8.5	0.3
Placebo (n=1649)	250	—	—	378	—	—	202	—	—

RRR = relative risk reduction compared to placebo.

- The reduction in occurrence of TIA amongst the treatment groups was similar to the effect on the stroke endpoint.
- Bleeding was more commonly reported in the groups receiving aspirin (ASA=8.2%, ASA/DP=8.7%) than those on dipyridamole alone or placebo (DP=4.7%, placebo=4.5%). There was also a higher proportion of severe/fatal haemorrhage within these groups.
- Withdrawal from the trial due to headache was more common in the groups receiving dipyridamole (DP=8.0%, ASA/DP=8.1%) than amongst those receiving aspirin alone or placebo (ASA=1.9%, placebo=2.4%).

Discussion

The results of this trial suggest that low dose aspirin and modified-release dipyridamole are equally effective in preventing recurrent TIA and ischaemic stroke, and that when used together, their effect is additive. However, there was no effect on all-cause mortality.

Problems

- The trial used a particularly low dose of aspirin (on the basis of *in vitro* evidence of pharmacological activity) in order to establish whether this would reduce the risk of bleeding. However, haemorrhagic complication rates remained similar to those previously reported. Subsequent meta-analysis (The Antiplatelet Trialists' Collaboration) suggests that the optimal dose of aspirin in secondary prevention of vascular events is slightly higher at 75mg od.
- Headache, although commonly reported by patients in all groups, was significantly more problematic in the DP-treated groups, with an associated withdrawal rate four times higher than that in the ASA-treated group. Headache is a common limiting side effect of DP in clinical practice
- Other trials have shown rather more modest benefits of dipyridamole, both alone and in combination with aspirin. The Cochrane review of evidence for dipyridamole in the prevention of stroke and other vascular events suggested that the combination of dipyridamole and aspirin had no advantage over aspirin alone in the prevention of vascular death.

Ischaemic stroke: aspirin and heparin

IST (International Stroke Trial): A randomised trial of aspirin, subcutaneous heparin, both, or neither among 19,435 patients with acute ischaemic stroke.

AUTHORS: International stroke trial collaborative group.
REFERENCE: Lancet (1997) 349, 1569–81.
STUDY DESIGN: RCT
EVIDENCE LEVEL: 1b

Key message

In patients with acute ischaemic stroke, subcutaneous heparin increases the risk of early haemorrhagic complications with no overall advantage at 6 months F/U. Aspirin offers a small advantage in preventing death or dependency at 6 months, and when used alone, is not associated with increased risk of early bleeding.

Impact

This trial demonstrated the safety and relative efficacy of early treatment with aspirin following acute ischaemic stroke, validating its widespread use. Heparin is not recommended for the treatment of most ischaemic strokes.

Aims

Most strokes are caused by acute occlusion of a cerebral artery. Both heparin and aspirin had been widely used for many years in the treatment of acute ischaemic stroke, but no large-scale trial had evaluated the safety or efficacy of either agent, either alone, or in combination. This study was undertaken to provide reliable evidence for this practice.

Methods

Patients: 19,435 patients at 467 hospitals in 36 countries.

Inclusion criteria:
- Any age, with clinical evidence of stroke within 48h (no evidence of intracranial haemorrhage);
- No clear indication or contraindication for aspirin or heparin.

Exclusion criteria:
- Only a small likelihood of worthwhile benefit (e.g. symptoms likely to resolve within few h or patient severely disabled pre-stroke);
- High risk of adverse bleeding events (i.e. contraindications or already on long-term anticoagulants).

Groups: At discharge clinicians to 'consider' giving long-term aspirin in all cases. Allocated using a factorial design:
- Aspirin 300mg od and heparin 12,500iu bd (n=2430);
- Aspirin 300mg od and heparin 5000iu bd (n=2432);
- Aspirin 300mg od and no heparin (n=4858);
- No aspirin and heparin 12,500iu bd (n=2426);

- No aspirin and heparin 5,000iu bd (n=2429);
- No aspirin and no heparin (n=4860).

Primary endpoint: Two main analyes: 'immediate heparin' (low or medium dose) vs 'avoid heparin' and 'immediate aspirin' vs 'avoid aspirin': death from any cause within 14d and death/dependency at 6 months.

Secondary endpoints:
- Symptomatic intracranial haemorrhage *or* ischaemic stroke within 14d;
- Major extracranial haemorrhage;
- Death from any cause by 6 months;
- Dependency or incomplete recovery from stroke at 6 months.

Follow-up: At 14d: clinical data gathered including final diagnosis of index event and treatment allocation. At 6 months: clinical data gathered at clinic F/U, by validated postal questionnaire or by telephone.

Results

- 'Heparin' vs 'no heparin': At 14d: no significant difference in number of deaths; fewer recurrent ischaemic strokes (2.9% vs 3.8%, $p<0.005$); more haemorrhagic strokes (1.2% vs 0.4%, $p<0.00001$); and more major extracranial haemorrhage (1.3% vs 0.4%, $p<0.00001$). At 6 months: no significant difference in proportion dead or dependent.
- Heparin dosage: 12,500iu bd associated with more haemorrhagic stroke and more major extracranial haemorrhage than 5000iu bd regimen, with no additional benefit in preventing recurrent ischaemic stroke.
- 'Aspirin' vs 'no aspirin': At 14d: no significant difference in deaths; fewer recurrent ischaemic strokes (2.8% vs 3.9%, $p<0.001$); no significant excess in haemorrhagic stroke; and significant increase in major extracranial haemorrhage (1.1% vs 0.6%, $p<0.0004$). At 6 months: no significant difference in deaths; proportion of patients dead or dependent only significantly different after adjustment for predicted prognosis.

Discussion

This large-scale trial provided evidence against the routine use of subcutaneous heparin at doses higher than 5000iu bd in the early treatment of acute ischaemic stroke, and confirmed a modest benefit from the early use of aspirin, with approximately 10 deaths or recurrent strokes prevented per 1000 patients treated.

Problems

- The trial was unblinded and there was no placebo control. However, at 6 months, most assessors were blinded to treatment allocation.
- The benefits from early aspirin treatment were modest; with such large numbers, it is unclear why adjustment for baseline characteristics was necessary.

Ischaemic stroke: thrombolysis

Tissue plasminogen activator for acute ischaemic stroke.

AUTHORS: The National Institute of Neurological Disorders and Stroke
r-TPA Study Group.
REFERENCE: N Engl J Med (1995) 333, 1581–87.
STUDY DESIGN: RCT
EVIDENCE LEVEL: 1b

Key message
Thrombolysis with recombinant tissue plasminogen activator (r-tPA) within
3h of onset of acute ischaemic stroke improves outcome at 3 months; this
benefit outweighs the increased incidence of intracranial haemorrhage.

Impact
Open-label thrombolysis with r-tPA within 3h of onset is now widely
used in the management of acute ischaemic stroke. Large-scale trials to
evaluate the risks and benefits of thrombolysis between 3 and 6h after
stroke onset are ongoing.

Aims
The findings of two previous open-label studies of thrombolysis for ischaemic stroke had indicated that early treatment maximised benefit and
reduced the risk of causing intracranial haemorrhage. This large-scale,
randomised, placebo-controlled trial was designed to assess the risks and
benefits of intravenous thrombolysis with r-tPA within 3h of onset of acute
ischaemic stroke.

Methods
Patients: 624 patients (291 in part 1; 333 in part 2) at multiple centres in
the USA.

Inclusion criteria: Acute ischaemic stroke:
• Clearly defined time of onset;
• Neurological deficit measurable by the National Institutes of Health
  Stroke Scale (NIHSS);
• Intracranial haemorrhage excluded by CT imaging.

Groups:
• Part 1: 144 patients randomised to tPA; 147 to placebo;
• Part 2: 168 patients randomised to tPA; 165 to placebo.

Endpoints:
• Part 1: clinical improvement of neurological deficit at 24h. 'Early clinical
  improvement' at 24h: either complete resolution of neurological deficit,
  or improvement of ≥4 points on the NIHSS;
• Part 2: minimal or no neurological deficit at 3 months. 'Favourable
  outcome' at 3 months: a score of 95 or 100 on the Barthel Index
  (0–100), 0 or 1 on the NIHSS, 0 or 1 on the Modified Rankin Scale, and
  1 on the Glasgow Outcome Scale. These four outcome measures were
  evaluated by means of a global test statistic (the Wald test), giving an
  overall odds ratio for favourable outcome.

- The groups were substratified according to the time from stroke onset to treatment (0–90min, 91–180min).

Follow-up: Both groups were assessed at 24h and at 3 months.

Results

- **Part 1:** At 24h after treatment, there was no statistically significant difference in the proportion of patients with early clinical improvement.
- **Part 2:**

Time from symptom onset to thrombolysis	Global test statistic. Odds ratio for favourable outcome tPA vs placebo (95% CI)	p
0–90min	1.9 (1.2 to 2.9)	0.05
91–180min	1.9 (1.3 to 2.9)	0.02

- Significantly more patients in the tPA groups suffered symptomatic (6.4% vs 0.65%) and fatal (2.9% vs 0.32%) intracranial haemorrhage in the first 36h after treatment.
- However, there was no significant difference in mortality between the two groups at 90d (54 of 312 (17%) of the tPA group and 64 of 312 (21%) of the placebo group (*p*=0.30)).

Discussion

Although part 1 of the study showed no significant advantage in the proportion of patients with clinical improvement at 24h, part 2 of the study showed clear advantage at 3 months with tPA-treated patients being at least 30% more likely to have minimal or no disability.

Problems

- The benefit of thombolysis in acute ischaemic stroke beyond 3h is still unknown. The practical difficulties involved in transporting patients rapidly to centres using thrombolysis, imaging, and treatment within this time mean that at present, only a small proportion of patients can be managed in this way. Time constraints also present difficulties in obtaining informed consent from patients (who may have language deficits).

Stroke: care in dedicated units

Alternative strategies for stroke care.

AUTHORS: Kalra L, Evans E, Perez I.
REFERENCE: Lancet (2000) 356, 894–9.
STUDY DESIGN: RCT
EVIDENCE LEVEL: 1b

Key message
Post-stroke care in a dedicated stroke unit improves outcomes of death and dependency compared to general ward and domiciliary care.

Impact
Early admission to a specialised stroke unit is now universally regarded as best practice in the care of patients following stroke. This large, randomised trial added weight to the evidence in favour of such organised inpatient care.

Aims
At the time that this trial was proposed, there was a growing body of evidence in favour of stroke unit care. However, up to 50% of stroke patients in the UK were cared for elsewhere with some evidence to suggest equivalent outcomes in patients with organised care at home. This trial set out to compare best care on a dedicated stroke unit, on the general ward, and at home.

Methods
Patients: 457 patients from 1 region of the UK.

Inclusion criteria:
- Stroke as diagnosed by World Health Organization criteria;
- Moderate severity, defined as persistent neurological deficit impairing mobility, continence, and ability to self-care;
- Onset of symptoms <72h.

Groups:
- Stroke unit care (n=152; 148 confirmed strokes);
- Stroke team care on general ward (n=153; 149 confirmed strokes);
- Domiciliary care (152 patients; 150 confirmed strokes).

Primary endpoint: Death or institutionalisation at 1y.

Secondary endpoints: Dependence assessed by Modified Rankin Scale (0–3=favourable outcome) and Barthel Index (15–20=favourable outcome).

Follow-up: Outcomes assessed at 3, 6, and 12 months.

Results

At 12 months	Stroke unit	Stroke team	Home care	Unit vs team OR (95% CI)	Unit vs home OR (95% CI)	Team vs home OR (95% CI)
Mortality	9%	23%	15%	0.37 (0.21 to 0.66)	0.59 (0.31 to 1.11)	1.56 (0.96 to 2.53)
Institution -isation	5%	7%	9%	0.71 (0.29 to 1.72)	0.58 (0.25 to 1.35)	0.82 (0.38 to 1.75)
Mortality or institution-alisation	14%	30%	24%	0.46 (0.30 to 0.72)	0.59 (0.37 to 0.95)	1.28 (0.87 to 1.87)
Modified Rankin 0–3	85%	66%	71%	1.29 (1.13 to 1.47)	1.21 (1.07 to 1.37)	0.94 (0.81 to 1.09)
Barthel index 15–20	87%	69%	71%	1.27 (1.12 to 1.44)	1.22 (1.09 to 1.37)	0.97 (0.85 to 1.11)

OR = odds ratio.

Discussion

This study showed significant advantage for specialised stroke unit care in the combined outcome of death or institutionalisation at 12 months over either stroke team management on general wards, or care at home. Regression analysis for baseline prognostic variables of age, Barthel index, and dysphasia strengthened this effect, giving a risk of death or dependency at 1y 3.2 times greater (95% CI 1.6 to 6.4) for the stroke team patients and 1.8 times greater (95% CI 1.1 to 3.8) for patients at home than for the stroke unit patients.

Problems

- Trials such as this have necessary limitations: the patients clearly cannot be blinded, and it is impossible to control for the inevitable human variability between medical and nursing teams in terms of application, engagement with patients, and assiduousness with basic care. However, the findings have been borne out by many other trials and meta-analyes.

Epilepsy: introduction of medication

MESS (MRC **M**ulticentre trial for **E**arly epilepsy and **S**ingle **S**eizures) **study:** Immediate vs deferred anti-epileptic drug treatment for early epilepsy and single seizures.

AUTHORS: Marson A, Jacoby A, Johnson A.
REFERENCE: Lancet (2005) 365, 2007–14.
STUDY DESIGN: RCT
EVIDENCE LEVEL: Ib

Key message

The first large-scale, randomised trial to provide data on the impact of early anti-epileptic drug treatment on short-term seizure recurrence and long-term seizure freedom. Its findings suggest that, whilst effective in preventing early seizure recurrence, early treatment does not affect long-term seizure control.

Impact

The findings of this trial have aided the decision-making process for clinician and patient when considering the introduction of anti-epileptic medication in early epilepsy.

Aims

Recurrence rates of anywhere between 23–71% have been reported after a single first seizure. Coupled with the risks of treatment as well as the variable natural history of the progression of the condition in individuals, it can be difficult to know when to commence anti-epileptic drug treatment. This study aimed to compare the effects of policies of immediate and deferred drug treatment on early seizure recurrence and long-term seizure freedom in patients suffering a single seizure or presenting with early epilepsy.

Methods

Patients: 1443 patients from multiple international centres.

Inclusion criteria:
- Age >1 month;
- At least one clinically definite, unprovoked epileptic seizure;
- Both patient and clinician uncertain whether to introduce anti-epileptic medication.

Exclusion criteria:
- Prior anti-epileptic drug treatment;
- Progressive neurological disease.

Groups:
- Immediate treatment (722 patients): Anti-epileptic drug selected by clinician and started 'as soon as possible';
- Deferred treatment (721 patients): Anti-epileptic drug treatment withheld until considered necessary by clinician and patient.

Primary outcomes:
- Time to first recurrent seizure of any type;
- Time to first recurrent tonic-clonic seizure;
- Time to second and fifth recurrent seizures of any type;
- Time to 2y remission;
- Proportion seizure-free for 2y: between 1 and 3y post-randomisation, and between 3 and 5y post-randomisation.

Secondary endpoints: Adverse events in each group.

Follow-up: At 3, 6, and 12 months, and yearly thereafter.

Results

		6 months	2y	5y	8y	p
Time to 1st recurrent seizure	Immediate treatment	22%	37%	48%	52%	<0.0001 (all)
	Deferred treatment	33%	48%	58%	61%	–
Time to 5th recurrent seizure	Immediate treatment	6%	12%	19%	26%	0.23 (all)
	Deferred treatment	7%	15%	22%	25%	–
Achieving 2y remission	Immediate treatment	–	64%	92%	95%	0.02 (at 2y)
	Deferred treatment	–	52%	90%	96%	–

Discussion

The findings of the trial clearly suggested that early treatment with anti-epileptic drugs prolonged the time to first and second recurrent seizures, and shortened the time to 2y remission. However, there was little difference between the two groups in longer-term seizure outcomes. Time to fifth seizure was similar in the immediate and deferred treatment groups, and the respective proportions achieving 2y seizure freedom at 5 and 8y were almost identical. This suggests that early treatment has little effect on long-term seizure control.

Problems

- The trial was unmasked, and the absence of a placebo in the non-treatment group might be expected to increase the number of self-reported events, particularly the subtle symptoms of partial seizures. However, the figures for more objectively verifiable tonic-clonic seizures were similar to those for 'any seizure', and suggest that bias was not significant.

Epilepsy: withdrawal of medication

> **MRC anti-epileptic drug withdrawal trial:** A randomised study of anti-epileptic drug withdrawal in patients in remission.
>
> **AUTHORS:** MRC AED withdrawal study group.
> **REFERENCE:** Lancet (1991) 337, 1175–80.
> **STUDY DESIGN:** RCT
> **EVIDENCE LEVEL:** Ib

Key message

Withdrawal of anti-epileptic drugs in seizure-free patients is associated with an increased risk of seizure recurrence in the subsequent 2y. Thereafter, the risk becomes similar to that of patients remaining on treatment. The most important prognostic factors for seizure recurrence are a history of tonic-clonic seizures, number of anti-epileptic drugs, and duration of seizure freedom.

Impact

This large-scale trial provided the first reliable data to guide decision-making in anti-epileptic drug withdrawal.

Aims

In most patients with epilepsy-associated seizures, treatment with anti-epileptic drugs (AEDs) leads to prompt remission of seizures. Despite both epilepsy and AED treatment being associated with medical risks as well as social consequences, there had been no clear consensus as to when and how treatment should be withdrawn in those likely to remain seizure free. This study aimed to compare the risks of seizure recurrence in patients with epilepsy in remission, using either slow drug withdrawal or maintenance of therapy, and to identify important prognostic factors in seizure recurrence.

Methods

Patients: 1013 patients from 40 centres in the UK and Europe. Additional 776 eligible, but non-randomised patients also followed up.

Inclusion criteria:
- Any age;
- ≥2 clinically definite partial or generalised epileptic seizures;
- Free of seizures for at least 2y;
- Taking ≥1 anti-epileptic drugs.

Exclusion criteria:
- Progressive neurological illness;
- Other condition likely to limit F/U to less than 2y.

Groups:
- Slow drug withdrawal (510 patients). Rates of withdrawal for particular drugs pre-specified, aiming for withdrawal over 6 month period;

- Continued drug therapy (503 patients). Maintained on existing doses unless clinical indication to change.

Primary endpoint: time to first recurrent seizure (of any type) or last seizure-free F/U.

Secondary endpoints: time to first recurrent, generalised, tonic-clonic seizure.

Follow-up: At 3, 6, and 12 months, and yearly thereafter.

Results

- **Seizure recurrence**

	0–6 months	6–12 months	18–24 months	2–3y	3–4y
No withdrawal	14%	11%	11%	9%	4%
Slow withdrawal	40%	37%	14%	6%	3%
OR (95% CI)	2.8 (1.8 to 4.3)	3.4 (2.2 to 5.2)	1.2 (0.6 to 2.2)	0.6 (0.3 to 1.3)	0.6 (0.1 to 2.5)

Discussion

There was a significant increase in the risk of seizure recurrence in the first 2y after drug withdrawal. The most important prognostic factors for seizure recurrence were; a history of tonic-clonic seizures (whether primary or secondary), duration of seizure freedom at randomisation (the shorter the period, the higher the risk of recurrence), and the number of initial anti-epileptic drugs prescribed (the higher the number of drugs, the greater the risk of recurrence).

Problems

- Analysis in this trial was by intention to treat. The design allowed for changes to be made to ongoing drug therapy on the basis of clinical indication, and in particular, children in the treatment group could withdraw from drugs after 1y. Overall, 35% of the treatment group withdrew during F/U.
- Although relatively large in scale, the trial detected few significant prognostic factors for seizure recurrence. A number of other factors seemed likely to be of prognostic value, but conclusions could not be drawn due to wide CIs.

Treatment of partial epilepsy

> **SANAD (Standard And New Anti-epileptic Drugs) study—Arm A:**
> The SANAD study of the effectiveness of carbamazepine, gabapentin, lamotrigine, oxcarbazepine, or topiramate for partial epilepsy.
>
> **AUTHORS:** SANAD study group.
> **REFERENCE:** Lancet (2007) 369, 1000–15.
> **STUDY DESIGN:** RCT
> **EVIDENCE LEVEL:** 1b

Key message

Lamotrigine is better tolerated than, and superior or non-inferior in efficacy to carbamazepine, the currently recommended first-line drug treatment of partial onset seizures.

Impact

The study group recommended that there should be a reassessment of the NICE guidelines for first-line anti-epileptic drug treatment of partial onset seizures on the basis of the study findings.

Aims

Carbamazepine had been established as the first-line anti-epileptic drug for patients with partial onset seizures. This was based upon previous meta-analysis of RCTs, which had demonstrated its relative efficacy over valproate. More recent RCTs had investigated the efficacy of several newer treatments; however, methodology had not been ideal (e.g. due to short F/U), and results had been variable, with limited analysis of quality of life variables. This large-scale, unblinded RCT was designed to assess the relative efficacy, tolerability, and cost-effectiveness of several newer anti-epileptic drugs compared with carbamazepine.

Methods

Patients: 1721 patients from multiple centres in the UK.

Inclusion criteria:
- Age >4y;
- 2 clinically definite partial onset seizures in past 12 months;
- Not previously treated with trial drug;
- Clinician judged carbamazepine to be a more appropriate standard treatment option than valproate.

Groups: Drug titration and maintenance dosage for all groups guided by treating clinician:
- Carbamazepine (n=378);
- Gabapentin (n=377);
- Lamotrigine (n=378);
- Topiramate (n=378);
- Oxcarbazepine (n=210, drug introduced later in trial).

Primary endpoints:
- Time from randomisation to treatment failure (due to inadequate seizure control, intolerable side effects, or addition of a second drug);
- Time from randomisation to first 12 months period of seizure freedom.

Secondary endpoints:
- Time from randomisation to first seizure;
- Time to achieve 2y remission;
- Incidence of significant adverse events and side effects.

Follow-up: At 3 and 6 months, 1y, and annually thereafter. Drug dosage, seizures, hospital admissions, and adverse drug effects recorded.

Results

- **Time to treatment failure:** Expressed as overall percentage of patients remaining on drug, lamotrigine proved superior to carbamazepine and to the other new anti-epileptic drugs at 6y F/U. Carbamazepine and topiramate were most frequently associated with withdrawal due to side effects, and gabapentin most frequently associated with withdrawal due to inadequate seizure control. Those taking carbamazepine were least likely to withdraw due to inadequate seizure control.
- **Time to 12 months seizure freedom:** Intention-to-treat analysis showed carbamazepine to be superior to the newer anti-epileptic drugs. However, per-protocol comparison suggested 'non-inferiority' of lamotrigine and carbamazepine.
- Carbamazepine was marginally superior to the newer drugs in time to first seizure and in time to 2y seizure freedom.
- 50% of patients reported side effects during the trial; differences between the drugs were small.

Discussion

This study demonstrated the superior or non-inferior efficacy of lamotrigine compared with the standard first-line drug treatment for partial onset seizures. Additional cost analysis and quality of life data suggested lamotrigine to be a viable alternative first-line therapy.

Problems

- The study was unblinded due to cost implications, potential drug interactions, and practical difficulties of supplying dummy medications.
- Newer anti-epileptic drugs have come into common use since the trial was designed, and were therefore not included. Of these, perhaps most significant is levetiracetam, which is now licensed monotherapy for partial and secondary generalised seizures, and adjunctive therapy in juvenile myoclonic epilepsy.

Treatment of generalised and unclassifiable epilepsy

> **SANAD (Standard And New Anti-epileptic Drugs) study—Arm B:**
> The SANAD study of the effectiveness of valproate, lamotrigine, or
> topiramate for generalised and unclassifiable epilepsy.
>
> **AUTHORS:** SANAD study group.
> **REFERENCE:** Lancet (2007) 369, 1016–1026.
> **STUDY DESIGN:** RCT
> **EVIDENCE LEVEL:** 1b

Key message
Valproate should remain the drug of first choice for many patients with
generalised epilepsy. It is more effective than lamotrigine and better tolerated than topiramate.

Impact
The first substantial evidence for efficacy and tolerability of valproate
in comparison to the newer anti-epileptic drugs for the treatment of
generalised epilepsy.

Aims
The relative efficacy of anti-epileptic drugs for generalised onset seizures
had been based upon a relatively poorer evidence base to those for partial
onset seizures. Despite valproate being established as the first-line treatment, meta-analysis had found few differences between outcomes with
this drug compared with carbamazepine or phenytoin. This large-scale,
unblinded RCT was designed to assess the relative efficacy, tolerability,
and cost-effectiveness of the newer anti-epileptic drugs compared to valproate, the current standard first-line treatment.

Methods
Patients: 716 patients from multiple centres in the UK.

Inclusion criteria:
- Age >4y;
- 2 clinically definite unprovoked generalised epileptic seizures in past
  12 months;
- Valproate regarded by clinician to be better standard treatment than
  carbamazepine.

Groups: Drug titration and maintenance dosage for all groups guided by
treating clinician:
- Lamotrigine (n=239);
- Topiramate (n=239);
- Valproate (n=238).

Primary endpoints:
- Time from randomisation to treatment failure (inadequate seizure control or side effects);
- Time from randomisation to first 12 months period of seizure freedom.

Secondary endpoints:
- Time from randomisation to first seizure;
- Time from randomisation to first 2y period of seizure freedom;
- Frequency of adverse effects.

Follow-up: At 3 and 6 months, 1y, and annually thereafter. Drug dosage, seizures, hospital admissions, and adverse drug effects recorded.

Results

- **Time to treatment failure (any reason):** Measured by cumulative incidence of treatment failure, valproate was superior to topiramate (hazard ratio (HR) 1.57, 95% CI 1.19 to 2.08), but not significantly superior to lamotrigine (HR 1.25, 95% CI 0.94 to 1.68). However, in *post hoc* analysis of subgroups with a diagnosis of generalised epilepsy (excluding unclassifiable epilepsy), valproate was significantly superior to both.
- **Time to treatment failure (adverse effects):** Topiramate was significantly inferior to both valproate (HR 1.55, 95% CI 1.07 to 2.26) and lamotrigine (HR 2.15, 95% CI 1.41 to 3.30), and lamotrigine was least likely to cause unacceptable side effects.
- **Time to treatment failure (inadequate seizure control):** Valproate was significantly superior to lamotrigine (HR 1.95, 95% CI 1.28 to 2.98), but its superiority over topiramate was not significant.
- **Time to 1y remission:** Valproate was significantly superior to lamotrigine (HR 0.76, 95% CI 0.62 to 0.94), but superiority over topiramate was not significant in the intention-to-treat analysis. However, per-protocol analysis suggested significant superiority of valproate over both lamotrigine and topiramate. The difference between these two analyses is likely to be due to patients switching to valproate following treatment failure on topiramate.
- **Time to first seizure:** Valproate was superior to both lamotrigine and topiramate.

Discussion

For patients with generalised epilepsies, valproate was better than both lamotrigine and topiramate for time to treatment failure. It was superior to lamotrigine, but not to topiramate for time to 1y remission. The current NICE and SIGN guidelines recommend valproate as the drug of first choice for generalised epilepsies, and on the basis of the SANAD findings, this guidance remains unchanged.

Problems

- As with arm A of the study, other anti-epileptic drugs have become available and widely used since the study was designed, and were not included.
- The issue of valproate teratogenicity remains a significant concern.

Migraine prophylaxis: propranolol

Long-acting propranolol in migraine prophylaxis: the results of a double-blind, placebo-controlled study.

AUTHORS: Pradalier A, Serratrice G, Collard M.
REFERENCE: Cephalalgia (1989) 9, 247–53.
STUDY DESIGN: RCT
EVIDENCE LEVEL: 1b

Key message
Propranolol reduces the frequency of classical migraine.

Impact
The first randomised trial to show efficacy of long-acting propranolol in the prevention of migraine attacks. Long-acting propranolol is now a standard prophylactic agent.

Aims
The use of propranolol in the prevention of migraine attacks had already been well established, more than 50 previous trials demonstrating efficacy in reducing attack frequency. The major drawback in the use of standard release preparations was the relatively short half-life and consequent dosage frequency. For the first time, this trial set out to assess the efficacy of long-acting propranolol in preventing migraine attacks.

Methods
Patients: 55 patients (19 of 74 excluded after 4wk placebo run-in) from multiple centres in France.

Inclusion criteria:
- Age 18–65y;
- >2y history of migraine (with or without aura);
- 2–8 attacks per month.

Groups:
- Long-acting propranolol 160mg od (n=31);
- Placebo (n=24).

Primary endpoint: Number of migraine attacks per month.

Follow-up: At baseline, 42, and 84d.

Results

Time from baseline (d)	Attacks per month (mean ± SD)	
	Propranolol (long-acting)	Placebo
0	6.11 ± 0.39	6.00 ± 1.37
42	5.89 ± 1.20	7.37 ± 1.20
84	3.15 ± 0.77	6.41 ± 1.70

Discussion

There was an overall reduction of 48% in the number of attacks per month in the treatment group by d84, whilst in the placebo group the number of attacks remained unchanged. Only 41 of the 55 patients completed the study, 5 patients withdrawing from the placebo group and 9 from the treatment group. Surprisingly, none of the patients withdrawing from the treatment group did so because of side effects, and there was no significant difference in safety and tolerability between the two groups.

Problems

- The patient numbers in the trial were small and the duration of treatment short.
- It is not possible to exclude the possibility that the reduction in attack frequency was at the cost of increased attack duration or severity, as these factors were not assessed during this trial.
- β-blockade cannot be used in all patients with migraine and is relatively contraindicated by a number of common conditions, including bronchial asthma, Raynaud's phenomenon, and peripheral vascular disease. Despite the tolerability data from this small trial, the use of propranolol and other β-blockers is limited by side effects in practice. In particular, reduced exercise tolerance and impotence may be a significant problem for younger patients.

Migraine prophylaxis: sodium valproate

Sodium valproate has a prophylactic effect in migraine without aura: a triple-blind, placebo-controlled, crossover study.

AUTHORS: Jensen R, Brinck T, Olesen J.
REFERENCE: Neurology (1994) 44, 647–651.
STUDY DESIGN: RCT
EVIDENCE LEVEL: 1b

Key message
The first randomised trial conducted according to International Headache Society guidelines to demonstrate efficacy of sodium valproate in preventing migraine attacks.

Impact
Valproate still has a role in migraine prophylaxis, but perhaps more significantly, the trial paved the way for the use of a series of newer anti-epileptic drugs in migraine prophylaxis (although a variety of newer agents are in use, only topiramate is licensed for this indication).

Aims
Previous trials of sodium valproate in migraine were compromised by methodological flaws. This trial was designed according to the International Headache Society guidelines on clinical trials in migraine and set out to assess the efficacy of valproate in preventing migraine attacks.

Methods
Patients: 43 patients randomised (34 completed the trial) from 1 centre in Denmark.

Inclusion criteria:
- Age 18–72y;
- >1y history of migraine without aura;
- Attacks on 2–10d per month.

Groups:
- Valproate-placebo sequence (n=22);
- Placebo-valproate sequence (n=21);
- During the 12wk valproate phase, patients were given valproate 1000mg daily, increased after 1wk to 1500mg according to serum levels. During the 12wk placebo phase and intervening 4wk washout phase, patients received identical placebo.

Primary endpoint: Treatment effect: the mean number of days with migraine during the valproate phase, as compared to the placebo phase.

Secondary endpoints:
- Responder rate: those patients for whom the mean number of migraine days during the valproate phase was 50% or less than during the baseline phase;
- Duration and intensity of headache.

Follow-up: At 10d, then at 4wk intervals during treatment.

Results

Primary endpoint: Treatment effect

	Baseline period	**Placebo phase**	**Valproate phase**
Migraine days in 4wk (95% CI)	6.1 (not reported)	6.1 (4.8 to 7.4)	3.5 (2.7 to 4.3)

Secondary endpoint: Responder rate

	Responders (>50% reduction in migraine days vs baseline) (%)	**Worse (increase in migraine days vs baseline) (%)**
Valproate	17/34 (50%)	4/34 (12%)
Placebo	6/34 (18%)	14/34 (41%)

- There was no significant change in either duration or intensity of headache between placebo and valproate phases.
- Side effects were reported by 14/43 (33%) during the valproate phase, and by 7/43 (16%) during the placebo phase. Six patients withdrew due to side effects, 4 during the valproate and 2 during the placebo phase.

Discussion

The results of this trial suggest that sodium valproate has a significant therapeutic effect in reducing the frequency of attacks in patients suffering frequent migraine without aura, but with no effect on duration or severity of the attack.

Problems

- The use of valproate in migraine is limited not only by the symptomatic side effects noted in this trial, but also by its potential teratogenicity in a predominantly young, female patient group.

Migraine treatment: sumatriptan

Oral sumatriptan for the acute treatment of migraine: evaluation of three dosage strengths.

AUTHORS: Cutler N, Mushet G, Davis R.
REFERENCE: Neurology (1995) 45, S5–S9.
STUDY DESIGN: RCT
EVIDENCE LEVEL: 1b

Key message
The first randomised trial to show equivalent efficacy of lower doses of oral sumatriptan for the acute treatment of migraine.

Impact
Oral triptans are now the standard first-line treatment for migraine attacks. Sumatriptan is prescribed as a 50mg oral dose.

Aims
Previous studies had demonstrated the efficacy of sumatriptan compared to placebo, whether administered by subcutaneous injection or in oral doses between 100mg and 300mg. This trial aimed to assess the efficacy of sumatriptan at lower doses.

Methods
Patients: 259 patients at 13 centres in the USA.

Inclusion criteria:
- Age 18–65y;
- >1y history of migraine with or without aura by International Headache Society criteria;
- 1–6 attacks per month during 2 months screening period.

Groups:
- Oral sumatriptan 25mg (n=66);
- Oral sumatriptan 50mg (n=62);
- Oral sumatriptan 100mg (n=66);
- Placebo (n=65).

Monitoring:
- Patients were randomised in the study clinic as soon as possible after the onset of a typical migraine attack.
- Headache severity rated on 4-point scale (0=none, 1=mild, 2=moderate, 3=severe) before treatment, and at 30min intervals thereafter for 4h. Presence of nausea, vomiting, and photophobia, and subjective rating of clinical disability on 4-point scale (0=none to 3=requiring bed rest) were recorded.

Primary endpoint: Proportion of patients with headache relief, defined as reduction in pain intensity score from 2 or 3 to 0 or 1.

Secondary endpoints:
- Proportion with no pain;
- Proportion with nausea, vomiting, photophobia;
- Proportion with reduction in clinical disability score from 2 or 3 to 0 or 1;
- Proportion reporting 'meaningful relief'.

Results

Primary endpoint: Proportion with pain relief.

	Placebo	25mg	50mg	100mg	p
2h	26%	52%	50%	56%	<0.05*
4h	38%	70%	68%	71%	<0.05*

* For all dosage strengths at 2 and 4h vs placebo.

Secondary endpoints: Proportion with no pain.

	Placebo	25mg	50mg	100mg	p
2h	8%	21%	16%	23%	<0.05*
4h	15%	45%	32%	52%	<0.05*

* Excluding 50mg dose at 2h vs placebo.

- Similar significant differences were seen between treatment and placebo groups at 2 and 4h in the proportion of patients free of photophobia and in the proportion with little or no clinical disability.
- The difference between treatment and placebo groups in the proportion of patients free of nausea only reached significance at 4h for the 50mg and 100mg treatment groups.

Discussion

This study was not powered to detect differences between the treatment groups, but demonstrated for the first time the efficacy and tolerability of oral sumatriptan at a low dose. The study is presented here as this was the first evidence for the first triptan at currently recommended dosage and in oral formulation. A series of other triptan drugs in a variety of dosages and formulations have followed. For a comprehensive meta-analysis of currently available triptans, see Ferrari and Goadsby (*Cephalalgia* (2002) 22, 633–58).

Problems

- It is surprising that oral treatment of migraine attacks in this trial was not precluded by nausea or vomiting, particularly as the trial design required patients to travel to the participating clinics before treatment. Oral treatment is clearly not possible in all patients, and in those suffering severe nausea/vomiting early in the attack, an alternative route (nasal or subcutaneous) should be used.
- All triptan preparations are considerably more expensive than simple analgesic medications, and given the high prevalence of migraine in the population, they represent a significant cost burden.

Multiple sclerosis: steroids

A double-blind, randomised, placebo-controlled study of oral high dose methylprednisolone in attacks of multiple sclerosis.

AUTHORS: Sellebjerg F, Frederiksen J, Nielsen P.
REFERENCE: Neurology (1998) 51, 529–34.
STUDY DESIGN: RCT
EVIDENCE LEVEL: 1b

Key message
The first RCT to demonstrate the efficacy of oral steroid treatment in attacks of multiple sclerosis (MS).

Impact
Oral steroid administration is widely used as an easier and cheaper alternative to the intravenous route in the treatment of MS relapse.

Aims
Previous trials had demonstrated the efficacy of high dose intravenous methylprednisolone in the management of attacks of MS, but suggested that intermediate dose oral steroids were no more effective than placebo. This trial set out to assess the efficacy of high dose oral steroid treatment on MS relapse.

Methods
Patients: 51 patients at 1 centre in Denmark.

Inclusion criteria:
- Age 18–59y;
- Relapsing-remitting MS;
- MS relapse: defined as new or recurrent previous symptoms of duration >24h and <4wk in the absence of systemic infection.

Groups:
- Oral methylprednisolone 500mg for 5d, followed by 10d tapered withdrawal (n=26);
- Placebo of identical appearance (n=25).

Primary endpoints:
- Scripps Neurological Rating Scale (SNRS; minimum score −10, maximum score 100, higher score means better function) at 1 and 3wk. Covariate analysis with baseline values;
- Patient assessment of symptom severity on visual analogue scale (VAS) at 1 and 3wk. Covariate analysis with baseline values;
- Change in SNRS between baseline and 8wk;
- Patient-subjective assessment of treatment determined by efficacy questionnaire.

Secondary endpoints:
- Response to treatment at 1, 3, and 8wk, defined as at least one point improvement on the Kurtzke Expanded Disability Status Scale;
- Change in SNRS and VAS at individual visits.

Follow-up: Patients assessed before treatment and after 1, 3, and 8wk of treatment. Thereafter, patients reviewed at the onset of a new attack up to 1y F/U.

Results

SNRS (increase=improvement):

	Score improvement (range)			
	Baseline score	At 1wk	At 3wk	At 8wk
Methylpred.	75 (55 to 83)	5 (2 to 8)	8 (3 to 12)	11 (3 to 15)
Placebo	69 (65 to 77)	1 (−1 to +3)	1 (−1 to +8)	0 (−5 to +6)
p	ns	0.006	0.01	0.0007

VAS (increase=improvement):

	Score improvement (range)			
	Baseline score	At 1wk	At 3wk	At 8wk
Methylpred.	71 (50 to 80)	4 (2 to 19)	15 (−1 to +24)	19 (6 to 26)
Placebo	67 (48 to 82)	1 (−8 to +7)	4 (−5 to +11)	0 (−5 to +6)
p	ns	0.03	0.06	0.0007

NB. Figures in brackets represent interquartile range.

- The difference in scores on the efficacy questionnaire at 8wk only reached significance as a secondary efficacy measure.
- The number of 'responders' after 1, 3, and 8wk, respectively, as judged by change in EDSS was significantly greater in the treatment group (8, 14, and 17) than the placebo group (1, 6, and 8).

Discussion

Previous trials had demonstrated the efficacy of high dose IV methylprednisolone vs placebo, and there was some small-scale trial evidence to suggest a similar efficacy of oral compared with intravenous administration. However, this trial provided the first clear evidence of the superiority of high dose oral steroids over placebo in MS relapse. High dose oral methylprednisolone is once more being widely used as an alternative to the intravenous route. Methylprednisolone 500mg is equivalent to prednisolone 625mg or dexamethasone 94mg.

Problems

- The main limitations of the trial are relatively small study numbers and a dramatic excess of side effects in the treatment group, which almost certainly introduced a degree of unblinding and may have influenced the self-reported outcomes.

Multiple sclerosis: β-interferon

> **PRISMS** (**P**revention of **R**elapses and disability by **I**nterferon β-1a **S**ubcutaneously in **M**ultiple **S**clerosis) study: Randomised, double-blind, placebo-controlled study of interferon β-1a in relapsing-remitting multiple sclerosis.
>
> **AUTHORS:** PRISMS study group.
> **REFERENCE:** Lancet (1998) 352, 1498–504.
> **STUDY DESIGN:** RCT
> **EVIDENCE LEVEL:** 1b

Key message

Subcutaneous interferon β-1a reduces relapse frequency and disease progression over a 2y period in patients with multiple sclerosis (MS).

Impact

Interferon β-1a is now widely used in patients with early MS and frequent relapses. Longer-term F/U of the PRISMS patients has suggested a rather more modest benefit at 4 and 8y than was suggested by this early trial, and the 2002 appraisal of β-interferon by the UK's National Institute of Health and Clinical Excellence (NICE) did not recommend its routine use in relapsing-remitting MS. However, more recent recommendations for its use made by the Association of British Neurologists have been approved by the Department of Health.

Aims

Earlier trials had suggested efficacy of interferon β in the short-term reduction of relapse rate and MRI lesion load in relapsing-remitting MS (*Neurology* (1993) 43, 655–61 and *Ann Neurol* (1996) 39, 285–94). However, evidence of efficacy had not been universally accepted due to the use of different types of interferon β, and a lack of clarity of significance of the results. This trial set out to definitively determine the effect of subcutaneous interferon β at two different doses in preventing relapse and limiting clinical progression of MS over a 2y period.

Methods

Patients: 560 patients at 22 centres in 9 countries.

Inclusion criteria:
- Adult;
- Clinically or laboratory-supported definite MS >1y duration;
- 2 relapses in past 2y;
- Kurtzke Expanded Disability Status Scale (EDSS) score 0–5 (where a higher score indicates greater disability).

Groups: All administered by subcutaneous injection 3 times wkly:
- Interferon β-1a 22mcg (6 million units) (n=189);
- Interferon β-1a 44mcg (12 million units) (n=184);
- Placebo (n=187).

Primary endpoint: Number of relapses during study

Secondary endpoints:
- Time to first and second relapse;
- Proportion of relapse-free patients;
- Progression of disability defined as 1 point increase on EDSS;
- Ambulation index;
- Arm function index;
- Requirement for hospital admission and steroid treatment;
- MRI findings.

Follow-up:
- Neurological assessment every 3 months and within 48h of MRI scans. MRI imaging twice yearly in all patients;
- Monthly MRI imaging for first 9 months of trial in 205 patients.

Results

	Placebo	Interferon (22mcg)	Interferon (44mcg)
Relapses	2.56	1.82	1.73
% reduction vs placebo	–	27 (14 to 39)	33 (21 to 44)
% relapse-free at 2y	16	27	32
OR (none vs any)	1.00	2.01 (1.21 to 3.21)	2.57 (1.56 to 2.45)

OR=odds ratio. Figures in brackets are 95% CI.

- Median time to first relapse was increased by 3 months in the 22mcg, and by 5 months in the 44mcg treatment groups compared with placebo.
- Time to sustained progression was prolonged by 6.5 months in the 22mcg, and by 9.4 months in the 44mcg treatment groups. Amongst patients with more severe disease, time to progression was only prolonged in the 44mcg treatment group.
- The median total MRI lesion load was increased by 11% in the placebo group. Median lesion load decreased by 1% in the 22mcg, and by 4% in the 44mcg treatment groups.

Discussion

This early interferon trial suggested significant benefits in terms of relapse prevention and delayed longer-term disease progression. A 2001 Cochrane review of the evidence for recombinant interferon in MS reported an overall reduction in relapse rate (relative risk 0.80, 95% CI 0.73 to 0.88) and disease progression (relative risk 0.69, 95% CI 0.55 to 0.87) at 2y. However, significant doubt was expressed over the strength of these results with regard to the number, assignment, and [unknown] clinical course of patients withdrawing from the trials. If all interferon-treated withdrawals suffered disease progression, the evidence that interferon prevents progression was no longer present.

Problems

- In 2002, the NICE appraisal of interferon β and glatiramer acetate for the treatment of MS reported that neither agent could be recommended on the basis of clinical and cost-effectiveness. This guidance led directly to the 'risk sharing scheme' agreement between the manufacturers and the Department of Health for the supply of interferon β and glatiramer acetate to the National Health Service (NHS).

Parkinson's disease: early treatment

A 5y study of the incidence of dyskinesia in patients with early Parkinson's disease treated with ropinirole or levodopa.

AUTHORS: Rascol O, Brooks D, Korczyn A.
REFERENCE: N Engl J Med (2000) 342, 1484–91.
STUDY DESIGN: RCT
EVIDENCE LEVEL: 1b

Key message
One of several RCTs to show a significantly reduced risk of dyskinesia in patients treated with a dopamine agonist compared to those treated with levodopa in early Parkinson's disease.

Impact
The trial supported the use of dopamine agonists as initial treatment for early Parkinson's disease.

Aims
This study aimed to resolve the longstanding controversy as to whether levodopa or a dopamine agonist should be the standard initial therapy in early Parkinson's disease, with particular reference to the incidence of treatment-induced dyskinesia. The trial also aimed to compare the efficacy and tolerability of the two drugs.

Methods
Patients: 268 patients at 30 centres in Europe, Israel, and Canada.

Inclusion criteria:
- Age ≥30y;
- Clinical diagnosis of Parkinson's disease;
- Hoen-Yahr stage 1–3 (unilateral early disease–more advanced bilateral disease);
- Requiring dopaminergic therapy;
- Maximum duration of prior treatment 6wk;
- Dopaminergic medication withdrawn 2wk before entry.

Groups: Open-label addition of levodopa available to patients in both groups if inadequate control on maximal doses of either study drug:
- **Ropinirole treatment** Introduced at 0.75mg od. Dose increments at wkly intervals according to clinical requirement to maximum 24mg od (n=179; 2 with dyskinesia at baseline).
- **Levodopa (+ benserazide) treatment** Introduced at 50mg od. Dose increments at wkly intervals according to clinical requirement to maximum 1200mg od (n=89; 1 with dyskinesia at baseline).

Primary outcome: Development of dyskinesia.

Secondary outcomes:
- Development of disabling dyskinesia;
- Measures of activities of daily living;

- Measures of motor function;
- 'Wearing off' with increasing symptom severity at end of dose.
- All primary and secondary outcomes assessed by means of the UPDRS (Universal Parkinson's Disease Rating Scale).

Follow-up: At wkly intervals for the first month; every 2wk for the next 2 months; monthly for the next 6 months; and every 2 months thereafter.

Results

- 85 patients (47%) in the ropinirole group and 45 patients in the levodopa group (51%) completed the study.
- Of these, 56 patients (66%) in the ropinirole group and 16 patients (35%) in the levodopa group received open-label supplementary levodopa.
- Overall, dyskinesia developed in 36 of 177 patients (20%) in the ropinirole group and in 40 of 88 patients (45%) in the levodopa group over the 5y F/U period.
- Before introduction of open-label levodopa, 9 of 177 patients (5%) in the ropinirole group and 32 of 88 patients (36%) had developed dyskinesia.
- Changes in mean UPDRS scores for activities of daily living did not differ significantly between the groups.
- There was a small but significant difference in the change from baseline in UPDRS motor scores between the two groups, with levodopa conferring a 4.5 point advantage (on a point score range of 0–108, 95% CI 1.25 to 7.72).

Discussion

Initial treatment of early Parkinson's disease with a dopamine agonist, ropinirole, significantly reduced the risk of developing dyskinesia compared to initial treatment with levodopa. Other motor complications were not significantly reduced in the ropinirole group. This effect on dyskinesia may reflect the difference in half-life between levodopa (1.5–2h) and ropinirole (6–8h), with levodopa giving pulsatile, and ropinirole more continuous dopamine receptor stimulation. Other trials suggest similar efficacy and tolerability of the other non-ergot-derived dopamine agonists in comparison with levodopa. The ergot-derived agents have now largely fallen out of favour due to concerns over the association with retroperitoneal, pulmonary, pericardial, and valvular fibrosis.

Problems

- The dropout rate in this trial was very high, with less than half of the randomised patients completing the study.
- There is a 7-fold cost difference between ropinirole and levodopa at the mean final doses reached in the study.

Parkinson's disease: timing of levodopa

ELLDOPA (Early vs Late LevoDOPA) study: Levodopa and the Progression of Parkinson's Disease.

AUTHORS: Fahn S, the Parkinson's Study Group.
REFERENCE: N Engl J Med (2004) 351, 2489–508.
STUDY DESIGN: RCT
EVIDENCE LEVEL: 1b

Key message
Levodopa does not accelerate, and may indeed slow the rate of decline in Parkinson's disease.

Impact
It has been common practice in the treatment of idiopathic Parkinson's disease to delay the introduction of levodopa for as long as possible, due to a belief that the drug is the cause of motor fluctuations and may accelerate disease progression. This practice was challenged by the findings of the ELLDOPA study.

Aims
The dopamine precursor, levodopa, remains an effective treatment for the symptoms of idiopathic Parkinson's disease. *In vitro* studies and more recent functional neuroimaging in Parkinson's disease patients have suggested that levodopa might have a neurotoxic effect, further depleting remaining dopaminergic neurons. This study set out to assess whether treatment with levodopa caused accelerated clinical decline compared with placebo.

Methods
Patients: 361 at 33 centres in the USA and 5 in Canada.

Inclusion criteria: Early idiopathic Parkinson's disease.
- >30y old;
- Diagnosed <2y previously;
- Unilateral or mild bilateral disease;
- Not on treatment and judged unlikely to require treatment within 9 months.

Groups: Double blind randomisation:
- Placebo (n=90);
- Carbidopa/levodopa 12.5/50mg tds (n=92);
- Carbidopa/levodopa 50/100mg tds (n=88);
- Carbidopa/levodopa 100/200mg tds (n=91);
- 40wk treatment including 9wk blinded dose titration, followed by medication withdrawal and 2wk 'washout' period.

Primary outcome measure: Change in Parkinson's disease severity between baseline and wk42 (2wk after withdrawal of study drug), as assessed by the total score on the universal Parkinson's disease rating scale (UPDRS).

Secondary outcome measure: Change in total UPDRS score at interim F/U visits.

Follow-up: At screening, baseline, and at wk 3, 9, 24, 40, 41, and 42.

Results

	Placebo	L-dopa 150mg	L-dopa 300mg	L-dopa 600mg	*p*
Change in UPDRS from baseline to 42wk (mean ± SD)	7.8±9.0	1.9±6.0	1.9±6.9	−1.4±7.7	<0.001 (all doses)

- In addition to the overall slowing of deterioration amongst those taking levodopa compared to the placebo group, there was a strong dose-response relationship beginning at wk9 (following dose titration).
- Those taking 600mg levodopa daily had lower UPDRS scores both during the treatment phase and after washout than those taking 300mg, who in turn fared better than those taking 150mg.

Discussion

Although not one of the stated aims of the trial, the interim treatment phase data did provide confirmation of the effectiveness of levodopa as a treatment for symptoms in idiopathic Parkinson's disease as compared to placebo. This had not been previously demonstrated in a randomised controlled trial. Within the relatively short timescale of the trial, the primary outcome data suggest that levodopa does not accelerate decline in early Parkinson's disease. The difference in UPDRS scores between treatment and placebo groups after washout could reflect either a prolonged therapeutic effect, or a neuroprotective effect of levodopa. The possibility that the washout period was simply too short and that levodopa was still having a therapeutic effect at the final assessment was considered. A small group of patients continued the washout period to 4wk; no further decline was observed, but the group was too small for these results to be meaningfully interpreted.

Problems

- The clinical course of idiopathic Parkinson's disease is long, often spanning decades. The trial duration of 9.5 months is short, and it is not clear that these results can be extrapolated to the longer term.

Motor neurone disease: riluzole

A controlled trial of riluzole in amyotrophic lateral sclerosis.

AUTHORS: Bensimon G, Lacomblez L, Meininger V.
REFERENCE: N Engl J Med (1994) 330, 585–91.
STUDY DESIGN: RCT
EVIDENCE LEVEL: 1b

Key message
Riluzole slows the progression of amyotrophic lateral sclerosis (ALS) and prolongs survival in patients with bulbar onset disease.

Impact
The use of riluzole in ALS is approved by the UK's National Institute for Health and Clinical Excellence (NICE), although its cost-effectiveness remains controversial.

Aims
The pathogenesis of ALS, a progressive motor neurone disease, remains unclear. It is a progressive and universally fatal neurodegenerative condition with a median survival from diagnosis of 37–49 months. Glutamate-mediated excitotoxicity has been mooted as an underlying cause, and therefore, drugs that modulate glutamatergic transmission had been proposed as potential therapeutic agents. This study aimed to evaluate the efficacy and safety of the antiglutamate agent, riluzole.

Methods
Patients: 155 patients at 7 centres in France.

Inclusion criteria:
- Clinically probable or definite ALS;
- Age 20–75y;
- 5y or less from symptom onset;
- Forced vital capacity (FVC) >60% predicted;
- No evidence of conduction block on nerve conduction studies.

Groups: Patients stratified according to limb or bulbar onset of disease:
- Riluzole: 100mg od (n=77; 62 limb onset, 15 bulbar onset);
- Placebo (n=78; 61 limb onset, 17 bulbar onset).

Primary endpoint: Survival and change in functional status after 12 months of treatment.

Secondary endpoints:
- Change in muscle power (22 muscle groups, MRC grading);
- Respiratory function (FVC);
- Clinical Global Impression of Change scale (CGIC);
- Patient assessment of fasciculations, cramps, stiffness, and tiredness (visual analogue scale).

Follow-up: Every 2 months from entry. Functional status assessed at each visit (limb and bulbar function evaluated by modified Norris scales, clinical examination and symptoms reported by patient).

Results

	Riluzole (n = 77)	Placebo (n = 78)	p
Alive at 12 months	57 (74%)	45 (58%)	0.01
Bulbar onset	15	17	not reported
Alive at 12 months	11 (73%)	6 (35%)	0.01
Limb onset	62	61	not reported
Alive at 12 months	46 (74%)	39 (64%)	0.17

- Overall median survival=449d (placebo group) and 532d (riluzole group).
- Amongst the bulbar onset patients, median survival=239d (placebo group) and 'not yet been reached after 476d of F/U' (riluzole group).
- Rates of decline in functional assessment scores were only significantly different for measures of muscle power (33% reduction in rate of deterioration over 12 months, p=0.03).

Discussion

Riluzole appeared to slow the rate of deterioration and prolong survival in patients with ALS. However, this effect was only significant in patients with bulbar onset disease, those with limb onset disease showing only a non-significant trend towards benefit. Therefore, it is perhaps surprising that in terms of specific functional assessment, the only significant effect appeared to be on the rate of progression of limb muscle weakness (the effect on rate of deterioration of bulbar function being non-significant). A 2007 Cochrane review of riluzole in ALS suggested a 2–3 months increase in median survival compared with placebo.

Problems

- The use of riluzole in ALS has been approved by NICE, but its cost-effectiveness remains controversial, with estimates of cost per quality adjusted life year (QALY) ranging from UK £18,000 to £43,000.

Peripheral neuropathy: gabapentin

Gabapentin for the treatment of painful neuropathy in patients with diabetes mellitus. A randomised controlled trial.

AUTHORS: Backonja M, Beydoun A, Edwards K.
REFERENCE: JAMA (1998) 280, 1831–36.
STUDY DESIGN: RCT
EVIDENCE LEVEL: 1b

Key message
Gabapentin significantly improves neuropathic pain and associated sleep disturbance in diabetic neuropathy.

Impact
Gabapentin is now widely used in the treatment of many forms of neuropathic pain, not just diabetic neuropathy.

Aims
Diabetic neuropathy can cause severe pain and is associated with sleep and mood disturbances. Its progress can be modified by improved glycaemic control. This trial aimed to assess the efficacy of gabapentin (normally used as an anti-convulsant) in the treatment of pain associated with diabetic peripheral neuropathy.

Methods
Patients: 165 patients at multiple centres in the USA.

Inclusion criteria:
- Types 1 or 2 diabetes mellitus (DM);
- Pain attributed to peripheral neuropathy of 1–5y duration;
- Pain rating score of at least 40mm on 100mm visual analogue scale of the Short Form McGill Pain Questionnaire (SF-MPQ).

Groups:
- **Gabapentin:** 4wk titration phase to max. 3600mg od, followed by 4wk fixed dose period at maximum tolerated dose (n=84);
- **Placebo:** Identical capsules (n=81).

Primary endpoint: Pain severity rating (range 0–10): recorded in daily diaries using 11 point Likert scale.

Secondary endpoints:
- SF-MPQ scores;
- Weekly mean sleep interference scores;
- Patient Global Impression of Change (PGIC);
- Clinical Global Impression of Change (CGIC).

Follow-up:
- Wk2 and 4: SF-MPQ completed;
- Wk8: SF-MPQ, Short-form 36 Quality of Life Questionnaire (SF-36 QoL), and Profile of Mood States (POMS) completed.

Results

Primary outcome measure:

	Gabapentin		Placebo		Difference	p
	Baseline	Wk8	Baseline	Wk8		
Mean pain score	6.4	3.9	6.5	5.1	−1.2	<0.001

Secondary outcome measures:
- Similar modest but significant differences were seen in the secondary outcome measures.
- Mean sleep interference scores (0–10) differed by 1.5 in favour of gabapentin (p=0.001).
- In the SF-MPQ total pain scores (0–45), there was a 6 point difference in favour of gabapentin (p=0.001).
- In the SF-MPQ visual analogue scale (100mm), there was a 17mm difference in favour of gabapentin (p=0.001).
- In the SF-MPQ present pain intensity scores (0–5), there was a 0.6 point difference in favour of gabapentin (p<0.001).
- Patients had significantly greater improvement in pain with gabapentin as compared with placebo on both PGIC and CGIC scales.

Discussion

This trial demonstrated modest but significant efficacy of gabapentin in the treatment of pain associated with diabetic neuropathy. Diabetes is a common cause of painful peripheral neuropathy, and restriction of the trial to this group produced a relatively homogeneous study population. It does not, of course, necessarily follow that all neuropathic pain will respond in the same way, but this has been widely assumed. A variety of other agents have efficacy in controlling neuropathic pain, including tricyclic antidepressants, the serotonin/noradrenaline reuptake inhibitor, duloxetine, and the newer anti-epileptic drug, pregabalin.

Problems

- Cost: the benefits of gabapentin demonstrated in this trial are of similar order to those of tricyclic antidepressant drugs. Gabapentin appears to work somewhat more rapidly and is slightly better tolerated, but there is a greater than 100-fold difference in price.

Bell's palsy: role of prednisolone and aciclovir

Early treatment with prednisolone or aciclovir in Bell's palsy.

AUTHORS: Sullivan F, Swan I, Donnan P *et al.*
REFERENCE: N Engl J Med (2007) 357, 1598–607.
STUDY DESIGN: RCT
EVIDENCE LEVEL: 1b

Key message
When prescribed within the first 3d of symptoms of Bell's palsy, complete recovery of facial function is more likely following treatment with prednisolone vs placebo. There is no added benefit of combining aciclovir with prednisolone.

Impact
This adequately powered study confirmed the previously held opinion that prednisolone is beneficial in treating Bell's palsy. As such, all patients should receive this treatment early (within 3d of symptoms).
For patients with risk factors for systemic steroid use, reassurance can be offered that around 85% will recover without treatment.

Aims
Bell's palsy has been proposed to have an association with herpes simplex virus (HSV). Corticosteroid treatment has been widely regarded as effective in improving prognosis. Antiviral agents such as aciclovir are also used; however, evidence for their efficacy is limited. Given the lack of level-1 evidence and a previously inconclusive Cochrane review, this study aimed to determine whether prednisolone or aciclovir used early in the course of Bell's palsy could improve the chances of recovery.

Methods
Patients: 551 patients at 17 centres in Scotland.

Inclusion criteria:
- Age >16y;
- Unilateral facial nerve weakness of no identifiable cause;
- Presenting to primary care or emergency department with referral for otorhinolaryngology opinion within 72h of onset.

Exclusion criteria:
- Pregnant or breastfeeding;
- Medical: uncontrolled diabetes mellitus, peptic ulcer disease, sarcoid;
- Infections: systemic, herpes zoster virus (HZV), middle ear infection.

Groups: Randomised twice to give 4 groups (2x2 factorial design):
- Prednisolone (25mg bd) and aciclovir (400mg 5x/d), for 10d (n=134);
- Placebo (lactose) and aciclovir (n=138);
- Prednisolone and placebo (n=138);
- Placebo and placebo (n=141).

Primary outcome: House-Brackmann grading system for facial nerve function (score 1–6, with 1=normal function). Function independently graded using photographs and blinded to study group assignments. The primary outcome was full recovery with a final score of 1.

Follow-up: Baseline visit at home/doctor's office at 3–5d, then at 3 months. If recovery incomplete, visit at 9 months performed.

Results

Full recovery	Pred.	No pred.	p	Aciclovir	No aciclovir	p
At 3 months	205/247 (83%)	152/239 (63.6%)	<0.001	173/243 (71.2%)	184/243 (75.7%)	0.5
At 9 months	237/251 (94.4%)	200/245 (81.6%)	<0.001	211/247 (85.4)	226/249 (90.8%)	0.1

Sample size calculation showed 236 per treatment, at 80% power, 0.05 significance level, to demonstrate a 10–12% difference in treatments.

Discussion

This study represents the strongest evidence available in answering how best to treat Bell's palsy. The fact that a previous Cochrane review was inconclusive did not mean there was 'no evidence', just that there was a lack of well-powered level-1 trials. That said, there has been weaker evidence also recommending aciclovir in Bell's palsy. In this RCT, aciclovir did not offer any benefit. A recent Japanese RCT (*Hato et al. Otology and Neurotology* (2007) 23, 408–13) recommended the use of valaciclovir in the treatment of Bell's palsy, but only for those patients with complete facial palsy. However, the study was not powered for subgroup analysis and facial function was not independently graded.

Problems

- Some may argue the ethics of offering placebo to patients, given that the majority of specialists already advocate the use of steroids.

Psychiatry

Introduction

The psychiatrist at the cinema: The popular image of psychiatry isn't great, and unhelped by films such as *'One Flew Over the Cuckoo's Nest'* (starring Jack Nicholson), *'Girl: Interrupted'* (Winona Ryder, Angelina Jolie), and *'A Beautiful Mind'* (Russell Crowe). But there are strongly positive models too, such as that of William Rivers in *'Regeneration'* (Jonathan Pryce), of Oliver Sacks in *'Awakenings'* (Robin Williams), and of the fictional Dr Powell in *'K-Pax'* (Jeff Bridges, Kevin Spacey). One of *K-Pax's* themes, the toll on psychiatrists of their work, is the focus of *'Face to Face'*, which makes for challenging viewing, as Liv Ullman portrays a fictional psychiatrist who inexorably declines with her own mental illness. If after watching that you need a pick-me-up (and you will), *'High Anxiety'* should help, as Mel Brooks plays the fictional Dr Thorndyke, medical superintendent at the 'Psychoneurotic Institute for the Very, VERY Nervous'.

The psychiatrist at parties: Responding to the party question 'what do you do?' is challenging for any doctor, but for a psychiatrist, it is particularly problematic. There are three likely responses to 'I'm a psychiatrist, actually' (the 'actually' immediately betraying nervousness about revealing this information). Some people are firmly dismissive, appearing to believe that the psychiatrist is expressing grandiose delusions, and is actually in need of psychiatric help himself or herself. Many will latch onto the poor psychiatrist for the rest of the night, sharing their neuroses and seeking advice, such that the party becomes an extension of the outpatient clinic. And others appear disconcerted—'oh, you've been analysing me, haven't you, why didn't you tell me that earlier?'. While the narcissistic among psychiatrists will relish these responses, most psychiatrists have unsurprisingly learnt the hard way to keep their occupation close to their chests, and some have developed elaborate alter egos in order to cope. Now, what did you say that you do … ?

Depression: antidepressants

Selective serotonin reuptake inhibitors vs tricyclic antidepressants: a meta-analysis of efficacy and tolerability.

AUTHORS: Anderson I.
REFERENCE: J Affective Disord (2000) 58, 19–36.
STUDY DESIGN: Meta-analysis
EVIDENCE LEVEL: 1a

Key message
Selective serotonin reuptake inhibitors (SSRIs) are better tolerated than tricyclic antidepressants (TCAs) with comparable efficacy.

Impact
Since this systematic review, TCAs have been replaced by SSRIs as first choice antidepressant agents.

Aims
SSRIs had become increasingly popular for the treatment of depression due to reported better side effect profiles and safety than TCAs. This study aimed to compare their efficacy and tolerability.

Methods
Patients: 102 RCTs (10,706 participants) included.

Inclusion criteria:
- RCTs;
- Unipolar major depressive illness;
- SSRI vs TCA (including the tetracyclic agent, maprotiline).

Search strategy:
- Previous meta-analyses and reviews;
- Medline search (to May 1997).

Outcomes:
- Reduction in scores on Hamilton Rating Scale for Depression (HAMD) or Montgomery and Asberg Depression Rating Scale (MADRS);
- Treatment discontinuation: overall/due to side effects.

Results
- Efficacy:
  - Overall, SSRIs and TCAs were of equal efficacy (effect size −0.03, 95% CI −0.09 to 0.03).
  - In a subgroup analysis, it appeared TCAs were more effective than SSRIs in the treatment of depressed inpatients, i.e. patients with severe depression (effect size −0.23, 95% CI −0.4 to −0.05; 25 trials, 1377 participants).
- Side effects:
  - More people discontinued TCAs due to side effects than SSRIs (17.3% vs 12.4%, $p < 0.0001$).

Discussion

The SSRIs have largely replaced TCAs as first-line agents for unipolar depression. This analysis provided a rational basis for this change in prescribing; the SSRIs were generally as effective and better tolerated.

Problems

- Subgroup analyses: Multiple subgroup analyses were performed, which may have increased the risk of finding erroneous differences.
- Newer antidepressants: The analysis did not address newer antidepressant agents, such as the selective serotonin-norepinephrine reuptake inhibitors (SNRIs), venlafaxine and duloxetine. Superior efficacy is claimed for some of these agents.
- Age: This evidence applies only to adults; there is active debate regarding the effectiveness and risks of antidepressants (SSRIs in particular) in children and adolescents.
- Risk of deliberate self-harm/suicide: There is an active debate regarding the risk of suicide following antidepressant prescription. Clearly, this is challenging epidemiology; depression is associated with both suicide and antidepressant prescription, and the emergence of suicidal ideation may trigger pharmacological treatment.

Depression: relapse prevention

Geddes' study: Relapse prevention with antidepressant drug treatment in depressive disorders.

AUTHORS: Geddes J, Carney S, Davies C et al.
REFERENCE: Lancet (2003) 361, 653–61.
STUDY DESIGN: Meta-analysis (systematic review)
EVIDENCE LEVEL: 1a

Key message
Antidepressant continuation substantially reduces the risk of relapse in depressive disorder.

Impact
The relapse prevention benefits of treatment underlie the standard recommendation to continue antidepressants for 6 months or more after recovery. Much more effort is now placed on educating patients about the likely benefits of continuing treatment with antidepressants beyond the point of recovery.

Aims
As depression often has a long-term course, patients remain at risk of relapse after successful treatment of acute episodes. Therefore, guidelines often recommend continuation of treatment for several months after recovery. However, there had been no consensus in practice. This review aimed to establish how long antidepressants should be continued to prevent relapse in depression.

Methods
Inclusion criteria:
- Study type: RCTs;
- Publication status: Published or unpublished, available at August 2000;
- Comparison: Continued antidepressant vs placebo;
- Participants: Already responded to acute antidepressant treatment.

Groups:
- Continued antidepressant;
- Placebo.

Search strategy:
- A Cochrane Collaboration Trials Register, which incorporated searches of Medline, EMBASE, Cinahl, PsycLIT, Psyndex, and Lilacs;
- Reference checking;
- Personal communications.
- Outcome: Relapse or recurrence of depression.

Results
- 31 trials (4410 participants) provided data for analyses.

- Trials compared placebo with most classes of antidepressant, although the majority involved a tricyclic antidepressant (TCA) or selective serotonin reuptake inhibitor (SSRI).
- Continued antidepressant treatment reduced the risk of relapse by roughly half (41% vs 19%, pooled OR 0.30, 95% CI 0.22 to 0.38). This reduction was similar for the antidepressant classes for which there was most evidence (15 TCA trials, 10 SSRI trials), and was also independent of treatment duration.

Discussion

This meta-analysis demonstrated the benefits of continuing antidepressant medication after recovery from an episode of depression. The large body of data and consistency of the findings allow for considerable confidence in interpretation. Most of the trials were of 12 months duration, although consistent benefits were seen even in those that extended to 3y follow-up. The magnitude of effect was so great to support speculation that anti-depressant medications are actually more effective at relapse prevention than promoting initial recovery.

Problems

- Lack of individual patient data analysis: The analyses were performed on the overall results of studies. Availability of individual patient data might have allowed identification of subgroups receiving different magnitudes of benefit.
- Applicability in primary care: The trials mainly recruited patients from secondary care. It is possible (although unproven) that the benefits may not apply to primary care populations with lower baseline risk of relapse.
- Duration of protective effects: From 3y onwards, the problem becomes a lack of evidence for efficacy rather than evidence of lack of efficacy. Given that antidepressants are often taken for several years, further studies extending the evidence over longer time periods would be of benefit.

Depression: electroconvulsive therapy (ECT)

> **The Northwick Park Electroconvulsive Therapy Trial**
>
> **AUTHORS:** Johnstone E, Deakin J, Lawler P et al.
> **REFERENCE:** Lancet (1980) 1317–20.
> **STUDY DESIGN:** RCT
> **EVIDENCE LEVEL:** 1b

Key message
Electroconvulsive therapy (ECT) is superior to sham therapy for acute depression. However, results are not sustained at long-term follow-up.

Impact
ECT remains the most controversial standard psychiatric treatment. Despite vehement opposition of some patients and patient groups, ECT remains a recommended treatment option for some people with severe depression. Indeed, in certain clinical situations, ECT remains an essential, life-saving treatment.

Aims
ECT was first introduced over 40y prior to this study. Its use had always been shrouded in controversy, not helped by a limited evidence base. With only a limited number of small studies, there was uncertainty whether the electric shock was the essential therapeutic element, or whether the anaesthetic itself might act as an antidepressant. Therefore, this study aimed to determine whether the electric shock and resulting convulsion is a required element.

Methods
Patients: 70 patients (52 female, 18 male) from 1 centre in the UK.

Inclusion criteria:
- Endogenous depression;
- Considered probable good response to ECT;
- Age 30–69y;
- Admitted to hospital for treatment and consent to ECT.

Groups:
- Real ECT (up to 8 treatments over 4wk);
- Sham ECT (anaesthesia without ECT).

Primary endpoint: Improvement in depressive symptoms (Hamilton rating scale).

Secondary endpoints:
- Other rating scales for depression severity;
- Tests of memory and concentration.

Follow-up: Weekly during study and subsequently at 1 and 6 months after completion.

Results

- Greater initial improvement in depression ratings was seen with real ECT than with sham treatment ($p<0.01$).
- The comparative benefit was no longer evident at 1 or 6 months F/U.
- Real ECT was associated with subjective and objective memory deficits during the course of treatment, but there was no evidence of sustained problems.

Discussion

This study showed that ECT is more effective than sham therapy for patients with severe depression, leading to rapid resolution of the severe depressive state. The difference between groups was smaller than the substantial improvement in both over the course of the study. The specific benefits of ECT over anaesthesia alone seen during treatment were not convincingly sustained in the longer term.

Problems

- Cognitive side effects: While this study did not find evidence of prolonged memory impairments after treatment, the tests used may not have been optimal. Tests of cognitive function have tended to be inconsistent between studies of ECT.
- Patient and carer attitudes: Acceptance of the need for this treatment is often low among patients and carers, perhaps fuelled by legitimate concerns about possible adverse effects (including cognitive side effects) and by potent media influences (such as alarming images seen in films like *'One Flew Over the Cuckoo's Nest'* starring Jack Nicholson).
- Consent to treatment: Many patients who fulfil criteria for ECT lack the capacity to consent to treatment.

Depression: collaborative care

Katon's study: Collaborative management to achieve treatment guidelines: impact on depression in primary care.

AUTHORS: Katon W, Von Korff M, Lin E *et al.*
REFERENCE: JAMA (1995) 273, 1026–31.
STUDY DESIGN: RCT
EVIDENCE LEVEL: 1b

Key message
Multifaceted collaborative care significantly improves the outcome of mild to moderate depression.

Impact
Until recently, the focus of treatment for depression was almost entirely on which treatment or treatments should be delivered, an antidepressant, and if so, which one, and for how long; or, if not, a psychological treatment, which one, and for how long? The Seattle group's ongoing work on 'collaborative care' shifted attention towards the broad context of treatment delivery, supporting explanation by clinician, video, or booklet; education of professionals; structured follow-up; and monitoring of adherence; to name but a few.

Aims
Much of depression treatment has focused on the nature of the treatment, as opposed to the multidisciplinary educational approaches required to provide 'holistic' care. This study aimed to compare the effectiveness of multifaceted collaborative care with usual care in patients with mild to moderate depression in the US primary care setting.

Methods
Patients: 217 patients from 1 primary care clinic in the USA.

Inclusion criteria:
- SCL-20 (depression) score ≥0.75;
- Age 18–80y;
- Willing to take an antidepressant;
- No alcohol dependence, psychosis, serious suicidal tendency, or dementia.

Groups:
- Collaborative care: patient booklet and video, symptom reporting, side effect reporting, structured follow-up of 2 physician and 2 psychiatrist appointments, pharmacy feedback on dispensing antidepressants (n=108);
- Usual care (n=109).

Endpoints:
- Antidepressant adherence at adequate dose for ≥30d/90d;

• Major or minor depression at 4 and 7 months;
• Improvement of ≥50% on SCL-20 at 4 and 7 months.

Follow-up: At baseline, then 1, 4, and 7 months.

Results

	Intervention	Usual care	*p*
Major depression:			
Adherence >90d	76%	50%	<0.01
Adherence >30d	88%	57%	<0.001
SCL improved at 4 months	74%	44%	<0.01
Minor depression:			
Adherence >30d	88%	48%	<0.001
SCL improved at 4 months	60%	68%	0.4

Discussion

The multifaceted approach to intervention led to much greater antidepressant adherence in both major and minor depression, and to significantly improved depression outcomes in the major depression group only. It has spawned many other trials (in the USA and elsewhere) of many variants (in content and intensity) of collaborative care, for depression in a variety of patient groups.

Problems

• Using the correct recipe: It is unclear which aspects of collaborative care were the effective ingredients; were all aspects essential or only some? Was the effect of the whole greater than that of the sum of the parts through synergistic effects, and if so, how could this be determined? Recently, attempts have been made to determine the effects of specific elements (Bower et al. *Br J Psychiatry* (2006) 189, 484–93).
• Applicability: This study was conducted in the US health care system, and it is likely that the effectiveness or otherwise of 'health care system' interventions is nation- and system-specific. However, there is growing evidence of the global effectiveness of such interventions.

Bipolar disorder: discontinuation of lithium therapy

> **Faedda's study:** Outcome after rapid vs gradual discontinuation of lithium treatment in bipolar disorders.
>
> **AUTHORS:** Faedda G, Tondo L, Baldessarini R *et al.*
> **REFERENCE:** Arch Gen Psych (1993) 50, 448–55.
> **STUDY DESIGN:** Cohort study
> **EVIDENCE LEVEL:** 2a

Key message
Gradual discontinuation of lithium is less likely to lead to early relapse than rapid discontinuation.

Impact
The need for gradual discontinuation is a key component of the effective and safe prescription of lithium. Patients need to be fully informed about the medicine, how to maximise its effectiveness, and minimise its side effects.

Aims
Long-term maintenance therapy with lithium is a common approach in the management of bipolar disorder. However, although there is now reasonable support for its effectiveness, there is relatively little evidence guiding its use. Patients stop their medicines for a variety of reasons, with or without the endorsement of their doctor. In chronic disorders, such as bipolar disorder, withdrawal of prophylactic treatment may be especially likely after a period of stability. At the time of this study, it was not known what advice regarding speed of withdrawal should be given to such patients.

Methods
Patients: 64 patients from 1 psychiatry outpatient clinic in Italy.

Inclusion criteria:
- DSM (Diagnostic and Statistical Manual of Mental Disorders)-III-R bipolar disorder;
- Stable on lithium monotherapy for ≥18 months;
- Stopped lithium for reason other than recurrence.

Groups:
- Gradual discontinuation (2–4wk) (n=30);
- Rapid discontinuation (<2wk) (n=34).

Primary endpoint: Relapse to episodes of mania or depression.

Follow-up: 5y.

Results

Endpoint	Gradual discontinuation	Rapid discontinuation	p
Recurrent episode	16/30 (53%)	32/34 (94%)	<0.001
Median time to recurrence	37 months	8 months	<0.001

Discussion

The excess of recurrent episodes of mood disorder was most apparent in the early months after discontinuation. After 2y, it was the same in both groups. The increased rate of relapse on rapid discontinuation was so great that prolonged treatment over several years was necessary for the benefit accrued by taking lithium to outweigh the harm caused by rapid discontinuation. The results of this study raised the concern that rapid discontinuation of lithium in patients with (apparently) unipolar mood disorder may trigger an episode of hypomania or mania and thereby a change of diagnosis to bipolar disorder.

Problems

- Study design: This was an observational study and not a randomised trial. Therefore, patient characteristics may have affected speed of discontinuation, biasing the results.
- Differences between study groups: Gender, age, and mean duration of lithium treatment were similar in the two groups. However, bipolar patients were more common in the rapid withdrawal group, and more likely to relapse earlier.
- Unplanned discontinuations: Compliance with prescribed medication is often poor, so discontinuations are unplanned and sudden. Patient education is pivotal.

Schizophrenia: atypical vs typical antipsychotics

CATIE (Clinical **A**ntipsychotic **T**rials of **I**ntervention **E**ffectiveness) **study:** Effectiveness of antipsychotic drugs in patients with chronic schizophrenia.

AUTHORS: Lieberman J, Stroup T, McEvoy J *et al.*
REFERENCE: N Engl J Med (2005) 353, 1209–23.
STUDY DESIGN: RCT
EVIDENCE LEVEL: 1b

Key message
Typical and atypical antipsychotics have similar efficacy in schizophrenia.

Impact
Atypical antipsychotics took psychiatric practice by storm in the late 1990s, and by 2000 were the dominant prescription in developed nations. This trial (and other evidence of adverse effects) is encouraging a return to older, typical antipsychotic medications as options in the treatment of psychosis.

Aims
The first generation of antipsychotic drugs (dopamine D2 receptor agonists) had high rates of neurological side effects, including extrapyramidal signs and tardive dyskinesia. Second generation (atypical) agents have lower affinity for D2 receptors and higher affinity for other receptors, including those for 5-hydroxytryptamine (serotonin) and norepinephrine. Although these increasingly popular agents had been proposed to have fewer side effects, there was no firm evidence as to their efficacy. Therefore, this study aimed to compare the effectiveness of atypical and conventional antipsychotic medications in schizophrenia.

Methods
Patients: 1460 patients from 57 clinical sites in the USA.

Inclusion criteria:
- Age 18–65y;
- Schizophrenia: DSM (Diagnostic and Statistical Manual of Mental Disorders)-IV criteria.

Groups:
- 4 'atypical' groups: olanzapine (n=336); quetiapine (n=337); risperidone (n=341); ziprasidone (n=185).
- 1 'typical' group: perphenazine (an older 'typical' or 'conventional' agent, that was not well known to clinical investigators; n=261).

Primary outcome: Discontinuation of treatment (any cause).

Secondary outcomes:
• Reason for discontinuation;
• Rating scale scores (Clinical Global Impression (CGI) and PANSS);
• Measures of safety and tolerability.

Follow-up: 18 months.

Results

• The majority (74%) of patients discontinued their assigned medication over the course of the 18 months study.
• Olanzapine was the agent least likely to be discontinued for any reason (hazard ratios≈0.7 vs other agents). It was also least likely to be discontinued because of lack of efficacy (hazard ratios≈0.45).
• The conventional and atypical agents had similar efficacy on the rating scale measures and on ratings of motor side effects.
• Olanzapine use was associated with a greater increase in weight, total cholesterol, triglycerides, and HbA1C than the other agents.

Discussion

The newer 'atypical' antipsychotics are now widely prescribed following the perception that they are both more effective and have fewer side effects than the older 'conventional' or 'typical' antipsychotics. Both these beliefs had come under question in the period leading up to this study. Meta-analysis had found that the newer and older agents were in fact of similar short-term efficacy and tolerability (see Geddes *et al. BMJ* (2000) 321, 1371–6), and there had been increasing awareness of the atypicals' specific side effect profiles. This well-powered study found that the typical antipsychotic, perphenazine, was not inferior to most of the atypical agents. Similar findings of equivalence between the classes have more recently come from the *UK CUTLASS 1* study (*Arch Gen Psych* (2006) 63, 1079–87). This study further suggests that there may be some specific benefit of olanzapine over other antipsychotics assessed, but at the cost of increased risk of metabolic side effects.

Problems

• Meaning of discontinuation: The primary outcome of discontinuation of treatment could be due to many causes, not simply differences in efficacy.
• Choice of typical antipsychotic: Perphenazine had not been widely used previously.
• Dose equivalence: The effective olanzapine dosage achieved in the study may have been higher than for comparator agents, contributing to apparent differences in effects.

Schizophrenia: relapse prevention

Carpenter's study: Continuous vs targeted mediation in schizophrenic outpatients: outcome results.

AUTHORS: Carpenter W, Hanlon T, Heinrichs D et al.
REFERENCE: Am J Psych (1990) 147, 1138–48.
STUDY DESIGN: RCT
EVIDENCE LEVEL: 1b

Key message
Continuous antipsychotic medication is more effective at preventing relapse in schizophrenia than intermittent use.

Impact
Continued antipsychotic medication is a key component of schizophrenia management. Therefore, a key function of Community Mental Health Teams is increasing patient adherence to antipsychotic medication. Indeed, a psychological treatment ('compliance therapy') has been developed with this aim in mind, although evaluation of its effectiveness has been limited to date.

Aims
Schizophrenia is a common mental disorder which can have a major and enduring impact on functional capacity. Antipsychotic medication has improved outcomes, but is associated with adverse effects in the short term and potentially the long term (tardive dyskinesia). This trial aimed to compare the effects of continued or intermittent antipsychotic use as a component of outpatient schizophrenia management.

Methods
Patients: 116 outpatients at 1 centre in the USA.

Inclusion criteria:
- Schizophrenia;
- Recent psychotic episode;
- Considered appropriate for long-term antipsychotic therapy.

Groups: Both groups received 'enriched psychosocial care', including weekly individual therapy:
- Continuous medication (n=59);
- Intermittent medication (drug-free unless symptomatic) (n=57).

Key outcomes:
- Admission to hospital;
- 'Decompensation' (worsening of functioning or symptoms);
- Total medication required.

Follow-up: 2y.

Results

Endpoint	Continuous	Intermittent	p
Admissions	36	60	<0.05
Decompensations (mean per patient)	2.75	4.21	<0.05

Discussion

Antipsychotic medications are not without side effects, so reducing their use is potentially desirable. This research group had previously found that intermittent medication in combination with enriched psychosocial care had been equivalent to care as usual. In this study, both groups received psychological intervention, so any differences should reflect the choice of medication strategy. While intermittent medication targeted to early signs of relapse did reduce the dose of antipsychotic received, it was at the cost of a worse clinical outcome with more recurrent episodes of illness. This was demonstrated not only in the numbers of 'decompensations' recorded by treating clinicians, but also in terms of the hard endpoint of need for hospital admission.

Problems

- Decision-making for individuals, not populations: Schizophrenia is a highly varied disease and one approach may not fit all patients. While intermittent antipsychotic medication may increase the risk of relapse, there may be patients for whom the reduction in dose, and presumably side effects, makes that a reasonable trade-off.
- Possibility of increased risks as well as reduced benefits: tardive dyskinesia is a chronic, irreversible neurological disorder associated with the prescription of antipsychotics. There has been some concern that it may be more likely when antipsychotics are prescribed intermittently.

Schizophrenia: management of treatment-resistant disease

Kane's study: Clozapine for treatment-resistant schizophrenia.

AUTHORS: Kane J, Honigfeld G, Singer J et al and the Clozaril Collaborative Study Group.
REFERENCE: Arch Gen Psych (1988) 45, 789–96.
STUDY DESIGN: RCT
EVIDENCE LEVEL: 1b

Key message
Clozapine is more effective than alternative antipsychotics in treatment-resistant schizophrenia.

Impact
This trial led to the reintroduction of clozapine into psychiatric practice. Clozapine is now the antipsychotic of choice in treatment-resistant schizophrenia (defined as a lack of response following the sequential use of the recommended doses for 6–8wk of at least 2 antipsychotics, at least 1 of which should be an 'atypical'). Mandatory blood monitoring is required in view of the small risk of agranulocytosis.

Aims
A number of studies had identified subgroups of patients who failed to respond to neuroleptic drug therapy, including a group that relapse despite initial successful therapy. Previous studies had reported efficacy in these patients from the atypical agent, clozapine, showing this to be superior to the dopamine receptor antagonist, chlorpromazine. Despite this, its use had been withdrawn due to case reports of agranulocytosis. This study aimed to evaluate the efficacy of clozapine in the treatment of schizophrenia that had already failed to respond to other antipsychotic agents.

Methods
Patients: 268 inpatients from 16 treatment centres in the USA.

Inclusion criteria:
• Schizophrenia: DSM (Diagnostic and Statistical Manual of Mental Disorders)-III criteria;
• Failure to respond to at least 3 different antipsychotics.

Groups:
• Clozapine (n=126);
• Chlorpromazine and benztropine (n=139).

Primary outcome: Improvement on Clinical Global Impression (CGI) and Brief Psychiatric Rating Scale (BPRS).

Secondary outcomes:
- Clinically significant improvement: defined as >20% reduction in BPRS score and either CGI rating as 'mild' or better, or BPRS score <36;
- Nurses' Observation Scale for Inpatient Evaluation (NOSIE-30);
- Assessment of adverse reactions and safety.

Follow-up: At 6wk.

Results
- Patients receiving clozapine showed greater improvement than those receiving chlorpromazine. This was evident on both the CGI (*p*<0.001) and BPRS (*p*<0.001).
- 30% of those receiving clozapine 'improved' to an extent that was clinically significant, compared to only 4% of those receiving chlorpromazine (*p*<0.001).
- Statistical superiority for clozapine was also seen for subscales of the BPRS (positive, negative, and general symptoms) and on the nurse-rated NOSIE.

Discussion
While many patients with schizophrenia receiving an antipsychotic agent experience benefit, failure to respond remains a major clinical problem. Use of clozapine was associated with particular risks (notably the increased rates of agranulocytosis), but this study established its particular place in the treatment of those who fail to respond to other antipsychotic medication.

Problems
- Uncertainty about pharmacological action: The pharmacological basis of clozapine's superiority remains unclear. Attempts to develop molecules with similar efficacy, but without serious side effects, have as yet been unsuccessful.
- Dose titration: Due to side effects, clozapine requires careful dose titration in the first month and daily dosing without breaks. Alongside the need for careful blood monitoring, this means that patient co-operation is essential.
- Extent and duration of response: Only 30% of participants receiving clozapine experienced clinically significant improvement at short-term follow-up; this trial did not tell us whether clozapine was more or less effective over longer periods of time that would have greater clinical relevance.

Panic disorder: cognitive therapy

> **Beck's study:** A crossover study of focused cognitive therapy for panic disorder.
>
> **AUTHORS:** Beck A, Sokol L, Clark D et al.
> **REFERENCE:** Am J Psych (1992) 149, 778–83.
> **STUDY DESIGN:** RCT
> **EVIDENCE LEVEL:** 1b

Key message
Cognitive therapy (CT) is an effective non-pharmacological treatment for panic disorder.

Impact
This trial was one of the first to demonstrate the effectiveness of CT for a common psychiatric disorder. The results have been reproduced several times, contributing to the emergence of CT (and the very closely related cognitive behaviour therapy, CBT) as the dominant psychotherapy with a strong and developing evidence base. Therefore, both pharmacological and non-pharmacological options are available for several common psychiatric disorders, including panic. Patients can be asked which approach they prefer.

Aims
In 1992, common pharmacological treatments for panic disorder included benzodiazepines and the tricyclic antidepressant, imipramine, both of which had significant adverse effects. Behavioural approaches and combined cognitive and behavioural approaches had started to emerge, but had not been rigorously evaluated in a randomised trial. This RCT aimed to compare the effectiveness of CT with that of brief, supportive psychotherapy (SP) in outpatients with panic disorder.

Methods
Patients: 33 patients at 1 outpatient clinic in the USA.

Inclusion criteria:
- Meeting DSM-III (Diagnostic and Statistical Manual of mental disorder) diagnostic criteria for panic disorder or agoraphobia with panic attacks;
- Age 18–65y.

Groups:
- CT: 12 weekly, individual sessions with a trained cognitive therapist (n=17);
- SP: 8 weekly, individual sessions of supportive contact with a trained therapist, based on client-centred therapy principles (n=16).

Primary endpoint: Clinician rating of absence of weekly panic attacks at 8wk.

Secondary endpoints:
- Self-rating of panic frequency at 8wk;
- Self-rating of panic intensity at 8wk;
- Beck Anxiety Inventory (BAI) score;
- Beck Depression Inventory (BDI) score.

Follow-up: Before treatment, then at 4 and 8wk.

Results

Primary endpoint	CT	SP	*p*
No weekly panic attacks, n (%)	12 (71%)	4 (25%)	<0.02
Secondary endpoints			**(group by time inter-action, linear trend)**
Panic frequency, mean (SD)	0.4 (0.6)	3.1 (4.1)	<0.01
Panic intensity, mean (SD)	1.2 (1.8)	2.5 (1.5)	<0.01
BAI score, mean (SD)	15 (13)	27 (14)	<0.03
BDI score, mean (SD)	7 (6)	14 (11)	<0.03

Discussion

These results provided convincing evidence of the short-term effectiveness of CT compared to a control intervention that was not expected to be effective.

Problems

- Long-term data: Unfortunately, in this trial, SP participants were able to choose to cross over to CT at 8wk, and all chose to do so. Therefore, long-term comparative data are unavailable from this trial.
- Cost: 12 sessions of individual therapy would be considered labour-intensive and expensive for such a common disorder. Group CT, computerised CT, and self-help CT via books or the internet offer ways of reducing therapist time and expense.
- Availability: CT is a specialised treatment; in the UK there is a shortage of staff appropriately trained to deliver it.
- Applicability: This trial was conducted at an innovative 'Center for Cognitive Therapy', and there is evidence that treatment effects at such centres are greater than in 'ordinary' health service settings.

Panic disorder: pharmacological and psychological treatment

> **Oehrberg's study:** Paroxetine in the treatment of panic disorder.
>
> **AUTHORS:** Oehrberg S, Christiansen P, Behnke K et al.
> **REFERENCE:** Br J Psych (1995) 167, 374–9.
> **STUDY DESIGN:** RCT
> **EVIDENCE LEVEL:** 1b

Key message

The combination of a selective serotonin reuptake inhibitor (SSRI) anti-depressant and cognitive therapy (CT) for the treatment of panic disorder is more effective than CT alone.

Impact

Combination therapy is now widely used for panic disorder. However, due to the limited availability of formal, individual CT, the usual psychological approach is an SSRI combined with cognitively informed self-help using written materials or computerised cognitive behaviour therapy (CBT).

Aims

Both pharmacological and psychological treatments had been shown to have efficacy in the treatment of panic disorder. Drug treatments had centred on higher dose benzodiazepines; however, adverse effects led to increased study of antidepressants, particularly SSRIs. Whilst these had been demonstrated to be successful, their use had not been compared to the mainstay of psychological therapy, CT. This study aimed to evaluate the efficacy and tolerability of combined paroxetine (SSRI) and CT vs CT alone in the treatment of panic disorder.

Methods

Patients: 120 patients from multiple Danish centres.

Inclusion criteria:
- DSM (Diagnostic and Statistical Manual of Mental Disorders)-III-R panic disorder;
- Age 18–70y;
- No significant depression (Hamilton Depression Scale ≤14);
- No psychosis, organic brain disease, alcohol or drug misuse.

Groups:
- CT and SSRI (paroxetine), dose titrated to low (20mg/d), or medium (40mg/d), or high (60mg/d) (n=60);
- CT and placebo (n=60).

Primary outcome: Frequency of panic attacks in 3wk periods.

Secondary outcomes:
- 50% reduction in Hamilton Anxiety Scale score (Ham-A);
- Clinical Global Impression (CGI) mildly ill or better;
- Mean reduction on Zung Self-Rating Scale for Anxiety.

Follow-up: At 3, 6, 9, and 12wk.

Results

Outcome (at 12wk)	CT and SSRI	CT and placebo	RR (95% CI)
Primary outcomes			
50% ↓ in panic attacks	42/60	25/60	1.68 (1.19 to 2.37)
0 or 1 panic attack in 3wk	19/60	8/60	2.38 (1.13 to 5.0)
Secondary outcomes			*p*
50% reduction in Ham-A	85%	51%	<0.001
CGI mildly ill or better	71%	40%	0.003
Zung mean change from baseline	−6.5	−4.3	0.04

Discussion

This trial demonstrated a clear benefit for the combination of SSRI and CT over CT alone. While other RCTs have not typically found such a striking magnitude of benefit, it has been shown overall that a combination of medication and psychological therapy is superior to either alone (e.g. see Furukawa *et al. B J Psych* (2006), 188, 305–12).

Problems

- Duration of effect: The duration of the study was only 12wk and it is uncertain whether differences would persist over the longer term. There is some evidence that the benefits of combination therapy over psychological interventions alone tend to be lost as medication is discontinued.
- Attitudes to treatment: Some patients are ambivalent or against taking medication, and especially reluctant to take 'antidepressants' when they are not depressed.
- Applicability: Many patients presenting with panic disorder have some depressive symptoms or will be misusing alcohol or street drugs. Application of the findings to these patients is uncertain.

Bulimia nervosa: cognitive vs standard behavioural therapy

Fairburn's study: Cognitive behaviour therapy (CBT) vs behavioural therapy (BT) vs interpersonal therapy for bulimia nervosa.

AUTHORS: Fairburn C, Jones R, Peveler R *et al.*
REFERENCE: Arch Gen Psych (1991) 48, 463–9.
STUDY DESIGN: RCT
EVIDENCE LEVEL: 1b

Key message

CBT is an effective psychological treatment for bulimia nervosa.

Impact

In the late 1980s, eating disorders were emerging as a major clinical problem, yet there was a dearth of evidence regarding the effectiveness of treatment. Cognitive interventions were just starting to be developed and assessed. This trial demonstrated the value of CBT above that of the simpler psychological treatment, BT. CBT has been endorsed in the UK as the preferred psychological treatment for patients with bulimia nervosa.

Aims

Both pharmacological and psychological treatments have been considered for bulimia nervosa. Most research into psychological therapies had focused on CBT, though many studies had found no differences in outcomes between this and other psychological therapies. This study aimed to determine whether: (a) CBT was more effective than control psychotherapy (interpersonal psychotherapy, IPT) and (b) the simpler, BT, was as effective as CBT.

Methods

Patients: 75 patients from multiple primary and secondary care centres in the UK.

Inclusion criteria: Bulimia nervosa, by DSM (Diagnostic and Statistical Manual of Mental Disorders)-III-R criteria:
• Age ≥17y;
• Body mass index >17kg/m^2.

Groups: Each intervention comprised outpatient psychotherapy (19 sessions over 18wk):
• CBT: combination of behavioural (eating normalisation) and cognitive (focus on patient's concerns regarding their shape and weight) (n=25);
• BT: focus only on normalisation of eating (n=25);
• IPT: modified for bulimia nervosa (n=25).

Endpoints: No primary endpoint was specified.

- Frequency of core symptoms, per 28d, including objective binge-eating episodes, self-induced vomiting, and laxative misuse;
- Eating Disorders Examination (EDE) subscales, including dietary restraint, attitudes to shape, and attitudes to weight;
- Eating Attitudes Test (EAT) score;
- Psychiatric symptoms, including the Beck Depression Inventory (BDI).

Follow-up: Before start of treatment and at end of treatment.

Results

Endpoint (means, at treatment end)	CBT	BT	IPT	p (3-way)	$p \leq 0.05$ (2-way)
Binge frequency	0.6	1.3	1.8	0.4	
Vomiting frequency	1.5	0.9	5.5	0.03	CBT>IPT
EDE restraint	1.3	2.3	2.1	0.05	CBT>IPT; CBT>BT
EDE shape	2.1	3.3	2.6	0.01	CBT>BT
EDE weight	1.7	2.9	2.4	0.01	CBT>IPT; CBT>BT
BDI	10.1	13.6	12.5	0.5	

Discussion

All 3 treatments helped; they were each associated with significant reductions in binge frequency. However, there were some notable differences in effectiveness. For example, frequency of vomiting was reduced by both CBT and BT, but not by IPT; and CBT was more effective on all the core endpoints, including measures of dietary restraint and attitudes to shape and weight.

Problems

- Applicability: The trial was conducted at a UK 'centre of excellence'. It is unclear whether these findings are applicable to 'ordinary' clinical settings.
- Availability of treatment: CBT is a specialist treatment and there is a dearth of qualified therapists. However, CBT for bulimia nervosa has been successfully delivered as a book and incorporated into stepped care guidelines (CBT self-help > group CBT > individual CBT).
- Acceptability of treatment: All psychotherapies, including CBT and BT, rely upon patient motivation in order to be effective. Therefore, engagement by the patient is crucial.
- Duration of effect: Participants were assessed only at the end of treatment rather than at intervals (e.g. 1 or 2y). It is not clear whether the beneficial effects of CBT endure and whether intermittent 'booster' CBT sessions help.

Eating disorders (anorexia and bulimia nervosa): family therapy

Russell's study: An evaluation of family therapy in anorexia nervosa and bulimia nervosa.

AUTHORS: Russell G, Szmukler G, Dare C et al.
REFERENCE: Arch Gen Psych (1987) 44, 1047–56.
STUDY DESIGN: RCT
EVIDENCE LEVEL: 1b

Key message

Family therapy (FT) has a role in the treatment of younger patients with severe eating disorders.

Impact

There is a paucity of randomised evidence to inform the management of anorexia nervosa. However, family therapy focused on the eating disorder remains a firm treatment option for younger patients with anorexia nervosa.

Aims

At the time of this trial, FT was frequently advocated for the treatment of anorexia nervosa despite a lack of good evidence. This trial aimed to compare the effectiveness of two therapies (family-oriented and non-family-oriented), which were matched for form, duration, and intensity in the treatment of severe (hospitalised) eating disorders.

Methods

Patients: 80 patients at 1 centre in the UK (57 had anorexia nervosa and 23 bulimia nervosa).

Inclusion criteria:
- Meet DSM (Diagnostic and Statistical Manual of Mental Disorders) criteria for anorexia nervosa and bulimia nervosa;
- Admitted to a specialist eating disorder treatment unit;
- Either gender.

Groups: All participants received inpatient care, focused on restoring weight, of an average 10wk. Patients were then randomised to the following treatments and treatment continued as an outpatient for 1y from discharge. Treatments were matched for therapist input.
- FT: involving all immediate family members; 3 defined tasks and 3 defined phases of treatment (n=41);
- Individual therapy (IT): with supportive, educational, cognitive, and problem-oriented elements (n=39).

Endpoints:
- General outcome, based on weight and menstrual status (good/ intermediate/poor);

- Morgan *and* Russell scales for anorexia nervosa;
- Need for readmission.

Follow-up: At discharge, 3, 6, and 9 months *and* (primary endpoint) at 1y.

Results

Good vs intermediate/poor outcomes (at 1y)	FT	IT	*p*
In AN onset <19, duration <3y	6/10	1/11	<0.02
In AN onset <19, duration >3y	2/10	2/9	ns
In AN onset >18	0/7	2/7	ns
In BN	0/9	1/10	ns

AN=anorexia nervosa; BN=bulimia nervosa.

Discussion

The study provided some evidence for the effectiveness of FT in young (age ≤18y) patients with anorexia nervosa of recent onset (<3y). However, there was no evidence for its effectiveness compared to IT in young, more chronic patients, in older patients, or in bulimia nervosa.

Problems

- Study complexity: The manuscript is complex, as is typical of RCTs from the 1980s. Additionally, the presentation of findings for each of the four subgroups complicates interpretation.
- Applicability: This trial was conducted in a 'centre of excellence'; it is unclear whether the findings can be generalised to other settings.
- Acceptability: There were dropouts from treatment in both groups, and dropouts had a worse outcome. This emphasises the crucial role of patient engagement in the management of eating disorders.
- Sample size: The study was small. However, there is a lack of randomised evidence on which to base treatment for this common disorder which has a high rate of suicide and medical complications.

Attention-Deficit/Hyperactivity Disorder (ADHD): medication

MTA (Multimodal Treatment study of children with ADHD) study: A 14 month RCT of treatment strategies for Attention-Deficit/Hyperactivity Disorder.
AUTHORS: The MTA Cooperative Group.
REFERENCE: Arch Gen Psych (1999) 56, 1073-86.
STUDY DESIGN: RCT
EVIDENCE LEVEL: 1b

Key message
Stimulant medications are superior to behavioural treatment in the management of attention-deficit/hyperactivity disorder (ADHD).

Impact
Stimulant medications (e.g. methylphenidate, atomoxetine, dexamfetamine) are now a mainstay of ADHD management. UK prescribing of stimulants for ADHD doubled between 1998 and 2004.

Aims
ADHD affects about 5% of children and adolescents, some of whom require treatment. At the time of this trial, there was poor evidence for the use of stimulants, especially regarding the duration and context of treatment, and the co-prescription of behavioural therapy. Therefore, this study aimed to compare the long-term efficacy of pharmacotherapy, behaviour therapy, and the combination compared to usual care in ADHD.

Methods
Patients: 579 children recruited through 6 teams at multiple centres in the USA (4541 potential participants screened for inclusion).

Inclusion criteria:
- Age 7 to 9.9y (school grade 1–4);
- Resident with same primary carer(s) for ≥past 6 months;
- DSM-IV Combined Type ADHD.

Exclusion criteria:
- Situations preventing family's full participation in assessment or treatment;
- Might require additional treatments incompatible with study regime.

Groups:
- Medication management (methylphenidate or alternatives) (n=144);
- Behavioural treatment (parent training, therapeutic summer camp, school-based interventions) (n=144);
- Combined treatment (n=145);
- Community care (treatment as usual) (n=146).

Outcome domains assessed: Teacher and parent assessments.
- ADHD symptoms, including inattention *and* hyperactivity-impulsivity;
- Other symptoms, including oppositional/aggressive *and* internalising;
- Social skills, parent-child relations.

Follow-up: At 14 months.

Results
- Medical management was superior to behavioural intervention/usual care for core ADHD symptoms of inattention, hyperactivity, and impulsivity (p=0.001).
- Combination treatment was superior to behavioural treatment alone, (but not better than medical management alone) for ADHD symptoms, oppositional/aggressive behaviours, internalising, and academic achievement.
- Combination treatment was better than usual care in all domains assessed.

Discussion
This landmark study convincingly demonstrated the key role of medication in the management of ADHD. The adequate sample size, duration, and broad range of outcomes assessed avoided some of the common pitfalls of such studies. The lack of substantial benefit from supplementing medical management with specific and intensive behavioural treatments was surprising at the time. However, it should be noted that medical management received by participants was not simply adjustment of prescriptions; it involved monthly half-hour reviews, including practical advice and support.

Problems
- Efficacy of specific medicines: The medication protocol involved several different agents, so any differences between them may have been obscured.
- Applicability: The time and resources to emulate this study may not be widely available.
- Use and abuse of stimulants: The increasing use of stimulants amongst children is controversial.

Chronic fatigue syndrome: cognitive behavioural therapy (CBT) vs medical care

> **Sharpe's study:** Cognitive behaviour therapy for chronic fatigue syndrome.
>
> **AUTHORS:** Sharpe M, Hawton K, Simkin S *et al.*
> **REFERENCE:** BMJ (1996) 312, 22–6.
> **STUDY DESIGN:** RCT
> **EVIDENCE LEVEL:** 1b

Key message

Cognitive behavioural therapy (CBT) is more effective than usual medical care for the treatment of people with chronic fatigue syndrome (CFS).

Impact

CFS was for many years an illness without an effective treatment. CBT is now a core option for CFS, alongside graded exercise therapy (GET). This trial demonstrated the role of CBT in the management of many medically unexplained symptoms and syndromes.

Aims

CFS is a common and disabling disorder. Yet, until recently, there had been few RCTs of possible treatments. In part, this has reflected uncertainty over the aetiology of this condition. The biopsychosocial model of CFS emerged in the 1990s as a possible explanation and led to the development of a structured psychological treatment, CBT. This trial was designed to compare the effectiveness of CBT with that of usual medical care, comprising diagnosis, reassurance, and encouragement.

Methods

Patients: 60 patients at 1 infectious diseases outpatient clinic in the UK.

Inclusion criteria:
- Age 18–60y with CFS (diagnosed by Oxford criteria);
- Main complaint of fatigue, worsened by activity, for ≥6 months;
- Impairment of activities of daily living (ADL) (Karnofsky score <80);
- No significant findings on physical examination or investigation.

Groups:
- Medical care only: Reassured no serious disease, told they had CFS, advised to increase activity as much as they felt able to (n=30);
- Medical care and CBT: as above; plus 16 × 1h, weekly, individual CBT sessions by qualified therapist (n=30).

Primary endpoint: 'Satisfactory functioning' (Karnofsky score ≥80) or 'clinically significant improvement' (of ≥10 Karnofsky points).

Secondary endpoints:
- Distance achieved in 6min walking test;
- Days in bed each week;
- Patient-rated fatigue severity (0–10).

Follow-up: At randomisation, 5 months (after CBT), 8 months, and 1y.

Results

Primary endpoint (at 1y)	Medical care alone	Medical care + CBT	*p*
Improvement	7 (23%)	22 (73%)	<0.001
Satisfactory functioning	8 (27%)	22 (73%)	<0.001
Secondary endpoints (change, baseline to 1y)			**Difference (95% CI)**
Distance walked (m)	+2	+57	55 (17 to 94)
Days in bed per wk	+0.5	−2.4	−2.8 (−1.7 to −4.0)
Fatigue severity	−1.6	−3.5	−1.9 (−0.5 to −3.3)

Discussion

There remains a lack of trial evidence for treatment of CFS. However, this trial and several subsequent RCTs have provided robust evidence for the role of CBT in 'typical' patients presenting to secondary care with chronic unexplained fatigue.

Problems

- Availability: CBT needs to be delivered by trained therapists (but not necessarily clinical psychologists). Unfortunately, there is a lack of appropriate expertise, resulting in long waits for treatment in the UK and elsewhere.
- Controversy: The use of a 'psychological' treatment for a 'physical' disorder is controversial, and not universally accepted by patients and patient groups. Persuading patients of the wisdom of this course takes time and skill.
- Possibility of differential response of subgroups: It is possible that CFS comprises different subgroups, some of which will respond well to CBT and others which may not. Indeed, some argue that CBT can be actively detrimental to well-being, although there is no evidence to support this.

Renal medicine

Introduction

Nephrology was a mid-20th century invention. Indeed, it is about as old or young as the present leaders in the field. There had long been an interest in renal physiology and post-mortem pathology, but they were not much use in isolation. A specialty needs a clientele, a useful product, a technique, and entrepreneurial doctors. For nephrology these were: patients with renal failure; dialysis, renal biopsy, and a remarkable cadre of determined, obsessional, and obstinately optimistic physicians and surgeons. They inhabited the worlds of general medicine, hypertension, and urology before creating niches for themselves as kidney failure doctors.

Although the Renal Association started in 1950, the International Society of Nephrology was only created in 1960. The success of dialysis and transplantation as treatments for 'terminal renal failure' (as it was once called) are among the outstanding achievements in medicine in the last 50 years. Their development bypassed business plans, risk assessments, protocols, and SWOT (Strengths, Weaknesses, Opportunities, and Threats) analyses that paralyse attempts at innovation today.

Treatment of renal disease with drugs such as corticosteroids and antimetabolites was empirical. Successful though these treatments may be, we do not really know whether we are applying them in the best way. Doing randomised trials of effective treatments is tricky, especially as many nephrologists are supremely confident they have identified the right way to do things. Slowly this mindset is being changed, prejudices are being challenged, and old as well as new treatments properly tested. The renal pharmacopoeia has and is being added to regularly with biologics such as the ESAs (Erythropoiesis Stimulating Agents), immunosuppressant monoclonals, and designer agonists such as calcimimetics. These are exciting times for clinical research and depressing ones for health economists.

This section describes some of the investigations that have persuaded some clinicians to change some of what they do some of the time.

Dopamine in renal failure

Low dose dopamine in patients with early renal dysfunction.

AUTHORS: Australian & New Zealand Intensive Care Society Clinical Trials Group.
REFERENCE: Lancet (2000) 356, 2139–43.
STUDY DESIGN: RCT
EVIDENCE LEVEL: 1b

Key message

Low dose dopamine provides no protection from renal failure in critically ill patients at risk of acute renal failure (ARF).

Impact

Low or 'renal' doses of dopamine (0.5–2.0mcg/kg/min) have been widely used in intensive care units to prevent the development of established ARF. This trial should stop such practice as the results are widely applicable and very clear.

Aims

Low dose dopamine increases renal blood flow in healthy volunteers and induces natriuresis and diuresis. With the assumption that these physiological changes would confer protection to critically ill patients (at risk of renal failure), it had been widely used in intensive care unit (ICU) settings, despite the absence of large RCTs confirming its efficacy and safety. This study aimed to investigate whether low dose dopamine could prevent the development of ARF.

Methods

Patients: 328 patients at 23 ICUs in Australia, New Zealand, and Hong Kong.
Inclusion criteria: Adult patients with early renal dysfunction:
- Presence of a central venous catheter;
- ≥2 signs of systemic inflammatory response syndrome (SIRS);
- 1 indicator of early renal dysfunction: either serum creatinine >150micromol/L in the absence of premorbid renal dysfunction, or urine output <0.5mL/kg/h over ≥4h, or rise in serum creatinine >80micromol/L in <24h in absence of CK >5000iu/L or myoglobinuria.

Groups:
- Dopamine: continuous infusion, at 2mcg/kg/min (n=163);
- Placebo: equivalent volume of vehicle solution infused continuously (n=165).

Primary endpoint: Peak serum creatinine concentration during trial infusion.

Secondary endpoints:
- Reason for cessation of trial infusion;
- Development of cardiac arrhythmia;
- Durations of mechanical ventilation, ICU stay, hospital stay;

- Peak plasma urea reached during trial infusion, change in serum urea and creatinine concentrations from baseline to peak value;
- Urine output (at predefined times);
- Number requiring renal replacement therapy (RRT) or creatinine >300 micromol/L;
- Survival to ICU discharge, survival to hospital discharge.

Follow-up: Infusion continued until: patient given RRT or patient died, or patient's SIRS and renal dysfunction resolved for at least 24h, or patient discharged from ICU. F/U until death or hospital discharge.

Results

	Dopamine	Placebo	Difference (95% CI)
Primary endpoint			
Peak serum creatinine (micromol/L; mean±SD)	245±144	249±147	4 (−28 to 36)
Secondary endpoints			
Number requiring RRT	35	40	5 (−10 to 20)
Survival to discharge	92	97	p=0.7

Discussion

Dopamine has favourable renal haemodynamic effects in animals and healthy volunteers, and these have been extrapolated to predict benefit for critically ill patients. This well-designed trial is the only appropriately powered study potentially able to demonstrate such a benefit and was resoundingly negative. The authors cited potential dangers of low dose dopamine (e.g. inadvertent exacerbation of medullary ischaemia secondary to its effects as a proximal tubular diuretic), although none were demonstrated in their study. Along with the lack of benefit, these should stop the use of low dose dopamine on ICUs as a nephroprotective agent.

Problems

- Mean urine output=37mL/h (treatment group) and 50mL/h (control group). Therefore, this was not a study of oliguric renal failure, although there is no physiological reason why the conclusions would differ.
- 50% patients received a loop diuretic, a controversial treatment in septic shock (although use of diuretics was the same in the two groups).
- Some advocate using dopamine with norepinephrine to 'protect' the kidney from the vasoconstrictive effect of norepinephrine. The original paper does not describe the effect on this subgroup, but a later letter clarifies that there was no benefit identified.

Acute renal failure: renal replacement therapy

Intensity of renal support in critically ill patients with acute kidney injury.

AUTHORS: The VA/NIH Acute Renal Failure Trial Network.
REFERENCE: N Engl J Med (2008) 359, 7-20.
STUDY DESIGN: RCT
EVIDENCE LEVEL: 1b

Key message
Outcome of acute kidney injury in the intensive care unit (ICU) setting is not improved by increasing the dose of renal replacement therapy.

Impact
The dose of renal replacement therapy does not appear to be a limiting factor in the survival of patients on ICU with acute kidney injury.

Aims
Acute renal failure (ARF), commonly part of multi-organ failure, occurs frequently in critically ill patients. It is characterised by a sustained decline in glomerular filtration rate (GFR). Renal replacement therapy (RRT) is the mainstay of treatment; however, method and dosing of RRT still remain a subject of debate, results of previous studies having been inconsistent. This study aimed to investigate whether an increased dose of RRT in the setting of acute kidney injury on ICU could improve patient survival.

Methods
Patients: 1,124 adult patients from 27 ICUs in the USA.

Inclusion criteria:
- Admission to ICU;
- Acute kidney injury requiring RRT;
- Failure of at least one other non-renal organ.

Groups:
- Group 1 assigned intensive RRT (6x per wk haemodialysis or 35mL/h/kg haemofiltration) (n=563);
- Group 2 assigned standard RRT (3x per week haemodialysis or 20mL/h/kg haemofiltration) (n=561).

Primary endpoint: Death from any cause by 60d after randomisation.

Secondary endpoints:
- Recovery of renal function by d28;
- Duration of RRT;
- Length of stay in ICU.

Follow-up: At 60d from randomisation.

Results

Primary endpoint	Group		p
	1	2	
Death from any cause by 60d	302/563 (53.6%)	289/561 (51.5%)	0.5
Secondary endpoints			
Complete recovery of renal function by 28d	85/553 (15.4%)	102/555 (18.4%)	Not reported
ICU-free days by 60d	18.7±0.9	20.1±0.9	0.3
Hospital-free days by 60d	11.0±0.7	13.0±0.7	0.005

Discussion

Previous studies had reported conflicting results on the benefits of higher doses of RRT on ICU. This study, the largest to date, used a modern optimum standard as the control arm did not show any benefit of increasing the dose. However, the control arm therapy is often not achieved on many ICUs, so this trial should not deter such units from attempting to increase the dose of RRT to this level.

Problems

- Patients with pre-existing chronic kidney disease (CKD) were excluded from this study, and there is some epidemiological evidence to suggest that acute kidney injury has a distinct natural history in this group.
- The timing of initiation of RRT was not standardised although this reflects current practice.
- The majority of patients were male although no heterogeneity was apparent on the basis of gender.

Chronic renal disease: protein restriction and blood pressure control

> **MDRD** (**M**odification of **D**iet in **R**enal **D**isease) **study:** The effects of dietary protein restriction and blood pressure control on the progression of chronic renal disease.
>
> **AUTHORS:** Klahr S, Levey A, Beck G *et al.*
> **REFERENCE:** N Engl J Med (1994) 330, 877–84.
> **STUDY DESIGN:** RCT
> **EVIDENCE LEVEL:** 1b

Key message
Protein restriction has no impact on progression of chronic renal disease, but clear benefits are seen from strict blood pressure (BP) control in patients with significant proteinuria.

Impact
Protein restriction is no longer recommended in the UK. This trial led the way in recommending aggressive BP control as a method of slowing progression of chronic kidney disease (CKD).

Aims
Animal models demonstrate a beneficial effect of dietary protein restriction and BP control on the progression of CKD. However, this had not been reliably demonstrated in humans. Similarly, very few trials prior to this study had investigated the effect of 'lower than usual' BP on the progression of CKD. This study included the results of RCTs in order to test the effects of dietary protein, phosphorus intake restriction, and tight BP control on the progression of CKD.

Methods
Patients: From multiple centres in the USA: 585 patients in study 1 (GFR 25–55mL/min), 255 patients in study 2 (GFR 13–24mL/min).

Inclusion criteria: CKD:
- Age 18–70y;
- Creatinine 106–619micromol/L (women), 124–619micromol/L (men);
- Mean arterial pressure (MAP) ≤125mmHg.

Groups:
- Study 1: low protein (n=291) vs usual protein diet (n=294),
  low BP (n=300) vs usual BP (n=285);
- Study 2: very low protein (n=126) vs low protein diet (n=129),
  low BP (n=132) vs usual BP (n=123);
- Usual protein diet=1.3g/kg/d protein; low protein diet=0.58g/kg/d; very low protein diet=0.28g/kg/d.
- Usual MAP ≤107mmHg (age 18–60) and ≤113mmHg (age ≥61); low MAP ≤92mmHg (age 18–60) and ≤98mmHg (age ≥61).

Primary endpoint: Rate of change of GFR.

Secondary endpoints: Rate of change of GFR in various pre-specified sub-groups (e.g. proteinuria <1g/d; 1–3g/d, >3g/d).

Follow-up: GFR measured (isotope method) at 2 and 4 months, and then every 4 months for a mean of 2.2y.

Results

Primary endpoint		Very low protein	Low protein	Usual protein	p
	Study 1	—	3.6 (3.1–4.2)	4.0 (3.5–4.6)	ns
Rate of decline of GFR (mL/min/y)	Study 2	3.6 (2.9–4.2)	4.4 (3.7–5.1)	—	ns
		Low BP	**Usual BP**		
	Study 1	3.6 (3.0–4.1)	4.1 (3.5–4.7)	—	ns
	Study 2	3.7 (3.1–4.3)	4.2 (3.6–4.9)	—	ns

Discussion

This trial, the largest study of protein restriction, failed to demonstrate a durable benefit of dietary protein restriction. There was no benefit of strict BP control overall, but there was when the patients were stratified according to urinary protein excretion (strict BP control slowed progression in patients with >3g/d proteinuria in study 1 and 2). The data from this study demonstrate a strong relationship between proteinuria and rate of progression, and contributed towards the development of strategies to reduce proteinuria as a method to slow progression of CKD. Furthermore, the MDRD formula for estimating GFR (now used throughout the UK) was developed from the results of this study.

Problems

- The significant results only came from (pre-specified) subgroup analysis. However, they have since been corroborated by other studies.
- The 'usual' BP target (equivalent to 140/90 and 160/90mmHg in patients under and over 60, respectively) is high by modern standards, and is no longer a valid comparator for patients with CKD.
- The rate of progression in this study was slower than expected and resulted in the study being underpowered to detect the expected difference between the groups.

Non-diabetic nephropathy: ACE inhibitors

> **REIN** (**R**amipril **E**fficacy **I**n **N**ephropathy) **study:** Randomised, placebo-controlled trial of the effect of ramipril on decline in glomerular filtration rate and risk of terminal renal failure in proteinuric, non-diabetic nephropathy.
>
> **AUTHORS:** GISEN Group (Gruppo Italiano di Studi Epidemiologici in Nefrologia).
> **REFERENCE:** Lancet (1997) 349, 1857–63.
> **STUDY DESIGN:** RCT
> **EVIDENCE LEVEL:** 1b

Key message
Ramipril slows the rate of decline of glomerular filtration rate (GFR) in patients with non-diabetic nephropathy and proteinuria of ≥3g/d.

Impact
The findings extended the indication for angiotensin-converting enzyme (ACE) inhibitors to all patients with proteinuria, not just those with diabetic nephropathy. The benefit of ACE inhibitors was more than expected for the degree of BP lowering.

Aims
GFR usually continues to decline despite treatment of the original causative factor in most forms of proteinuric chronic renal disease. Hypertension is likely to have the largest contribution to this renal dysfunction. ACE inhibitors are known to reduce both urinary protein excretion and BP. However, the differential contribution of these two effects towards slowing the decline in GFR had been unclear. This study was designed to investigate this further.

Methods
Patients: 352 patients at 14 Italian centres.
Inclusion criteria: Non-diabetic proteinuric nephropathy:
- Age 18–70y;
- Measured GFR 15–70mL/min per 1.73m^2;
- Urinary protein excretion >1g/24h for at least 3 months.

Groups:
- Stratum 1: proteinuria 1–2.9g/24h (results not published);
- Stratum 2: proteinuria ≥3g/24h:
  - Ramipril (n=78);
  - Placebo (n=88).

Primary endpoint: Effect of allocation to ramipril or placebo on rate of decline in GFR.

Secondary endpoints:

- Degree of proteinuria;
- Time to doubling of serum creatinine or progression to end-stage renal failure (ESRF);
- Major cardiovascular complications;
- Total and cardiovascular mortality rate.

Follow-up: GFR measured (by iohexol clearance) at 1, 3, and 6 months after randomisation, and then 6 monthly. Stratum 2 was stopped early (after mean F/U of 16 months) and published in this report.

Results

Primary endpoint	Ramipril	Placebo	*p*
GFR/month (mL/min)	−0.53 (±0.08)	−0.88 (±0.13)	0.03
Secondary endpoints			
Urinary protein excretion (g/24h)	Not adequately reported		
Doubling serum creatinine or ESRF	18	40	0.02
Systolic BP (mean) (mmHg)	144.0 (±1.8)	144.6 (±1.5)	0.9
Diastolic BP (mean) (mmHg)	88.2 (±0.9)	88.9 (±0.9)	0.6

Discussion

This study demonstrated a benefit of ACE inhibitors on proteinuric non-diabetic nephropathy independent of their BP-lowering effect. However, this report only related to the strata of patients with more marked proteinuria (≥3g/24h) as the benefit was only apparent in the interim analysis of this population. The study also demonstrated that ACE inhibitors were safe in this population with hyperkalaemia only being reported in 2 patients (1 in ramipril group, 1 in placebo group).

Problems

- The study was stopped early based on an interim analysis of only 87 patients, which increased the risk of chance affecting the results.
- Data concerning the effect of ramipril on urinary protein excretion were inadequately reported. Although the change in protein excretion in the ramipril group was significant (and was not significant in the placebo group), it is the difference in the change between the two groups that is critical. This was not reported.
- A later publication of the data from patients in stratum 1 did not demonstrate a benefit in terms of the primary outcome, but did demonstrate a benefit in terms of progression to ESRF.

Haemodialysis: statins and cardiovascular risk

4D (Die Deutsche Diabetes Dialyse) study: Atorvastatin in patients with type 2 diabetes mellitus undergoing haemodialysis.

AUTHORS: Wanner C, Krane V, März W *et al.*
REFERENCE: N Engl J Med (2005) 353, 238–48.
STUDY DESIGN: RCT
EVIDENCE LEVEL: 1b

Key message
Statin therapy has no benefits in high-risk dialysis patients with diabetes mellitus (DM).

Impact
The efficacy of lipid-lowering therapy in dialysis patients remains uncertain.

Aims
Haemodialysis patients are at very high risk of cardiovascular disease and death (approximately 100 times that of the age-matched population, for patients 45y old). Observational data had shown a negative association between blood cholesterol and mortality in dialysis patients (compared with a log-linear relationship in the normal population), although this may be due to 'reverse causality' (the outcome/effect having predated the cause/exposure, i.e. the outcome (disease/mortality) having caused individuals to change their behaviour (exposure). Since benefits of statins are well established, particularly in patients with DM, this RCT aimed to investigate the efficacy of lipid-lowering therapy in a diabetic group of haemodialysis patients.

Methods
Patients: 1255 patients at 178 dialysis centres in Germany.
Inclusion criteria: Type 2 DM and on long-term haemodialysis:
• Age 18–80y;
• On haemodialysis for <2y;
• Low-density lipoprotein (LDL) cholesterol 2.1–4.9mmol/L.

Groups:
• Placebo (n=636);
• Statin (atorvastatin, 20mg PO od) (n=619).

Primary endpoint: Composite endpoint of coronary death, fatal stroke, non-fatal myocardial infarction (MI), or non-fatal stroke.

Secondary endpoints:
• Death from all causes;
• All cardiac events combined;
• All cerebrovascular events combined.

Follow-up: At 4wk, then 6 monthly. Median F/U=4y.

Results

Primary endpoint	Placebo	Atorvastatin	RR (95% CI)	p
Coronary death, fatal stroke, non-fatal MI, or stroke	243 (38%)	226 (37%)	0.92 (0.77 to 1.10)	0.4
Secondary endpoints				
All cardiac events	246 (39%)	205 (33%)	0.82 (0.68 to 0.99)	0.03
Death from all causes	320 (50%)	297 (48%)	0.93 (0.79 to 1.08)	0.3
All cerebrovascular events	70 (11%)	79 (13%)	1.12 (0.81 to 1.55)	0.5

Discussion

The study failed to demonstrate a benefit in terms of its primary endpoint. The unexpected finding of more ischaemic strokes in the statin group contributed significantly to this outcome. This observation was unexpected when considered in the context of all other statin trials where clear reduction in the incidence of stroke had been demonstrated. The results of ongoing larger studies should be awaited before lipid-lowering therapy is abandoned in dialysis patients.

Problems

- It is likely that much of the cardiovascular risk associated with end-stage renal disease is unrelated to atherosclerosis. Therefore, the benefits of lipid-lowering therapy may be less than expected. This study did not seem to incorporate this fact in its design.
- By the time that patients with type 2 DM come to haemodialysis, much vascular disease has already accrued, and the effect of 4y of statin therapy may not be significant. However, the trial did not exclude benefit with longer-term treatment.

Haemodialysis: target haemoglobin concentration

The effects of normal as compared with low haematocrit values in patients with cardiac disease who are receiving haemodialysis and erythropoietin.

AUTHORS: Besarab A, Bolton K, Browne J *et al.*
REFERENCE: N Engl J Med (1998) 339, 584–90.
STUDY DESIGN: RCT
EVIDENCE LEVEL: 1b

Key message

It may be harmful to target a 'normal' haemoglobin (Hb) in patients on haemodialysis who are receiving erythropoietin (EPO).

Impact

This was the first study to demonstrate a possible detrimental effect of raising haemoglobin into the healthy population's normal range and supported guidelines that recommended a lower target.

Aims

The majority of patients on haemodialysis are anaemic and require exogenous EPO and intravenous iron to correct anaemia. Such correction of anaemia can ameliorate left ventricular hypertrophy which predisposes patients to cardiac death. However, most patients still have Hb concentrations of 9–11g/dL. This study aimed to investigate whether raising Hb into the 'normal' range (13–15g/dL) would provide additional benefit.

Methods

Patients: 1233 patients at 51 centres in the USA.

Inclusion criteria:
• Undergoing chronic haemodialysis;
• Documented congestive cardiac failure or ischaemic heart disease;
• Iron replete (transferrin saturation >20%).

Groups: Both groups received intravenous iron if required:
• Normal (13–15g/dL) target haemoglobin (n=618);
• Low (9–11g/dL) target haemoglobin (n=615).

Primary endpoint: Time to death or non-fatal myocardial infarction (MI).

Secondary endpoints:
• Hospitalisation for congestive heart failure;
• Hospitalisation for ischaemic heart disease;
• Coronary revascularisation (coronary artery bypass graft, CABG; percutaneous coronary intervention, PCI);
• Red cell transfusion;
• Change in quality of life score.

Follow-up: Planned 3y F/U, but study stopped after median of 14 months due to results of interim analysis.

Results

	Normal Hb	Low Hb	Relative risk (95% CI)
Primary endpoint			
Death or non-fatal MI	202	164	1.3 (0.9–1.9)
Secondary endpoints			*p*
Hospitalisation for all causes	445	425	0.3
Red cell transfusion	129	192	<0.001
Non-fatal MI	19	14	0.5

Discussion

This study did not bear out the expectation that further correction of anaemia would lead to improved morbidity and mortality. In fact, it was stopped early because it was thought that the chances of demonstrating a benefit of the normal Hb strategy were very slight. Furthermore, the study had almost demonstrated a significant harm with this strategy. Interestingly, when achieved Hb was used in place of group assignment, the results showed a reduced risk of death in patients with a higher Hb. This might suggest it is the dose of EPO, not the target Hb, that is harmful, although the report said this was not the case (data not shown). More patients in the normal Hb group received intravenous iron (526 vs 464, *p*<0.001), but this analysis was *post hoc* and potentially confounded, as this therapy was not randomised.

Problems

- 32 patients died in the normal Hb group after stopping study therapy and were included appropriately in the intention-to-treat analysis. However, the number of patients who died after withdrawing from the low Hb arm was not reported.
- Although similar at baseline, the adequacy of dialysis became significantly lower in the normal Hb group than in the low Hb group. This was not explored in the analysis, although results from other studies suggest it was probably not significant.

Dose of peritoneal dialysis

> **ADEMEX** (**ADE**quacy of peritoneal dialysis in **MEX**ico) study:
> Effects of increased peritoneal clearances on mortality rates in perito-
> neal dialysis.
>
> **AUTHORS:** Paniagua R, Amato D, Vonesh E *et al.*
> **REFERENCE:** J Am Soc Nephrol (2002) 13, 1307–20.
> **STUDY DESIGN:** RCT
> **EVIDENCE LEVEL:** 1b

Key message
The largest RCT of dialysis regimes in peritoneal dialysis (PD), which
fails to demonstrate a change in overall mortality with increased dialysis
dose.

Impact
Although controversial to some, this study has led to changes in guidelines regarding targets of dialysis adequacy measures in PD.

Aims
Clinical guidelines often emphasise the importance of small solute clearance as a marker of adequacy of renal replacement therapy based upon
observational studies, which suggested that increased total clearance
(residual renal function plus peritoneal clearance) in PD was associated
with better outcomes. It was assumed that as renal clearance declined, it
could be replaced with peritoneal clearance. However, no RCT evidence
existed to support this hypothesis. This study aimed to clarify this issue.

Methods
Patients: 965 patients at 24 centres in Mexico.

Inclusion criteria: patients on PD:
- Age 18–70y;
- Measured peritoneal clearance (pCrCl) <60L/wk/1.73m^2.

Exclusion criteria:
- HIV or hepatitis B virus (HBV) seropositive;
- Active malignancy;
- Cardiac failure.

Groups:
- Control: remained on standard 4x2L chronic ambulatory peritoneal
  dialysis (CAPD) regimen (only available regimen in Mexico) (n=484);
- Intervention group: had prescription changed to achieve peritoneal
  clearance of 60L/wk/1.73m^2 (n=481).

Primary endpoint: Death from any cause.

Secondary endpoints:
- Hospitalisation;
- Therapy-related complications (e.g. peritonitis);
- Correction of anaemia;
- Effects on nutritional status.

Follow-up: Planned F/U for 2y after last patient randomised. Mean F/U=22 months.

Results

Primary endpoint	Control	Intervention	*p*
Deaths (n)	157	159	1.0
Secondary endpoints			
Hospitalisation rate (admissions per patient per y)	1.03	1.17	0.2
Peritonitis rate (patient months per episode)	24.4	23.3	0.6
nPNA (measure of nutrition) (g/kg/d)	0.78	0.77	ns

Discussion

Some retrospective studies had suggested that increased dose of PD would result in reduced mortality: this study did not support this assertion. However, a reduced rate of death due to uraemia and congestive heart failure seen in the intervention group, and a higher rate of drop-out from the study due to uraemia in the control group did suggest that there were some benefits to increased dialysis dose, and that the dialysis prescription should still be tailored to the individual patient.

Problems

- 58% patients were prevalent PD patients, who were 'technique survivors' (i.e. established users of PD). There may be reasons why such patients do not respond in the same way as patients new to PD.
- The study population differs from the current PD population. For example, congestive heart failure (which affects 25% of PD patients in North America) was an exclusion criterion. Similarly, the patients were younger than the current average North American PD population.

Membranous nephropathy: steroids and chlorambucil

Methylprednisolone plus chlorambucil as compared with methylprednisolone alone for the treatment of idiopathic membranous nephropathy.

AUTHORS: Ponticelli C, Zucchelli P, Passerini P *et al.*
(Italian Idiopathic Membranous Nephropathy Study Group).
REFERENCE: N Engl J Med (1992) 327, 599–603.
STUDY DESIGN: RCT
EVIDENCE LEVEL: 1b

Key message
Combined treatment with chlorambucil and methylprednisolone induces earlier, but not more, remissions of nephrotic syndrome caused by idiopathic membranous nephropathy.

Impact
This trial was essentially negative and led to many nephrologists ceasing to employ chlorambucil in their management of membranous nephropathy.

Aims
Idiopathic membranous nephropathy is a primary glomerulonephritis that usually causes nephrotic syndrome. The benefit of any treatment in membranous nephropathy is uncertain, especially since some patients remit spontaneously. Previous uncontrolled trials had suggested a potential benefit of chlorambucil and this study aimed to elucidate whether this was a necessary addition.

Methods
Patients: 92 patients at multiple centres in Italy.

Inclusion criteria:
- Nephrotic syndrome (urinary protein excretion >3.5g/d and serum albumin <25g/L);
- Histological diagnosis of membranous nephropathy;
- No other cause of membranous nephropathy apparent.

Groups:
- 1: Methylprednisolone and chlorambucil: 3 cycles of 1 month methylprednisolone followed by 1 month of chlorambucil (n=45);
- 2: Methylprednisolone alone (n=47).

Primary endpoint: Clinical response (complete remission defined as <0.2g/d urinary protein excretion; partial remission defined as 0.21–2g/d urinary protein excretion).

Follow-up: Mean F/U=54 months in both groups (all patients followed up for at least 2y).

Results

Primary endpoint	Group 1	Group 2	RR (95% CI)	p
Clinical response				
Year 1	26/45	12/47	2.26 (1.23 to 4.17)	0.002
Year 2	24/44	15/47	1.71 (0.97 to 3.02)	0.03
Year 3	27/41	17/43	1.67 (1.0 to 2.8)	0.01
Year 4	20/32	13/31	1.49 (0.83 to 2.7)	0.1

Discussion

Previous trials had suggested a potential benefit with chlorambucil and methylprednisolone, but it was not clear whether chlorambucil was a necessary ingredient for this effect *(N Engl J M (1989) 320, 8–13)*. This trial concluded that the addition of chlorambucil caused earlier, but not more, remissions from the nephrotic syndrome. Furthermore, there was no difference between the two groups in terms of renal function at 4y. Therefore, there is little to justify the additional hazard of chlorambucil in the treatment of idiopathic membranous nephropathy.

Problems

- The control arm in this study was methylprednisolone rather than placebo, so it could not assess whether steroids were superior to placebo in the management of this condition.
- The very small numbers of events meant that there was a genuine chance of random error explaining the results of this study (despite the small p value), as demonstrated by the width of the 95% confidence intervals.

Severe renal vasculitis: plasma exchange vs methylprednisolone

MEPEX (<u>ME</u>thyl Prednisolone or plasma <u>EX</u>change) study: Randomised trial of plasma exchange or high dosage methylprednisolone as adjunctive therapy for severe renal vasculitis.

AUTHORS: Jayne D, Gaskin G, Rasmussen N *et al.*
REFERENCE: J Am Soc Nephrol (2007) 18, 2180–8.
STUDY DESIGN: RCT
EVIDENCE LEVEL: 1b

Key message
Plasma exchange is more effective than high-dose methylprednisolone in achieving renal recovery in patients with severe acute renal failure due to anti-neutrophil cytoplasmic antigen (ANCA)-associated vasculitis.

Impact
Plasma exchange is now the standard of care for patients with severe acute renal failure due to ANCA-positive vasculitis, in addition to standard chemotherapy with cyclophosphamide and oral steroids.

Aims
ANCA-positive systemic vasculitis (Wegener's granulomatosis or microscopic polyangiitis) is the commonest cause of rapidly progressive glomerulonephritis. Although combination therapy with cyclophosphamide and prednisolone can achieve remission in 80–90% of cases, those presenting with severe renal failure (creatinine >500micromol/L) have poorer outcomes, only 50% having independent renal function at one year. Therefore, this study assessed additional therapies to see if they could improve the prognosis in this group of patients.

Methods
Patients: 137 patients at 28 centres in 9 European countries.

Inclusion criteria:
- Diagnosis of Wegener's granulomatosis or microscopic polyangiitis (based on standard diagnostic criteria);
- Biopsy-proven pauci-immune necrotising glomerulonephritis;
- Serum creatinine >500micromol/L.

Groups:
- Intravenous methylprednisolone (1g/d, for 3 consecutive days) (n=67);
- Plasma exchange (7 exchanges of 60mL/kg within 14d of study entry) (n=70);
- All patients also received oral cyclophosphamide (2.5mg/kg/d, reduced to 1.5mg/kg/d at 3 months) and converted to azathioprine (2mg/kg) at 6 months, and oral prednisolone (starting 1mg/kg/d and tapered to 5–10mg/d) from 5–12 months.

Primary endpoint: Renal recovery at 3 months (defined by patient survival, dialysis independence and serum creatinine <500micromol/L).

Secondary endpoints:
- Patient survival at 1y;
- End-stage renal disease (ESRD) (defined as ≥6wk dialysis without subsequent recovery);
- Serum creatinine in recovering patients at 1y.

Follow-up: At 6wk, then 3, 6, and 9 months, and 1y. All patients had F/U for at least 1y.

Results

Primary endpoint	Methylprednisolone	Plasma exchange	p
Renal recovery at 3 months	33/67 (49%)	48/70 (69%)	0.02
Secondary endpoints			
Patient survival at 1y	51/67 (76%)	51/70 (73%)	0.7
ESRD at 1y	22/51 (43%)	10/51 (19%)	0.03
Serum creatinine at 1y	198 micromol/L	199 micromol/L	0.9

Discussion

The benefits of plasma exchange had only previously been demonstrated by subgroup analysis of trials in patients with rapidly progressive glomerulonephritis and advanced renal failure. This trial demonstrated both a statistically significant and clinical reduction in dialysis dependence. Although plasma exchange is not inexpensive, it was certainly cost-effective, given that it halved the risk of ESRD at 12 months.

Problems

- Although this trial demonstrated the superiority of plasma exchange over intravenous methylprednisolone, it is possible that the combination would be even more efficacious.

Treatment of lupus nephritis

Mycophenolate mofetil or intravenous cyclophosphamide for lupus nephritis.

AUTHORS: Ginzler E, Dooley M, Aranow C *et al.*
REFERENCE: N Engl J Med (2005) 353, 2219–28.
STUDY DESIGN: RCT
EVIDENCE LEVEL: 1b

Key message

In lupus glomerulonephritis mycophenolate mofetil is more effective in inducing remission and has a more favourable safety profile than intravenous (IV) cyclophosphamide.

Impact

Mycophenolate mofetil is now used routinely in the treatment of lupus glomerulonephritis.

Aims

Anecdotal series and small trials had suggested a benefit of the immunosuppressant, mycophenolate mofetil, in the treatment of lupus nephritis. This larger trial aimed to show non-inferiority of oral mycophenolate mofetil compared with IV cyclophosphamide as part of induction therapy for active lupus nephritis.

Methods

Patients: 140 patients from 19 study centres.

Inclusion criteria:
- Diagnosis of systemic lupus erythematosus (American College of Rheumatology criteria);
- Lupus nephritis: World Health Organization classification of proliferative glomerulonephritis class III (focal), IV (diffuse), or V (membranous);
- ≥1 of the following markers of disease activity:
  - Decrease in renal function (creatinine 88 micromol/L);
  - Proteinuria (>500mg/24h);
  - Microscopic haematuria (>5 RBC per high power field) or presence of red cell casts;
  - Serological abnormalities (anti-ds-DNA antibodies or hypocomplementaemia).

Exclusion criteria:
- Creatinine clearance <30mL/min; serum creatinine >3mg/dl.
- Severe coexisting morbidities or conditions requiring intravenous antibiotics;
- Prior treatment with mycophenolate mofetil;
- Treatment with IV cyclophosphamide within the previous 12 months;
- Monoclonal antibody therapy within the previous 30d;
- Pregnancy or lactation.

Groups: All patients received 1mg/kg prednisolone, tapered by 10 to 20% at 1 to 2 weekly intervals dependent upon clinical improvement:

- Mycophenolate mofetil (500mg bd, increased to 750mg bd at wk2, and advanced weekly to a maximum dose of 1000mg tds) (n=71);
- Intravenous cyclophosphamide monthly ($0.5g/m^2$ of body surface increased to $1g/m^2$ of body surface) (n=69).

Primary endpoint: Complete remission at 24wk defined as return of creatinine, proteinuria, or urine sediment to within 10% of normal values.

Secondary endpoints:

- Partial remission at 24wk defined as a 50% improvement in all abnormal renal measurements;
- Changes in renal function, complement, anti-ds-DNA titre, and serum albumin.

Follow-up: At 12wk and 24wk.

Results

	Response at 24wk (n)		
	None	**Partial**	**Complete**
Mycophenolate	19	21	16
Cyclophosphamide	21	17	4

- 52.1% in the mycophenolate group and 30.4% in the IV cyclophosphamide group had either complete or partial remission ($p=0.009$).
- 8 patients in the mycophenolate group did not have an early response at wk12, and 6 of these patients received IV cyclophosphamide.
- 12 patients in the IV cyclophosphamide group did not have an early response at wk12 and went on to receive mycophenolate mofetil.

Discussion

Intravenous cyclophosphamide was previously the standard treatment for severe lupus nephritis, but it had a very serious toxic side effect profile. In this study, mycophenolate mofetil was superior to IV cyclophosphamide in inducing complete remission of lupus nephritis. Additionally, mycophenolate appeared to be better tolerated than cyclophosphamide.

Problems

- Treatment assignment was not blinded, which could have led to potential bias in patient recruitment and interpretation of the results.
- The study was short in duration and looked primarily at the induction of remission. It would be important to determine whether the effects of mycophenolate were maintained during longer F/U.

Respiratory medicine

Introduction

Respiratory medicine traces its origins back to chest clinics and sanatoria, which were established to cope with the epidemic killer tuberculosis. This became curable in the mid-late 1950s involving some of the very first large-scale clinical trials. The development of lung function testing followed important advances in respiratory physiology. Radiological, cross-sectional imaging and nuclear medicine techniques have long been applied to the lungs. Immunological, pharmacological, molecular, and genetic advances have followed.

Today, respiratory medicine is a very diverse specialty involving common chronic diseases, rarer conditions, pulmonary involvement in systemic disorders, lung infections, tumours, and adverse drug effects. It is also an important component of general internal medicine. Respiratory medicine has been prominent in producing clinical guidelines, many of which are now evidence-based, and hence a good source of information and reference.

Asthma is the most common chronic medical condition in the Western world, affecting all ages. Unlike most others, it is increasing in prevalence. Smoking is well established as the cause of both chronic obstructive pulmonary disease (COPD) and lung cancer, the most frequent cause of cancer death (in both sexes). Although declining, lag effects mean both conditions are increasing in prevalence and will continue to be of major importance for decades to come, particularly in the emerging Third World. Sleep medicine has long been neglected, but is beginning to receive attention, and respiratory infections remain regrettably common.

Respiratory research is broad-based but the level of government and major charity funding is scandalously low. We summarise important recent clinical papers under the subheadings asthma, COPD, infection, lung cancer, and smoking, with contributions from pulmonary vascular disease and sleep.

Asthma: self-management

Randomised comparison of guided self-management and traditional treatment of asthma over one year.

AUTHORS: Lahdensuo A, Haahtela T, Herala J et al.
REFERENCE: BMJ (1996) 312, 748–52.
STUDY DESIGN: RCT
EVIDENCE LEVEL: 1b

Key message
Guided self-management using peak expiratory flow (PEF) monitoring reduces asthma events and improves overall quality of life.

Impact
Self-management of asthma is now considered standard and recommended by the UK's British Thoracic Society and other international asthma management guidelines.

Aims
Some studies had reported that >70% admissions for acute attacks of asthma could be avoided by proper prior medical care. A major problem is that patients do not react appropriately to worsening symptoms, greater than 50% leaving these untreated for over a week prior to admission. Guidelines do recommend self-management, although consensus on the optimal approach had yet to be reached. This study aimed to compare the efficacy of guided self-management of asthma using PEF monitoring with traditional asthma treatment over one year in a multicentre, prospective, single-blind study.

Methods
Patients: 115 patients at 3 centres in Finland.

Inclusion criteria: Mild to moderate asthma:
- Adults ≥18y;
- Variation of morning to evening PEF >15% on 2d in 1wk in past 6 months;
- Optimal PEF ≥250L/min;
- Baseline inhaled corticosteroid (ICS) treatment, becolmetasone dipropriate (BDP) 500–2000mcg/d or budesonide 400–1600mcg/d over past 6 months.

Exclusion criteria: Last course of prednisolone within 4wks.

Groups:
- Self-management group (SMG): Received education about asthma, their medication, principles of self-management, and physiotherapy techniques (over 2.5h), and their ability to monitor PEF was checked over a 1 month run-in (n=56);
- Traditional asthma treatment (TAT): Shown how to use inhalers and given general asthma information (over 1h) (n=59).

Primary endpoints: Asthma events, including hospital admissions, unscheduled emergency visits, days off work, courses of antibiotics and prednisolone.

Secondary endpoints: Quality of life focusing on asthma symptoms and sickness impact using the third part of the St George's Questionnaire (25 items), assessed at the beginning of the trial and at 4 monthly visits.

Follow-up: All patients completed at least 4 months F/U. Both groups seen at 4 month intervals for 1y. SMG patients recorded daily am PEF, symptom score (0–3), and medication use. (1) Budesonide dose was doubled if PEF fell to <85% of optimal value. (2) Prednisolone started if PEF was <70% optimal value.

Results

Primary endpoints, mean (95% CI)	SMG (n=56)	TAT (n=59)	*p*
Unscheduled emergency visits	0.5 (0 to 4)	1.0 (0 to 4)	0.04
Days off work	2.8 (0 to 62)	4.8 (0 to 27)	0.02
Courses of prednisolone	0.4 (0 to 4)	1.0 (0 to 5)	0.006
Secondary endpoints			
Quality of life (−50 to +50) at 1y	16.6 (15.9)	8.4 (18.4)	0.009*

*ANOVA repeated measures over 12 months.
Baseline: Mean age=42y; 63%=female; mean FEV_1=2.9L (82% predicted).

Discussion

Guided self-management reduced asthma events by about 50% compared to traditional treatment. The difference became apparent early on and increased over 1y of F/U. ICS treatment dosage and spirometry did not differ in the two groups. The thresholds of reduction from optimum PEF (15% fall for doubling ICS and 30% for 7d course of prednisolone) were lower than previously employed. Adherence to doubling ICS was 62%, while it was 77% to starting prednisolone. Although the SMG plan was based on changes in PEF, adherence was closely related to severity of symptoms.

Problems

- The main therapeutic intervention of doubling ICS to prevent asthma exacerbations has been shown to be ineffective in double-blind, controlled trials, yet self-management has been shown to be effective in many (but not all) studies.
- No objective measure of treatment adherence in either group was available, and it is possible that self-management works by increasing compliance.
- The respective contributions of PEF measurement and the other components and the mechanisms of benefit are unclear.
- Patients with severe asthma were not included.

Asthma: early inhaled steroid

> **START (inhaled Steroid Treatment As Regular Therapy in early asthma) study:** Early intervention with budesonide in mild persistent asthma.
>
> **AUTHORS:** Pauwels R, Pedersen S, Busse W et al.
> **REFERENCE:** Lancet (2003) 361, 1071–76.
> **STUDY DESIGN:** RCT
> **EVIDENCE LEVEL:** 1b

Key message

Long-term, once-daily, inhaled low-dose budesonide decreases severe exacerbations and improves symptom control in recent onset, mild, persistent asthma.

Impact

National and international asthma guidelines recommend the use of low dose inhaled steroids in persistent asthma, even of recent onset and in patients with mild disease.

Aims

Airway inflammation is a major determinant of symptoms and abnormal physiology in asthma, even in mild disease. Inhaled corticosteroids (ICS) are beneficial in reducing inflammation as well as in improving symptoms, lung function, morbidity, and mortality in chronic persistent asthma over a range of severity. However, the effectiveness of early intervention in mild persistent asthma (of recent onset) had not been established. This study aimed to evaluate the merits of early intervention.

Methods

Patients: 7241 patients at 499 centres in 32 countries.

Inclusion criteria:

- Mild asthma with symptoms ≥once weekly and <daily.
- Reversible airflow obstruction; post-bronchodilator increase in forced expiratory volume in 1 second (FEV_1) >12% *or* peak expiratory flow (PEF) variation of >15% on two occasions over 2wk.

Exclusion criteria:

- Asthma >2y or >30days previous steroid treatment;
- Pre-bronchodilator FEV_1 <60% or post-bronchodilator FEV_1 <80% predicted.

Groups:

- Inhaled budesonide (400mcg od) from a Turbohaler for 3y (n=3597), including 1000 children (<11y) who had 200mcg od;
- Inhaled placebo (n=3568), including 974 children (<11y).

Primary endpoint: Time to first severe asthma-related event defined as hospital admission, emergency treatment (systemic steroids and nebulised/parenteral bronchodilators), or death.

Secondary endpoints:

- Asthma symptoms, asthma-free days, life restriction in previous 2wk;
- Time to introduction of inhaled or oral steroid treatment;

- Spirometry; pre- and post-bronchodilator FEV_1;
- Adverse events.

Follow-up: At 6 and 12wk; then every 3 months for 3y.

Results

Primary endpoint	Budesonide (n=3597)	Placebo (n=3568)	*p*
Risk of 1st severe asthma-related event at 3y	117 (3.5%)	198 (6.5%)	<0.0001
Secondary endpoints			
Symptom-free days	93%	90%	<0.0001
ICS or oral steroids by 3y	1121 (31%)	1599 (45%)	<0.0001
Number requiring at least 1 course of prednisolone	547 (15%)	825 (23%)	<0.0001
Change in pre-bronchodilator FEV_1 at 3y (% predicted)	+3.49	+1.77	<0.0001

Discussion

This study showed substantial morbidity associated with mild asthma in the first few years after diagnosis. Early intervention with once daily budesonide reduced the risk of a severe asthma exacerbation by nearly 50% and the risk of a life-threatening attack by >60%. Effectiveness was independent of all baseline characteristics, including lung function and treatment. Delayed introduction of inhaled steroids may reduce benefit.

Problems

- Effects of budesonide were probably reduced by the study design, which allowed patients to start inhaled steroids throughout the trial in order to reduce dropouts (29% on placebo and 27% on budesonide) and differential withdrawal. About half the placebo patients received steroids at some time during the study and about 30% were taking an ICS during the first year.
- Post-bronchodilator FEV_1 in adolescents was not improved by budesonide though there was less reduction over time compared to placebo. This has not been seen in other studies, but it may be that loss of lung function occurs early after initial diagnosis of asthma. Adherence to treatment may also have an effect.
- The most frequent adverse effects (in >5% patients) were similar in the two groups: respiratory infections, rhinitis, pharyngitis, bronchitis, sinusitis, conjunctivitis, headache, fever, and accidental injury. Eleven patients died (3 on budesonide, 8 on placebo); only one case was asthma-related.
- Growth rate in children aged 5–15y at randomisation who took budesonide was reduced by –0.43cm/y (CI –0.54 to –0.32) compared with placebo. There was no difference between 200mcg (in children <11y) and 400mcg doses. The effect was greater during the 1st and 2nd y but amounted to 1.3cm at 3y. No later measurements were made though other studies suggest no long-term effect on final height.

Asthma: long-acting β₂ agonist and inhaled steroid

Added salmeterol vs higher dose corticosteroid in asthma patients with symptoms on existing inhaled corticosteroid.

AUTHORS: Greening A, Ind P, Northfield M *et al.* (on behalf of Allen & Hanburys Ltd. UK Study Group).
REFERENCE: Lancet (1994) 344, 219–24.
STUDY DESIGN: RCT
EVIDENCE LEVEL: 1b

Key message

Addition of salmeterol to a standard dose of becolmetasone improves lung function and asthma control more rapidly and effectively than increasing the dose of inhaled corticosteroid (ICS).

Impact

This was the first study of an alternative strategy for asthma management, and was the forerunner of many other studies examining differing severities of asthma and baseline ICS doses. The approach of adding a long-acting β₂ agonist instead of increasing ICS dose has now been adopted in national and international asthma guidelines.

Aims

The recognition of underlying airway inflammation in even mild asthma encouraged early use of ICS. Guidelines previously recommended doubling the ICS dose in uncontrolled asthma. However, there is little controlled evidence regarding stepwise increases in ICS. This study aimed to compare two strategies: increasing ICS dose or addition of salmeterol (a long-acting β₂ agonist, LABA) in adult patients with asthma suboptimally controlled on becolmetasone dipropionate (BDP, 400mcg od).

Aims

Patients: 426 patients at 99 general practice centres in the UK.

Inclusion criteria: Adult patients with asthma:
- Taking BDP by metered dose inhaler (MDI, 200mcg bd);
- Symptomatic on ≥4d out of last 7 during 2wk run-in;
- Variation in peak expiratory flow (PEF) of ≥15% over 1wk.

Exclusion criteria No prednisolone in previous 6wk and ≤4 courses in previous year.

Groups: Patients matched for age, gender, morning (am) and evening (pm) PEF, and asthma exacerbations in the previous year:
- BDP (200mcg bd by MDI) and salmeterol (50mcg bd by diskhaler, DKH) (n=220);
- BDP (500mcg bd by MDI) and placebo (by DKH) (n=206).

Primary endpoint: Mean am PEF as change from baseline.

Secondary endpoints:
- Mean pm PEF as change from baseline at wk1;
- Proportion of symptom-free days and nights;
- Mean daily and nightly use of salbutamol relief.

Follow-up: Patients recorded medication use, am/pm PEF, asthma symptoms (scored 0–4 on diary card daily during 2nd week of run-in and last week of each month), and were assessed at 1, 3, and 6 monthly visits.

Results

Primary endpoint (mean change in am PEF)	Salmeterol + BDP 200mcg bd (n=220)	BDP 500mcg bd (n=206)	*p*
At wk1	20L/min	3L/min	<0.001
At wk21	28L/min	6L/min	<0.01
Secondary endpoints			
Mean change in pm PEF from baseline at wk1	+15L/min	–5L/min	<0.01
Symptom-free days at wk21	44%	39%	ns
Daytime relief salbutamol use (puffs/d) at wk21	2.1	2.4	ns

Baseline: Mean age=48y; mean am PEF=349L/min (74% predicted).

Discussion

Addition of salmeterol to patients symptomatic on BDP 400mcg/d was significantly better than increasing the BDP dose 2½-fold, with am and pm PEF at wk1 maintained throughout the period of study. Favourable responses were more common with salmeterol than increasing BDP dose. Salmeterol also rapidly improved symptom control, reduced rescue salbutamol use (statistically significant at certain timepoints), and produced no increase in exacerbations of asthma. In patients with stable persistent asthma, addition of formoterol (another LABA) to steroid (budesonide) has also been shown to improve symptoms and lung function, and to reduce the rate of severe exacerbations, more than increasing the dose of steroid alone (FACET Study: *N Engl J Med* (1997) 337, 1405–11).

Problems

- Salmeterol might be expected to produce greater bronchodilatation than an increase in ICS dosage; however, the 6 months study should have allowed time for improved airway calibre with anti-inflammatory therapy.
- There were large numbers of patient withdrawals (n=136, 32%), reflecting the unrestricted, 'real world' design in general practice. Withdrawals were equally distributed between the two groups.
- The response to increasing BDP dose was disappointing; pm PEF was unchanged over 21wk (though am PEF did increase). There was no suggestion of differential non-compliance (patients in both groups recorded >90% for DKH and MDI), and the study was double-dummy (all given treatment or placebo at some stage) and double-blinded.
- Adverse effects were predictable, with both treatments well tolerated.

Asthma: leukotriene receptor antagonists

Montelukast, a once-daily leukotriene receptor antagonist, in the treatment of chronic asthma.

AUTHORS: Reiss T, Chervinsky P, Dockhorn R et al.
REFERENCE: Arch Intern Med (1998) 158,1213–20.
STUDY DESIGN: RCT
EVIDENCE LEVEL: 1b

Key message
Montelukast improves asthma control and is generally well tolerated.

Impact
Montelukast, an oral leukotriene receptor antagonist, has an additive role in the management of chronic asthma.

Aims
Cysteinyl leukotrienes are involved in the pathogenesis of asthma. Montelukast is a potent, specific, once-daily leukotriene receptor antagonist. This trial was designed to assess the efficacy and tolerability of oral monte-lukast in patients with asthma.

Methods
Patients: 681 patients randomised (607 patients completed 12wk study) at 50 centres in the USA.

Inclusion criteria: Non-smokers with:
- Intermittent or persistent stable asthma for >1y;
- Forced expiratory volume-1 second (FEV_1) 50–85% predicted at baseline;
- ≥15% increase in FEV_1 post-salbutamol;
- 2wk asthma daytime symptom score >64 (out of 336);
- Daily average use of ≥1 puff of salbutamol.

Groups: Groups matched for age, gender, race, asthma duration, inhaled corticosteroid (ICS) usage (23%), FEV_1, peak expiratory flow (PEF), daytime and nocturnal symptoms, and rescue salbutamol use:
- Oral montelukast (10mg nocte) (n=408);
- Placebo (n=273).

Primary endpoint: FEV_1, daytime asthma symptom score.

Secondary endpoints:
- Morning and evening PEF;
- Daily salbutamol use;
- Nocturnal wakenings/wk;
- Asthma specific quality of life;
- Change in peripheral blood eosinophil count;
- Asthma control.

Follow-up: Study duration=12wk.

Results

Primary endpoint	Placebo (n=273)	Montelukast 10mg (n=408)	p
Change in FEV_1 at 12wk	+4.2%	+13.1%	<0.001
Secondary endpoints			
Change in morning PEF	+4.6L/min	+24.0L/min	<0.001
Change in evening PEF	+4.2L/min	+15.9L/min	<0.001
Nocturnal wakenings/wk	−0.80	−1.66	<0.001
Peripheral eosinophils $\times 10^9$/L	−0.03	−0.092	<0.001

Baseline: Median age=31y; 55%=female; 94% had exercise-induced asthma; 90% had allergic rhinitis; 23% used ICS. Baseline FEV_1=2.5L (67% predicted).

Discussion

Montelukast provided clinical benefit with significant improvement in all asthma control variables compared with placebo, maintained over 12wk. Near maximal benefit occurred on the first day of treatment. There was no evidence of rebound deterioration on discontinuation of treatment. An electronic, centralised spirometry system provided quality control, thus ensuring accuracy. Treatment was discontinued because of adverse effects in 12 patients on placebo (4.4%) and 9 on montelukast (2.2%). Increased ALT occurred in 2.5% patients on montelukast and in 1.5% on placebo (ns).

Problems

- Benefits were relatively modest in this group of patients with quite severe chronic asthma (baseline FEV_1 67% predicted), but were similar in patients taking ICS (dose not specified) and those not on ICS.
- Montelukast reduced prednisolone courses (6.9%) compared with placebo (9.6%), but this was not significant.
- This was a short-term study of only 12wk duration; longer studies are required to assess chronic changes.
- Comparisons with more conventional treatment regimes, including higher dose inhaled steroids and concomitant treatment with long-acting β_2 agonists, are required.

COPD: pulmonary rehabilitation

Results at 1 year of outpatient multidisciplinary pulmonary rehabilitation.

AUTHORS: Griffiths T, Burr M, Campbell I *et al.*
REFERENCE: Lancet (2000) 355, 362–68.
STUDY DESIGN: RCT
EVIDENCE LEVEL: 1b

Key message
An intensive, multidisciplinary, outpatient rehabilitation programme is an effective short- and long-term intervention in patients with severe chronic obstructive pulmonary disease (COPD), and has the potential to reduce the use of health services.

Impact
Pulmonary rehabilitation is now considered standard therapy for patients with severe COPD and is recommended by the UK's British Thoracic Society and National Institute for Health and Clinical Excellence (NICE).

Aims
Pulmonary rehabilitation had been suggested as beneficial in the short term in controlled trials of patients with COPD. This study aimed to evaluate both short- and long-term benefits, particularly with regard to health status and health service usage as well as walking distance.

Methods
Patients: 200 patients from multiple hospital consultants and general practitioners (GPs) in the UK.

Inclusion criteria: Referred for pulmonary rehabilitation with:
- Chronic disabling lung disease, clinically stable over 2 months;
- Forced expiratory volume-1 second (FEV_1) <60% predicted with <20% bronchodilator reversibility.

Exclusion criteria:
- Unable to walk;
- Severe sensory or cognitive impairment;
- Symptomatic ischaemic heart disease.

Groups: Stratified by gender and obstructive lung disease (>97%):
- Multidisciplinary pulmonary rehabilitation: over 3 half days (2h sessions) per wk, for 6wk (n=99);
- Usual outpatient or primary care F/U over 12 months (n=101).

Primary endpoints: Hospital admissions, days in hospital with respiratory and non-respiratory illness.

Secondary endpoints:
- GP consultations, home visits, contacts with primary care (PC) staff;
- Walking ability: 10m shuttle walk test;
- Generic health status: SF36 questionnaire, hospital anxiety and depression (HAD) score;
- Disease-specific health status: St George's Respiratory Questionnaire (SGRQ), chronic respiratory disease questionnaire (CRDQ).

Results

Primary endpoints	Pulmonary rehab (n=99)	Usual treatment (n=101)	p
Patients admitted to hospital	40 (40%)	41 (41%)	ns
Hospital admissions/patient	1.4	1.9	0.04
Resp. illness mean days in hospital	9.4	18.1	0.02
Secondary endpoints			
GP consultations resp. illness	4.7	4.5	0.21
GP consults all cause	8.6	7.3	0.03
Resp. PC home visits	1.3	1.8	0.34
All cause PC home visits	1.5	2.8	0.04
Walking distance (m) at 1y	148	113	0.002

Baseline: Mean age=68y; mean FEV_1=0.9L (39% predicted); mean transfer coefficient (KCO)=81% predicted.

Discussion

Pulmonary rehabilitation did not affect the numbers of patients admitted to hospital, but did reduce the number of admissions per patient and the number of days spent in hospital (whether for respiratory illness or all causes) by about 50%. Although numbers of consultations in general practice (for all causes) increased though in the pulmonary rehabilitation group, home visits were reduced. The multidisciplinary rehabilitation programme produced large health status improvements in disease-specific and general questionnaires as well as in walking distance; statistically and clinically significant differences were persistent, if diminished at one year.

Problems

- The pulmonary rehabilitation programme had many components and the contribution of each is unclear. One of the aims was to change a patient's behaviour and attitude to their chronic disability and handicap, which may have occurred though a general increase in fitness. This could also explain reduced overall primary care attendances.
- The programme did not include a clinical psychologist, who might have increased the 'emotionally-based' benefits (anxiety component of HAD and CRDQ), which appeared less robust than the physical measures.
- The decrease in average bed occupancy was equivalent to 4d for each patient who attended pulmonary rehabilitation. Together with more efficient use of PC services, this implies large potential cost savings. A full health economic analysis is necessary.
- Treatment effects waned over the 12 months F/U; it is unclear whether this was due to disease progression, exacerbations causing deconditioning, or loss of effect due to failure to continue home exercise. Only 25% attended patient-led post-rehabilitation support sessions.
- 138 (41%) of 338 patients originally referred did not fit the entry criteria or refused to participate.

COPD: long-acting anticholinergic

Improved health outcomes in patients with COPD during 1 year's treatment with tiotropium.

AUTHORS: Vincken W, van Noord J, Greefhorst A *et al.* (on behalf of the Dutch/Belgian Tiotropium Study Group).
REFERENCE: Eur Resp J (2002) 19, 209–16.
STUDY DESIGN: RCT
EVIDENCE LEVEL: 1b

Key message

Tiotropium once daily is superior to multidosed ipratropium in improving dyspnoea and health-related quality of life, in reducing exacerbations, and in producing long-lasting bronchodilatation in patients with chronic obstructive pulmonary disease (COPD).

Impact

Tiotropium should replace ipratropium in severe COPD. Reduced rates of exacerbation and hospital admission have beneficial economic implications. The long-acting bronchodilators, salmeterol and formoterol, are alternatives for those having ≥2 exacerbations per year.

Aims

Inhaled anticholinergics are effective bronchodilators, acting by reversing the increased cholinergic airway tone present in COPD. Ipratropium had long been used in COPD, but tiotropium had several advantages, including longer duration of action and lack of taste. The aim of this study was to compare tiotropium with standard ipratropium therapy, evaluating dyspnoea, exacerbation rate, health-related quality of life (HRQOL), and lung function.

Methods

Patients: 535 patients at 29 centres in the Netherlands and Belgium.

Inclusion criteria: COPD with:
- Age ≥40y and forced expiratory volume-1 second (FEV_1) ≤65% predicted, and FEV_1/forced vital capacity (FVC) ratio of ≤70%;
- Smoking history of >10 pack years (i.e. 20 cigarettes/d for 10y).

Exclusion criteria:
- Asthma, atopy, allergic rhinitis, or raised total blood eosinophil count;
- On regular oxygen therapy or recent upper respiratory tract infection.

Groups: Double-blind and double-dummy. Matched for age, sex, concomitant inhaled β_2 agonist/steroid, theophylline, and prednisolone (<10mg/d) usage:
- Tiotropium (18mcg od mane as dry powder capsule via Handihaler) (n=356);
- Ipratropium (40mcg qds [2 puffs of 20mcg] by metered dose inhaler) (n=179).

Primary endpoint: Trough FEV_1 and FVC (defined as mean FEV_1 and FVC on subsequent clinic visits, 23–24h after last tiotropium dose *or* 8–9h after last ipratropium dose).

Secondary endpoints:
- Breathlessness: Transition Dyspnoea Index (TDI). Focal score ≥1 unit considered clinically meaningful;
- HRQOL using St George's Respiratory Questionnaire (SGRQ) and SF36. Increase in SGRQ ≥4 units considered clinically meaningful;
- Exacerbation rate and safety.

Follow up: At 1, 7, 13, 26, 39, and 52wk.

Results

Primary endpoint	Tiotropium od (n=302)	Ipratropium qds (n=141)	*p*
Trough FEV$_1$ change from baseline at 1y	+120mL	−30mL	<0.001
Trough FVC change from baseline at 1y	+320mL	+110mL	<0.05
Secondary endpoints			
Change in TDI focal score at 1y	+0.46	−0.441	<0.05
Change in SGRQ score at 1y	−3.74	−0.44	0.004
% having ≥1 exacerbation over 1y	35%	46%	0.01
Number of exacerbations/patient/y	0.73	0.96	0.006

Baseline: 85%=male; mean age=64y; mean FEV$_1$=1.23L (41% predicted); mean FEV$_1$/FVC ratio=46%.

Discussion

This paper summarised the results of two studies (both of identical design), one of which was an extension of a previously published study. Tiotropium od was significantly more effective than low dose ipratropium qds, with outcomes sustained over 12 months F/U. Lung function improved more significantly, and rescue salbutamol usage and dyspnoea were reduced more significantly by tiotropium. Furthermore, more patients achieved clinically meaningful improvement in HRQOL. Exacerbation rates, duration of exacerbation, hospital admissions, days in hospital, and time to admission were also reduced further by tiotropium. These are important issues with potentially beneficial economic implications.

Problems

- Tiotropium and ipratropium doses may not have been equivalent, though for 1h after the first dose, FEV$_1$ was marginally (but non-significantly) higher after ipratropium. 'Non-bronchodilator' effects may have different dose-response; ipratropium 80mcg qds may have been a better comparator.
- Tiotropium caused significantly more dry mouth (12.1%) than ipratropium (6.1%, *p*=0.03), suggesting greater anticholinergic efficacy.
- 92 patients were withdrawn from the study, adverse effects including worsening of COPD in 10.1% on tiotropium and 12.8% on ipratropium.
- The mechanism behind exacerbation reduction remains unclear; it is possible that sustained bronchodilatation raises the threshold of symptom awareness.
- Compliance, which might favour the od medication, was not assessed, but the study was randomised, double-blind, and double-dummy.

COPD: inhaled steroids and long-acting β_2 agonists

TORCH (<u>T</u>owards a <u>R</u>evolution in <u>C</u>OPD <u>H</u>ealth) study: Salmeterol and fluticasone propionate and survival in chronic obstructive pulmonary disease.

AUTHORS: Calverley P, Anderson J, Celli B *et al.*
REFERENCE: N Engl J Med (2007) 356, 775–89.
STUDY DESIGN: RCT
EVIDENCE LEVEL: 1b

Key message
In chronic obstructive pulmonary disease (COPD), there are significant benefits from single inhaler combination therapy of inhaled steroid and long-acting β_2 agonist (LABA), over inhaled steroid or LABA alone. However, overall mortality at 3y is not significantly reduced.

Impact
Combination therapy, with inhaled steroid and LABA in a single inhaler, is recommended for the treatment of moderate to severe COPD. Evidence is provided for the cardiovascular safety of salmeterol alone. Inhaled steroid monotherapy in COPD cannot be recommended though further study is warranted.

Aims
The UK's National Institute for Health and Clinical Excellence (NICE) recommends the use of an inhaled steroid for those patients with COPD and forced expiratory volume-1 second (FEV_1) <50% predicted, with ≥2 exacerbations per year. This trial was designed to investigate the effects of a LABA, an inhaled steroid, and the combination, on overall mortality over 3y.

Methods
Patients: 6184 patients at 444 centres in 42 countries.

Inclusion criteria:
- Age 40–80y with at least 10 pack years of smoking history;
- Pre-bronchodilator FEV_1<60% predicted;
- FEV_1/forced vital capacity (FVC) ≤70%;
- <10% increase in predicted FEV_1 with salbutamol 400mcg.

Groups: Groups matched for age, sex, body mass index (BMI), geographic location, smoking status, previous treatment, prior exacerbation rate, FEV_1, and St George's Respiratory Questionnaire (SGRQ) score:
- Salmeterol plus fluticasone (50mcg/500mcg bd) (n=1533);
- Fluticasone (500mcg bd) (n=1534);
- Salmeterol (50mcg bd) (n=1521);
- Placebo (n=1524).

Primary endpoint: Time to death from any cause at 3y, regardless of whether the patients continued to take study medication.

Secondary endpoints:
- Frequency of exacerbations;
- Health status according to the SGRQ;
- Post bronchodilator FEV_1.

Follow-up: All patients were assessed every 3 months.

Results

Primary endpoint	Placebo	Combination salmeterol and fluticasone	p
No. of deaths from any cause	231 (15.2%)	193 (12.6%)	0.05
Secondary endpoints			
Annual exacerbation rate	1.13	0.85	<0.001
SGRQ change from baseline	+0.2 units	−3.0 units	<0.001
Mean change in FEV_1 over 3y	−0.062L	+0.029L	<0.001

Baseline: Mean FEV_1 in all groups was 1.1L (44% predicted).

Discussion

The study provided excellent epidemiological data, showing that 35% of deaths in patients with COPD were due to pulmonary causes, 27% to cardiovascular disease, and 21% to cancer. The combination of salmeterol and fluticasone did not meet the pre-defined criteria for improved survival, but did demonstrate significant improvement in exacerbation rates, health status, and lung function over placebo, fluticasone, and salmeterol alone. The study also demonstrated salmeterol alone to offer similar advantages over placebo, with no excess of cardiovascular events; it can be recommended in the management of COPD.

Problems

- The failure to achieve a significant reduction in overall mortality with combination treatment may have been due to a lower than expected mortality on placebo; the study was powered to detect a 25% reduction in mortality at 3y.
- There were a high number of dropouts (approximately 40%, greatest on placebo) and this is likely to have led to an underestimate of benefit from the active drugs.
- Although patients with moderate to severe disease were included, potential recruitment to placebo may have mitigated against more severe cases, particularly those with frequent exacerbations.
- As expected, the study showed an increase in oropharyngeal side effects, but there was no difference between the groups in the numbers of fractures or cataracts. However, three years may be insufficient to detect significant differences in the incidence of these important problems.
- There was a significant excess of patients with pneumonia in the groups that received fluticasone, either alone, or in combination. Although pneumonia deaths were not significantly increased in these groups, this finding warrants further investigation.

COPD: long-term oxygen therapy

Long-term domiciliary oxygen therapy in chronic hypoxic cor pulmonale complicating chronic bronchitis and emphysema. Report of the Medical Research Council Working Party.

AUTHORS: Stuart-Harris C, Bishop J, Clark T *et al.*
REFERENCE: Lancet (1981) 1, 681–6.
STUDY DESIGN: RCT
EVIDENCE LEVEL: 1b

Key message

In patients with hypoxaemic cor pulmonale due to severe chronic obstructive pulmonary disease (COPD), oxygen therapy (for at least 15h/d) prolongs life. However, this effect is not seen until after 500 days of treatment in male patients.

Impact

This was the first RCT of long-term oxygen therapy (LTOT) in cor pulmonale due to severe COPD, and the first to show a reduction in mortality in this condition from a treatment other than smoking cessation. It was the foundation study for all guidelines on the use of LTOT.

Aims

Severe COPD complicated by hypoxic cor pulmonale and CO_2 retention carries a grave prognosis. Correction of hypoxaemia can reverse pulmonary hypertension and secondary polycythaemia. The aim of this study was to examine O_2 therapy in these patients (for 15h/d, over 3y), to determine whether it could reduce mortality, and improve exercise tolerance and working capacity.

Methods

Patients: 87 patients at 3 centres in the UK.

Inclusion criteria:
- Age <70y;
- Irreversible airflow obstruction with chronic bronchitis or emphysema;
- Forced expiratory volume-1 second (FEV_1) <1.2L;
- P_aO_2 5.33–8.0 kPa (breathing air at rest), clinically stable over 3wk;
- ≥1 episode of heart failure with ankle oedema.

Exclusion criteria: Restrictive lung disease, severe hypertension, proven coronary heart disease.

Groups: Matched for age, P_aO_2, P_aCO_2, pulmonary artery pressure (PAP), cardiac output, and red cell mass (RCM):
- LTOT: at least 15h/d, 2L/min via nasal prongs (n=42; 33 men and 9 women);
- Standard therapy (chosen by physician): included diuretics, bronchodilators, digoxin, antibiotics, and prednisolone (n=45; 33 men and 12 women).

Primary endpoint: Survival up to 5y.

Secondary endpoints: Arterial blood gases, annual red cell mass (RCM) (using [51]chromium tagged red cells), and annual PAP (by right heart catheter).

Follow-up: Clinic review every 2 months for 3y. Occasional home visits.

Results

Primary endpoint	LTOT (n=42)	Standard therapy (n=45)	p
Deaths up to 5y	19 (45%)	30 (67%)	<0.05
Secondary endpoints	**(n=22)**	**(n=18)**	
P_aO_2 on air fall in mmHg/y in survivors >500d	+0.11	−0.96	<0.05
P_aCO_2 on air increase in mmHg/y in survivors >500 d	−0.96	+1.2	0.05
PAP on air mmHg/y (n=21)	−0.06	+2.79	<0.05
RCM mL/kg/y	−1.25	+0.12	<0.05

Baseline means: age=57y; FEV_1=0.68L; P_aO_2=6.7kPa; P_aCO_2=7.23kPa.

Discussion

O_2 for 15h overnight produced significant survival benefits. Benefit was only seen in men after 500d, when a linear risk of dying of 29% per annum in controls was significantly reduced to 12% by LTOT (p=0.04). Surprisingly, PAP was not reduced by O_2 therapy. Risk of early death was predicted by female gender, high initial RCM, and raised P_aCO_2. In these patients, there was a fall in P_aO_2 and a rise in P_aCO_2 over time, with O_2 failing to prevent disease progression. Patients with high P_aCO_2 or mood disturbance who survived long-term benefited the most from LTOT.

Problems

- Not placebo-controlled and O_2 provided as concentrator, liquid O_2, or cylinders by different centres. Compliance was unproven, though treatment proved generally acceptable, with only 1 patient withdrawal. Cylinder weighing, time records from concentrators, and home visits suggested O_2 usage was at least 15h/d.
- Despite similar physiology, women died more rapidly than men (in a linear fashion from enrolment). This did not appear to be due to more severe disease and remains unexplained. Mortality in men followed an unusual pattern, with no divergence between treated and untreated patients until 500d. A likely explanation is that severely ill patients (too advanced to obtain benefit from O_2) were included, and it was not until they had died that benefit in the remainder was observed.
- No information is available for longer O_2 usage (>15h/d). The NOTT US study showed greater benefit from O_2 over 24h vs O_2 at night only (12h) in patients having severe COPD with hypoxaemia and pulmonary hypertension but no CO_2 retention.
- No reduction in hospital admissions or improved work record was seen with LTOT, but many of the patients were elderly and/or disabled. No cost/benefit analysis was undertaken.
- Improved well-being was reported in some patients on O_2, but not formally quantified. Although assessment of quality of life and exercise capacity are now central to such trials, simple measurement tools were not available when this study was planned and performed.

COPD: non-invasive ventilation

Early use of non-invasive ventilation for acute exacerbations of chronic obstructive pulmonary disease on general respiratory wards.

AUTHORS: Plant P, Owen J, Elliott M.
REFERENCE: Lancet (2000) 355, 1931–5.
STUDY DESIGN: RCT
EVIDENCE LEVEL: 1b

Key message

Compared with standard therapy, non-invasive ventilation (NIV) leads to more rapid improvement and reduces mortality in exacerbations of chronic obstructive pulmonary disease (COPD) when used in a general ward setting for patients with respiratory failure (mild to moderate acidosis). It also reduces the need for invasive mechanical ventilation.

Impact

Recommended by the UK's British Thoracic Society for acidotic patients, NIV is considered standard therapy for acute exacerbations of COPD. It should be used in emergency departments and medical wards to reduce the need for intubation and intensive care.

Aims

Prospective RCTs of NIV in intensive care unit (ICU) settings had shown reductions in the need for intubation and in-hospital mortality in patients with acute exacerbations of COPD. Other studies, in non-ICU settings, had produced mixed evidence. The aim of this study was to determine whether NIV was feasible in a ward (non-specialised) environment, and whether it could reduce intubation and mortality compared with standard treatment in mild to moderate, acute acidotic exacerbations of COPD.

Methods

Patients: 236 patients in general respiratory wards at 14 UK hospitals.

Inclusion criteria: Adults admitted as emergency with acute exacerbations of COPD (respiratory rate (RR) >23/min, pH 7.25–7.35, and P_aCO_2 >6kPa on ward arrival, and <12h since admission).

Exclusion criteria: pH <7.25; Glasgow Coma Scale (GCS) <8; pneumothorax.

Groups: Intention-to-treat analysis:
- *Standard treatment:* Controlled O_2 aiming for SaO_2 85–90%; nebulised salbutamol/terbutaline and ipratropium; prednisolone and antibiotic. Aminophylline and doxapram at discretion of attending medical staff (n=118);
- *NIV:* Standard treatment and nurse/physiotherapist initiated NIV via face/nasal mask with expiratory pressure 4cmH$_2$O and inspiratory pressure 10cmH$_2$O, then 15–20cmH$_2$O (or max. tolerated over 1h). O_2 to keep SaO_2 85–90%. NIV for: as long as possible (d1); 16h (d2); 12h (d3); then discontinued routinely (d4) (n=118).

Primary outcome: 'Need for intubation' (defined by any of the following within 14d of admission: pH <7.20; pH 7.20–7.25 twice, 1h apart;

hypercapnic coma (GCS <8 and P_aCO_2 >8kPa); P_aO_2 <6kPa despite max. tolerated O_2; cardiorespiratory arrest).

Secondary endpoints: RR, P_aO_2 and P_aCO_2 (at 1 and 4h; on d3; on/within 3 months of discharge). Also: mobility, nutritional status, mask comfort, breathlessness, and nursing workload (daily).

Results

Primary endpoint	NIV	Standard	p
Failed	18 (15%)	32 (27%)	0.02
Died	12 (10%)	24 (20%)	0.05
Secondary endpoints*	**(n=101)**	**(n=106)**	
Correction of acidosis at 1h	pH 7.342	pH 7.324	0.02
Median time to relief of breathlessness	4d	7d	0.03

*pH and RR improved after 4h, but acidosis and breathlessness improved more rapidly with NIV.
Baseline: Mean FEV_1=26.7% predicted; Mean TLCO=28.4% predicted. Well matched groups.
Mean: RR=28/min; pH=7.32; P_aCO_2=8.75kPa. Most (93%) tolerated NIV, which took an additional 26min of nursing time.

Subgroup	Outcome	NIV	Standard	p
pH <7.30	Need for intubation	13/36 (36%)	16/38 (42%)	0.64
	Died in hospital	8/36 (22%)	13/38 (34%)	0.31
pH ≥7.30	Need for intubation	5/82 (6%)	16/80 (20%)	0.01
	Died in hospital	4/82 (5%)	11/80 (14%)	0.06

Patients with pH <7.25 excluded as poor prognosis without ventilation (randomisation unethical).

Discussion

NIV was feasible on general wards. It produced more rapid correction of acidosis, greater fall in RR, and a trend towards more rapid correction of P_aCO_2, suggesting it increased minute ventilation by increasing tidal volume; the RR reduction offloaded the respiratory muscles, leading to faster relief of breathlessness. 'Need for intubation' was defined and used as the primary endpoint to avoid confounding effects of ICU bed availability and different doctors' views about indications for intubation/ventilation.

Problems

- A difficulty in generalising the findings is that they apply only to the use of a simple ventilator, standardised protocol, and a limited range of masks (4 types) in wards staffed by nurses who received a mean 7.6h training (first 3 months) and 0.9h (per subsequent month).
- Not all patients tolerate NIV, often due to discomfort from tight masks.
- Subgroup with pH <7.30 (n=74) did not significantly benefit from NIV in terms of treatment failure or mortality, although the study was not powered for this analysis; more sophisticated NIV, endotracheal intubation, or intensive care may be needed in this group.
- Physiological changes due to NIV appear small (no difference between groups at 4h). However, this, in part, reflected the removal of data for 'treatment failures' (more common in the standard group).

Severe emphysema: lung volume reduction surgery

NETT (National Emphysema Treatment Trial): A randomised trial comparing lung volume reduction surgery with medical therapy for severe emphysema.

AUTHORS: NETT research group.
REFERENCE: N Engl J Med (2003) 348, 2059–73.
STUDY DESIGN: RCT
EVIDENCE LEVEL: 1b

Key message
Lung volume reduction surgery (LVRS) improves exercise capacity, but not survival, compared with maximal medical therapy in selected patients.

Impact
The UK's National Institute for Health and Clinical Excellence (NICE) now recommends consideration of LVRS for breathless patients with marked restriction of their activities despite maximal medical therapy and with forced expiratory volume-1 second (FEV_1) >20%, P_aCO_2 <7.3, diffusion capacity (TLCO) >20%, and predominantly upper lobe emphysema.

Aims
Prior to this trial, LVRS was proposed as a palliative treatment for emphysema. This study aimed to investigate the effect of LVRS on mortality, the magnitude, and durability of improvement in breathlessness, and to identify patient selection criteria.

Methods
Patients: 1218 patients from 17 clinics in the USA.

Inclusion criteria:
- Evidence of emphysema on history, examination, and CT scan;
- Pre-rehabilitation FEV_1 ≤45%, total lung capacity (TLC) ≥100%, residual volume (RV) ≥150% predicted;
- Pre-rehabilitation P_aO_2 ≥6kPa and P_aCO_2 ≤8kPa;
- Non-smoker for at least 4 months before and during the study;
- Body mass index (BMI) <32.3kg/m² and approval by cardiologist, respiratory physician, and thoracic surgeon for surgery;
- Completion of rehabilitation programme.

Exclusion criteria:
- Post-rehabilitation FEV_1 ≤20%, and either TLCO ≤20% or non-heterogenous emphysema on CT scan;
- Bronchiectasis, previous LVRS, lobectomy, sternotomy, or giant bullae;
- Pulmonary hypertension, unexplained weight loss, daily use of 20mg of prednisolone (or greater), or cardiac arrhythmia;
- 6min walking distance (6MWD) ≤140m post-rehabilitation.

Groups: Matched for age, race, distribution of emphysema, and 6MWD:
- LVRS: bilateral, stapled, wedge resection of 20–35% of each lung by video-assisted thoracoscopic surgery or median sternotomy (n=608);
- Maximal medical therapy only (n=610).

Primary endpoint: Mortality and maximal exercise capacity after 2y (on cycle ergometry).

Secondary endpoints:
- Pulmonary function tests;
- 6MWD;
- Results on St George's Respiratory Questionnaire (SGRQ), Quality of Well-Being Scale, and a Shortness of Breath Questionnaire.

Follow-up: At 6 months, 1y, and annually thereafter.

Results

Primary endpoint (No. of deaths/total)	LVRS	Medical	*p*
Overall mortality	157/608 (26%)	160/610 (26%)	0.9
Upper lobe emphysema and low exercise capacity	26/139 (19%)	51/151 (34%)	0.005
Secondary endpoints *(No./total)*			
Improvement in FEV_1	134/313 (43%)	62/330 (19%)	<0.001
Improvement in exercise capacity at 24 months	54/371 (15%)	10/378 (2.6%)	<0.001
Improvement in health-related quality of life	121/371 (33%)	34/378 (9%)	<0.001

Baseline: Mean FEV_1=26.7% predicted; Mean TLCO=28.4% predicted.

Discussion

This study provided reliable data on the risks and benefits of LVRS for severe emphysema. LVRS was associated with greater improvement in lung function, exercise capacity, quality of life, and dyspnoea compared with medical therapy. Subgroup analysis demonstrated that surgery might reduce the risk of death among patients with upper lobe emphysema and low exercise capacity at 36 months, but could increase the risk in others.

Problems

- After exclusion of 140 patients at high risk of death from surgery (according to an interim analysis), the 538 patients randomly assigned to surgery were more likely than the 540 assigned to medical therapy to have improvements in exercise capacity and quality of life; however, there was no reduction in mortality over an average of 29 months F/U.
- Overall 90d mortality was greater in the surgical group. No reduction in mortality was seen at 90d, even in the group of patients with upper lobe emphysema and low exercise capacity.
- The significant finding of late mortality reduction following surgery in patients with low exercise capacity and upper lobe emphysema was only demonstrated by subgroup analysis. Confirmatory prospective studies using these results as entry criteria are required.

Treatments for smoking cessation

A controlled trial of sustained-release bupropion, a nicotine patch, or both for smoking cessation.

AUTHORS: Jorenby D, Leischow S, Nides M *et al.*
REFERENCE: N Engl J Med (1999) 340, 685–91.
STUDY DESIGN: RCT
EVIDENCE LEVEL: 1b

Key message

Treatment with bupropion significantly improves rates of smoking cessation compared to nicotine patches or placebo. The combination of bupropion and a nicotine patch is not significantly more effective.

Impact

One of the first studies to confirm the benefit of bupropion in smoking cessation and to compare it with nicotine replacement therapy (NRT). Bupropion now plays an important part in smoking cessation programmes.

Aims

Only a small proportion of those who attempt to stop smoking are successful. Studies have shown NRT to boost the rate of smoking cessation by a factor of up to 2.6. With mood and affect known to play an important role in motivation to use nicotine, this study aimed to determine whether bupropion, an antidepressant, was useful in helping people to stop smoking.

Methods

Subjects: 893 subjects at 4 centres in the USA.

Inclusion criteria: Motivated to quit smoking:
- Age >18y and weight ≥45.4kg;
- Smoking >15 cigarettes/d.

Exclusion criteria:
- Significant medical condition as assessed by the study site physician;
- Current psychiatric disorder, including depression;
- Dependence upon any other drug within the previous year.

Groups: All subjects received brief counselling and weekly assessments.
- Bupropion: 150mg sustained-release (Zyban®) for 9wk (n=244);
- Nicotine patch: 21mg (7wk); 14mg (1wk); 7mg (1wk) (n=244);
- Bupropion plus nicotine patch: for 9wk (n=245);
- Matched placebo tablets and patches (n=160).

Primary endpoints: Point prevalence abstinence rate at 6 and 12 months, judged by history and expired carbon monoxide concentration of ≤10ppm. Continuous abstinence at all visits throughout the 12 months.

Secondary endpoints: Withdrawal symptoms, body weight, and Beck depression inventory scores.

Follow-up: Assessments and relapse prevention counselling at 10, 12, 26, and 53wk. Counsellor also telephoned at 3, 4, 5, 7, and 11 months.

Results

Primary endpoints (at 12 months)	Placebo (n=82)	Nicotine patch (n=152)	Bupropion (n=169)	p
Abstinent	25 (15.6%)	40 (16.4%)	74 (30.3%)	<0.001*+
Continuously abstinent	4 (5.6%)	15 (9.8%)	31 (18.4%)	<0.001*+
Secondary endpoints				
Mean change in withdrawal symptoms: d14	+0.76	+0.52	+0.55	ns
Weight change: 7wk	+2.1kg	+1.6kg	+1.7kg	ns

*Nicotine patch vs placebo; + Bupropion vs nicotine patch; Baseline means: Age=44y; 53% female; 93% Caucasian. Consumption=27 cigarettes/d over 26y. Previous attempts to quit=2.8.

- Bupropion adverse effects: 42.4%=insomnia (19.5% on placebo); 11.9%= discontinued (3.8% on placebo). 5 serious adverse events reported.

Discussion

Previous trials had shown that people with negative affect were more likely to start smoking and to find it more difficult to abstain. This study showed that bupropion treatment resulted in higher rates of abstinence at 1y compared with placebo or nicotine patches. There were no significant differences between bupropion alone and bupropion-nicotine patch combination, and the UK's National Institute for Health and Clinical Excellence (NICE) does not recommend combination treatment. The study also demonstrated that improvements in smoking cessation were independent of depression and withdrawal scores, which were unaltered by NRT or bupropion. NICE recommends the use of bupropion (or NRT) for smokers who have expressed a desire to quit, and as part of an abstinence contingent treatment (ACT) in which the smoker makes a commitment to stop smoking on a particular target date.

Problems

- All subjects received rigorous counselling in addition to study medication. It would be useful to determine the effect of this intervention alone, although considerable health care resources would be required to provide this service for all patients who wish to stop smoking.
- Enrolled volunteers may not represent the majority of smokers. Nevertheless, there was a high dropout rate (20% overall).
- The overall efficacy of bupropion was limited; more than two thirds of subjects in the trial were still smoking at 1y. It will be important to know if the benefits of bupropion translate into significant savings in health care costs and improved clinical endpoints in long-term prospective trials.
- The study did not assess smoking cessation in patients with proven smoking-related diseases, e.g. ischaemic heart disease or chronic obstructive pulmonary disease (COPD), in whom smoking cessation may be most beneficial and cost-effective.

Pulmonary embolism: postoperative prophylaxis

Prevention of fatal postoperative pulmonary embolism by low doses of heparin.

AUTHORS: Kakkar V, Corrigan T, Fossard D *et al.*
REFERENCE: Lancet (1975) 2, 45–51, Lancet (1977) 1, 567–9.
STUDY DESIGN: RCT
EVIDENCE LEVEL: 1b

Key message

Subcutaneous heparin significantly reduces postoperative mortality from pulmonary embolism (PE) as well as incidence and extent of deep venous thrombosis (DVT) without a significant rise in haemorrhagic risk.

Impact

Thromboprophylaxis with unfractionated heparin, or more recently, low molecular weight heparin, is now standard practice for all patients undergoing surgical procedures and for other clinical episodes associated with a high risk of venous thromboembolic disease.

Aims

Venous thromboembolic (VTE) disease was, and still is, the cause of significant morbidity and mortality. Before routine thromboprophylaxis was introduced, studies proposed a 20–30% incidence of DVT following general surgery, rising to 40–60% after orthopaedic surgery. PE was reported to occur in around 5–10% of cases, being fatal in 1–2%. Although there had been several good quality trials showing low dose subcutaneous heparin to be highly effective at reducing the incidence of postoperative DVT, these trials did not produce a widespread change in practice since the impact of heparin on the incidence of PE was not defined and concerns remained about the risk of haemorrhage. This study attempted to answer these questions.

Methods

Patients: 4031 patients at 27 international centres.

Inclusion criteria:

- Age >40y;
- Elective major surgical procedures only (i.e. requiring general anaesthesia, lasting >30min, requiring inpatient postoperative stay >5d).

Exclusion criteria:

- In centres using radioactive fibrinogen test: emergency procedures, and patients having procedures on thyroid, left breast, and lower limbs (other than hip surgery);
- Patients receiving anticoagulant therapy.

Groups: 440 patients excluded from analysis, leaving 4,031 patients:
- Control group: no specific thromboprophylaxis (n=2033);
- Heparin group: 5000 units of calcium heparin (2h preoperatively and every 8h thereafter, for 7d, or until ambulant) (n=1998).

Primary endpoint: Death from PE (as defined by presence of fresh emboli in the pulmonary trunk, main pulmonary artery, or in ≥2 lobar arteries at postmortem (PM), where no other cause of death was found).

Secondary endpoints:
- Diagnosis of DVT/PE;
- Operative and postoperative haemorrhage.

Follow-up: Until discharge or death in hospital.

Results

Data from 1977 paper*	Postop Deaths	PM examinations	Deaths from PE (at PM)
Control (n=2033)	94 (4.6%)	66 (70.2%)	15 (21% of PMs, 0.74% overall)
Heparin (n=1998)	76 (3.8%)	50 (65.7%)	0
p	Not reported	>0.7	<0.001

* Lancet (1977) **1**, 567–9.

Discussion

The data quoted above derive from the 1977 F/U study (which excluded unreliable data from one centre) with unaltered conclusions. PE was the most common cause of death in the control group, followed by pneumonia and myocardial infarction. There were no deaths from PE in the heparin group. However, of the patients who died of PE, two thirds were diagnosed postmortem, reflecting the acute and potentially catastrophic nature of the condition. Incidence of DVT was also found to be significantly less in the heparin group, in keeping with results from other trials. However, there were significantly fewer cases of bilateral/extensive DVT in the heparin group. There was no increase in haemorrhage, haemoglobin drop or transfusion requirement, although more wound haematomas were noted.

Problems

- No randomisation to compression stockings.
- The high-risk period for VTE persists for 4–6wk postoperatively, particularly after orthopaedic procedures. This paper might have underestimated the number of deaths from PE and the subsequent impact of heparin.

Pulmonary embolism: type of heparin

A comparison of low molecular weight heparin with unfractionated heparin for acute pulmonary embolism.

AUTHORS: Simonneau G, Sors H, Charbonnier B et al.
REFERENCE: N Engl J Med (1997) 337, 663–9.
STUDY DESIGN: RCT
EVIDENCE LEVEL: 1b

Key message

Initial subcutaneous therapy with the low molecular weight heparin (LWMH), tinzaparin, is as effective and safe as intravenous (IV) unfractionated heparin (UFH) in symptomatic patients with acute pulmonary embolism (PE).

Impact

LMWH is now considered standard therapy and recommended by the UK's British Thoracic Society for patients with PE who do not require thrombolysis or embolectomy.

Aims

The efficacy and safety of LMWH in the initial management of patients with deep venous thrombosis (DVT) is established. This study was designed to determine whether subcutaneous LMWH (tinzaparin) was superior to continuous IV UFH in consecutive patients with symptomatic PE, with regard to efficacy and safety.

Methods

Patients: 612 patients at 57 centres in France, Belgium, and Switzerland.

Inclusion criteria: PE confirmed by: (1) positive angiography, (2) high probability ventilation-perfusion (VQ) scan, *or* (3) indeterminate VQ scan combined with DVT confirmed by venography or compression ultrasonography (USS).

Exclusion criteria:
- Massive PE requiring thrombolysis or embolectomy (judged by the attendant physician);
- Active bleeding or contraindications to anticoagulation;
- Received therapeutic anticoagulation for >24h before study entry;
- Life expectancy of <3 months, hepatic or renal failure, pregnancy.

Groups: Matched for age, gender, weight, predisposing factors, and DVT:
- LMWH: Tinzaparin (175iu/kg od SC) (n=304);
- UFH: Heparin (50iu/kg bolus IV), then initial infusion rate of 500iu/kg/d, subsequently adjusted so that APTT ratio was 2–3 (n=308).

Primary endpoints: Combined outcome event of death, recurrent VTE, or major bleeding within the first 8d and at d90.

Secondary endpoint: Change from d1 to d8 in % of detectable pulmonary vascular obstruction.

Follow-up: Oral anticoagulation begun between the first and third days of initial heparin therapy (both groups) and continued for at least 3 months, aiming for INR 2–3. Heparin continued until INR ≥2.0 on 2 measurements made 24h apart, at least 5d after commencing heparin treatment.

Results

Primary endpoints	UFH (n=308)	LMWH (n=304)	p
Death, recurrent VTE, or bleeding at 8d	9 (2.9%)	9 (3%)	ns
Death, recurrent VTE, or bleeding at 90d	22 (7.1%)	18 (5.9%)	ns
Secondary endpoints	**(n=260)**	**(n=258)**	
% decrease in pulmonary vascular obstruction at d8	9.09±13.9	18.4±13.5	ns
% of patients with improvement in VQ scan	81%	80%	ns

Baseline: Mean age=67y; 45%=male; 72% had DVT. Mean pulmonary vascular obstruction=47% on VQ scan.

Discussion

This study suggested that tinzaparin, a LMWH, can be used safely and effectively with a once-daily regime in the management of patients with acute PE who do not require thrombolysis or embolectomy. During 3 months F/U, there was a non-significant trend towards better outcomes with LMWH over UFH. The trial confirmed previous studies which validated the use of LMWH in DVT, and extended the role of LMWH into the management of PE. Given the simplicity of once-daily subcutaneous administration, LMWH is established as the treatment of choice for acute PE without haemodynamic instability.

Problems

- 222 patients in the LMWH group and 201 in the UFH group received therapeutic doses of UFH before randomisation (for <24h, allowing their inclusion in the study). This makes the validation of LMWH in the first 24h of acute PE less clear-cut.
- 52% of the initial 1482 patients who met the enrolment criteria were excluded for a variety of reasons. However, only 15% of suitable patients then declined participation.
- The authors acknowledge that their selection criteria excluded patients who were at highest risk of death (232 requiring thrombolysis or inferior vena caval umbrella), recurrent VTE, and haemorrhage. In the initial 8 days of treatment, incidence of critical events was only 3%. This unexpectedly low event rate markedly reduced the power of the study to detect a significant difference between the two treatment groups.
- The study was not blinded, though the independent committee assessing the critical events was unaware of treatment group.

Pulmonary embolism: thrombolysis

Heparin plus alteplase compared with heparin alone in patients with submassive pulmonary embolism.

AUTHORS: Konstantinides S, Geibel A, Heusel G *et al.*
REFERENCE: N Engl J Med (2002) 347, 1143–50.
STUDY DESIGN: RCT
EVIDENCE LEVEL: 1b

Key message

Alteplase (recombinant tissue plasminogen activator) with heparin improves the clinical course of stable patients with submassive pulmonary embolism (PE) in comparison with heparin alone.

Impact

Following this study, thrombolysis should be considered for normotensive patients with PE who have moderate to severe right ventricular (RV) dysfunction.

Aims

Thrombolysis is established therapy for patients with acute massive PE and haemodynamic instability or cardiogenic shock. Patients with RV dysfunction due to PE have increased rates of in-hospital death, even in the absence of hypotension or shock. This study aimed to investigate the benefits of thrombolysis in patients with RV dysfunction but preserved haemodynamic status.

Methods

Patients: 256 patients at 49 centres in Germany.

Inclusion criteria: Confirmed PE and at least one of the following:
- Echocardiographically detected RV dysfunction (enlarged RV with loss of inspiratory collapse of the IVC without left ventricular (LV) or mitral valve disease);
- Echocardiographically detected pulmonary arterial hypertension (PAH, tricuspid regurgitant jet >2.8m/s);
- Precapillary PAH defined by right heart catheter mean pulmonary artery pressure (PAP) >20mmHg with wedge <18mmHg;
- New ECG evidence of RV strain: complete or incomplete right bundle branch block (RBBB) or S wave in lead I combined with Q wave in lead III or inverted T waves in V_1–V_3.

Exclusion Criteria:
- Age >80y;
- Haemodynamic instability defined as systolic BP <90mmHg;
- Onset of symptoms >96h before diagnosis;
- Contraindications to thrombolysis.

Groups: Groups matched for age, gender, weight, heart rate, BP, severity of dyspnoea, hypoxaemia, and comorbidity. Unfractionated heparin given

as a 5000U bolus, then 1000 u/h adjusted to maintain the APTT at 2.5–3x upper limit of normal, with warfarin started on d3:
- Heparin + alteplase (100mg: 10mg bolus + 90mg infusion over 2h) (n=118);
- Heparin + placebo (n=138).

Primary endpoint: In-hospital death or deterioration requiring escalation of treatment; inotropes, rescue thrombolysis, intubation, resuscitation, catheter fragmentation, or embolectomy.

Secondary endpoints:
- Recurrent PE;
- Major bleeding (Hb drop of >4g/dL);
- Haemorrhagic or ischaemic stroke.

Follow-up: At end of hospital stay or on d30, whichever occurred first.

Results

Primary endpoint	Heparin + placebo (n=138)	Heparin + alteplase (n=118)	p
Death or escalation	34 (24.6%)	13 (11.0%)	0.006
Secondary endpoints			
Recurrent PE	4 (2.9%)	4 (3.4%)	ns
Major bleeding	5 (3.6%)	1 (0.8%)	<0.001
Ischaemic stroke	1 (0.7)	No cases	ns

Baseline: Mean age=62y; 52%=female; mean P_aO_2=8.2kPa; mean P_aCO_2=3.9kPa; 31% had RV dysfunction on echocardiogram.

Discussion

This study demonstrated a role for thrombolysis in the management of PE with RV dysfunction, preventing the need for escalation of treatment during the hospital stay, independent of heparin effect on APTT. This may result in improved patient experience and a reduction in overall health care costs. It also highlighted the importance of echocardiography in PE and showed that thrombolysis with alteplase was very safe, with only one major bleed in the thrombolysis group vs five with placebo.

Problems

- Thrombolysis significantly improved the need for escalation of therapy in this study, but did not affect survival despite being the largest trial of thrombolysis. This reflected the low mortality: only 3 deaths in the placebo group and 4 in the thrombolysis group.
- The primary endpoint of clinical deterioration requiring escalation of therapy may be inadequately objective. No information was available regarding rates of recurrence, long-term consequences, quality of life, or pharmacoeconomics.
- Current treatment of PE commonly employs subcutaneous low molecular weight heparin (LMWH, which also has some thrombolytic properties) rather than IV unfractionated heparin. It would be useful to compare thrombolysis and LMWH vs LMWH alone in patients with submassive PE to guide best management.

Empyema: intrapleural streptokinase

MIST1 (Multicentre Intrapleural Sepsis Trial): UK controlled trial of intrapleural streptokinase for pleural infection.

AUTHORS: Maskell N, Davies C, Nunn A *et al.*
REFERENCE: N Engl J Med (2005) 352, 865–74.
STUDY DESIGN: RCT
EVIDENCE LEVEL: 1b

Key message
Intrapleural streptokinase does not improve mortality, rate of surgery, or length of hospital stay among patients with pleural infection.

Impact
Prior to this trial, intrapleural fibrinolytics were routinely used to aid drainage of infected pleural fluid collections. The data from this study suggested no benefit over saline placebo, and streptokinase is now seldom used in empyema.

Aims
Infected pleural fluid contains fibrous septae which result from the process of inflammation. Intrapleural fibrinolytic agents were thought to disrupt the fibrin loculations, enhancing the effectiveness of percutaneous drainage and avoiding the need for surgery. This trial was designed to clarify the role of intrapleural streptokinase in pleural infection.

Methods
Patients: 430 patients at 52 centres in the UK (included 27 teaching hospitals and 18 centres with on-site thoracic surgery).

Inclusion criteria: Pleural infection:
• Macroscopically purulent pleural fluid;
• Positive on culture or Gram staining for bacteria;
• Pleural fluid pH <7.2 with clinical evidence of infection.

Groups: All patients underwent small bore chest tube drainage and received IV antibiotics.
• Streptokinase (250,000iu in 30mL normal saline every 12h for 6 doses via intercostal drain) (n=208);
• Placebo (also in 30mL normal saline every 12h for 3d) (n=222).

Primary endpoint: Number of patients who died or required surgical drainage of the infected pleural fluid during the 3 months after randomisation.

Secondary endpoints: Included:
• Rates of death and surgery, analysed separately at 3 and 12 months;
• Duration of hospital stay;
• Residual abnormality on CXR after 3 months.

Results

Primary endpoint	Placebo (n=221)	Streptokinase (n=206)	p
No. of patients who died or required surgical drainage	60 (27%)	64 (31%)	0.4
Secondary endpoints			
Mortality at 3 months	30 (14%)	32 (16%)	0.7
Surgery at 3 months	32 (14%)	32 (16%)	0.9
Median hospital stay (range)	12d (2–152)	13d (1–271)	0.2

Baseline: Mean age=61y; 69%=male; 68% had coexisting illness. Effusion was visibly purulent in 83 patients; median duration of symptoms=15d pre-randomisation.

Discussion

Previous small trials and case series had suggested that fibrinolytics improved drainage of pleural fluid, possibly also reducing the need for surgery. These data suggested, for the first time, that routine administration of streptokinase to patients after chest tube insertion did not improve mortality, need for surgery, length of hospital stay, X-ray appearances, or lung function at 3 months. In addition, serious adverse events were more common with streptokinase (7%) than placebo (3%) (p=0.08).

Problems

- The study's inclusion criteria may have led to enrolment of patients at varying pathological stages of empyema formation. Patients with organised effusions are less likely to respond to fibrinolysis.
- The trial may not have entirely reflected current clinical practice, in which ultrasound or cross-sectional imaging are commonly employed to aid drain placement and determine the presence of loculations. The study was unable to identify multi-loculated parapneumonic pleural effusions where streptokinase may still have a role.
- The duration of hospital stay may have been influenced by patients' relatively high age and the fact that 68% of patients had significant comorbidities.
- Streptokinase may still play a role in patients who are poor surgical candidates with very large chest drain-resistant pleural collections, or in health care settings where surgery is unavailable.
- The study raises several questions about the role of medical and surgical thoracoscopy, ultrasound, and drain size in the management of empyema.

Pulmonary arterial hypertension: endothelin antagonist

BREATHE-1 (Bosentan Randomised trial of Endothelin Antagonist THErapy): Bosentan therapy for pulmonary arterial hypertension.

AUTHORS: Rubin L, Badesch D, Barst R *et al.*
REFERENCE: N Engl J Med (2002) 346, 896–903.
STUDY DESIGN: RCT
EVIDENCE LEVEL: 1b

Key message
Bosentan, an oral endothelin receptor antagonist, improves exercise capacity in patients with pulmonary arterial hypertension (PAH).

Impact
Bosentan now forms part of the pharmacological treatment of patients with PAH, previously a condition with limited management options.

Aims
Endothelin-1, a powerful vasoconstrictor, plays a pathogenetic role in PAH. This study was designed to investigate the effects of two separate doses (125mg and 250mg bd) of bosentan (an oral antagonist of both endothelin receptors) on exercise capacity in patients with PAH (including patients in World Health Organization (WHO) functional class IV).

Methods
Patients: 213 patients from 27 centres in Europe, USA, Israel, and Australia.

Inclusion criteria:
- Resting mean pulmonary artery pressure (PAP) >25mmHg;
- Pulmonary wedge pressure <15mmHg and pulmonary vascular resistance >249dyn.sec.cm^{-5};
- Baseline 6 minute walk distance (6MWD) between 150 and 450m;
- PAH either primary or associated with scleroderma or systemic lupus erythematosus (SLE);
- Clinically stable and not scheduled to receive epoprostenol within 3 months before inclusion;
- Not receiving glibenclamide or ciclosporin in view of potential interaction with the study medication.

Groups: Groups matched for age, gender, weight, race, cause of PAH, previous treatment, baseline 6MWD, and cardiac index. Patients recruited during the first 2 months continued for an additional 12wk of double-blind treatment (period 2). All patients were eligible to continue an open-label extension:
- 62.5mg bd for 4wk, then 125mg bd for 12wk (n=74);
- 62.5mg bd for 4wk, then 250mg bd for 12wk (n=70);
- Placebo (n=69).

Primary endpoint: Change in exercise capacity from baseline to wk16, as indicated by 6MWD.

Secondary endpoints:
- Change in the Borg dyspnoea score (0–10, higher values indicating more breathlessness) from baseline to wk16;
- Change in WHO functional class (higher class indicating more severe disease) from baseline to wk16;
- Time from randomisation to clinical deterioration.

Results

Primary endpoint	Placebo	Bosentan 250mg bd	p
Change in 6MWD (0–16wk)	– 8m	+46m	<0.001
Secondary endpoints			
Change in Borg score (0–16wk)	+0.3 (±0.2)	–0.6 (±0.2)	0.01
WHO class improvement from III to II	28%	34%	Not reported
Clinical deterioration up to wk28	14 (20%)	4 (6%)	0.01

Baseline: Mean age=48y; 70% had primary pulmonary hypertension and 65% were functional class III; mean PAP=54mmHg; mean 6MWD=334m.

Discussion

Before this study, prostaglandin analogues were the only approved treatment for PAH. This trial suggested that bosentan significantly improved 6MWD, Borg score, WHO functional class, and also prolonged time to clinical deterioration. There were no significant differences in tolerance of the two treatment doses or their efficacy, although increased aminotransferase levels were seen with the higher dose regime. More recent studies have also demonstrated the efficacy of the oral phosphodiesterase (PDE) type 5 inhibitor, sildenafil, in improving exercise capacity and WHO class (*N Engl J Med* (2005) 353, 2148–57).

Problems

- Effects on exercise capacity were small but clinically significant (and comparable with prostaglandin analogues). Although symptoms were improved, bosentan failed to improve mean PAP and survival.
- There was an unacceptable incidence of abnormal liver function tests with the 250mg dose. Adverse events led to discontinuation of study medication in 9 (6%) patients in the bosentan groups and 5 (7%) in the placebo group (lack of efficacy).
- The trial included patients with PAH of varying aetiology; the majority (70%) had primary pulmonary hypertension in which exercise capacity was improved by bosentan. However, in PAH associated with systemic sclerosis and SLE, bosentan only prevented deterioration in exercise capacity, possibly reflecting an alternative pathogenesis.
- Further studies will clarify the duration of the effects of bosentan, potential complications of treatment, and responses in subgroups of patients, thereby determining the precise role of endothelin antagonists in PAH.

Obstructive sleep apnoea: nasal CPAP

Comparison of therapeutic and subtherapeutic nasal continuous positive airway pressure for obstructive sleep apnoea: a randomised prospective parallel trial.

AUTHORS: Jenkinson C, Davies R, Mullins R et al.
REFERENCE: Lancet (1999) 353, 2100–5.
STUDY DESIGN: RCT
EVIDENCE LEVEL: 1b

Key message

Therapeutic nasal CPAP (nCPAP) improves daytime somnolence and health status in patients with obstructive sleep apnoea (OSA).

Impact

nCPAP is now established as standard therapy for symptomatic OSA and recommended by the Scottish Intercollegiate Guidelines Network (SIGN) as first-line therapy for moderate to severe OSA.

Aims

OSA is caused by airway occlusion during sleep, secondary to pharyngeal collapse. Each episode is terminated by transient arousal, which restores pharyngeal muscle tone, re-opening the airway. Recurrent obstructive and arousal episodes lead to sleep disturbance and daytime somnolence. This study aimed to assess whether therapeutic nCPAP reduces daytime sleepiness and improves overall health status in comparison with sub-therapeutic nCPAP.

Methods

Patients: 172 patients referred to 1 sleep unit in the UK.

Inclusion criteria:
- Men aged 30–75y;
- Epworth Sleepiness Score ≥10 out of 24;
- Patients with OSA (defined as >10 episodes of desaturation/h (>4% fall in arterial oxygen saturation (SaO_2) during a sleep study, with confirmation that these episodes were caused by pharyngeal collapse).

Exclusion criteria:
- Patients preferring alternative therapy (e.g. weight loss, tonsillectomy);
- Urgent CPAP required for respiratory failure;
- Patient about to lose their job due to sleepiness.

Groups: Groups matched for all baseline characteristics e.g. SF36 score, Epworth Score, age, weight, BMI, neck size, SaO_2 dips:
- Subtherapeutic control group: received nCPAP at about $1cmH_2O$ (using the lowest machine pressure with restricted flow) for 4wk (n=53);
- Therapeutic autotitrated nCPAP (n=54).

Primary endpoints: at 4wk:
- Epworth Sleepiness Score (0–24, with 24 most sleepy);
- Objective sleepiness, as judged by maintenance of wakefulness test (MWT): patients asked to resist sleep whilst semi-recumbent in a dark room, then instructed to tap in response to a dim light flashing every 3s. Sleep defined as a failure to tap for 21s. Patient then immediately woken up and mean time to sleep onset over 160 daytime min calculated;
- Energy and vitality as measured by the SF36 questionnaire;
- Self-reported health status as judged by the mental component of the SF36 questionnaire, a higher score representing better mental health.

Results

Primary endpoint	Subtherapeutic nCPAP (n=53)	Therapeutic nCPAP (n=54)	p
Change from baseline in Epworth Score	−2.0	−8.5	<0.0001
MWT	+3.5min	+10.4min	0.002
Change in energy and vitality score on SF36 (score 0–100)	+17	+37.6	<0.0001
Change in mental component of SF36	+4.3	+10.6	<0.0001

Baseline: Mean age=49y; mean BMI=35; mean nocturnal desaturation=31 dips >4% SaO_2/h; mean Epworth score=16.5.

Discussion

Prior to this study, trials attempting to establish the benefit of CPAP in OSA were insufficiently blinded or used a tablet as placebo in the control group. The inclusion of a subtherapeutic nCPAP control arm in a double-blind fashion demonstrated large improvements in sleepiness measures with therapeutic nCPAP that were significantly greater than with subtherapeutic control treatment. The trial also provided data on nCPAP usage: patients in the therapeutic group used a mean of 5.4h/night, use correlating with improved Epworth Score.

Problems

- The subtherapeutic nCPAP control group demonstrated some statistically significant improvements in Epworth Sleepiness Score and SF36 scores, implying a positive placebo effect or possible actual benefit, and underestimation of the actual benefits of nCPAP. Reassuringly, patients were not worse on sham treatment.
- Longer-term studies with other outcomes and comparison of nCPAP with other treatment modalities, e.g. tonsillectomy and weight loss, would be useful. It is also unclear whether patients with lower Epworth Scores would benefit from nCPAP.
- It would be useful to know about comorbidities in the groups (e.g. ischaemic heart disease, previous cerebrovascular accident, hypertension) and whether these affect the response to CPAP.

Small cell lung cancer: radiotherapy

Twice-daily compared with once-daily thoracic radiotherapy in limited small cell lung cancer treated concurrently with cisplatin and etoposide.

AUTHORS: Turrisi A, Kyungmann K, Blum R *et al.*
REFERENCE: N Engl J Med (1999) 340, 265–71.
STUDY DESIGN: RCT
EVIDENCE LEVEL: 1b

Key message
Given concurrently with chemotherapy, twice-daily thoracic radiotherapy improves survival compared with a once-daily regime.

Impact
The addition of early, concurrent radiotherapy to standard chemotherapy for treatment of limited stage small cell lung cancer improves survival; a twice-daily regimen improves outcome still further. Whether this is due to an increase in the biological dose or the acceleration of treatment is under further evaluation.

Aims
Small cell lung cancers can be divided into two categories: limited (clinically confined to one side of the chest) and extensive. For small cell lung cancer contained within a radical radiotherapy portal (limited stage small cell lung cancer), radiotherapy had been demonstrated to improve survival. This study aimed to define the optimal radiotherapy regimen.

Methods
Patients: 417 patients from multiple centres in the USA.

Inclusion criteria:
- Histologically confirmed small cell lung cancer;
- Confined to one hemithorax ± ipsilateral supraclavicular fossa;
- Staging by CT or MRI of chest, abdomen, and brain; bone scan; bilateral iliac crest bone marrow aspiration; and biopsy-limited stage disease;
- Adequate organ function.

Treatment:
- 4 cycles of cisplatin 60mg/m^2 on d1 + etoposide 120mg/m^2 on d1–3;
- Radiotherapy dose 45Gy, starting with 1st cycle chemotherapy with either:
  - Once-daily group: 1.8Gy daily in 25 fractions over 5wk (n=206);
  - Twice-daily group: 1.5Gy in 30 fractions over 3wk (n=211);
- Prophylactic cranial irradiation offered to patients with complete response (2.5Gy in 10 fractions over 2wk).

Primary endpoint: Overall survival from date of trial entry to date of death.

Statistical analysis:
- Target enrolment 400 patients;
- 82% power to detect 15% improvement in 2y survival;
- Patients randomised according to performance status and weight loss in 6 months before trial entry.

Follow-up: Median F/U=8y.

Results

	Twice-daily group (n=196)	Once-daily group (n=185)	p
Median survival	23 months	19 months	Not reported
2y survival	47%	41%	ns
5y survival	26%	16%	0.04
Grade 3 oesophagitis	27%	11%	Not reported

Median age 62y, 59% male, 90% white, there were 11 treatment-related deaths.

Discussion

The survival rate obtained in this trial exceeded that in any previous large, randomised trial of chemotherapy and radiotherapy in small cell lung cancer. 353 deaths had been anticipated at 2y but after 5y, only 335 deaths had been reported. Previous studies of concurrent treatment had used cyclophosphamide- or doxorubicin-based chemotherapy with increased toxicity. The newer cisplatin/etoposide regimen used here was better tolerated in combination with radiotherapy, allowing the delivery of full systemic doses of chemotherapy. In addition, commencing radiotherapy early with the first cycle of chemotherapy was thought to be advantageous.

Problems

- Patients in the twice-daily group received a biologically higher dose of radiotherapy. Would the difference in survival be lost if the once-daily group were treated with an equivalent dose?
- In practice, it is difficult to deliver radiotherapy along with the first chemotherapy cycle due to treatment planning delay. The second cycle may be a more realistic aim.
- Rates of grade 3 oesophagitis could be decreased by delivering modern 3D conformal radiotherapy.

Non-small cell lung cancer: chemotherapy

The Big Lung Trial: Chemotherapy vs supportive care in advanced non-small cell lung cancer: improved survival without detriment to quality of life.

AUTHORS: Spiro S, Rudd R, Souhami R *et al.*
REFERENCE: Thorax (2004) 59, 828–36.
STUDY DESIGN: RCT
EVIDENCE LEVEL: 1b

Key message

Cisplatin–based chemotherapy improves survival without detriment to quality of life and is cost-effective in advanced non-small cell lung cancer (NSCLC).

Impact

Platinum-based chemotherapy is recommended for patients with advanced NSCLC and now forms part of standard therapy, alongside a third generation drug, e.g. gemcitabine.

Aims

A meta-analysis of over 50 RCTs (over 9,000 patients) by the NSCLC Collaborative group *(BMJ* (1995) 311, 899–909) had shown survival benefits from cisplatin-based cytotoxic chemotherapy when used alongside surgery (± radiotherapy, RT), radical RT, and supportive care; the clearest evidence of positive effect was for regimens containing cisplatin in non-surgical (i.e. relatively advanced) disease. However, the individual studies used differing patient selection criteria and treatment regimens, with limited analysis of quality of life (QoL) and costs. With uncertainty surrounding whether the limited survival benefits had positive impacts on QoL, this study was designed to evaluate the survival benefits of chemotherapy, as well as assessing QoL and costs of treatment.

Methods

Patients: 725 patients from 57 UK and 5 non-UK centres.

Inclusion criteria: Patients of all stages and performance status for whom supportive care was considered the treatment of choice included:
- Histological or cytological diagnosis of NSCLC;
- Medically unsuitable for (or declined) radical RT or surgery;
- Fit to receive chemotherapy;
- No concurrent or recent significant malignancy.

Groups: Groups matched for gender, age, clinical stage, histology, centre, chemotherapy, and performance status:
- No chemotherapy (NoC) (n=361);
- 3 cycles of 3 weekly chemotherapy (C): with cisplatin, mitomycin, and ifosfamide; or cisplatin, mitomycin, vinblastine; or cisplatin, vinorelbine; or cisplatin, vindesine (n=364).

Primary endpoint: Overall survival.

Sub-studies:
- QoL as judged by validated questionnaires at baseline, 6–8wk, 12, 18, and 24wk (n=273, 135 C). Primary endpoint: global QoL at 12wk;
- Costs, collected retrospectively from randomisation to death or 2y F/U. Included inpatient stays, investigations, chemotherapy, radiotherapy, procedures, and hospice care (n=194, 99 C).

Results

Primary endpoint	No chemotherapy	Chemotherapy	*p*
1y survival	20%	29%	Not reported
2y survival	5%	10%	Not reported
Sub-studies			
QoL score (0–100) at 12wk	48.2	52.1	0.4
Cost per wk of life	£149	£157	ns

Baseline: Median age=65y, 74% male; stage III or IV=95% disease: squamous histology=53%; WHO performance status 0 or 1=78%.

Discussion

This study demonstrated chemotherapy to improve median survival from 5.7 months to 8 months. The probability of survival increased almost 50% at 1y and doubled at 2y. Importantly, it showed that this increase in survival was not associated with worse QoL and was cost-effective. The trial confirmed the results of previous meta-analyses in a setting applicable to clinical practice and is consistent with subsequent prospective studies of chemotherapy in NSCLC.

Problems

- The study included various chemotherapy regimens which were combined in the analysis. Supportive care was determined locally. More recent studies have shown that newer third generation agents combined with platinum-based drugs (e.g. gemcitabine and carboplatin) offer superior survival to those included in this trial.
- The authors point out that despite the lack of change to overall QoL in the chemotherapy group, treatment was associated with a 5% risk of death from drug-related toxicity.
- Despite the clear survival benefit demonstrated, the absolute improvement in median survival following chemotherapy was only 9wk (equal to 3 cycles of chemotherapy). More recent chemotherapy regimens may offer improved survival or QoL.

Non-small cell lung cancer: epidermal growth factor receptor inhibitors

BR.21 study: Erlotinib in previously treated non-small cell lung cancer.

AUTHORS: Shepherd F, Pereira J, Ciuleanu T *et al.*
(National Cancer Institute of Canada Clinical Trials Group).
REFERENCE: N Engl J Med (2005) 353, 123–32.
STUDY DESIGN: RCT
EVIDENCE LEVEL: 1b

Key message
Erlotinib, an epidermal growth factor receptor (EGFR) inhibitor, prolongs survival (compared with placebo) in patients with non-small cell lung cancer (NSCLC) after first- or second-line chemotherapy.

Impact
Lung cancer is the leading cause of cancer death in the Western world and survival from NSCLC remains poor. This study demonstrated that non-cytotoxic chemotherapy is useful in the management of NSCLC. EGFR inhibitors offer a novel modality of treatment which may be particularly effective in certain patient groups, sparking great interest in the molecular pathogenesis of lung cancer.

Aims
The USA's Food and Drug Administration (FDA) had approved the use of EGFR inhibitors for the treatment of NSCLC. This trial was designed to investigate any survival advantage for erlotinib over placebo in patients who had received prior chemotherapy.

Methods
Patients: 731 patients at 72 centres worldwide (National Cancer Institute of Canada Clinical Trials Group).

Inclusion criteria:
• Pathological evidence of NSCLC;
• Previously received 1 or 2 regimens of chemotherapy;
• Eastern Cooperative Oncology Group (ECOG) performance status 0–3.

Exclusion criteria:
• Cerebral metastases;
• Other malignant disease within 5y;
• Cardiac, ophthalmic or gastrointestinal disease.

Groups: Patients stratified according to centre, performance status, response to prior chemotherapy, number of prior regimens, and previous platinum-based chemotherapy:
• Erlotinib (150mg od) (n=488);
• Placebo (n=243);
• 22 patients were subsequently ineligible.

Primary endpoint: Overall survival.

Secondary endpoints included:
- Progression-free survival;
- Response rate (complete and partial) and duration of response;
- Toxic effects;
- Quality of life.

Follow-up: History, examination, and blood tests were performed every 4wk, and radiological investigations every 8wk for 6 months.

Results

Primary endpoint	Placebo	Erlotinib	*p*
Median overall survival	4.7 months	6.7 months	<0.001
Secondary endpoints			
Progression-free survival	1.8 months	2.2 months	<0.001
Response rate	<1%	8.9%	<0.001

Baseline: Median age=61y; 65%=male; 50% tumours were adenocarcinomas, 30% squamous cell carcinomas. 49% had received 2 prior chemotherapy regimes, 93% had received cisplatin-based therapy.

Discussion

These data suggested that erlotinib improved survival in patients with NSCLC who had already received first- or second-line chemotherapy. Overall, 9% of patients responded to erlotinib, but the likelihood of response was much higher among women (p=0.006), lifelong non-smokers (p<0.001), East Asians (p<0.02), and patients with adenocarcinoma (p<0.001). Erlotinib also improved quality of life in patients with NSCLC, an important outcome.

Problems

- 19% of patients on erlotinib (vs 2% on placebo) required dose reductions due to adverse effects. A total of 12% experienced a rash and 5% diarrhoea. Overall, 5% of patients discontinued erlotinib because of toxic effects.
- The study did not address the role of the EGFR inhibitor in the most vulnerable patients (performance status 4).
- To date there have been no head-to-head trials of docetaxel vs erlotinib although the INTEREST trial (*Lancet* 2008; 372: 1809–18) showed non-inferior survival on gefitinib (a related EGFR inhibitor) compared with docetaxel as 2nd line treatment in patients with NSCLC. The UK's National Institute of Health and Clinical Excellence (NICE) now recommends erlotinib as an alternative to docetaxel after failure of first-line chemotherapy, if the manufacturer provides erlotinib at the same cost as docetaxel.

Rheumatology

Introduction

In the fourth century B.C., the Greek physician, Hippocrates, developed a medical theory called humoralism, which held that four humors (liquids) coursing through the human body determined a person's temperament and state of health. He used the term rheuma, which literally means 'flowing', to describe an excess of the watery humor thought to flow down from the brain. The words rheuma and catarrhos ('flowing down') were used interchangeably by ancient Greeks to describe a variety of illnesses including joint problems. The French physician, Ballonius, in 1642 coined the term 'rheumatism' and distinguished noxious humors that affected joints from those that caused catarrh (hay fever, head colds, and sinusitis).

Thomas Sydenham (1624–89), a London physician who himself suffered from gout, distinguished the acute arthritis that attacked young people (probably rheumatic fever) from a chronic, crippling arthritis (probably rheumatoid arthritis) that came to be called rheumatic gout. Another British physician, AB Garrod, whose practice was devoted to studying 'articular affections', introduced the term 'rheumatoid arthritis' (from the Greek arthron, 'joint') in 1858 because, he insisted, the majority of patients said to have 'rheumatic gout' had an affliction that was related 'neither to true gout nor to true rheumatism.' Osteoarthritis (from the Greek osteon, 'bone') was commonly used as a synonym for rheumatoid arthritis. A clear distinction between the two ailments emerged at the beginning of the 20th century. In 1904, a Boston physician, Joel E Goldthwait, described the differences he saw using X-rays. In 1909, physicians, Edward H Nichols and Frank L Richardson of New York, reported on the pathological differences between osteoarthritis and rheumatoid arthritis. Today, there are clear criteria established for the clinical manifestations of rheumatic diseases, but there is still a long way to go in terms of establishing a clear understanding of their pathogenesis.

Rheumatoid arthritis: TNF-α antagonists

PREMIER study: A multicentre randomised, double-blind, clinical trial of combination therapy with adalimumab plus methotrexate vs methotrexate alone or adalimumab alone in patients with early, aggressive rheumatoid arthritis who had not had previous methotrexate treatment.

AUTHORS: Breedveld F, Weisman M, Kavanaugh A *et al.*
REFERENCE: Arthritis Rheum (2006) 54, 26–37.
STUDY DESIGN: RCT
EVIDENCE LEVEL: 1b

Key message

In patients with early (<3y), aggressive rheumatoid arthritis (RA), combination therapy with adalimumab and methotrexate is significantly superior to either methotrexate alone or adalimumab alone in improving signs, and symptoms, inhibiting radiographic progression, and effecting clinical remission.

Impact

Tumour necrosis factor-α (TNF-α) antagonists are now routinely used in the treatment of RA in patients who have active disease. The best efficacy is achieved when they are used in combination with methotrexate.

Aims

Both TNF-α antagonist, adalimumab, and methotrexate had previously been shown to be effective in the treatment of RA. However, no trial had assessed their use in combination. This trial explored the effectiveness of combination therapy in the treatment of early, aggressive RA.

Methods

Patients: 799 patients recruited from 133 international centres.

Inclusion criteria:
- Diagnosis of RA (according to the 1987 American College of Rheumatology (ACR) criteria);
- Disease duration <3y;
- Age ≥18y;
- Active disease with ≥8 swollen joints and ≥10 tender joints, plus 1 of: early morning stiffness for >45min; ESR >28mm/h; CRP >15mg/L;
- Rheumatoid factor +ve or erosion of at least 1 joint.

Exclusion criteria:
- Previous immunosuppressant/disease-modifying anti-rheumatic drug (DMARD) therapy.
- Active infections, including tuberculosis.

Groups: All patients received concomitant folic acid 5-10mg/wk;
- Adalimumab 40mg SC fortnightly + methotrexate 20mg/wk (n=268);

- Adalimumab 40mg SC fortnightly + placebo (n=274);
- Placebo SC fortnightly + methotrexate 20mg/wk (n=257).

Primary endpoints: 50% improvement (ACR50) at 1y and mean change in baseline of the modified Sharp score (a measure of joint damage assessed radiographically, based on joint space narrowing and erosions).

Secondary endpoints: Percentage of patients achieving clinical remission (28 joint Disease Activity Score (DAS-28) <2.6), improvement in physical function measured by the health assessment questionnaire, and ACR20, ACR50, ACR70, and ACR90 responses at 2y.

Follow-up: 2y.

Results

- At 1y, 62% of patients receiving combination therapy exhibited an ACR50 response vs 46% receiving methotrexate alone or 41% receiving adalimumab alone (p=0.001). Similar effects on ACR20, ACR70, and ACR 90 response rates were observed at 2y.
- There was also significantly less radiographic progression among patients on combination treatment after 1 and 2y (1.3 and 1.9 Sharp units, respectively) when compared with patients on methotrexate alone (5.7 and 10.4 Sharp units) or adalimumab alone (3 and 5.5 Sharp units) (p≤0.002).
- 49% of patients on combination therapy displayed disease remission (DAS20<2.6) at 2y whilst only 25% displayed remission in the methotrexate alone or adalimumab alone groups.

Discussion

This study provided evidence that early use of a TNF-α antagonist could induce remission in almost half the patients treated with adalimumab in combination with concomitant methotrexate.

Problems

- Further long-term data are required to establish the durability of remission on this drug combination as well as long-term cost-effectiveness.
- Despite impressive data from this study illustrating better outcomes in poor prognosis patients with RA treated early with combination therapy, the current UK National Institute for Health and Clinical Excellence (NICE) guidelines state that patients have to 'fail' with 2 DMARDs prior to anti-TNF-α therapy, thereby delaying the widespread introduction of TNF inhibitors.

Rheumatoid arthritis: comparison of TNF-α antagonists

TEMPO (**T**rial of **E**tanercept and **M**ethotrexate with radiographic **P**atient **O**utcomes) **study:** Therapeutic effect of the combination of etanercept and methotrexate compared with each treatment alone in patients with rheumatoid arthritis.

AUTHORS: Klareskog L, van der Heijde D, Jager J et al.
REFERENCE: Lancet (2004) 363, 675–81.
STUDY DESIGN: RCT
EVIDENCE LEVEL: 1b

Key message

Treatment with a combination of etanercept and methotrexate is superior in the treatment of rheumatoid arthritis (RA) than either agent alone.

Impact

Tumour necrosis factor-α (TNF-α) antagonists are now routinely used in the treatment of RA in patients who have active disease.

Aims

Etanercept is a human, soluble dimeric, TNF type II receptor fusion protein, linked to the IgG1-Fc fragment. It binds to and inactivates TNF. Both etanercept and methotrexate have previously been shown to be effective in the treatment of RA. This trial aimed to explore their effectiveness when used in combination.

Methods

Patients: 686 patients from numerous international centres.

Inclusion criteria:
- Diagnosis of RA (according to the 1987 American College of Rheumatology (ACR) criteria);
- Age ≥18y with disease duration 6 months to 20y;
- Active disease with ≥10 swollen joints and ≥12 tender joints plus one of: early morning stiffness for >45min; ESR>28mm/h; CRP>20mg/L;
- Failure of at least 1 disease-modifying anti-rheumatic drug (DMARD) other than methotrexate;
- Not treated with methotrexate in the previous 6 months.

Exclusion criteria:
- Immunosupressant therapy in the preceding 6 months;
- Previous treatment with any anti-TNF-α agent;
- Treatment with an investigational or biologic agent in the preceding 3 months;
- Treatment with DMARD or corticosteroid in the preceding 4wk;
- Active infections.

Groups: All patients received 5mg folic acid twice a week:
- Methotrexate 7.5mg weekly escalated to 20mg weekly within 8wk if patient had painful or swollen joints + SC placebo twice a week (n=228);
- Etanercept 25mg SC twice a week plus oral placebo tablet weekly (n=223);
- Methotrexate + etanercept (n=231).

Primary endpoint: Numeric index of the ACR response (ACR-N) area under the curve (AUC) over the first 24wk. Radiographic endpoint was change in total joint damage score (modified total Sharp score=joint erosion + joint space narrowing score) over 52wk.

Follow-up: Every 4wk for 30wk.

Results
- ACR-N AUC at 24wk was greater for the combination group vs etanercept or methotrexate alone (18.3%-y [95% CI 17.1 to 19.6] vs 14.7%-y [13.5 to 16], $p<0.0001$, and 12.2%-y [11.0 to 13.4], $p<0.0001$, respectively).
- The combination was more efficacious than methotrexate or etanercept alone in retardation of joint damage (mean total Sharp score −0.54 [95% CI −1.00 to −0.07] vs 2.8 [1.08 to 4.51], $p<0.0001$, and 0.52 [−0.1 to 1.15], $p=0.0006$, respectively).
- The number of patients reporting infections or adverse events was similar in all groups.

Discussion
This study added another therapeutic option in the treatment of active RA. It showed that combination therapy with etanercept and methotrexate was superior to either agent alone. This observation emphasised the importance of co-prescribing methotrexate, when tolerated, even at modest doses, in order to achieve synergy with an anti-TNF-α agent such as etanercept.

Problems
- Use of anti-TNF-α agents is expensive (in the UK, costs are ≈£8000/y compared with methotrexate at ≈£20/y). Use of anti-TNF therapies has significant economic implications which may result in some degree of rationing.
- The study population comprised an unusually high proportion of patients in the established phase of disease without prior exposure to methotrexate. Such a population does not reflect the typical DMARD refractory patient considered for anti-TNF therapy in routine clinical practice.

Rheumatoid arthritis: infliximab

ATTRACT (Anti-TNF Trial in Rheumatoid Arthritis with Concomitant Therapy): Infliximab (chimeric anti-tumour necrosis factor alpha monoclonal antibody) vs placebo in rheumatoid arthritis patients receiving concomitant methotrexate.

AUTHORS: Maini R, St Clair W, Breedveld F et al. (ATTRACT study group).
REFERENCE: Lancet (1999) 354, 1932–9.
STUDY DESIGN: RCT
EVIDENCE LEVEL: 1b

Key message
Treatment with infliximab and methotrexate is more effective than methotrexate alone in patients with uncontrolled active rheumatoid arthritis (RA).

Impact
Tumour necrosis factor-α (TNF-α) antagonists are now routinely used in the treatment of RA in patients who have active disease despite the use of conventional disease-modifying drugs.

Aims
Many patients with RA fail to respond to or are unable to tolerate conventional disease-modifying therapy such as methotrexate. This study aimed to investigate whether a chimeric human-mouse monoclonal antibody to TNF-α (infliximab) provided clinical benefit in patients with active disease.

Methods
Patients: 428 patients from 34 international centres.

Inclusion criteria: Active RA:
- Diagnosis of RA (according to the 1987 American College of Rheumatology criteria);
- Active disease with ≥6 swollen joints, plus 2 of: early morning stiffness for >45min; ESR >28mm/h; CRP >2mg/dL;
- Stable dose of methotrexate (at least 12.5mg/week PO/IM);
- Stable dose of folic acid for at least 4wk;
- Receiving both drugs for at least 3 months;
- If oral corticosteroids (dose of 10mg/kg or less) or NSAIDs were used, then the dose must have been stable for 4wk prior to screening;
- Hb >5.3mmol/L, WBC >3.5x10⁹/L, neutrophils >1.5x10⁹/L, AST and ALP less than twice the upper limit of normal, creatinine <150micromol/L.

Groups: All patients received IV infusions at wk 0, 2, and 6:
- Infliximab 3mg/kg every 4wk (n=86) or 8wk (n=85);
- Infliximab 10mg/kg every 4wk (n=81) or 8wk (n=87);
- Placebo (n=88).

Primary endpoint: 20% improvement as defined by the American College of Rheumatology (ACR20) at wk30.

Secondary endpoints:
- 50% and 70% improvement as defined by the American College of Rheumatology (ACR50 and ACR70);
- Reduction in individual measurements of disease severity;
- General health assessment.

Follow-up: Every 4wk for 30wk.

Results

Primary endpoint	Placebo	Infliximab 3mg/kg every 8wk	Infliximab 3mg/kg every 4wk	Infliximab 10mg/kg every 8wk	Infliximab 10mg/kg every 4wk
ACR20	20%	50%	53%	52%	58%
p	–	<0.001	<0.001	<0.001	<0.001
Secondary endpoints					
ACR50	5%	27%	29%	31%	26%
p	-	<0.001	<0.001	<0.001	<0.001
ACR70	0%	8%	11%	18%	11%
p	-	0.007	0.002	<0.001	0.002

Discussion

Whilst conventional treatments such as methotrexate are effective, some patients develop adverse reactions and others maintain disease activity with resultant erosive destruction and deformation of joints. Uncontrolled RA also leads to an increase in mortality. TNF-α antagonists have revolutionised treatment of these patients, improving symptoms and inhibiting joint destruction. More recent studies *(Arthritis Rheum* (2003) 48, 35–45) have demonstrated the efficacy of the fully human anti-TNF-α monoclonal antibody, adalimumab. This has the advantage of being administered by subcutaneous injection.

Problems

- Although there was no difference in the number of serious adverse events between placebo and infliximab groups in this trial, subsequent experience indicates that infliximab may predispose to unusual infections, including reactivation of tuberculosis (TB).
- In this study, low levels of double-stranded DNA were induced in a small proportion of patients. Drug-induced lupus is rare, resolving with cessation of infliximab and treatment with steroids as required.
- Infliximab is contraindicated in patients with multiple sclerosis as it may precipitate demyelinating episodes.
- The efficacy of infliximab may decrease with repeated infusions over time because of the formation of human antichimeric antibodies.

Rheumatoid arthritis: early treatment

BeSt ('BEhandel STrategieën' – Dutch acronym for 'best strategy') study: Clinical and radiographic outcomes of four different treatment strategies in patients with early rheumatoid arthritis.

AUTHORS: Goekoop-Ruiterman Y, de Vries-Bouwstra J, Allart C *et al.*
REFERENCE: Arthritis Rheum (2005) 52, 3381–90.
STUDY DESIGN: RCT
EVIDENCE LEVEL: 1b

Key message

Patients with early rheumatoid arthritis (RA) show faster improvement of function and inhibition of radiographic joint damage when treated with combination disease-modifying therapy, including either prednisolone or infliximab.

Impact

Optimised suppression of synovitis at the onset of RA leads to superior outcomes.

Aims

The approach to RA management has changed from just symptom relief to prevention of long-term complications. This study aimed to establish whether combination drugs provided more clinical and radiographic benefit than single agents in the treatment of early RA. Additionally, it aimed to establish whether corticosteroids and tumour necrosis factor-α (TNF-α) agents should be part of this early aggressive treatment.

Methods

Patients: 508 patients from 18 peripheral and 2 university hospitals in the western Netherlands.

Inclusion criteria: Active RA:
- Diagnosis of RA (according to the 1987 American College of Rheumatology (ACR) criteria);
- Age >18y;
- Disease duration ≤2y;
- Active disease: ≥6/68 tender joints and either ESR ≥28mm/h or global health score ≥20mm.

Groups:
- Group 1 (sequential monotherapy): 1 drug at a time, starting with methotrexate, switching to other drugs if no improvement (sulfasalazine, leflunomide, then methotrexate with infliximab, if necessary) (n=126);
- Group 2 (step-up combination regimen): beginning on methotrexate, with more drugs added as necessary (sulfasalazine, then hydroxychloroquine, then prednisolone, then switching to methotrexate with infliximab) (n=121);

- Group 3 (combination therapy with prednisolone): started immediately on a combination of methotrexate, sulfasalazine, and tapered high-dose prednisolone (switching sulfasalazine for ciclosporin if necessary, and then to methotrexate with infliximab) (n=133);
- Group 4 (combination therapy with infliximab): combination therapy from the beginning with methotrexate and infliximab (and then, if necessary, leflunomide, sulfasalazine, ciclosporin, and prednisolone) (n=128).

Primary endpoint: Functional ability, measured by the Dutch version of the Health Assessment Questionnaire (D-HAQ) and radiographic damage according to the modified Sharp/Van der Heijde score. The latter was assessed on radiographs of the hands and feet obtained at baseline and 1y.

Follow-up: Every 3 months and treatment adjusted according to disease activity score (DAS) 44. Therapy intensified if DAS44 ≤2.4.

Results

	Mean D-HAQ score		
	Groups 1+2	Groups 3+4	*p*
3 months	1.0	0.6	1+2 vs 3+4; *p*<0.001
1 year	0.5	0.5	1 vs 3; *p*=0.01
			1 vs 4; *p*=0.003

- In the first year of F/U, patients treated with initial combination therapy, including prednisolone (group 3) or infliximab (group 4), had less progression of radiographic joint damage.

Discussion

Patients treated by initial combination therapy with either prednisolone or infliximab had more functional improvement than patients treated with sequential monotherapy or step-up combination therapy. Patients were less likely to progress to joint erosions after initial combination therapy with either prednisolone or infliximab. There were no benefits of step-up combination therapy over sequential monotherapy in terms of symptom improvement or inhibition of radiographic damage.

Problems

- Despite the favourable outcomes achieved with step-down combination therapy using a tapered prednisolone regime, many patients dislike the side effects associated with steroids.

Rheumatoid arthritis: B cell targeted therapy

> Efficacy of B cell targeted therapy with rituximab in patients with rheumatoid arthritis.
>
> **AUTHORS:** Edwards J, Szczepanski L, Szechinski J *et al.*
> **REFERENCE:** N Engl J Med (2004) 350, 2572–81.
> **STUDY DESIGN:** RCT
> **EVIDENCE LEVEL:** 1b

Key message
Treatment with the anti-CD20 monoclonal antibody, rituximab, is effective in patients with uncontrolled active rheumatoid arthritis (RA), despite treatment with methotrexate.

Impact
Rituximab is now approved in the treatment of severe uncontrolled active RA when tumour necrosis factor (TNF)-α antagonists have failed.

Aims
Rituximab is an anti-CD20 monoclonal antibody used in the treatment of CD20$^+$ B cell non-Hodgkin's lymphoma. CD20 is a B cell surface antigen that is expressed only on pre-B and mature B cells. The aim of this trial was to confirm previous (non-RCT) observations that selective depletion of B cells with the use of rituximab leads to sustained clinical improvements for patients with rheumatoid arthritis.

Methods
Patients: 161 patients from 26 rheumatology centres in 11 countries.

Inclusion criteria: Active RA despite treatment with methotrexate:
- Diagnosis of RA (according to the 1987 American College of Rheumatology (ACR) criteria).
- Age >21y;
- Seropositive rheumatoid factor ≥20iu/mL;
- Active disease defined by ≥8 swollen joints, 8 tender joints on ≥10mg methotrexate, and ≥2 of the following:
  - CRP level ≥15mg/L;
  - ESR ≥28mm/h;
  - Early morning stiffness >45min.

Exclusion criteria:
- Diagnosis of autoimmune disease other than RA;
- American Rheumatism Association functional class IV disease;
- Rheumatoid vasculitis; active infection; immunodeficiency; history of malignancy.

Groups: All patients received a 17d course of steroids and one dose of folinic acid:
- Methotrexate alone ≥10mg/wk (n=40);

- Rituximab alone 1g on d1 and 15 (n=40);
- Rituximab on d1 and 15 + cyclophosphamide 750mg on d3 and 17 (n=41);
- Rituximab on d1 and 15 + methotrexate ≥10mg/wk (n=40).

Primary endpoint: Proportion of patients with an ACR50 response (50% improvement) at wk24.

Secondary endpoints:
- 20% and 70% improvement defined by ACR20 and ACR70;
- Change in disease activity score (DAS28).

Follow-up: Clinical assessments at baseline and wk12, 16, 20, and 24.

Results

	% attaining score at wk24		Change in score at wk24
	ACR 50	**ACR 20**	**DAS 28**
Methotrexate	13	38	−1.3±−1.2
Rituximab	33 (*p*=0.005)	65 (*p*=0.03)	−2.2±−1.4 (*p*=0.002)
Rituximab + cyclophosphamide	41 (*p*=0.005)	76 (*p*=0.001)	−2.6±−1.5 (*p*=0.002)
Rituximab + methotrexate	43 (*p*=0.005)	73 (*p*=0.003)	−2.6±−1.3 (*p*=0.001)

p values compared with methotrexate alone

Discussion

This trial demonstrated that two doses of rituximab, alone or in combination with cyclophosphamide or methotrexate, provided a significant and enduring improvement in the symptoms of RA. Additionally, this effect was sustained for up to 48wk. The study also identified B cells as a key contributor to the immunopathogenesis of RA.

Problems

- Depletion of B cells may result in long-term effects on the acquired immune system and careful monitoring is required. However, this study showed a similar incidence of infection in rituximab treated and control groups at wk24 and 48.

Arthritis: cardiovascular outcomes with drug therapies

MEDAL (<u>M</u>ultinational <u>E</u>toricoxib and <u>D</u>iclofenac <u>A</u>rthritis <u>L</u>ong-term**) programme:** Cardiovascular outcomes with etoricoxib and diclofenac in patients with osteoarthritis and rheumatoid arthritis.

AUTHORS: Cannon C, Curtis S, FitzGerald G et al.
REFERENCE: Lancet (2006) 368, 1771–81.
STUDY DESIGN: Meta-analysis
EVIDENCE LEVEL: 1a

Key message
Rates of thrombotic cardiovascular events in patients with osteoarthritis or rheumatoid arthritis on the cyclooxygenase-2 (COX-2) inhibitor, etoricoxib, are similar to those in patients on long-term diclofenac.

Impact
Etoricoxib can be used with caution in patients at risk of thrombotic vascular events.

Aims
Studies had shown increased rates of thrombotic cardiovascular complications with COX-2 inhibitors. However, comparable data for the use of non-steroidal anti-inflammatory drugs (NSAIDs) were not present. This study aimed to compare the relative risk of thrombotic cardiovascular events with etoricoxib and diclofenac using a non-inferiority trial design.

Methods
Patients: 34,701 patients from 1,380 sites in 46 countries (patients combined from 3 trials: MEDAL, EDGE, and EDGE II).

Inclusion criteria:
• Diagnosis of rheumatoid arthritis according to the 1987 American College of Rheumatology;
• Diagnosis of osteoarthritis of the knee, hip, hand, or spine;
• Age ≥50y;
• Low dose aspirin was recommended for prophylaxis in patients with established cardiovascular, peripheral arterial, or cerebrovascular disease.

Groups:
• Etoricoxib (n=17412);
• Diclofenac (n=17289).

Primary endpoint: Comparison of thrombotic cardiovascular events with etoricoxib and diclofenac.

Follow-up: Every 4 months for 3.5y.

Results

The hazard ratio of thrombotic events in the two groups was 0.95 (95% CI 0.81–1.11), showing non-inferiority of etoricoxib to diclofenac.

Discussion

This large study showed no difference in the cardiovascular thrombotic rates of diclofenac and etoricoxib treatment in patients with osteoarthritis and rheumatoid arthritis.

Problems

- This study did not have a placebo group; hence, it was not possible to estimate absolute cardiovascular risks associated with etoricoxib and diclofenac.
- Increased cardiovascular risk has been demonstrated with other similar agents, including rofecoxib and valdecoxib. However, in the light of the findings in the MEDAL programme it cannot be assumed that this is a class effect.
- In the VIGOR study, the COX-2 inhibitor, rofecoxib, was compared with naproxen when more cardiovascular events were observed in the rofecoxib group. The explanation for this could be 3-fold. Firstly, rofecoxib promotes intravascular thrombosis. Secondly, naproxen is protective against these thromboses, or thirdly, both the previous considerations might apply. It would be interesting to compare etoricoxib with naproxen in terms of cardiovascular outcomes.

Ankylosing spondylitis: TNF-α antagonists

Treatment of active ankylosing spondylitis with infliximab: a randomised, controlled, multicentre trial.

AUTHORS: Braun J, Brandt J, Listing J, *et al.*
REFERENCE: Lancet (2002) 359, 1187–93.
STUDY DESIGN: RCT
EVIDENCE LEVEL: 1b

Key message

Infliximab improves the disease activity index in patients with active anky-losing spondylitis despite treatment with non-steroidal anti-inflammatory drugs.

Impact

The first trial to show the effectiveness of tumour necrosis factor-α (TNF-α) antagonists in the treatment of ankylosing spondylitis, providing a therapeutic option for patients with uncontrolled pain and inflammation.

Aims

There are few treatment options for ankylosing spondylitis. Infliximab, a monoclonal antibody to TNF-α, had already been used with great success in other chronic inflammatory conditions such as rheumatoid arthritis. This trial aimed to assess the role of infliximab in the treatment of anky-losing spondylitis.

Methods

Patients: 70 patients recruited from multiple centres in Germany.

Inclusion criteria:
- Diagnosis of ankylosing spondylitis as defined by New York criteria (1984);
- Bath ankylosing spondylitis disease activity index (BASDAI) ≥4;
- Spinal pain as assessed on 10cm visual analogue scale.

Exclusion criteria:
- Active tuberculosis within the previous 3y;
- Specific chest X-ray changes;
- Serious infections in the previous 2 months;
- History of malignant disease in the previous 5y.

Groups: Drugs were administered at 0, 2, and 6wk:
- Infliximab (n=34);
- Placebo (n=35).

Primary endpoint: 50% improvement in BASDAI.

Secondary endpoints: Improvement in visual analogue score for spinal pain, Bath ankylosing spondylitis functional index (BASFI), Bath ankylosing spondylitis metrology index (BASMI), short form (SF)-36, CRP, and ESR.

Follow-up: At 2, 6, and 12wk.

Results

	50% BASDAI improvement at wk12	95% CI	Baseline BASDAI	Wk12 BASDAI
Infliximab	53%	37–69%	6.5	3.3
Placebo	9%	3–22%	6.3	5.7
		$p < 0.0001$		

- BASFI and BASMI showed similar differences.

Discussion

There have been very few randomised studies of disease-modifying drugs in the treatment of ankylosing spondylitis. This study showed infliximab to significantly reduce disease activity, and improve function and quality of life in patients who were chronically ill and partly disabled by ankylosing spondylitis.

Problems

- This was a short-term trial. Therefore, long-term effectiveness of infliximab and its effects on radiographic progression of disease could not be assessed. Subsequent studies show sustained improvement in function although TNF blockade does not arrest progression of radiographic axial damage.

Gout: NSAIDs and COX-2 inhibitors

Safety and effectiveness study: Randomised, double-blind trial of etoricoxib and indometacin in treatment of acute gouty arthritis.

AUTHORS: Schumacher H, Boice J, Daikh D et al.
REFERENCE: BMJ (2002) 324, 1488–92.
STUDY DESIGN: RCT
EVIDENCE LEVEL: 1b

Key message
The cyclooxygenase-2 (COX-2) inhibitor, etoricoxib, is comparable to indometacin in the effective and rapid treatment of gouty arthritis.

Impact
Etoricoxib is now used in the treatment of gout where classical non-steroidal anti-inflammatory drugs (NSAIDs) are contraindicated.

Aims
The NSAID, indometacin, had been established as the most commonly used treatment for gout, despite limited studies demonstrating its efficacy. COX-2 inhibitors had been proposed to have efficacy in treating acute inflammatory conditions without some of the gastrointestinal side effects of NSAIDs. This study aimed to assess the safety and efficacy of a selective COX-2 inhibitor compared with the gold standard treatment, indometacin, in the treatment of acute gouty arthritis.

Methods
Patients: 142 men and 8 women from 43 outpatient centres in 11 countries.

Inclusion criteria:
- Age ≥18y;
- Diagnosis of acute gout (onset within 48h) associated with moderate or severe pain;
- Sum score ≥5 for pain (0–4 point scale), tenderness (0–3 point scale) and swelling (0–3 point scale);
- No clinically significant abnormalities of blood count, chemistry, and urinalysis.

Exclusion criteria:
- Polyarticular gout involving more than 4 joints;
- Concurrent medical or arthritic disease;
- Unstable medical condition;
- Cerebrovascular accident or myocardial infarction in the preceding year;
- Patients on antiplatelet or anticoagulant therapy, digoxin, or corticosteroids (1 month previously).

Groups:
- Indometacin (50mg tds) (n=75);
- Etoricoxib (120mg od) (n=75).

Primary endpoint: Patient's assessment of pain in the study joint (0–4 point scale: none/mild/moderate/severe/extreme) 4h after initial dose on d1, and then 4h after the first dose on d2 to 8.

Secondary endpoints: Investigator's assessment of the study joint on the basis of palpation or passive movement, swelling and erythema, and the patient's and investigator's global assessment of response to treatment.

Follow-up: d2, 5, 8, and 14.

Results

- Patient's assessment of pain in the study joint over d2 to 5 showed a mean change from baseline of −1.72 (95% CI −1.9 to −1.55) for etoricoxib and −1.83 (−2.01 to −1.65) for indometacin.
- Etoricoxib showed efficacy similar to indometacin for all secondary efficacy endpoints.

Discussion

This was the largest controlled trial in gout reported to date. It found that the efficacy of etoricoxib was comparable to that of indometacin with significantly less drug-related adverse effects in the etoricoxib group. In practice, it may be more convenient for patients to take a once-daily formulation, and etoricoxib is likely to be a popular choice in the treatment of acute gout. The study was well designed because emphasis was placed on drug effects during the initial days of the acute gouty attack. This is important because acute gout is usually a self-limiting condition.

Problems

- One limitation of the study was that patients with polyarticular gout were excluded. Therefore, it is difficult to conclude whether the efficacy of the COX-2 inhibitor, etoricoxib, was equivalent to indometacin in this patient population.
- Many patients with gout are also at risk of cardiovascular complications, and such patients were excluded from this study. Given the concern about COX-2 inhibitors' association with thrombotic events, further safety evaluation studies should be undertaken.

Scleroderma lung disease: cyclophosphamide

Cyclophosphamide vs placebo in scleroderma lung disease.

AUTHORS: Tashkin D, Elashoff R, Clements P et al.
REFERENCE: N Engl J Med (2006) 354, 2655–66.
STUDY DESIGN: RCT
EVIDENCE LEVEL: 1b

Key message
Oral cyclophosphamide has some beneficial effect on lung function, dyspnoea, skin thickening, and health-related quality of life in patients with symptomatic scleroderma-related interstitial lung disease.

Impact
Cyclophosphamide is used to improve quality of life in the treatment of scleroderma-related lung disease.

Aims
Cyclophosphamide had been the only treatment to date to show promise in the treatment of scleroderma-related interstitial lung disease in a number of retrospective studies. This study aimed to provide definitive evidence regarding cyclophosphamide's efficacy, toxicity, and risk-benefit ratio in sclerodermalung disease.

Methods
Patients: 158 patients from 13 clinical centres in the USA.

Inclusion criteria:
- Diagnosis of limited or diffuse systemic scleroderma with evidence of active alveolitis on examination of bronchoalveolar lavage fluid or high resolution CT;
- Forced vital capacity (FVC) between 45% and 85% of predicted;
- Grade 2 exertional dyspnoea (according to the baseline instrument of the Mahler Dyspnoea Index).

Exclusion criteria:
- Single breath carbon monoxide diffusion capacity less than 30% predicted;
- History of smoking in preceding 6 months;
- Clinically significant pulmonary hypertension requiring treatment;
- Patients taking prednisolone more than 10mg/d, previous cyclophosphamide treatment and previous potentially disease-modifying treatment.

Groups:
- Oral cyclophosphamide (1mg/kg/d, increased monthly up to 2mg/kg/d) (n=79);
- Placebo (n=79).

Primary endpoint: FVC expressed as a percentage of predicted at 12 months.

Secondary endpoints:
- Health Assessment Questionnaire (HAQ) disability index;
- Skin thickening.

Follow-up: 3 monthly for 12 months.

Results

- 145 patients completed at least 6 months of treatment.
- The mean absolute difference in adjusted 12 months FVC percent predicted between the cyclophosphamide and placebo groups was 2.53% (95% CI, 0.28 to 4.79%), favouring cyclophosphamide ($p<0.03$).
- There was no effect on measures of gas transfer, but there was a significant improvement in dyspnoea, skin thickening, and HAQ disability index in the cyclophosphamide-treated group.

Discussion

Whilst the effect of cyclophosphamide was modest in scleroderma-related interstitial lung disease, there was a marked improvement in quality of life. Therefore, this double-blinded study concluded that this agent should be considered in the treatment of inflammatory lung disease secondary to scleroderma.

Problems

- It would have been interesting to follow up these patients over a longer period in order to determine whether benefit was also seen in mortality, and also to assess the long-term side effect profile of cyclophosphamide.

Painful shoulder: corticosteroid injection vs physiotherapy

Effectiveness of corticosteroid injection vs physiotherapy for treatment of painful stiff shoulder in primary care

AUTHORS: van der Windt D, Koes B, Devillé W *et al.*
REFERENCE: BMJ (1998) 317, 1292–6.
STUDY DESIGN: RCT
EVIDENCE LEVEL: 1b

Key message

Intra-articular corticosteroid injections are superior to physiotherapy in the treatment of painful stiff shoulder syndromes.

Impact

Corticosteroid injections could be used as an early treatment in the management of painful shoulder syndrome.

Aims

Painful stiff shoulder (or capsular) syndrome is characterised by painful restriction of passive motion, particularly lateral rotation and abduction. With limited comparative data, this trial aimed to compare two common interventions in the treatment of this syndrome: intra-articular steroid injection and physiotherapy.

Methods

Patients: 109 patients consulting general practitioners from 40 practices in The Netherlands.

Inclusion criteria:
• Age ≥18y;
• Painful passive glenohumeral mobility with limited lateral rotation more restricted than abduction and medial rotation.

Exclusion criteria:
• Bilateral symptoms;
• Positive painful arc or resistance tests or loss of power;
• Corticosteroid or physiotherapy in the preceding 6 months;
• Contraindications to treatment;
• Type 1 diabetes.

Groups:
• Physiotherapy (n=56);
• Corticosteroid injection (40mg triamcinolone acetate via the posterior approach) (n=53).

Primary endpoint: Outcome at 3 and 7wk as assessed by patient on a 6-point Likert scale and 100mm visual analogue scale (100=very severe pain). Functional disability was evaluated with a shoulder disability questionnaire (a 16-item scale consisting of common situations that might cause shoulder pain).

Secondary endpoints: An independent observer scored the overall clinical severity of the disorder on a visual analogue scale after a physical examination of the patient.

Follow-up: At baseline, then 3, 7, 13, 26, 52wk.

Results

- At 7wk, 77% treated with injections were deemed to be improved compared with 46% treated with physiotherapy.
- However, by 52wk, the differences between the two interventions were relatively small.

Discussion

Intra-articular steroid injections may be preferable to physiotherapy in the initial treatment of painful stiff shoulder because they provide comparatively quick relief of symptoms. However, long-term effects of the two treatments were demonstrated to be similar.

Problems

- Little is known about the long-term effectiveness and adverse event profile of the two interventions. Specifically, more data are required regarding the likelihood of recurrence and the effects of repeated steroid injections on tendon integrity.

Part 2

Surgical specialties

Anaesthetics

Introduction

William Morton was the first person to publicly administer an anaesthetic, ether, on the 16th October 1846 at Massachusetts General Hospital, Boston, although nitrous oxide had earlier been used as an analgesic by Gardner Colton and Horace Wells in 1844. The first anaesthetic performed in the UK was on the 19th December 1846 by a dental surgeon James Robinson. Two days later, at University College Hospital, Robert Liston performed surgery, while a medical student, William Squire, administered the anaesthetic.

Prior to the introduction of anaesthesia, surgery had to be performed as a last resort and on patients who had to be restrained in order to complete the procedure. Professor James Simpson introduced chloroform in November 1847 which was easier to administer than ether but had more side effects. Modern anaesthesia has been based on agents such as halothane, enflurane, isoflurane, sevoflurane, and desflurane.

1878 saw the first use of endotracheal tubes as an airway while local anaesthetic agents were introduced in 1892, making regional anaesthesia possible. 1894 saw the development of the first anaesthetic chart. It took until the 1920s for intravenous anaesthetic induction agents (in the form of barbiturates) to be introduced, with the first muscle relaxant (d-tubocurarine) used in 1942 by Griffiths and Johnson.

Although analgesics such as morphine date back to early times, short-acting opioids were first invented in 1960 and were commercially used from 1963, in the form of fentanyl. With the introduction of propofol in 1986, the concept of total intravenous anaesthesia (TIVA) was made possible in conjunction with the short-acting opioids such as alfentanil or sufentanil, and more recently the ultrashort acting opioid (remifentanil).

With the advent of newer anaesthetic agents capable of rapid onset and better recovery profiles, premedication is used less frequently. As a result, daycase surgery rates are increasing. One key facet to modern anaesthesia has been the recognition of the need to prevent post-operative nausea and vomiting. Antiemetics have stayed as they were in the last few decades apart from the addition of the hydroxytryptamine antagonists.

In today's world, the anaesthetist is involved in >65% of the clinical areas in the hospital including the anaesthetic room, endoscopy, accident and emergency, pain clinics, and intensive care. Anaesthetics have come a long way from just a whiff of ether. With safer anaesthetic agents and techniques, boundaries have been pushed in the type of operations being carried out and the pre-operative morbidity of the patients on whom they are performed.

Pre-operative optimisation

> Reducing the risk of major elective surgery: RCT of pre-operative optimisation of oxygen delivery.
>
> **AUTHORS:** Wilson J, Woods I, Fawcett J et al.
> **REFERENCE:** BMJ (1999) 318, 1099–103.
> **STUDY DESIGN:** RCT
> **EVIDENCE LEVEL:** 1b

Key message
Pre-optimisation of high-risk elective patients using fluids and inotropes reduces mortality and morbidity.

Impact
Although pre-optimisation of patients may save lives and subsequently reduce costs, the initial high costs of implementing this for routine practice have so far precluded its regular use.

Aims
The extent of pre-and post-operative monitoring following major elective surgery is variable, depending upon a number of factors, including anticipation of development of complications, and intensive care unit (ICU) or high dependency unit (HDU) bed availability. Measures that optimise the cardiac index and enhance O_2 delivery to tissues, including the use of fluid and inotropes, have been proposed to improve outcomes in those at high risk. This study aimed to determine whether improving O_2 delivery pre-operatively improved overall outcomes, and whether the choice of inotrope used made a difference.

Methods
Patients: 138 patients at 1 UK centre.

Inclusion criteria: At high risk of developing peri-operative complications (based upon type of surgery or presence of specified comorbidities).

Primary endpoints: Hospital mortality and morbidity.

Secondary endpoints:
- Length of stay in hospital;
- Use of intensive care or high dependency care;
- Haemodynamic measurements.

Groups:
- Control group (received treatment as preferred by the surgeon and anaesthetist, according to routine practice) (n=46);
- Treatment groups: adrenaline (n=46) and dopexamine (n=46):
  - Admitted to HDU/ICU 4h pre-operatively;
  - Large-bore IV cannula, arterial line, and pulmonary artery catheter (PAC) inserted;

- Fluid and inotropes optimised until O_2 delivery (DO_2) >600mL/min/m^2 achieved. DO_2=cardiac index x blood O_2 saturation x blood O_2 content (Hb) x 1.34;
- Intra-operative treatment was at the discretion of the anaesthetist;
- Post-operatively, treatment groups and those from the control group deemed to need ICU, went to ICU, where inotropes were continued for 12–24h.

Results

	Adrenaline (n=46)	Dopexamine (n=46)	Control (n=46)
Hospital survival	98% (n=45)	96% (n=44)	83% (n=38)
Actual mortality	2%	4%	17%
Predicted mortality	12%	15%	13%
Standardised morbidity ratio (95% CI)	0.19 (0 to 1.05)	0.28 (0.04 to 1.08)	1.36 (0.6 to 2.75)
Actual morbidity	52%	30%	61%
Predicted morbidity	54%	61%	57%
Standardised mortality ratio (95% CI)	0.96 (0.62 to 1.44)	0.50 (0.27 to 0.84)	1.07 (0.71 to 1.54)

Fisher's test for combined treatment groups vs control, p=0.007.

Discussion

This study showed lower mortality and morbidity in the pre-optimised patients in whom dopexamine was used. Although lower mortality was demonstrated in the adrenaline group, there was no improvement in morbidity. Therefore, pre-optimisation demonstrated clear mortality benefits (treatment group mortality 3% vs control group mortality 17%) and reduced length of hospital stay; however, these results will have a major impact on need for resources such as HDU/ICU beds.

Problems

- A meta-analysis of improving O_2 delivery measured by PAC in ICU patients failed to show a positive result (*Crit Care Med* 2002: 30, 1686–92). Studies with larger numbers are needed.
- A cost analysis would be useful to determine whether pre-optimisation would cost more or save money in the long-term.

Antibiotic prophylaxis in colorectal surgery

Randomised multicentre trial of antibiotic prophylaxis in elective colorectal surgery: single dose vs. 3 doses of a second-generation cephalosporin without metroniadazole and oral antibiotics.

AUTHORS: Fujita S, Saito N, Yamada T *et al.*
REFERENCE: Arch Surg (2007) 142, 657–61.
STUDY DESIGN: RCT
EVIDENCE LEVEL: 1b

Key message
A single dose of prophylactic antibiotic produces comparable results to multiple (3) doses in most cases, but there is a significant decrease in surgical site infections with 3 doses.

Impact
Local policy needs to dictate prophylactic antibiotic regimens as the risk of infections such as methicillin-resistant *Staphylococcus aureus* (MRSA) and *Clostridium difficile* need to be weighed up against the need for multiple prophylactic antibiotic doses.

Aims
Antibiotic prophylaxis has become standard practice for patients undergoing colorectal surgery. However, the choice of antibiotic as well as the optimal route and dose continue to be the subject of debate. This study aimed to establish differences in surgical site infections after using a single vs a 3-dose prophylactic antibiotic regimen in patients undergoing colorectal surgery.

Methods
Patients: 384 patients at 7 centres in Japan.

Inclusion criteria:
- Age 20–80y;
- Undergoing elective colorectal surgery.

Exclusion criteria:
- Emergency operations;
- Small bowel obstruction;
- Stomal or bypass surgery;
- Pre-operative infectious disease;
- Penicillin or cephalosporin allergy;
- Antibiotic administration pre-admission;
- Inflammatory bowel diseases;
- Angina or myocardial infarction;
- Mild or severe renal dysfunction;
- Mild or severe diabetes mellitus;
- Steroid administration before surgery.

Groups: All patients underwent similar bowel preparation 1d pre-surgery:
- Single-dose: 1x dose of 1g cefmetazole IV pre-incision (n=190);
- 3-dose: 1x dose of 1g cefmetazole IV pre-incision and 2x post-operative 1g doses at 8h and 16h after first dose (n=187).

Primary endpoint:
- Incisional surgical site infection (SSI).

Secondary endpoints:
- Organ or space SSI;
- All other infectious complications within 30d (e.g. urinary tract infection).

Results

Primary endpoint	Single-dose (n=190)	3-doses (n=187)	*p*
Incisional SSI	27 (14.2%)	8 (4.3%)	0.009
Secondary endpoints			
Organ/space SSI	5 (2.6%)	9 (4.8%)	0.3
Other infectious complication	12 (6.3%)	9 (4.8%)	0.5

Discussion
There is good evidence to show that antibiotic prophylaxis is essential in abdominal surgery. However, there is no consensus as to the optimal dose and duration of prophylactic treatment. This study showed a decrease in incisional infections post-operatively, but no other significant differences in infectious complications, between single and multiple (3) doses of antibiotic.

Problems
- In the current climate, every intervention needs to be justified. If a longer course of antibiotics is to be common practice, it will need to be justified and weighed against the risk of more resistant infections, e.g. MRSA and *Clostridium difficile*.

Laryngoscopy: use of cricoid pressure

The effect of cricoid pressure and neck support on the view at laryngoscopy.

AUTHORS: Vanner R, Clarke P, Moore W *et al.*
REFERENCE: Anaesthesia (1997) 52, 896–913.
STUDY DESIGN: RCT
EVIDENCE LEVEL: 1b

Key message
Cricoid pressure provides improved views at laryngoscopy, particularly if applied upwards and backwards.

Impact
Correctly applied cricoid pressure can usually improve poor laryngoscopic views, facilitating easier intubation.

Aims
Cricoid pressure is routinely used during 'crash' induction to prevent regurgitation of gastric contents (i.e. in emergency cases with patients who have not been starved). However, some reports indicate that it may make tracheal intubation more difficult and that there is a lack of evidence to substantiate the use of adjunct techniques, including foam neck support and bimanual cricoid pressure. This study aimed to investigate the views at laryngoscopy with and without application of cricoid pressure, as well as views obtained with standard upward pressure vs backward and upward pressure.

Methods
Patients: 50 patients at 1 centre in the UK.

Inclusion criteria:
● Female;
● Not pregnant;
● Gynaecological operation requiring tracheal intubation.

Exclusion criteria:
● Cardiovascular disease;
● Symptoms of reflux.

Conditions:
● 6 conditions: no cricoid pressure, standard cricoid pressure, and upward and backward cricoid pressure, all with and without neck support;
● Larynx view grading 1–3: as proposed by Cormack and Lehane (*Anaesthesia* (1984) 39, 1105–11). Grade 1 represents a better view of the glottis, grade 3 represents no clear views of the glottis.

Results

(With neck support)	Laryngoscopy view			Probability of best view
	1	**2**	**3**	
No pressure	44	5	1	6% (CI 2 to 12%)
Upward and backward pressure	50	0	0	44% (CI 34 to 54%)
Standard pressure	48	2	0	11% (CI 6 to 19%)

- Results with and without neck support=no significant difference.
- Laryngoscopy view: $p=0.02$ (not significant, as inadequate grade 2/3 views for Chi-square or other statistical tests to be valid).

	Best view		Best view	
Up and back	n=51	With support	n=9
Standard pressure	n=13	No support	n=20
No difference	n=36	No difference	n=21
CONCLUSION	Up and back better than standard ($p<0.01$)	CONCLUSION	No significant difference ($p=0.1$)

Discussion

This study formally confirmed what was anecdotally noted by most ana-esthetists in practice: correctly applied cricoid pressure of optimal force helps improve poor laryngoscopy views. Backward and upward pressure gave better views than standard cricoid pressure. However, there was no significant improvement obtained by the use of a supporting neck pillow. Note that this technique is very 'UK and colonies' specific. In most anaesthetists' minds, the Sellick manoeuvre remains the optimal technique (*Lancet* (1961) 2, 404–6).

Problems

- Potential for observer bias (as it was not possible to blind a study of this nature).
- Small numbers.

Depth of anaesthesia: bispectral monitoring

> **B-AWARE!:** Bispectral index monitoring to prevent awareness during anaesthesia.
>
> **AUTHORS:** Myles P, Leslie K, McNeil J et al.
> **REFERENCE:** Lancet (2004) 363, 1757–63.
> **STUDY DESIGN:** RCT
> **EVIDENCE LEVEL:** 1b

Key message

Using bispectral index (BIS) monitoring in high-risk patients reduces the incidence of awareness under anaesthesia.

Impact

BIS monitoring should ideally be used for high-risk anaesthesia to prevent patient awareness of the procedure. Cost and other resource issues persist in limiting its adoption into mainstream practice in the UK; however, medico-legal considerations related to the detection of intra-operative awareness have led to its wider use in some populations (e.g. USA and Australia).

Aims

Awareness under anaesthesia is a distressing complication, quoted to occur in <0.2% of surgical patients. Incidence is reportedly higher during caesarean section and cardiac/trauma surgery. Although depth of anaesthesia is classically monitored by clinical measures, including blood pressure (BP) and heart rate, these are unreliable. BIS monitoring involves time and frequency domain, and bispectral analysis of the electroencephalogram (EEG). This trial aimed to assess whether BIS could reduce the incidence of awareness under anaesthesia.

Methods

Patients: 2463 patients at multiple centres in Australia and New Zealand.

Inclusion criteria:

- Age ≥18y, undergoing relaxant general anaesthesia;
- ≥1 risk factor for awareness:
  - Caesarean section, high-risk cardiac surgery (ejection fraction <30%, cardiac index <2.1L/min/m^2, severe aortic stenosis, pulmonary hypertension, undergoing off-pump coronary artery bypass graft surgery), acute trauma with hypovolaemia, rigid bronchoscopy, significant impairment of cardiovascular status and expectant intra-operative hypotension, severe end-stage lung disease, history of awareness, anticipated difficult intubation, known/suspected heavy alcohol intake, chronic benzodiazepine/opiate use, current protease inhibitor use.

Exclusion criteria:
- Traumatic brain injury, memory impairment, or psychosis;
- Known EEG abnormality.

Groups:
- BIS monitoring (n=1225);
- Control (n=1238).

Primary endpoint: Patient-confirmed awareness under anaesthesia at any time (structured questionnaire).

Secondary endpoints:
- Possible awareness;
- Recovery time;
- Hypnotic drug administration;
- Marked hypotension (systolic BP <90mmHg requiring drug treatment);
- Anxiety and depression (hospital anxiety and depression validated scale);
- Patient satisfaction (1–5 scale, at 30/7);
- Major complications;
- 30d mortality.

Follow-up: Post-operative interviews at 2–6h, 24–36h, and 30d.

Results

Primary endpoint	BIS (n=1225)	Control (n=1238)	p
Awareness	2 (0.2%)	11 (0.9%)	0.02
Secondary endpoints			
Possible awareness	22 (1.8%)	27 (2.2%)	0.5
Recovery time	63 (40–95) min	66 (40–100) min	0.3
Hypnotic drug given	91 (7%)	80 (6%)	0.3
Marked hypotension	717 (58%)	694 (56%)	0.2
Anxiety (A) and depression (D) score	3 and 3	3 and 3	1.0A 0.7D
Patient 'very satisfied'	751 (67%)	781 (68%)	0.5
Major complications	283 (23.2%)	288 (23.4%)	0.9
Mortality at 30 days	51 (4.2%)	50 (4.1%)	0.9

Discussion

A well designed trial with a very specific primary outcome. Reduction in awareness was the only positive trial outcome. Number needed to treat (NNT) to prevent one episode of awareness in high-risk patients was 138.

Problems

- Only patients at high-risk for awareness were included; the cost of using a BIS monitor for all patients may not be justified. However, this must be balanced against the considerable cost of awareness.

Peri-operative β-blockade

POISE (Peri-Operative ISchaemic Evaluation): Effects of extended-release metoprolol succinate in patients undergoing non-cardiac surgery.

AUTHORS: Devereaux P, Yang H, Yusuf S *et al.* (POISE study group).
REFERENCE: Lancet (2008) 370, 1839–47.
STUDY DESIGN: RCT
EVIDENCE LEVEL: 1b

Key message

Peri-operative β-blocker decreases the incidence of cardiac death, myocardial infarction (MI), and cardiac arrest; but increases overall all-cause mortality and strokes in high-risk patients undergoing non-cardiac surgery.

Impact

Peri-operative β-blockade continues to be the subject of much debate.

Aims

Small non-cardiac surgery trials had suggested β-blockers might reduce the incidence of major cardiovascular events *(New Engl J Med (1999) 335, 1713–20 and (1999) 341, 1789–94)*. However, more recent moderate-sized RCTs had not demonstrated such a benefit *(e.g. BMJ (2006)332, 1482–88)*. With a meta-analysis of non-cardiac RCTs also suggesting a positive effect of β-blockade, but at the cost of an increased risk of hypotension and bradycardia *(BMJ (2005) 331, 313–21)*, there remained no clear consensus. This study aimed to evaluate the effect of peri-operative β-blockade on mortality and morbidity in patients undergoing non-cardiac surgery.

Methods

Patients: 8351 patients from 190 centres in 23 countries.

Inclusion criteria: Undergoing non-cardiac surgery, and:
- Age >45y, with expected length of hospital stay ≥24h;
- Any of: coronary artery disease, peripheral vascular disease, stroke, hospitalisation for congestive cardiac failure (CCF) in past 3y, undergoing major vascular surgery (except arteriovenous shunt, vein stripping, or carotid endarterectomy);
- Any 3 of 7 risk criteria: undergoing (1) intrathoracic/intraperitoneal or (2) emergency/urgent surgery; (3) history of CCF, (4) transient ischaemic attacks; (5) diabetes mellitus; (6) serum creatinine >175micromol/L; (7) age >70y.

Exclusion criteria:
- HR <50beats/min or second/third degree heart block;
- Asthma or prior adverse reaction to β-blocker or taking verapamil;
- Receiving β-blocker or physician plan to start one peri-operatively;
- Coronary artery bypass graft (past 5y) and no ischaemia since revascularisation;
- Low-risk surgical procedure (based on physicians' judgement).

Groups:
- Extended-release metoprolol succinate (n=4174; 482 withdrew);
- Placebo (n=4177; 485 withdrew).

- Initial dose of metoprolol (100mg PO)/placebo, 2–4h pre-surgery; then 0–6h post-op. 12h after first post-op dose, daily metoprolol (200mg)/placebo started (continued for 30d). If oral route unsuitable, 6hourly IV metoprolol (15mg)/saline (placebo) until oral resumed.

Primary endpoint: Composite of cardiovascular (CV) death, non-fatal MI, and non-fatal cardiac arrest, at 30d.

Secondary endpoints: See table below.

Follow-up: Morbidity and mortality data at 30d after randomisation.

Results

Primary endpoints	Metoprolol (n=4174)	Placebo (n=4177)	HR (95% CI)	*p*
CV death, arrest, MI	243 (5.8%)	290 (6.9%)	0.83 (0.7 to 0.99)	0.04
Non-fatal MI	151 (3.6%)	215 (5.1%)	0.7 (0.57 to 0.86)	0.0007
Secondary endpoints				
All cause mortality	129 (3.1%)	97 (2.3%)	1.33 (1.03 to 1.74)	0.03
Coronary revascularisation	11 (0.3%)	27 (0.6%)	0.41 (0.20 to 0.82)	0.01
*Atrial fibrillation	91 (2.2%)	120 (2.9%)	0.76 (0.58 to 0.99)	0.04
Non-fatal stroke	41 (1%)	19 (0.5%)	2.17 (1.26 to 3.74)	0.005
*Hypotension	626 (15%)	404 (9.7%)	1.55 (1.38 to 1.74)	<0.0001
*Bradycardia	274 (6.6%)	101 (2.4%)	2.71 (2.19 to 3.43)	<0.001

* Clinically significant symptoms/signs.

Discussion

Fewer in the metoprolol group reached the primary composite endpoint, and fewer had MI; however, there were more deaths, strokes, and clinically significant hypotension and bradycardia. With regard to cardiac mortality/morbidity, these findings are at variance with the smaller early studies and are more in keeping with larger trials such as POBBLE (*J Vasc Surg* (2005) 41, 602–9), MaVS (*Am Heart J* (2006) 152, 983–90) and DIPOM *(BMJ* (2006) 332, 1482). Although post-operative cardiac morbidity/mortality is high in patients with DM, DIPOM was the only study to specifically examine β-blockade in diabetics; however, high numbers of withdrawals meant that a meaningful answer was not achieved. Overall, these results are contrary to the present guidelines of the American Heart Association (AHA) and American College of Cardiology (ACC). In many ways, POISE was disappointing, as the role of β-blockade in peri-operative care remained undetermined; however, in those already taking β-blockers, it has been proven that the drugs should not be discontinued peri-operatively.

Problems

- The increased incidence of relative hypotension could have contributed to the increase in strokes; it is worrying that the BP was allowed to fall to such an extent (<100mmHg) in a group at high risk for carotid artery atherosclerosis, who require higher driving pressures to prevent stroke.

Safety of nitrous oxide

ENIGMA: AvoidancE of NItrous oxide for patients underGoing MAjor surgery.

AUTHORS: Myles P, Leslie K, Chan M *et al.* (ENIGMA trial group).
REFERENCE: Anesthesiology (2007) 107, 221–31.
STUDY DESIGN: RCT
EVIDENCE LEVEL: 1b

Key message
Patients who do not receive nitrous oxide (N_2O) have fewer complications after major surgery. Hospital stay remains unchanged.

Impact
N_2O use remains a matter of debate and its routine use can be questioned. There are no studies to date comparing the safety of different inspired N_2O concentrations.

Aims
Although a commonly used anaesthetic agent, N_2O has several reported adverse effects. Furthermore, its weak anaesthetic properties require it to be administered at high concentrations, thereby reducing the delivery of supplemental oxygen. The aim of this trial was to assess whether using N_2O as part of an anaesthetic increased complication rates and length of stay.

Methods
Patients: 2050 patients, at 19 centres in Australia.

Inclusion criteria:
- Age ≥18y;
- Surgery lasting ≥2h;
- Expected to be in hospital for at least 3d.

Exclusion criteria:
- Cardiac or thoracic surgery;
- Single lung ventilation;
- N_2O considered contraindicated by the anaesthetist.

Groups:
- N_2O group (n=1015; 9 did not receive N_2O);
- N_2O-free group (n=997; 5 received N_2O).

Primary endpoint: Duration of inpatient hospital stay.

Secondary endpoints:
- Duration of intensive care stay;
- Post-operative complications within 30d, including:
  - Any respiratory complication (pneumonia, pulmonary atelectasis, pneumothorax, pulmonary embolism);

- Any major complication (pneumonia, pneumothorax, pulmonary embolism, wound infection, myocardial infarction (MI), venous thromboembolism, stroke, awareness, and death;
- Other (fever, severe nausea and vomiting, blood transfusion, and quality of recovery at 24h after surgery).

Results

Primary endpoint	N_2O	N_2O-free	p
Length of hospital stay[+](d)	7.1 (4–11.8)	7 (4–10.9)	0.06
Secondary endpoints			
Length of stay ICU[++](d)	1	1	0.02
Post-operative complications	21%	16%	0.003

[*] Although quoted in this way in the paper, there is clearly skewing of this outcome measure. The choice of median values in the table reflects the marked right (positive) skew of the outcome data.

[+] Values = median (range)

Discussion

This study showed no differences in primary outcome or length of hospital stay, but did show decreases in post-operative complications such as severe nausea and vomiting in the N_2O-free group. Although incidence of MI or death was reduced in this group, differences were not significant. The effects of increased inspired oxygen were found to have no statistical impact on primary outcome, length of intensive care unit (ICU) stay, wound infection, or severe nausea and vomiting. Whether this is a consequence of increased oxygen or reduced N_2O delivery remains debatable.

Problems

- This was, in a sense, a negative study, of which the subject still remains a much debated field in anaesthesia. The perceived benefits of N_2O include analgesia, reduced requirement of other anaesthetic components; reduction in risk of awareness in paralysed patients; and its safe use in concentrations up to 50% by non-medical practitioners (e.g. midwives, paramedics).
- Authors claim lack of significance for decreased MI/death in the N_2O-free group may be due to study being underpowered. F/U study (ENIGMA II) is underway.

Safety of epidural analgesia

> **MASTER** (**M**ulticentre **A**ustralian **ST**udy of **E**pidu**R**al anaesthesia)
> **trial:** Epidural anaesthesia and analgesia and outcome of major surgery:
> a randomised trial.
>
> **AUTHORS:** Rigg J, Jamrozik K, Myles P *et al.* *(*MASTER Study Group).
> **REFERENCE:** Lancet (2002) 359, 1276–82.
> **STUDY DESIGN:** RCT
> **EVIDENCE LEVEL:** 1b

Key message

Epidural anaesthesia does not affect post-operative mortality or major
complication rates, but does decrease respiratory complications.

Impact

Epidural anaesthesia as post-operative analgesia for high-risk patients has
the desirable potential of reducing respiratory complications, a factor
that may improve post-operative recovery.

Aims

The benefits of epidural analgesia have been long debated. Whilst it can
reduce the peri-operative stress response, epidural catheter insertion is
not without its risks. This trial aimed to compare outcomes in high-risk
patients in whom epidural anaesthesia or alternative regimes had been
used for post-operative analgesia.

Methods

Patients: 888 patients, at 25 centres in 6 countries (Australia, East Asia, and
the Middle East).

Inclusion criteria:
- High-risk patients, i.e. ≥1 risk factor for adverse events:
  - Morbid obesity, diabetes mellitus, chronic renal failure, respiratory
    insufficiency, major hepatocellular disease, cardiac failure, acute
    myocardial infarction (MI), myocardial ischaemia, *or* age ≥75 and ≥2
    of: significant respiratory disease, cardiac dysrhythmia, hypertension,
    moderate obesity, frailty, previous MI;
- Elective non-laparoscopic surgery of the abdomen, or oesophagectomy;
- Operations lasting >1h.

Exclusion criteria:
- Cardiac or pulmonary surgery;
- Age <18y;
- Patients undergoing surgery within 12h of admission to hospital;
- Contraindications for epidural insertion.

Groups:
- Epidural group (n=461). Only 225 fully compliant with protocol of 72h
  of post-operative epidural analgesia);
- Control group (n=454).

Primary endpoint: Combined endpoint of mortality or major post-operative complication within 30d.

Secondary endpoint: Visual analogue pain score.

Results

	Control	Epidural	*p*
Combined endpoint	60.7%	57.1%	0.3
Respiratory failure	30.2%	23.3%	0.02
10cm visual analogue pain score (after coughing, morning of day 3)	3.5 (SD 2.6)	2.8 (SD 2.5)	0.0007

Discussion

Although no difference in mortality or major post-operative complication rate was demonstrated in this study, the post-operative respiratory failure rate was less in the epidural group. This was supported by lower pain scores in patients having epidural analgesia, which allowed better physiotherapy, deep breathing, and coughing to be performed post-operatively. Although this study demonstrated a non-significant benefit for the defined primary endpoint of mortality or major complication within 30d, it is reassuring to know that epidurals do decrease respiratory complications.

Problems

- The study was too small to perform subset analysis of any specific group of patients. Repeating this trial using a more defined group of high-risk surgical patients might demonstrate a significant benefit in the primary endpoint.

Post-epidural headache

Postdural puncture headache: a randomised comparison of five spinal needles in obstetric patients.

AUTHORS: Vallejo M, Mandell G, Sabo D et al.
REFERENCE: Anesth Analg (2000) 91, 916–20.
STUDY DESIGN: RCT
EVIDENCE LEVEL: 1b

Key message
Pencil-point spinal needles significantly reduce the incidence of post-dural puncture headache in the obstetric population.

Impact
This study highlighted the need for increased availability and use of pencil-point non-cutting needles in obstetric anaesthesia.

Aims
Postdural puncture headache (PDPH) is an established complication of spinal anaesthesia and is associated with a variety of factors, including age, sex, pregnancy, previous history of PDPH, and needle characteristics (size, tip shape, bevel orientation, approach). This study aimed to compare the incidence of PDPH and need for epidural blood patch (EBP) treatment rates after the use of five different spinal needles.

Methods
Patients: 1002 women at 1 centre in the USA.

Inclusion criteria: All women bookers for elective lower segment caesarean section (LSCS) under spinal anaesthesia.

Groups:
Randomised into receiving spinal analgesia with 1 of 5 needle types: 2x cutting (26-Gauge (G) Atraucan, and 25-G Quincke) and 3x non-cutting (24-G Gertie Marx, 24-G Sprotte, and 25-G Whitacre).

Procedure:
• Patients pre-hydrated with 1.5L Ringer's lactate IV;
• All spinal procedures done in sitting position;
• Standard dose of hyperbaric bupivacaine (12–14mg), as well as fentanyl (25mcg) and morphine (0.25mg).
• PDPH treatment: PDPH treated conservatively for 24h;
• EBP undertaken if intensity unchanged after 24h. EBP performed with 10–20mL of autologous blood, at same site as spinal.

Follow-up: Recruitment period Jan 1993–Dec 1998. Patients seen daily by a blinded assessor. PDPH defined as occipital/frontal headache relieved by supine position. Patients with PDPH assessed daily until discharge. All patients had F/U by telephone 1wk post-discharge.

Results

Needle type	n	PDPH	EBP
Atraucan	180	9 (5%)	5 (55%)
Quincke	172	15 (8.7%)	10 (66%)
Gertie Marx	201	8 (4%)	1 (12.5%)
Sprotte	211	6 (2.8%)	0
Whitacre	201	6 (3.1%)	0

- EBP rate: significantly lower in Gertie Marx, Sprotte, and Whitacre groups, compared with Quincke; and also in Sprotte and Whitacre groups compared with Atraucan.
- 37 patients excluded as no information on bevel orientation available.

Discussion

The pencil-point, non-cutting Sprotte and Whitacre needles were associated with significantly lower incidences of PDPH. The Quincke needle had the highest rates of PDPH and EBP use. Although pencil-point needles are more expensive, the added costs of EBP should also be considered.

Problems

- Although the study took place between 1993–1998, its implications on practice remain relevant today. There have since been studies that show performing spinal anaesthesia in the sitting position increases the chance of having PDPH (although this should not affect the overall conclusions of this study as all of the spinal needles were inserted with patients in the same position).

Post-operative nausea and vomiting

> **IMPACT** (**I**nternational **M**ulticentre **P**rotocol to **A**ssess the single and **C**ombined benefits of anti-emetic medication in a controlled clinical **T**rial): A factorial trial of six interventions for the prevention of post-operative nausea and vomiting.
>
> **AUTHORS:** Apfel C, Korttila K, Abdalla M *et al.* (IMPACT investigators).
> **REFERENCE:** N Engl J Med (2004) 350, 2441–51.
> **STUDY DESIGN:** RCT
> **EVIDENCE LEVEL:** 1b

Key message

Several treatment strategies reduce the relative risk of post-operative nausea and vomiting (PONV). Prophylaxis for low-risk patients is not deemed cost-effective; however, moderate-risk patients may benefit from a single intervention and high-risk patients may need multiple interventions.

Impact

Patients should be risk stratified in order to tailor treatment.

Aims

PONV is a common complication, often secondary to anaesthetic use. Aside from being unpleasant for patients, vomiting increases the risks of aspiration and other complications, subsequently delaying discharge and increasing costs of patient care. This 2^6 factorial study aimed to compare adverse outcomes in high-risk patients in whom epidural anaesthesia or an alternative was used for post-operative analgesia.

Methods

Patients: 5199 patients at 28 international centres.

Inclusion criteria:

- Elective surgery lasting ≥1h;
- ≥40% risk of PONV (presence of ≥2 risk factors: female, non-smoker, previous PONV, motion sickness, anticipated post-operative opioid use).

Exclusion criteria:

- Study drug contraindicated;
- Emetogenic/anti-emetic use in previous 24h;
- Expected to require post-operative ventilation;
- Pregnant or lactating.

Groups:

- Anti-emetic drug (vs no treatment):
  - Ondansetron (n=5161);
  - Droperidol (n=5161).
- Maintenance with propofol (vs inhalational anaesthetic, n=5161);
- Nitrogen as carrier gas (vs N_2O, n=4277);
- Remifentanil (vs fentanyl, n=4789).

Primary endpoint: Incidence of any nausea, emetic episodes (retching or vomiting), or both during first 24 post-operative hours.

Results

Intervention	Received intervention		% relative risk	p
	YES	**NO**	**(95% CI)**	
Ondansetron	735/2576 (28.5%)	996/2585 (38.5%)	−26 (−31.5 to −19.9)	<0.001
Dexamethasone	739/2596 (28.5%)	992/2565 (38.7%)	−26.4 (−31.9 to −20.4)	<0.001
Droperidol	742/2573 (28.8%)	989/2588 (38.2%)	−24.5 (−30.2 to−18.4)	<0.001
Propofol*	1066/3427 (31.1%)	665/1734 (38.4%)	−18.9 (−25 to −12.3)	<0.001
Nitrogen carrier†	668/2146 (31.1%)	755/2131 (35.4%)	−12 (−19.3 to −4.3)	0.003
Remifentanil‡	827/2386 (34.7%)	792/2403 (33%)	5.2 (−2.9 to 13.8)	0.2

* vs inhalational anaesthetic / † vs N_2O as carrier gas / ‡ vs fentanyl.

Discussion

This was the biggest study of prophylaxis for PONV. All of the anti-emetic drugs were equally effective. Relative risk reduction was approximately equal to that seen when using total intravenous anaesthesia (i.e. a combination of substituting a volatile inhalational anaesthetic with propofol for maintenance and substituting N_2O with nitrogen as a carrier gas). Whilst a maximum relative reduction in risk of PONV of 70% can be achieved by combination of options, this must be offset against the costs and risks of adverse events.

Problems

- Application of the results to a general surgical population relies upon patients being stratified into being at high risk of PONV. The risk factors for PONV can be ranked as: high-dose opioid use**, history of PONV**, history of motion sickness, non-smokers**, female patients**, type of surgery (high risk associated with gynaecological surgery; middle ear surgery; gastrointestinal distension; passage of blood into stomach following ear, nose, and throat or dental surgery; thyroid and sinus surgery; laparoscopic surgery), early ambulation, and anaesthetic drugs—induction of anaesthesia with etomidate or ketamine; use of N_2O; volatile agents (especially if used for induction of anaesthesia).

** main factors

Breast surgery

Introduction

The background to the development of the specialty of breast cancer in England came with surgeons such as Dr David Patey of Middlesex Hospital, who first described a simple mastectomy in the 1940s. In Scandinavia, multidisciplinary working emerged in the early 1970s, leading to the development of the concept of breast screening and a more collaborative approach towards patient management. Subsequently, in 1985, Professor Forrest recommended breast screening to be established nationally in the UK, a policy later adopted by Mrs Thatcher's government. The initiation of breast screening in 1990 led to multidisciplinary working of surgeons, radiologists, pathologists, and oncologists, and has improved breast cancer survival significantly across the UK.

The emergence of guidelines for the management of breast cancer and targets for its early diagnosis have ensured that breast cancer treatment and management remains one of the most heavily policed and regulated treatments by the government. Breast cancer trials started in the early 1930s and have made major contributions to the field of EBM. The first major trials involved the use of radiotherapy after mastectomy and were carried out in the UK; those were followed by tamoxifen treatment trials, which have majorly impacted on the management of breast cancer. The UK continues to play a major role in trial development and delivery.

Breast cancer: lymph node involvement

A randomised comparison of sentinel node biopsy with routine axillary dissection in breast cancer.

AUTHORS: Veronesi U, Paganelli G, Viale G *et al.*
REFERENCE: N Engl J Med (2003) 349, 546–53.
STUDY DESIGN: RCT
EVIDENCE LEVEL: 1b

Key message

70% of breast cancer patients are node negative. Axillary surgery, in the form of axillary dissection, leads to arm swelling, lymphoedema, and loss of sensation. Which patients are node-negative can be predicted by sentinel node biopsy; this can avoid axillary clearance while preventing morbidity associated with the procedure.

Impact

Sentinel node biopsy is now accepted as the treatment of choice for women with small breast cancers, including screening detected breast cancers.

Aims

Breast cancer screening allows the diagnosis of cancer to be made at an early stage, and at a time when the axillary nodes are likely to be free of disease. Axillary dissection is a procedure that can be associated with considerable morbidity. Furthermore, the cost to the UK's National Health Service (NHS) of treatment for complications such as arm swelling and lymphoedema associated with axillary clearance surgery is approximately £200m per year. Therefore reducing these complications by more conservative sentinel node biopsy is a priority. The aim of this study was to determine the safety and morbidity from sentinel node biopsy when used to stage breast cancer.

Methods

Patients: 516 women at 1 centre in Italy.

Inclusion criteria:
- Tumour ≤2cm in diameter;
- Clinically node negative.

Exclusion criteria:
- Previous invasive breast cancer;
- Previous treatment for invasive breast cancer;
- Clinically node-positive cancers;

Groups:
- Sentinel node biopsy (n=259);
- Axillary clearance (n=257).

Primary endpoint: Prediction of the status of sentinel node, measured in terms of the % cases of axillary involvement detected by sentinel node biopsy in relation to the % found by axillary dissection.

Secondary endpoints:
- Indicators of quality of life;
- Number of axillary node metastasis appearing during F/U;
- Disease-free and overall survival.

Results

	Sentinel node biopsy (n=259)	Axillary clearance (n=257)	*p*
Positive sentinel node	n=92 (35.5%) (95% CI 29.7 to 41.7)	n=83 (32.3%) (95% CI 26.6 to 38.4)	ns
Axillary pain (at 24 months)	8%	39%	<0.001
Arm swelling (at 24 months)	1%	37%	<0.001
Recurrence	n=13	n=21	ns
Deaths	n=1	n=2	ns

Discussion

This, and the subsequent ALMANAC trial (*J Natl Cancer Inst* (2006) 98, 599–609) demonstrated that sentinel node biopsy was an appropriate method for staging the axilla. Sentinel node biopsy was carried out using a radioisotope and a colloid-linked blue dye injected either around the tumour or underneath the ipsilateral areola, allowing tracking of the isotope and dye to the first (sentinel) node in the axilla. This was removed at axillary surgery and where it was clear, no further axillary dissection was required. For those patients in whom nodes were involved, further dissection of the axilla was required.

Problems

- F/U was short and therefore the risk of axillary recurrence was unclear (although it did appear to be low).
- Study morbidity was only examined in detail in 200 of the total patients recruited (100 in each group), but was clearly lower in the sentinel node biopsy group.
- It is unclear whether optimal treatment for patients who were sentinel node positive was axillary clearance or radiotherapy to the axilla. This is the basis for further trials ongoing in both the USA and Europe.

Breast cancer: breast-conserving surgery

Eight-year results of a RCT comparing total mastectomy and lumpectomy with or without irradiation in the treatment of breast cancer.

AUTHORS: Fisher B, Redmond C, Poisson R et al.
REFERENCE: N Engl J Med (1989) 320, 822–8.
STUDY DESIGN: RCT
EVIDENCE LEVEL: 1b

Key message

Breast-conserving surgery (lumpectomy or local excision) combined with radiotherapy (RT) is equal to mastectomy in terms of local control and overall survival.

Impact

Following this study, breast-conserving surgery followed by RT has become widely accepted as the treatment of choice for most women with small (<4cm) breast cancers that are unifocal. The omission of RT after breast-conserving surgery is considered substandard.

Aims

The initial results of this study (published in 1985, by the same group) had suggested women undergoing 'segmental mastectomy' and irradiation for breast cancer had comparable disease-free survival to those undergoing total mastectomy with axillary node dissection. This trial aimed to provide longer-term (over 8y F/U) data in the assessment of whether breast-conserving surgery followed by RT provided equivalent local and distant disease control to mastectomy.

Methods

Patients: 1843 patients from multiple centres across the USA.

Inclusion criteria:
- Stage I or II breast cancer (tumour size <4cm);
- Margins of receptor specimen free of tumour;
- No metastasis.

Exclusion criteria:
- Women in whom the margin was involved after breast-conserving surgery subsequently underwent mastectomy and were excluded from the results of the breast-conserving surgery group;
- Patients not suitable for RT.

Groups:
- Breast-conserving surgery (n=636);
- Breast-conserving surgery and RT (n=629);
- Mastectomy (n=590).

Primary endpoint: Local recurrence.

Secondary endpoints:
- Distant disease-free survival;
- Overall survival.

Results

Event	Mastectomy (n=590)	BCS (n=636)	BCS and RT (n=629)
		n. (%)	
1st treatment failure	187 (31.7%)	239 (37.6%)	184 (29.3%)
Local recurrence	48 (8.1%)	46 (7.2%)	7 (1.1%)
Distant (metastasis)	111 (18.8%)	139 (21.9%)	143 (22.7%)
2nd cancer	15 (2.5%)	14 (2.2%)	17 (2.7%)
Death from another cause	15 (2.5%)	12 (1.9%)	16 (2.5%)
Alive, no evidence of disease	373 (63.2%)	371 (58.3%)	412 (65.5%)

BCS = Breast-conserving surgery

- Equivalent local and distant recurrence was achieved with breast-conserving surgejry (lumpectomy and RT) compared with mastectomy for patients with stage I/II breast cancer.
- Local control was significantly better for patients undergoing breast-conserving surgery and RT vs breast-conserving surgery alone. Overall survival did not differ ($p=0.3$, ns).
- Local recurrence rate in patients receiving no RT was significantly worse than those receiving breast-conserving surgery and RT ($p=0.01$).

Discussion

This trial confirmed the efficacy of wide local excision (lumpectomy) with irradiation and ushered in an era of breast-conserving surgery for the treatment of stage I/II breast cancer. Subsequently, other trials comparing wide local excision and RT vs mastectomy have shown no difference, and a meta-analysis of the two treatments has shown equal recurrence rates and survival in both groups at 5y.

Problems

- The trial ensured mastectomy for all patients whose initial conservative surgery did not clear margins, whereas today most people undergo re-excision.
- The inclusion of patients who had margins involved in the mastectomy group may have biased the recurrence rate in this arm.

Breast cancer: radiotherapy and breast-conserving surgery

Breast-conserving surgery with or without radiotherapy: pooled analysis for risks of ipsilateral breast tumour recurrence and mortality.

AUTHORS: Vinh-Hung V, Verschraegen C.
REFERENCE: J Natl Cancer Inst (2004) 96, 115–21.
STUDY DESIGN: Meta-analysis
EVIDENCE LEVEL: 1a

Key message
Radiotherapy (RT) is required after breast-conserving surgery to prevent local recurrence and improve overall survival.

Impact
RT is now considered essential after breast-conserving surgery for both invasive and *in situ* cancer.

Aims
RT had been considered a necessary adjunct to breast-conserving surgery as this had been demonstrated to confer similar survival rates to mastectomy. However, RT is not without its own risks and complications. For this reason, several RCTs had been conducted to compare outcomes following breast-conserving surgery with and without RT. These had conflicting conclusions, this meta-analysis therefore aimed to pool the individual RCT results in order to evaluate the effects of omitting RT on local recurrence and overall survival after breast-conserving surgery for invasive cancer.

Methods
Patients: 9422 women from 15 RCTs.

Inclusion criteria:
- All RCTs comparing RT vs no RT after breast-conserving surgery (lumpectomy or local excision);
- Patients undergoing breast-conserving surgery.

Exclusion criteria:
- Patients with metastatic disease;
- Patients not in an RCT;
- Size of tumour variation either <1cm or <5cm;
- Resection margins either free or >2cm.

Primary endpoint: Local recurrence.

Secondary endpoints:
- Distant recurrence;
- Overall survival.

Results
- Omission of RT was associated with a 3x increased risk of local recurrence and an 8.6% increase in mortality, both of which were significant.

	BCS without RT	BCS with RT
Deaths	824/4097	755/4109 1.086* (95% CI 1.003 to 1.175)
Recurrence	875/4731	279/4691 2.32* (95% CI 1.56 to 3.45)

BCS=breast-conserving surgery.
* Relative risk of mortality.

Discussion

These results are similar to other meta-analyses of RT and surgery (*N Engl J Med* (1995) 333, 1444–56; *Lancet* (2000) 355, 1757–70), in which RT reduced the risk of recurrence and after 10y also reduced the risk of death from breast cancer, when applied after breast-conserving surgery. It should be recognised that the benefit of RT in every situation is dependent on the risk of relapse. Therefore, for a 65y old woman with a 1cm oestrogen receptor positive tumour and negative lymph nodes, the benefit from RT in terms of improved survival would be 8.6%. This amounts to 0.5% at 5y and 1.5% survival benefit at 10y. Thus in selected elderly patients, RT may not add greatly to the value of treatment. However, for the majority of patients treated with breast-conserving surgery, RT should be mandatory following surgery.

Problems

• This was a pooled analysis, which may therefore be subjective to publication bias or lack of transparency in patient allocation.

Breast cancer: radiotherapy for *in situ* disease

> **EORTC (European Organisation for Research and Treatment of Cancer) study:** Radiotherapy in breast-conserving treatment for ductal carcinoma *in situ*: first results of the EORTC randomised phase III trial 10853.
>
> **AUTHORS:** Julien J, Bijker N, Fentiman I *et al.*
> **REFERENCE:** Lancet (2000) 355, 528–33.
> **STUDY DESIGN:** RCT
> **EVIDENCE LEVEL:** 1b

Key message

Radiotherapy (RT) after local excision (breast-conserving surgery) for ductal carcinoma *in situ* (DCIS) confers benefits over local excision alone in preventing local recurrence. RT reduces the overall number of both invasive and non-invasive cancers in the ipsilateral breast at a median of 4.25y.

Impact

Although RT reduced local recurrence (both invasive and *in situ*), no effects on overall survival were seen, with deaths from breast cancer similar in both groups due to the failure of RT to prevent metastasis. RT is still used in women at high risk of local recurrence after breast-conserving surgery with DCIS.

Aims

Breast-conserving surgery has become an increasingly popular option for patients with DCIS, providing a more satisfactory cosmetic appearance than mastectomy. Studies had demonstrated breast-conserving therapy to be as effective as mastectomy. However, with an increasing incidence of DCIS detection due to breast cancer screening programmes, the risk of residual disease with breast-conserving treatment remained a concern. This study aimed to determine optimal adjuvant RT after local excision of DCIS of the breast.

Methods

Patients: 1010 women from 46 centres in 13 European countries.

Inclusion criteria: Locally excised DCIS with intent-to-remove the whole lesion.

Exclusion criteria:
- Incompletely excised DCIS *or* DCIS >4cm in size;
- Age >70y;

Groups: Allocated after breast-conserving wide local resection surgery:
- Radiotherapy: external beam, within 12wk of surgery (n=507; 502 completed study);
- No further treatment (n=503; 500 analysed).

Primary endpoint: Invasive and non-invasive recurrence in the treated breast.

Secondary endpoints:
- Regional recurrence, contralateral breast cancer *or* metastasis;
- Death.

Follow-up: At 6 monthly intervals until the 10th post-operative year, and then at annual intervals. Bilateral mammograms annually.

Results

	Number of events	4-year recurrence free rates	Hazard ratio (95% CI)	*p*
All local recurrence				
No treatment	83	84%	0.62 (0.44 to 0.87)	0.005
Treatment	53	91%		
DCIS recurrence*				
No treatment	44	92%	0.65 (0.41 to 1.03)	0.06
Treatment	29	95%		
Invasive recurrence*				
No treatment	40	92%	0.60 (0.37 to 0.97)	0.04
Treatment	24	96%		
Distant metastasis				
No treatment	12	98%	0.98 (0.44 to 2.18)	1.0
Treatment	12	99%		
Death				
No treatment	12	99%	0.97 (0.44 to 2.16)	0.4
Treatment	12	99%		
Contralateral breast cancer				
No treatment	8	99%	2.57 (1.24 to 5.33)	0.01
Treatment	21	97%		
Event-free survival				
No treatment	93	82%	0.82 (0.61 to 1.10)	0.2
Treatment	78	86%		

*1 patient with recurrence of DCIS had a second local recurrence that was invasive.

Discussion

This trial confirmed previous data from the USA, that RT prevented local recurrence. However, 30% of patients were subsequently shown to have margin involvement on histopathological review. No effect on overall survival was seen due to the frequency of distant metastasis being similar in both groups. Contralateral breast cancers were seen more frequently in the group given RT, but subsequent F/U has failed to substantiate this finding and the numbers were originally small.

Problems

- Numbers with involved margins limit the strength of the findings.
- The lack of overall effect on survival has left considerable argument as to the value of adjuvant RT.
- The trial confirmed the benefit of using RT after breast-conserving surgery for DCIS, although the magnitude of the benefit and value in preventing local recurrence remains contentious.

Breast cancer: radiotherapy for early disease

EBCTG (**E**arly **B**reast **C**ancer **T**rialist's collaborative **G**roup): Effects of radiotherapy and of differences in the extent of surgery for early breast cancer on local recurrence and 15year survival: an overview of the randomised trials.

AUTHORS: Early Breast Cancer Trialist's Collaborative Group.
REFERENCE: Lancet (2005) 366, 2087–106.
STUDY DESIGN: Meta-analysis
EVIDENCE LEVEL: 1a

Key message
A two-third reduction in local recurrence is seen across all trials of radiotherapy (RT) after breast-conserving surgery, with a reduction in breast cancer mortality. However, high rates of toxicity in terms of lung cancer and cardiovascular mortality are seen at 20y in patients treated with RT.

Impact
RT is now standard treatment for all patients undergoing breast-conserving surgery to reduce local recurrence and improve overall survival.

Aims
Following the proven advantage conferred by breast-conserving surgery, several trials have attempted to compare the benefit of RT after breast-conserving surgery vs breast-conserving surgery alone or mastectomy. This meta-analysis analysed 10 and 15y results from 78 RCTs of RT for early breast cancer.

Methods
Patients: 42,400 patients involved in total across these trials.

Protocol: Meta-analysis of 78 trials to determine the overall effects of RT on local control and overall survival in early breast cancer. Trials included RT after mastectomy alone or with axillary sampling, and breast-conserving surgery with or without RT.

Inclusion criteria: Any trial involving post-operative RT for early breast cancer.

Primary endpoint: Breast cancer recurrence and mortality.

Secondary endpoints:
- Second cancers;
- Cardiovascular complications.

Results
- In 7300 women undergoing breast-conserving surgery, RT reduced local recurrence by two thirds at 10y (from 27.2% to 8.8%) and mortality by 5.3% ($p=0.005$) at 15y.

- In 8500 women undergoing mastectomy for node-positive disease, 5y local recurrence rates were reduced to 6% by RT (from 23%) and mortality at 15y by 4.4% (p=0.005).
- An increase in non-breast cancer deaths was seen at 20y, with a 4.3% increase in mortality seen in patients undergoing RT. These were a combination of lung cancer and vascular deaths, including stroke from irradiation of the carotid arteries in the supraclavicular fossa.
- Benefits of chest wall RT or RT after breast-conserving surgery were greatest in node-positive patients and those who were younger.

Discussion

Differences in local treatment affect local recurrence rates and in the hypothetical absence of any other cause of death would avoid one breast cancer-related death for every four local recurrences prevented at 15y following treatment. RT is mandatory after breast-conserving surgery, and post-mastectomy in node-positive breast cancers.

Problems

- Many RT trials were over 20y old and used megavoltage RT. Late toxicity may diminish with newer RT regimes and planning.

Breast cancer: tamoxifen

P-1 study: Tamoxifen for the prevention of breast cancer: current status of the national surgical adjuvant breast and bowel project.

AUTHORS: Fisher B, Constantino J, Wickerham D *et al.*
REFERENCE: J Natl Cancer Inst (2005) 97, 1652–62.
STUDY DESIGN: RCT
EVIDENCE LEVEL: 1b

Key message
Tamoxifen prevents the development of breast cancer, but increases the risk of thromboembolic events and endometrial cancer.

Impact
This and the IBIS-1 study both indicate that apart from in very high-risk women, the value of tamoxifen as preventative treatment is unconvincing. Therefore, tamoxifen is now only used in high-risk patients with breast cancer.

Aims
The study was aimed at devising progressively better regimens for the systemic treatment of detectable diseases and improving methods of detection so as to identify breast cancer at an earlier stage of development. With tamoxifen known to decrease the incidence of contralateral cancers following its administration as adjuvant therapy, it was proposed that it may play a role in breast cancer prevention. This study aimed to test this hypothesis in women at high risk for the development of breast cancer.

Methods
Patients: 57,641 high-risk women screened for participation (13,175 participated) at multiple centres across the USA.

Inclusion criteria: Women at high risk for breast cancer:
- Age >60 *or* age 35–59y with 5y predicted risk of breast cancer of at least 1.66% (i.e. at high risk);
- Past history of Lobular Carcinoma *in situ* (LCIS) or atypical hyperplasia;
- Normal mammogram.

Exclusion criteria:
- Low risk of breast cancer;
- Age <35y;
- Previous thromboembolism.

Groups:
- Placebo (n=6707);
- Tamoxifen (n=6681).

Primary endpoint: Reduction in invasive and non-invasive breast cancer.

Secondary endpoints:
- Adverse events;
- Non-breast cancer deaths;

- Thromboembolic disease;
- Other cancers.

Follow-up: Median follow-up=7y.

Results

Primary endpoint (all women)	Placebo (n=6599)	Tamoxifen (n=6576)	p (risk reduction)
Breast cancer			
– Total	244	124	
– Invasive	175	89	<0.00001 (49%)
– Non-invasive	69	35	<0.002 (50%)
Breast cancer (average annual rate/1000 women)	6.76	3.43	RR 0.51 (95% CI 0.39 to 0.66)
Secondary endpoints			**RR (95% CI)**
Endometrial cancer (average annual rate/1000 women)	0.91	2.30	2.53 (1.35 to 4.97)
Pulmonary embolism (average annual rate/1000 women)	0.23	0.69	3.01 (1.15 to 9.27)
Osteoporotic fractures (n)	137	111	0.81 (0.63 to 1.05)
Deaths (n)	71	57	0.81 (0.56 to 1.16)

- 9 deaths attributable to breast cancer (6 in placebo group, 3 in tamoxifen; ns)

Discussion

This study, as well as the IBIS-1 trial in Europe (*Lancet* (2002) 360, 817–24), both showed a reduction in breast cancer incidence among high-risk women treated with tamoxifen. However, there was no effect seen on breast cancer mortality and critics have argued that if one is not reducing deaths from breast cancer, then there is no value in the treatment. In the IBIS-1 trial, increased pulmonary embolic events were seen that led to an increase in mortality in the tamoxifen-treated patients.

Problems

- These trials were powered for reduction in breast cancer events, whereas the treatment is only of benefit if it prevents deaths from breast cancer in a population. From the data in these trials, it is unlikely that tamoxifen will prevent breast cancer deaths.

Breast cancer: tamoxifen for early disease

EBCTG (**E**arly **B**reast **C**ancer **T**rialist's collaborative **G**roup): Tamoxifen for early breast cancer: an overview of the randomised trials.

AUTHORS: Early Breast Cancer Trialist's Collaborative Group.
REFERENCE: Lancet (1998) 351, 1451–67.
STUDY DESIGN: Meta-analysis
EVIDENCE LEVEL: 1a

Key message

The use of tamoxifen in oestrogen receptor (ER) positive or unknown primary breast tumours is associated with a significant reduction in the risk of recurrence and improvement in overall 10y survival. However, there is an increase in incidence of endometrial cancer.

Impact

This is one of a series of 5yearly systematic reviews started in 1984 by this group. They have provided solid data on which to base breast cancer treatment, revolutionising practice. Endocrine therapy with agents such as tamoxifen is now standard treatment for all patients with ER-positive breast cancer. The benefit of the treatment depends on the level of ER expression, but up to a 40% reduction in recurrence is achieved with treatment for 5y.

Aims

The aims of the studies incorporated into this meta-analysis were to determine the benefit of tamoxifen in women with early breast cancer, after surgical and local treatment had been conducted. Initial trials did not select patients by the presence of ER positivity, but subsequently all trials selected patients by ER type. This updated overview consolidated the information obtained from previous studies on adjuvant tamoxifen use.

Methods

Patients: 36,689 women from 55 RCTs that began before 1990 (87% of worldwide evidence). Data collected/finalised from 1995–6 were analysed.

Inclusion criteria: Patients aged between 18–70y, with early breast cancer (restricted to the breast), and no distant disease.

Exclusion criteria:
• Metastatic breast cancer;
• Previous venous thromboembolism;
• Pregnancy.

Data collected:
• Age and menopausal status;
• Nodal involvement; ER and progesterone receptor (PR) status;
• Treatments (1, 2, or 5y of tamoxifen) and outcomes.

Statistics: Comparisons based on intention-to-treat principle. Each trial analysed separately and then combined. Two-sided significance tests used.

Groups: Adjuvant tamoxifen 20mg/d for 1, 2, or 5y.

Primary endpoint: Breast cancer mortality.

Secondary endpoints: Breast cancer recurrence and adverse events.

Follow-up: Median F/U=10y.

Results

	Reduction in recurrence (vs placebo)	Reduction in all cause mortality
Tamoxifen (1y)	18%, SD3 ($p<0.0001$)	10%, SD3
Tamoxifen (2y)	25%, SD2 ($p<0.0001$)	15%, SD2
Tamoxifen (3y+)	42%, SD3 ($p<0.01$)	22%, SD4
Overall	26.4%, SD1.5 ($p<0.001$)	14.5%, SD1.5
ER-poor	6%, SD11	−3%, SD11
ER-unknown	37%, SD8	21%, SD9
ER-rich	43%, SD3 ($p<0.0001$)	23%, SD4 ($p<0.0001$)

SD=standard deviation.

Discussion

This meta-analysis concluded that 5y tamoxifen provided the optimal standard of care for ER-positive cancers. The greatest benefit was found in those at highest risk (i.e. node-positive tumours). Both pre- and post-menopausal women benefited. Although recurrence reductions occurred early in the first 5y period, mortality reductions commenced after 3y and continued to increase up to 10y. Thus, 5y treatment had a longer impact on recurrence and mortality, even once the drug was stopped. There was an absolute decrease of 50% in contralateral breast cancer, but coincidentally, there was a 2.58 times higher incidence of endometrial cancer, with an annual excess of deaths of 0.2 per 1,000. The reduction in contralateral breast cancer was maximal for ER-rich patients, with a 47% reduction (SD9); whereas for ER-poor patients, there was a non-significant reduction in contralateral breast cancer. The effects were seen regardless of age at diagnosis. There was no increase in the incidence of colorectal cancer. Tamoxifen should not be used concurrently with chemotherapy due to an increased risk of venous thromboembolism. The 4th cycle (presented in 2000) included data from 200,000 women (400 RCTs from 250 groups). This demonstrated the benefits (for 15y survival) of treatment with chemotherapy (e.g. FAC: 5-fluorouracil, adriamycin, cyclophosphamide) and hormonal therapy (e.g. tamoxifen in ER-positive disease). There was also some benefit on mortality from improved local disease control by surgery and radiotherapy.

Breast cancer: hormonal therapy

> **ATAC** (**A**rimidex, **T**amoxifen, **A**lone or in **C**ombination) study:
> Anastrozole alone or in combination with tamoxifen versus tamoxifen
> alone for adjuvant treatment of post-menopausal women with early
> breast cancer.
>
> **AUTHORS:** The ATAC Trialists' Group.
> **REFERENCE:** Lancet (2002) 359, 2131–39.
> **STUDY DESIGN:** RCT
> **EVIDENCE LEVEL:** 1b

Key message

In post-menopausal patients with hormone receptor positive early breast
cancer, there is 3.7% absolute reduction in risk of cancer recurrence and
50% reduction in relative risk of contralateral breast cancer compared
to tamoxifen. There are no effects on breast cancer mortality.

Impact

Aromatase inhibitors are now an integral part of adjuvant therapy for
breast cancer.

Aims

Many breast cancers are dependent upon oestrogens for their growth.
Adjuvant tamoxifen is an established treatment in those with oestrogen
receptor positive tumours, demonstrated to improve disease-free and
overall survival. However, long-term survival has been associated with
the development of complications, including an increased incidence of
endometrial cancer. Aromatase inhibitors (AIs) inhibit the synthesis of
oestrogen from androgens in post-menopausal women, with anastrozole
reported to be a well-tolerated agent demonstrated to confer a survival
advantage. This study aimed to evaluate and compare the effects of anastrozole with tamoxifen, or combination therapy, on disease recurrence
and breast cancer mortality in post-menopausal women with hormone
receptor positive early breast cancer.

Methods

Patients: 9366 women at 381 international centres.

Inclusion criteria:
- Post-menopausal women;
- Early breast cancer;
- Oestrogen receptor positive or unknown;
- Completed primary surgery and chemotherapy.

Exclusion criteria:
- Oestrogen receptor negative cancer;
- Previous tamoxifen use;
- Previous invasive cancer.

Groups:
- Anastrozole (n=3125);
- Tamoxifen (n=3125);
- Combination (n=3125).

Primary endpoint: Breast cancer disease-free survival.

Secondary endpoints:
- Time to recurrence;
- Incidence of contralateral breast cancer;
- Adverse effect rates for each drug;
- Health-related quality of life;
- Bone and lipid effects of each drug.

Results

	Anastrozole (n=3125)	Tamoxifen (n=3125)	Combination (n=3125)
Recurrence-free survival	89.4%	87.4%	87.2%
	HR 0.83 (95% CI 0.78 to 0.97) p=0.01		
All-cause mortality	200 (6.4%)	203 (6.5%)	215 (6.9%)
	0.97 (0.85 to 1.12) p=0.7 (HR)		
Endometrial cancer	3 (0.1%)	13 (0.5%)	6 (0.3%)
	p=0.001		
Venous thromboembolism	87 (2.8%)	140 (4.5%)	124 (4.0%)
Fractures	340 (11.0%)	237 (7.7%)	*
	HR 1.49 (95% CI 1.27 to 1.77) p=0.001		

*Closed in view of lack of efficacy. HR=hazard ratio.

Discussion

Anastrozole reduced recurrence of breast cancer (mainly local and contralateral breast cancer), and was associated with significantly reduced venous thrombosis and endometrial cancer. Compared with tamoxifen, anastrozole, an aromatase inhibitor (AI), offered no advantage with respect to all-cause mortality. Anastrozole also induced bone loss and premature osteoporotic fractures. Anastrozole is one of several new AIs. Whether it should be given upfront as in ATAC, or sequentially after 2y tamoxifen is not yet clear, but is the focus of further ongoing trials.

Breast cancer: herceptin

HERA (**HER**ceptin **A**djuvant trial): Trastuzumab after adjuvant chemotherapy in HER2-positive breast cancer.

AUTHORS: Piccart–Gebhart M, Procter M, Leyland–Jones B et al.
REFERENCE: N Engl J Med (2005) 353, 1659–72.
STUDY DESIGN: RCT
EVIDENCE LEVEL: 1b

Key message
First RCT to demonstrate that the use of a monoclonal antibody directed against the extracellular domain of the HER2 oncoprotein receptor prevents relapse in HER2-positive breast cancer and improves overall survival by 30%.

Impact
Trastuzumab is now the treatment of choice after adjuvant chemotherapy for the 15–25% of patients with early HER2-positive breast cancer. It carries a small risk (<2%) of causing congestive heart failure. It has confronted publicly funded health systems with a major challenge of affordability.

Aims
Self-sufficiency in growth signals is one of six molecular 'hallmarks of cancer' identified in the late 20th century. The transmembrane receptor tyrosine kinase, HER2/neu, is overexpressed in up to a quarter of breast cancers where it mediates growth signals and increases the risk of cancer relapse and death. Trastuzumab (Herceptin®) is a monoclonal anti-HER2 antibody that slows progression of advanced HER2-positive disease. This trial aimed to show that taking trastuzumab for 1–2y after standard chemotherapy could reduce relapse in early disease.

Methods
Patients: 5081 women from 26 groups and 91 independent international centres.

Inclusion criteria: Quite broad compared to USA-based trials:
• Well women with completely excised HER2-positive early breast cancer;
• HER2/neu 3+ tumour immunohistochemistry or 2+ and FISH-positive;
• 6 months (≥4 cycles) of (neo)adjuvant chemotherapy pre-randomisation;
• Either axillary node positive or node negative with primary >1cm;
• Adequate cardiac function (left ventricular ejection fraction >55%).

Exclusion criteria: HER2-negative disease or metastatic cancer.

Groups: Trastuzumab dosing=8mg/kg, then 6mg/kg 3-weekly infusions.
• Observation only (no treatment) (n=1693);
• 1y of trastuzumab (n=1694);
• 2y of treatment after adjuvant chemotherapy (n=1694).

Primary endpoint: Disease-free survival (DFS).

Secondary endpoints:
- Contralateral breast cancer; 2nd non-breast malignant disease;
- Overall survival (OS);
- Cardiac morbidity (congestive heart failure (CHF) or cardiac death).

Follow-up: Every 3 months for 1st 2y, then annually from years 2–10. Comprised clinical review and periodic blood tests, chest X-ray, mammogram, electrocardiogram, and echocardiogram or multiple-gated acquisition (MUGA) scan for left ventricular ejection fraction.

Results

Primary endpoint	Observation	1y trastuzumab	p
2y DFS	77%	86%	<0.0001
Secondary endpoints			
2y OS	95%	96%	ns
Symptomatic CHF	0.1%	1.7%	<0.001
Contralateral breast cancer	0.4%	0.4%	ns
Breast cancer related deaths	2.2%	1.7%	ns

Discussion

The first HERA results were released after only 12 months median F/U, due to a strongly positive gain in DFS for 1y trastuzumab vs observation. On release, around half the women in the control arm chose to switch to delayed adjuvant trastuzumab. This will confound future analyses of the HERA data, and there will always be some doubt as to the durability of the survival benefit. In a later analysis at around 2y, the OS endpoint reached significance (HR of 0.66, p=0.01). The HERA authors point out that the only other agent found to improve OS after 2y was tamoxifen, 'the most successful [systemic] treatment ever developed for breast cancer'. Trastuzumab was associated with cardiac morbidity, with 1.7% experiencing cardiac toxicity vs 0.1% on placebo. The cardiac side effects were accentuated when given with anthracycline chemotherapy and require cardiac monitoring for all women. The trial's third arm of 2y trastuzumab had not yet been reported.

Problems

- F/U was short; it is unclear whether survival benefits will remain at 10y.
- The UK cost of therapy at £25,000 per patient is expensive, particularly when only ≈40% of patients will benefit.
- Several large RCTs (e.g. *NSABP-B31, N9831,* and *BCIRG-006*) have suggested trastuzumab is more effective if given *concurrently* with chemotherapy (as well as following it).
- The *FinHer (Finland Herceptin)* RCT *(N Engl J Med (2006) 354, 809–20)* (n=232), found a strong DFS benefit for *short-course* concurrent trastuzumab (stops at end of chemotherapy, hence is quarter of the expense). This is being looked at further by the short-or-long-duration (SOLD) trial.

Breast cancer: timing of chemotherapy

Neoadjuvant vs adjuvant systemic treatment in breast cancer: a meta-analysis.

AUTHORS: Mauri D, Pavlidis N, Ioannidis J.
REFERENCE: J Natl Cancer Inst (2005) 97, 188–94.
STUDY DESIGN: Meta-analysis
EVIDENCE LEVEL: 1a

Key message
Compared with standard post-operative adjuvant therapy, neoadjuvant chemotherapy showed no improvement in survival. However, where radiotherapy (RT) was given without surgery, increased loco-regional recurrence was seen.

Impact
Primary neoadjuvant chemotherapy is now an accepted treatment modality for large primary cancers.

Aims
Increasing consideration of non-metastatic breast cancer as a systemic (rather than local) disease has led to an interest in the role of neoadjuvant chemotherapy to treat the early systemic signs of the disease. Local chemotherapy response can range from tumour regression to a complete pathological response. This meta-analysis aimed to determine the benefits of pre-operative chemotherapy in early breast cancer on local/distant recurrence and overall survival.

Methods
Patients: 3946 women from 9 trials of primary systemic chemotherapy vs post-operative adjuvant chemotherapy.

Inclusion criteria:
- Large invasive breast cancers unsuitable for breast-conserving surgery;
- Suitable for chemotherapy;
- No prior treatment.

Exclusion criteria:
- Patients unsuitable for chemotherapy;
- Prior surgical treatment;
- Metastatic breast cancer.

Primary endpoint: Overall survival.

Secondary endpoints:
- Loco-regional recurrence;
- Distant recurrence;
- Clinical and pathological response rate to chemotherapy.

Results

- Of 3,946 randomised patients (1,972 neoadjuvant arm, 1,074 adjuvant arm), there were 1,310 occurrences of disease progression and 966 deaths.

	(RR = Relative Risk)
Primary measurable outcome	RR 1.00, 95% CI=0.90 to 1.12
Disease progression	RR 0.99, 95% CI=0.91 to 1.07
Disease recurrences	RR 0.94, 95% CI=0.83 to 1.06
Loco-regional recurrence	RR 1.22, 95% CI=1.03 to 1.44

- No differences in overall survival between primary systemic therapy and adjuvant therapy.
- In those patients given primary systemic therapy and in whom surgery was subsequently omitted because of an incomplete response, there was increased loco-regional recurrence despite RT.

Discussion

Primary systemic therapy conferred no survival difference, although it did reduce the need for mastectomy. A good prognosis was achieved for those patients who achieved complete tumour remission with chemotherapy. But for those in whom no response was seen, prognosis remained poor. Altogether, one third of patients had died by the time of this meta-analysis, indicating a generally poor response to treatment whether given before or after surgery in this group of patients.

Problems

- This meta-analysis of 9 trials included significant variation between treatments offered, and subsequently, between whether or not surgery and RT or RT alone was given. Nonetheless, the study indicated clearly that neoadjuvant therapy was as safe as systemic therapy in terms of overall survival.

Breast cancer: bisphophonates for bone metastases

Efficacy of pamidronate in reducing skeletal complications in patients with breast cancer and lytic bone metastases.

AUTHORS: Hortobagyi G, Theriault R, Porter L *et al.*
REFERENCE: N Engl J Med (1996) 335, 1785–91.
STUDY DESIGN: RCT
EVIDENCE LEVEL: 1b

Key message
Monthly infusions of pamidronate given in addition to chemotherapy can reduce skeletal complications in women with lytic bone metastases from breast cancer.

Impact
Bisphosphonates are now a well established treatment for women with bone metastases from breast cancer, with newer generation agents providing even better results.

Aims
Bone metastases occur in most women with advanced breast cancer. The skeletal destruction that develops can lead to pain, immobility, and reduction in quality of life. Bisphosphonates inhibit bone resorption by osteoclasts and are often used to treat cancer-related hypercalcaemia. Early trials had suggested that they may reduce skeletal complications in women with breast cancer. This trial aimed to confirm these findings.

Methods
Patients: 382 patients from 97 centres in the USA, Canada, Australia, and New Zealand.

Inclusion criteria:
- Stage IV breast cancer and receiving chemotherapy;
- At least one lytic bone metastases (≥1cm diameter);
- Eastern Cooperative Oncology Group (ECOG) performance score 0–3.

Exclusion criteria:
- Skeletal complications (pathological fracture, need for radiation to bone or bone surgery, spinal cord compression due to vertebral collapse);
- Corrected serum calcium >3mmol/L in 2wk pre-enrolment;
- Serum creatinine >220micromol/L;
- Ascites;
- Serum bilirubin >43micromol/L;
- Heart failure of New York Heart Association (NYHA) Class III/IV;
- Treatment with bisphosphonate in 60d pre-study;
- Treatment with radiation, corticosteroids (except as part of chemotherapy), calcitonin, or plicamycin during 2wk pre-enrolment.

Groups:
- Monthly pamidronate 90mg (n=185);
- Placebo (n=197 patients; 2 not evaluable).

Primary endpoint: Time to first skeletal complication.

Secondary endpoints:
- Proportion of patients with skeletal complications;
- Bone pain;
- Performance status.

Follow-up: Monthly clinical review and serum calcium measurement. X-ray skeletal surveys at 3, 6, and 12 months.

Results

	Pamidronate	Placebo	*p*
Median time to 1st skeletal complication	13.1 months	7 months	0.005
Proportion of patients developing skeletal complications	43%	56%	0.008

- Pamidronate significantly reduced bone pain progression, compared with placebo (decreased scores in 44% vs 32%, *p*=0.03).
- Significantly less deterioration in performance status with pamidronate compared with placebo (*p*=0.03).

Discussion

The response of bone disease to chemotherapy ranged from 0 to 30%. The addition of bisphosphonate had clear benefits, particularly after 6 cycles of treatment. Hypercalcaemia rates were reduced after 3 cycles, need for radiotherapy after 6, need for surgery after 9, and rate of non-vertebral pathological fractures after 12 cycles. The treatment was well tolerated. Bisphosphonates are now an integral part of the management of breast cancer with bone metastases. Newer bisphosphonates developed since this trial was performed may deliver improved results and can be infused over shorter periods, with oral agents also being available.

Problems

- Fairly stringent exclusion criteria were present. For example, patients with skeletal complications were excluded; this should be considered when extrapolating the significance of these results to patients with complications of their malignancy or pre-existing conditions.

Mastalgia: tamoxifen

Double-blind controlled trial of tamoxifen therapy for mastalgia.

AUTHORS: Fentiman I, Caleffi M, Brame K *et al.*
REFERENCE: Lancet (1986) 8, 287–8.
STUDY DESIGN: RCT
EVIDENCE LEVEL: 1b

Key message
Tamoxifen relieves cyclical mastalgia, when given as a 3 months course.

Impact
Tamoxifen therapy (low dose) is now routinely used in the treatment of mastalgia.

Aims
Mastalgia (breast pain) is a common symptom. The exact aetiology of cyclical mastalgia has not yet been established; however, it is thought to be due, in part, to elevated oestrogen levels. Often spontaneously resolving, the therapeutic efficacy of treatments can be difficult to evaluate. The aim of the study was to determine whether tamoxifen (20mg/d), compared with placebo, relieved symptoms in women with severe cyclical mastalgia.

Methods
Patients: 60 women at 1 centre in the UK.

Inclusion criteria:
- Severe cyclical mastalgia for more than 7d;
- Age 20–70y;
- No clinical breast lumps.

Exclusion criteria:
- Patients whose pain did not continue over a 6wk rolling period.

Groups:
- Tamoxifen (n=31);
- Placebo (n=29).

Primary endpoint: Relief in the linear analogue breast pain scores at 6 months.

Secondary endpoints:
- Side effects on treatment;
- Patient assessed scoring.

Follow-up: Weekly self-administered linear analogue breast pain cards and menstrual calendars (pre-menopausal women). Side effect review and clinical examination at 1, 3, 4, and 6 months.

Results

	Tamoxifen (n=31)	Placebo (n=29)	p
Success	22 (71%)	11 (38%)	0.03
Side effects	23 (74%)	10 (34%)	0.01

- Primary outcome event: >30% reduction in mean pain score (p=<0.03).
- Pain score/minor side effects: 71% showed decrease in pain score using tamoxifen vs placebo, but there was a high incidence of side effects (which were mainly minor). No venous thromboembolism recorded.
- Major side effects: hot flushes (26%) and vaginal discharge (16%). Compared with placebo, tamoxifen showed a significant reduction in cyclical breast pain at 6 months.

Discussion

Tamoxifen appeared to be of value in relieving both cyclical and non-cyclical symptoms. Although the results of this study were not as dramatic as those of previous investigations, this study did exclude those with very short duration symptoms (<6 months), hence potentially excluding a greater proportion of patients with spontaneously resolving symptoms. Two further studies have since been conducted. The first compared tamoxifen 20mg/d with a 10mg/d dose (from day 15–25 in the menstrual cycle for 3 months) and found the 10mg/d dose to be equally as effective as 20mg/d. A further trial that compared tamoxifen 10mg vs 20mg for 3 months vs 6 months found no significant difference between both groups in terms of pain relief. Tamoxifen is not licensed for mastalgia in the UK or the USA, but is now used at a dose of 10mg/d from day 10–25 of the cycle, over a 6 months period for patients with severe cyclical mastalgia. Tamoxifen is contraindicated in pregnancy because of potential teratogenicity. More recent studies have also demonstrated the efficacy of leutenising hormone releasing hormone (LHRH) analogues such as goserelin in providing short-term relief in cases of severe cyclical mastalgia *(Am J Obstet Gynecol* (2004) 191, 1942–9). However, long-term therapy with these agents can lead to bone loss, and therefore, treatment periods should not exceed 6 months at a time.

Problems

- This study and the two subsequent RCTs were small and conducted over 20y ago. Nonetheless, a 10mg dose of tamoxifen from d15–25 of the menstrual cycle significantly relieves breast pain and is widely used.

Cardiac surgery

Introduction

At the end of the 19th century, the pre-eminent surgeon of his time, Stephen Paget, stated that '*surgery of the heart has reached the limit set by nature to all surgery; no new discovery can overcome the natural difficulties that attend a wound of the heart.*' Such conventional wisdom would have stifled uninspired minds. However, a handful of surgical pioneers who were willing to think 'out of the box' and challenge perceived limitations continued to dream that the impossible would one day become a reality.

A little over 50 years later, the era of modern heart surgery began in earnest. Stories about pioneering procedures such as the Blalock–Taussig shunt, crossover circulation by Lillehei, deep hypothermia by Bigelow, and the heart-lung machine by Gibbon, to name a few, are now treasured classics. The second half of the 20th century saw advancements in the correction of complex congenital cardiac defects, heart-lung transplantation, and surgery for ischaemic and valvular heart disease.

The establishment of what is now almost regarded as 'routine' cardiac surgery rests not only on the shoulders of surgical giants, but equally on the courage of patients and the trust that they place into the hands of their physicians. It is to these people that we owe our salute.

Coronary artery disease: surgery vs best medical therapy

Eleven-year survival in the Veterans Administration randomised trial of coronary bypass surgery for stable angina.

AUTHORS: The Veterans Administration Coronary Artery Bypass Surgery Cooperative Study Group.
REFERENCE: N Engl J Med (1984) 311, 1333–9.
STUDY DESIGN: RCT
EVIDENCE LEVEL: 1b

Key message

Compared to best medical therapy, coronary artery bypass graft (CABG) improves prognosis in two subgroups of patients with stable angina without left main stem stenosis. The first group (technically high risk based upon angiograms) includes those with triple vessel disease and/or impaired left ventricular function on angiography. The second group (clinically high risk) includes patients with at least 2 out of 3 risk factors (including previous myocardial infarction (MI), resting ST depression, and history of hypertension). The survival advantage is even more pronounced in patients with combinations of the above risks.

Impact

This is the earliest, large-scale RCT to demonstrate the superiority of CABG over best medical treatment in selected patient groups. This refinement in the selection of patients who would benefit most from CABG is crucial in ensuring that patients with stable angina receive the most appropriate therapy.

Aims

Coronary artery disease is subject to varied management. The study was designed to ascertain whether CABG improved survival in patients with chronic stable angina compared to best medical therapy. The aim was to allocate patients on an intention-to-treat basis, thus mimicking real life clinical decision more closely.

Methods

Patients: 686 patients at 13 centres in the USA.

Inclusion criteria:
- Stable angina for >6 months;
- On medical therapy for >3 months;
- >50% stenosis in ≥1 coronary arteries;
- Resting or exercise ECG changes.

Groups:
- CABG (n=332; includes 20 patients who did not have the operation);
- Best medical practice (n=354; including 133 who proceeded to CABG).

Primary endpoint: Death from all causes.

Follow-up: Minimum of 107 months. Mean F/U=11.2y.

Results

	CABG	**Best medical practice**	**p**
High risk based on angiography	76% (50%)	52% (38%)	0.002 (0.03)
Clinically high risk	72% (49%)	52% (36%)	0.003 (0.02)
Combination	76% (54%)	36% (24%)	0.002 (0.005)

Survival at 7y (in brackets=survival at 11y).

Discussion

CABG was superior to best medical therapy in terms of long-term prognosis in patients with triple vessel disease. The 7 and 11y survival rates were similar across the three categories for patients post-CABG, whereas survival was dramatically lower for patients in the combination category who were treated medically. These results provide the first steps towards a risk stratification model for different patients under consideration for CABG and are extremely useful for patient counselling.

Problems

- This trial was conducted in the 1970s. Patients undergoing CABG now are considerably older with greater comorbidities.
- The large numbers of patient crossover from the medical to the surgical group dilutes the advantages of the original CABG group.

Coronary artery disease: surgery vs angioplasty (1)

CABRI (Coronary Angioplasty vs Bypass Revascularisation Investigation): First-year results of CABRI.

AUTHORS: CABRI trial participants.
REFERENCE: Lancet (1995) 346, 1179–84.
STUDY DESIGN: RCT
EVIDENCE LEVEL: 1b

Key message

At 1y, there is no significant difference in survival between patients with multivessel disease who undergo percutaneous transluminal coronary angioplasty (PTCA), compared to coronary artery bypass graft (CABG). However, the patients in the PTCA group have significantly higher rates of angina, medication requirements, and repeat intervention.

Impact

Although PTCA can produce equivalent survival rates to CABG in the short term, patients should be cautioned on the high risks of angina recurrence and requirement for re-intervention. Being less invasive, insertion of either a bare metal or drug eluting stent, in conjunction with PTCA, is an acceptable initial approach in non-diabetic patients.

Aims

Whether to use percutaneous transluminal coronary angioplasty (PTCA) or coronary artery bypass graft (CABG) in patients with multivessel coronary artery disease amenable to either treatment remained a matter of debate. This study aimed to compare the clinical outcomes of PTCA and CABG as the initial treatment option in patients with multivessel disease.

Methods

Patients: 1054 patients at 26 centres in Europe.

Inclusion criteria:
- Age <76y;
- Symptoms of 'typical angina pectoris' or 'unstable angina' (pain at rest with ST segment change in the absence of myocardial infarction, MI);
- Atypical angina/asymptomatic patients included only if unequivocal evidence of myocardial ischaemia on ECG or isotope scintigraphy;
- Left ventricular ejection fraction >0.35.

Exclusion criteria:
- Single vessel disease;
- Left main coronary artery disease;
- Severe triple vessel disease (defined as 'last remaining vessel', equivalent to two occluded main epicardial vessels);
- Overt cardiac failure or other severe concomitant cardiac disease (e.g. valvular disease, aortic aneurysm, etc.);
- MI within previous 10d or recent cerebrovascular event;
- Previous CABG or PTCA.

Groups:
- CABG (n=513);
- PTCA (n=541).

Primary endpoints:
- All-cause mortality;
- Angina status.

Secondary endpoints:
- Re-intervention rate;
- Medication requirements.

Follow-up: Minimum 28 months. Last patient randomised at 65 months.

Results

	CABG	PTCA	*p*
Initial intervention as randomised	93.2%	96.3%	–
Mortality at 1y	2.7%	3.9%	0.3
Angina at 1y	10.1%	13.9%	0.01
Re-intervention rate	3.5%	36.5%	<0.001

- Crossover: 20 patients randomised to CABG had primary PTCA; 15 patients randomised to PTCA had primary CABG (mainly for clinical reasons).

Discussion

Comparable 1y survival rates were noted between PTCA and CABG. PTCA did confer some obvious advantages, including a less invasive procedure and shorter initial hospitalisation times. However, it was also associated with the necessity for more repeat interventions and repeated hospitalisations in the future. In addition, a high proportion of these patients are likely to require a CABG in the medium term.

Problems

- This trial did not require complete revascularisation in the PTCA arm; other trials have demonstrated complete revascularisation to confer both symptomatic and prognostic benefits.
- 15.7% of patients randomised to PTCA had CABG within the first year. This high rate of crossover may dilute the advantages of the original CABG group, in terms of survival.
- Only looking at F/U to 1y, hence would not be expected to pick up the survival advantage of CABG, which accrues with time.
- Patients included in the study are very different from the current population undergoing PCI, most of whom have at least one contraindication which would have prevented them from being included in this study. Patients currently undergoing PCI are higher risk and consequently would be expected to show more of a survival advantage from CABG.

Coronary artery disease: surgery vs angioplasty (2)

> **BARI (Bypass Angioplasty Revascularisation Investigation):** Comparison of coronary bypass surgery with angioplasty in patients with multivessel disease.
>
> **AUTHORS:** BARI investigators.
> **REFERENCE:** N Engl J Med (1996) 335, 217–25.
> **STUDY DESIGN:** RCT
> **EVIDENCE LEVEL:** 1b

Key message

In non-diabetic patients with triple vessel disease, percutaneous transluminal coronary angioplasty (PTCA) provides an acceptable alternative to coronary artery bypass graft (CABG) in terms of 5y survival. However, re-intervention rates in the PTCA group are significantly higher. In patients with diabetes mellitus (DM) and multivessel disease, CABG is superior to PTCA in terms of 5y prognosis.

Impact

This is the largest randomised study to compare PTCA vs CABG in patients with multivessel disease. 5y results suggest that patients with DM should be referred for CABG, whereas PTCA is a potentially acceptable alternative for suitable non-diabetic patients, although they should be informed of the higher likelihood of need for re-intervention.

Aims

CABG had been demonstrated to result in improved survival for certain subgroups of patients with multivessel coronary artery disease. Although initially used for single vessel disease, less invasive PTCA had been increasingly used in these patients with multivessel disease. This study was designed to ascertain whether PTCA, as an initial treatment in patients with multivessel disease, was comparable to CABG.

Methods

Patients: 1829 patients at 18 centres in the USA and Canada.

Inclusion criteria:
- Multivessel disease suitable for both PTCA and CABG;
- Severe angina or evidence of ischaemia.

Exclusion criteria:
- Emergency revascularisation;
- Left main stem stenosis;
- Prior CABG or PTCA;
- Age >80y;

- Need for concomitant major surgery (e.g. aortic/mitral valve surgery, abdominal aortic aneurysm (AAA) surgery, carotid endarterectomy).

Groups:
- CABG (n=914);
- PTCA (n=915).

Primary endpoint: All-cause mortality.

Secondary endpoints:
- Q wave myocardial infarction (MI);
- Need for revascularisation.

Follow-up: Average of 5.4y (range 3.8–6.8y).

Results

	CABG	PTCA	p
5y survival (all patients)	89.3%	86.3%	0.2
5y survival (patients with DM)	80.6%	65.5%	0.003
5y survival (non-diabetic patients)	91.4%	91.1%	0.7
Re-intervention rate	8%	54%	<0.001
5y cumulative rate of MI	11.7%	10.9%	0.5

Discussion

For patients with DM and multivessel disease, CABG was the procedure of choice. In non-diabetic patients with triple vessel disease, PTCA was an acceptable alternative to CABG in terms of 5y survival rates. However, PTCA was associated with high rates of repeat revascularisation (54%), with approximately 31% of patients subsequently requiring CABG within 5y.

Problems

- The high re-intervention rate in the PTCA group was largely attributable to coronary re-stenosis following the procedure. With the advent of coronary stents, this study is now largely of historical value as most percutaneous coronary interventions now are accompanied by stent insertions.
- It is conceivable that with a longer period of F/U, more patients in either group would require repeat procedures, although it is not known whether the increase would be greater in the PTCA or the CABG group. Also, the survival advantages of CABG accrue with time.
- See final bullet point of CABRI study (re: different patient mix).

Coronary artery disease: surgery vs bare metal stent

SoS (**S**tent **O**r **S**urgery) **trial:** Coronary artery bypass surgery vs percutaneous coronary intervention with stent implantation in patients with multivessel coronary artery disease.

AUTHORS: SoS trial investigators.
REFERENCE: Lancet (2002) 360, 965–70.
STUDY DESIGN: RCT
EVIDENCE LEVEL: 1b

Key message

At a median F/U of 2y, patients with multivessel coronary artery disease (CAD) treated with bare metal stent (BMS) have a significantly higher repeat revascularisation and mortality rate than those undergoing coronary artery bypass graft (CABG).

Impact

Although angioplasty and stent play an important role in management, CABG ultimately remains the gold standard in the treatment of patients with multivessel CAD.

Aims

Previous RCTs had shown no difference in outcome (in terms of subsequent myocardial infarction (MI) or death) between percutaneous transluminal coronary angioplasty (PTCA) and CABG. However, it is likely these studies were underpowered. Subsequent meta-analysis of these early studies concluded PTCA to be associated with poorer outcomes, with both poorer resolution of symptoms and an increased need for repeat procedure. With the use of coronary stent implantation as an adjunct to balloon dilatation reported to improve outcomes of percutaneous coronary intervention (PCI), this trial aimed to compare the clinical outcomes of patients with multivessel CAD treated with either initial BMS or CABG.

Methods

Patients: 988 patients at 53 centres in Europe and Canada.

Inclusion criteria:

- Consensus view of trial surgeon and interventionist that revascularisation clinically indicated and appropriate by either strategy;
- Interventionist identified ≥1 lesion suitable for stent implantation.

Exclusion criteria:

- Previous thoracotomy;
- Previous coronary revascularisation;
- Requiring intervention for pathology of the valves, great vessels, or aorta.

Groups:
- CABG (n=500);
- BMS (n=488).

Primary endpoint: Rate of repeat revascularisation.

Secondary endpoints:
- All-cause mortality;
- Death or Q wave MI;
- Symptoms of angina;
- Cardiac medication requirements;
- Left ventricular function.

Follow-up: Median of 2y (range 1–4y).

Results

(At 2y)	CABG	BMS	*p*
Revascularisation rate	6%	21%	<0.001
Mortality	2%	5%	0.01
Q wave MI	8%	5%	Not stated
Composite mortality and Q wave MI	10%	9%	0.8
Left ventricular ejection fraction (mean at 1y)	54.8% (SE 0.6)	55.3% (SE 0.6)	0.6 (95%CI −1.1 to 2.1)

Discussion

CABG was superior to BMS for the treatment of patients with multivessel CAD. Patients that underwent CABG had lower incidences of repeat revascularisation and lower overall mortality. The higher incidence of MI in the CABG group was mainly observed in the peri-operative period.

Problems

- It is estimated that only 3–6% of the eligible patient population were randomised, leading to an inherent selection bias. Therefore, it might be difficult to extrapolate the findings to the general patient population.
- As in the ARTS trial (*N Engl J Med* (2001) 344, 1117–24), the majority of patients in the trial had double vessel disease. It is known from other studies that the patient population benefiting the most from CABG are those with triple vessel disease. If the trial population contained only patients with triple vessel disease, the margin of benefit might be even more pronounced in favour of CABG.

Coronary bypass grafts: comparison of arterial vs venous graft

> **Cleveland Clinic Study:** Influence of the internal mammary artery graft on 10year survival and other cardiac events.
>
> **AUTHORS:** Loop F, Lytle B, Cosgrove D *et al.*
> **REFERENCE:** N Engl J Med (1986) 1, 1–6.
> **STUDY DESIGN:** Observational, retrospective
> **EVIDENCE LEVEL:** 2b

Key message

The use of the internal mammary artery (IMA) graft to the left anterior descending (LAD) artery confers superior long-term survival and reduces major adverse cardiac events, compared to the use of vein grafts.

Impact

This landmark paper caused a monumental shift towards the use of the left IMA as the conduit of choice for coronary artery bypass graft (CABG).

Aims

The conduits used in coronary artery bypass grafting have different degradation rates. The aim of this study was to determine the influence of the IMA, as compared to a vein graft, on long-term morbidity and mortality after CABG.

Methods

Patients: 5,931 patients at 1 centre in the USA (first 1,000 patients annually undergoing isolated CABG between 1971–9 were analysed),

Groups:
- IMA group: IMA to anterior descending coronary artery either alone or with ≥1 saphenous vein graft(s) (n=2306);
- Non-IMA group: saphenous vein graft(s) only (n=3625).

Inclusion criteria:
- >50% stenosis of LAD artery ± disease in other coronary arteries;
- Use of either IMA or vein grafts to LAD ± grafts to other coronary arteries.

Exclusion criteria:
- Left main stem stenosis >70%;
- Emergency surgery;
- Previous cardiac surgery;
- Bilateral/sequential/free IMA grafts;
- IMA graft to other coronary arteries;
- Peri-operative deaths.

Primary endpoint: Survival at follow-up.

Secondary endpoints:
- Cardiac re-operations;
- Late myocardial infarction (MI);
- Hospitalisation for cardiac events.

Follow-up: Mean of 8.7y (IMA group: 8.5y, non-IMA group: 8.8y).

Results

	IMA group	Non-IMA group	*p*
Primary endpoints (actuarial survival at 10y)			
Single vessel disease	93.4%	88%	0.05
Double vessel disease	90%	79.5%	<0.0001
Triple vessel disease	82.6%	71.0%	<0.0001
Secondary endpoints (risk ratios)			
Cardiac re-operations	1	2.00	<0.0001
Hospitalisation for cardiac events	1	1.25	<0.0001
Late MI	1	1.41	<0.0001

Discussion

Patients with IMA to LAD grafts had superior 10y survival, as compared to patients receiving vein grafts to the LAD artery. This was especially pronounced in patients with triple vessel disease. There was also a significant reduction in risk of major adverse cardiac events.

Problems

- This was an observational study and therefore carried inherent limitations. The authors attempted to correct for patient differences by using statistical modelling to even out potential confounding variables.
- This study was based upon patients operated on in the 1970s. Patient demographics have changed considerably since then.
- The superior results of the IMA graft were based on increased long-term patency. However, with the now routine post-operative use of statins, ACE inhibitors, antiplatelet agents and anti-hypertensive medications, vein graft patency rates may be higher.

Coronary artery bypass graft: off-pump vs on-pump bypass

Octopus trial: A multicentre, randomised study comparing outcomes among patients who underwent coronary artery bypass grafting without the aid of the cardiopulmonary bypass machine (off-pump) vs those who did (on-pump).

AUTHORS: Dijk D, Nierich A, Jansen E *et al.*
REFERENCE: Circulation (2001) 104, 1761–6.
STUDY DESIGN: RCT
EVIDENCE LEVEL: 1b

Key message
At 1 month F/U off-pump surgery produces equivalent rates of operative survival, freedom from coronary re-intervention, stroke, myocardial infarction (MI), and quality of life as compared to on-pump surgery.

Impact
Off-pump surgery for coronary artery bypass grafting is an acceptable alternative to on-pump surgery.

Aims
This study aimed to investigate whether off-pump surgery was safe, with minimal complications and satisfactory early outcomes, as compared to on-pump surgery.

Methods
Patients: 281 patients at 3 centres in The Netherlands.

Inclusion criteria:
- First time isolated CABG;
- Off-pump deemed technically feasible.

Exclusion criteria:
- Emergency/concomitant major surgery;
- Poor left ventricular function;
- Q wave MI in the previous 6wk.

Groups: At randomisation:
- Off-pump (n=142; 10 converted to on-pump and 1 had angioplasty instead);
- On-pump (n=139; 5 underwent off-pump).

Primary endpoint: Post-operative mortality.

Secondary endpoints: Stroke, MI, coronary re-intervention, and quality of life.

Follow-up: Minimum 1 month post-operative F/U

Results

At 1 month	Off-pump	On-pump	p
Primary endpoint			
Overall mortality	0%	0%	ns
Secondary endpoints			
MI	4.9%	4.3%	ns
Re-intervention	1.4%	0%	ns
Stroke	0.7%	1.4%	ns
Overall quality of Life	0.69	0.71	ns

Discussion

Off-pump surgery has gained acceptance as a safe and viable alternative to conventional on-pump surgery. It has distinct advantages in minimising ascending aorta manipulation during surgery, therefore potentially minimising atherosclerotic embolisation and peri-operative stroke. The avoidance of cardiopulmonary bypass may reduce systemic inflammatory responses, potentially avoiding end-organ complications. However, continuous quality improvements have ensured that coronary artery bypass surgery remains low in complications either with the on- or off-pump techniques.

Problems

- The patients enrolled in this study had predominantly one-to-two vessel disease. The majority of patients referred for surgery these days have triple vessel disease. The technical difficulty of the procedure escalates with an increasing number of grafts.
- The patients in this study had normal ejection fraction and would therefore be more tolerant of cardiac manipulation with the off-pump technique. Patients with poor left ventricular function are more prone to haemodynamic instability and less likely to tolerate the off-pump procedures.
- Off-pump CABG might potentially be associated with poor quality anastomosis due to the need to suture a moving target. The study only had follow-up to 1 month, and mid- to late-term complications such as graft stenosis or occlusions might not have been picked up.

Valve replacement: mechanical vs biological valve (1)

> **Veterans Affairs Study:** Outcomes 15 years after valve replacement with a mechanical vs a bioprosthetic valve: final report of the Veterans Affairs randomised trial.
>
> **AUTHORS:** Hammermeister K, Sethi G, Henderson W et al.
> **REFERENCE:** J Am Coll Cardiol (2000) 36,1152–8.
> **STUDY DESIGN:** RCT
> **EVIDENCE LEVEL:** 1b

Key message
At 15y, patients receiving biological prosthesis have a higher incidence of structural valvular degeneration, and subsequently a greater necessity for re-operation. However, they have a lower incidence of bleeding compared to patients receiving mechanical prosthesis.

Impact
The choice of valve to implant is a complex interaction of several factors (see impact message for 'Edinburgh Valve Study').

Aims
Thromboembolism is a major problem with mechanical heart valves. Although the risk is significantly lower with biological valves, early data had shown them to have limited durability due to valve degeneration. With no direct comparisons of the use of these two types of valve, this study aimed to compare morbidity and mortality of mechanical and biological valves, for mitral and aortic valve replacement (MVR and AVR, respectively).

Methods
Patients: 575 patients (all male) at 13 Veterans Affairs medical centres in the USA.

Inclusion criteria:
- No previous history of valve replacement;
- Life expectancy >3y;
- Implanted aortic prosthesis ≥21mm in diameter *or* implanted mitral prosthesis ≥37mm in diameter.

Exclusion criteria:
- Active endocarditis;
- Contraindication to warfarin.

Groups:
- Mechanical (n=286: 198 AVR, 88 MVR);
- Biological (n=289: 196 AVR, 93 MVR).

Primary endpoints: Time to death (from any cause) and time to occurrence of any of the following valve-related complications: systemic embolism, clinically important bleeding, prosthetic valve endocarditis, valve thrombosis, re-operation on randomly assigned valve, and primary valve failure (non-thrombotic valve obstruction or prosthetic valve regurgitation-perivalvular vs central).

Follow-up: For an average of 15y.

Results

(At 15y)	Mechanical	Biological	p
AVR: Mortality (all-cause)	66%	79%	0.02
MVR: Mortality (all-cause)	81%	79%	0.3
AVR: Valve re-operation	10%	29%	0.004
MVR: Valve re-operation	25%	50%	0.2
AVR: Bleeding	51%	30%	0.0001
MVR: Bleeding	53%	31%	0.01
AVR: Primary valve failure	0%	23%	0.0001
MVR: Primary valve failure	5%	44%	0.0002

Discussion

This landmark trial served to provide quantitative data on the relative morbidity and mortality associated with mechanical and biological valves. The overall survival of patients that underwent aortic valve replacement with a mechanical prosthesis was superior to that of those receiving a biological prosthesis. However, a subgroup analysis did not demonstrate this advantage in those aged >65y. Therefore, the choice of prosthesis used needs to consider three factors: whether the patient's post-operative life expectancy is likely to outlast the prosthesis, warfarin usage and its associated bleeding complications/monitoring, and the patient's view on the potential need for re-operation.

Problems

- The patients in this trial were all male and significantly younger than currently encountered patient populations.
- New generations of bio-prosthesis are predicted to provide an increased period of freedom from structural deterioration, thus potentially averting the need for re-operation.
- The incidence of bleeding complications associated with warfarin usage can be decreased by maintaining a lower level (INR) of warfarin anticoagulation without increasing thrombotic/embolic episodes, as demonstrated by several RCTs (e.g. *N Engl J Med* (1990) 322, 428–32).

Valve replacement: mechanical vs biological valve (2)

Edinburgh Valve Study: 20-year comparison of a Bjork–Shiley mechanical heart valve with porcine bio-prostheses.

AUTHORS: Oxenham H, Bloomfield P, Wheatley D et al.
REFERENCE: Heart (2003) 89, 715–21.
STUDY DESIGN: RCT
EVIDENCE LEVEL: 1b

Key message

There are no differences in overall survival at 20y between patients receiving either mechanical or biological valves. However, patients receiving mechanical valves are less likely to require re-operation due to valve failure. This is tempered by the fact that these patients are subject to elevated risks of bleeding from anticoagulation.

Impact

In general, patients are recommended to have a biological valve if they are either aged >65y and require aortic valve replacement, or are >70y and require mitral valve replacement. However, individual patient factors (e.g. pre-operative warfarin use, comorbidities, and personal preference) must be considered.

Aims

A previous long-term comparison of mechanical with porcine prosthetic heart valves by the same group had reported significantly higher survival with the Bjork–Shiley (mechanical) prosthesis at a median F/U of 12y, largely due to an increased risk of re-operation due to porcine valve failure beyond 7y. Although the improved survival trend with mechanical valves remained beyond 12y, it was no longer significant. Furthermore, mechanical valves carry the risk associated with long-term anticoagulant use. This paper reported 20y F/U comparisons of morbidity and mortality outcomes in patients receiving either biological or mechanical valve prosthesis for either mitral or aortic valve replacement (MVR and AVR, respectively).

Methods

Patients: 533 patients (excluding 8 patients with tricuspid valve replacement) at 1 centre in Scotland.

Inclusion criteria: All patients requiring heart valve replacement.

Exclusion criteria: Long-term anticoagulation contraindicated or patient reluctance to take anticoagulation over the long term.

Groups:
- Mechanical prosthesis (n=267: 129 MVR, 109 AVR, 29 AVR and MVR);
- Biological prosthesis (n=266: 132 MVR, 102 AVR, 32 AVR and MVR).

Primary endpoint: Survival (at 20y).

Secondary endpoints:
- Re-operation;
- Bleeding;
- Embolism;
- Endocarditis.

Follow-up: Mean F/U = 20.4y. F/U at regular intervals with either clinic visits or mailed questionnaires.

Results

- Demographics:
  - Mean age=53.9y (mechanical group=54.4y; biological group=53.4y);
  - 6 patients lost to F/U;
  - 56% (n=296) female;
  - 7.5% (n=40) had previous valve replacement.

At 20y	Mechanical	Biological	*p*
AVR survival	28.4%	31.3%	0.6
MVR survival	22.4%	18.4%	0.4
Re-operation	12.2%	67.8%	<0.0001
Bleeding (major episodes)	40.7%	27.9%	0.008
Embolism	36.6%	37.9%	0.8
Endocarditis	7.5%	10.3%	0.6

Discussion

This trial served to provide quantitative data with which to inform patients undergoing valve replacement, with regards to choice of prosthesis. Although mechanical valves are known to be practically free from structural deterioration over a patient's lifetime, there was a cumulative risk of major bleeding episodes of 1% per year. Biological prostheses are prone to structural deterioration over time (mitral>aortic). The death from re-operation has progressively improved over the years and, for first-time aortic valve re-operation, was observed as approaching an acceptable 5%. Therefore, individual patient factors must be considered for the choice of prosthesis.

Problems

- Patient demographics have changed considerably since the initiation of this trial in the 1970s. Patients are now older when they undergo valve replacement (mean age >65y). There are also fewer patients with rheumatic mitral valve disease requiring replacement. The majority of mitral valve surgery repairs follow myxomatous valve changes.
- There have been advances in the fixation and anti-calcification technologies of newer generation biological prostheses, with longer freedom from structural deterioration. Therefore there is a lower likelihood of need for re-operation in this group.

Gastrointestinal and hepatobiliary surgery

Introduction

Over the last century, general surgery has evolved from an extremely broad specialty to one with multiple sub-specialties based on anatomical site. Vascular, urological, and breast surgery no longer fall within the repertoire of the general surgeon and even gastrointestinal surgery itself has specific upper and lower divisions. These include well defined anatomical areas such as the pancreas, liver, and luminal oesophago-gastric surgery, as well as colorectal and pelvic floor surgical specialties. These changes have been driven by a variety of factors, but technological advances and acknowledgement of the benefits of subspecialism on post-operative morbidity and mortality—particularly for major resections—have been fundamental. Many are disappointed that we do not see the archetypal general surgical consultant patrolling the Nightingale wards any more. Operating lists consisting of breast, thyroid, vascular, and gastrointestinal surgery, which inspired generations of general surgeons to train in that specialty, are frequently recalled in coffee room conversations but now have little place in modern practice.

Advances in anaesthesia and intensive care, cross-sectional and interventional radiology, and oncological treatments have also been significant. Their influence in the trials selected in this chapter will be clearly evident. Multimodality treatment for malignancy is increasingly seen with pre-operative (neo-adjuvant) treatments, often followed by radical and often technically exacting surgery. However, nowhere has there been such a quantum change in practice as in the development of minimally invasive surgery (laparoscopic and endoscopic). These techniques allow technically advanced procedures to be performed without the morbidity and discomfort of large incisions. Early mobilisation is encouraged, with return to normal functional status recognised as an important parameter in assessing therapies in clinical trials.

This chapter reviews some of these important new developments in gastrointestinal and hepatobiliary surgery.

Gastro-oesophageal reflux: medical vs surgical management

Seven-year follow-up of an RCT comparing proton pump inhibition with surgical therapy for reflux oesophagitis.

AUTHORS: Lundell L, Miettinen P, Myrvold H *et al.*
REFERENCE: Br J Surg (2007) 94, 198–203.
STUDY DESIGN: RCT
EVIDENCE LEVEL: 1b

Key message
First RCT to show that the long-term outcome of anti-reflux surgery is superior to continuous treatment with the proton pump inhibitor (PPI), omeprazole, in terms of control of reflux symptoms.

Impact
Many upper gastrointestinal surgeons (particularly in continental Europe and Australia) recommend anti-reflux surgery as an alternative to PPIs in the primary management of gastro-oesophageal reflux disease (GORD).

Aims
Following the introduction of PPIs, anti-reflux surgery fell into disrepute. However, it soon became apparent that a significant number of patients with GORD relapsed, even on high doses of PPIs. Interest in surgical treatments was renewed, particularly since the advent of laparoscopic surgery. This trial was designed to compare long-term omeprazole therapy with anti-reflux surgery, in managing patients with reflux oesophagitis.

Methods
Patients: 298 patients from multiple Scandinavian centres.

Inclusion criteria:
- Chronic symptoms consistent with GORD;
- Evidence of erosive oesophagitis at endoscopy.

Groups:
- Omeprazole (20mg od, adjustable to 40 or 60mg od in patients who had relapse of their symptoms on 20mg) (n=154);
- Open posterior fundoplication 360° or 180° (n=144).

Primary endpoint: Failure of treatment defined as relapse of symptoms or evidence of oesophagitis at endoscopy.

Secondary endpoints:
- Failure of treatment following adjustment of the dose of omeprazole;
- Incidence of obstructive symptoms such as dysphagia, inability to belch, and flatulence, which sometimes complicate anti-reflux surgery.

Follow-up: At 1, 3, 5, and 7y, with endoscopy, to check for evidence of erosive oesophagitis. Analysis conducted on intention-to-treat basis.

Results
- The proportion of patients in whom treatment was successful (did not fail) during 7y of F/U was significantly higher in the surgical than the medical group (66.7% vs 46.7%, respectively; $p=0.002$). A smaller but significant difference remained following adjustment of the dose of omeprazole ($p=0.045$).
- A higher proportion of patients in the surgical group reported obstructive symptoms ($p<0.001$). The incidence of these symptoms remained relatively stable throughout the study period.

Discussion
Previous studies had demonstrated that anti-reflux surgery (both open and laparoscopic) was effective in controlling reflux symptoms in the short term. These data showed that the results of surgery were durable and superior to best medical treatment in the longer term, suggesting that anti-reflux surgery could emerge as the primary treatment of choice in the management of GORD.

Problems
- This and other studies have shown that a small but significant proportion of patients have persistent complaints such as dysphagia and flatulence following anti-reflux surgery, whereas PPIs are generally tolerated very well. This should be taken into account when counselling patients regarding treatment options for GORD.
- Open fundoplication was used in this study, which has now largely been replaced by its laparoscopic counterpart. However, there is good evidence that laparoscopic anti-reflux procedures are equally effective and durable in the management of GORD.
- The costs of the two treatments were not evaluated in this trial. However, there is evidence from other studies that anti-reflux surgery is also cost-effective compared with long-term use of PPIs.

Gastro-oesophageal reflux: type of anti-reflux surgery

RCT of laparoscopic vs open fundoplication: blind evaluation of recovery and discharge period.

AUTHORS: Nilsson G, Larsson S, Johnsson F.
REFERENCE: Br J Surg (2000) 87, 873–8.
STUDY DESIGN: RCT
EVIDENCE LEVEL: 1b

Key message
First double-blind RCT to show an improved short-term outcome following laparoscopic fundoplication compared with an open procedure in patients with gastro-oesophageal reflux disease (GORD).

Impact
Laparoscopic fundoplication is now considered the procedure of choice for patients with refractory GORD who require surgery.

Aims
GORD is the commonest upper gastrointestinal disease in the West, and open anti-reflux surgery has been shown to have good and long-lasting results. This trial was designed to determine whether laparoscopic fundoplication had any advantages over the open procedure in terms of speed of post-operative recovery and time for return to work.

Methods
Patients: 60 patients from 1 centre in Sweden.

Inclusion criteria:
- Refractory GORD confirmed with 24h pH monitoring;
- No previous upper abdominal surgery.

Groups:
- Laparoscopic 360° posterior fundoplication (n=30);
- Open 360° posterior fundoplication (n=30);

5 patients assigned to the laparoscopic group underwent conversion to an open procedure (4 of them due to intra-operative complications) and they were analysed separately (not an intention-to-treat analysis).

Endpoints:
- Operating time;
- Pain scores and requirement of analgesics;
- Nausea scores and requirement of anti-emetics;
- Respiratory function (forced expiratory volume, FEV; and forced vital capacity, FVC);
- Length of hospital stay;
- Duration of sick leave.

Follow-up: Twice a day until discharge from hospital and once a week after discharge until the patient returned to work. The type of operation was unknown to the patients and hospital staff.

Results

Endpoints	Laparoscopic* (n=25)	Open* (n=30)	p
Operating time (min)	148 (99–208)	109 (75–174)	<0.0001
Morphine (mg/hosp. stay)	34 (0–216.4)	67 (25–360)	<0.001
Antiemetics (doses/hosp. stay)	0 (0–3)	1 (0–9)	0.1
FEV at d1 (L)	2.6 (1.1–5.2)	2 (0.9–3.4)	0.008
Hospital stay (d)	3 (2–6)	3 (2–10)	0.02
Sick leave (d)	27 (13–139)	32 (7–126)	ns

* Values represent medians (range); NB. 5 patients in laparoscopic group converted to open procedure.

Discussion

Laparoscopic anti-reflux surgery has gained popularity based on the results of observational studies published by specialist centres. This was one of the first RCTs to show that the laparoscopic approach had some modest, short-term benefits compared with open anti-reflux surgery. In the UK, laparoscopic fundoplication is now widely accepted as the procedure of choice for severe GORD that does not respond to medical treatment.

Problems

- Small numbers: designed to include only 30 patients in each arm. The analysis was not performed on an intention-to-treat basis.
- In this trial, the advantages of the laparoscopic approach in terms of post-operative pain, and duration of hospital stay/sick leave, were more modest than expected. Indeed, other randomised studies have failed to demonstrate any benefits at all compared with the open procedure.
- Only the short-term outcome of laparoscopic fundoplication was assessed in this trial. Other studies have since shown that laparoscopic anti-reflux surgery is at least as effective and durable as its open counterpart in terms of reflux control, and is associated with a good functional outcome overall.
- 4 patients assigned to the laparoscopic group in this study suffered significant intra-operative complications. Other non-randomised studies have also reported some rare but serious complications, including major vascular injuries and oesophageal perforations. However, the overall operative morbidity of laparoscopic fundoplication remains low and reduces further with increasing experience of the procedure.

Oesophageal cancer: neoadjuvant chemotherapy

Surgical resection with or without pre-operative chemotherapy in oesophageal cancer.

AUTHORS: Medical Research Council Oesophageal Cancer Working Party.
REFERENCE: Lancet (2002) 359, 1727–33.
STUDY DESIGN: RCT
EVIDENCE LEVEL: 1b

Key message
First large RCT to show that pre-operative chemotherapy improves survival in patients with resectable oesophageal cancer.

Impact
In the UK, pre-operative chemotherapy is now routinely considered for the majority of patients with resectable oesophageal cancer.

Aims
In spite of recent advances in the diagnosis and management of oesophageal cancer, the majority of patients who undergo surgery with curative intent develop loco-regional recurrences or distant metastases within 2y of surgery. This trial was designed to determine whether a combination of systemic pre-operative chemotherapy and surgery could improve the outcome of these patients compared with surgical resection alone.

Methods
Patients: 802 patients from 42 European centres.

Inclusion criteria:
- Resectable, histologically confirmed carcinoma of the oesophagus (regardless of histological type or anatomical site);
- No other previous or concomitant malignancy;
- No evidence of cervical lymphadenopathy or other metastases;
- No contraindication to surgery or chemotherapy.

Groups:
- CS group: Immediate pre-operative chemotherapy (two 4d cycles, 3wk apart, of cisplatin and fluorouracil) followed by surgical resection (n=400);
- S group: Immediate surgical resection (n=402).

Local clinicians decided type of surgical procedure and could choose to give pre-operative radiotherapy to all their patients, irrespective of randomisation.

Primary endpoint: Survival time.

Secondary endpoints: Dysphagia and performance status.

Follow-up: On completion of treatment; at 3, 6, 9, and 12 months from randomisation; then 6 monthly until death. Analysis by intention-to-treat. Median F/U for survivors=36.9 months (CS) and 37.9 months (S).

Results

Primary endpoint	CS group	S group	*p*
Survival rate at 2y	43%	34%	0.004*
Median survival	512d (16.8 months)	405d (13.3 months)	95% CI 30 to 196
Secondary endpoints			
Worsened dysphagia	8%	5%	>0.05
Worsened performance status	24%	17%	>0.05

* For overall survival.

Discussion

This trial was the first to demonstrate that two cycles of neoadjuvant cisplatin and fluorouracil significantly improved survival in patients with localised oesophageal cancer who underwent surgical resection. Subgroup analysis also showed that chemotherapy was equally effective regardless of histology, tumour site, age, or sex. Pre-operative chemotherapy is now considered actively for the majority of patients with resectable oesophageal cancer in the UK.

Problems

• Modest doses of cisplatin and fluorouracil were used in this trial in an attempt to reduce toxicity and morbidity prior to major surgery and in order to increase compliance. There is evidence that higher doses of these agents and addition of other chemotherapeutics such as epirubicin can improve survival even further.

• No specific surgical protocol was prescribed in this trial. It has been argued that at least part of the apparent beneficial effect of chemotherapy may be due to sub-optimal surgery (e.g. lack of systematic lymphadenectomy). Indeed, a large North American trial of similar design that used a stricter surgical protocol and the same chemotherapeutic agents in higher doses, failed to demonstrate survival benefit in the chemotherapy plus surgery group.

• This trial recruited patients with resectable oesophageal cancer regardless of their pre-operative staging, and subgroup analysis by tumour stage was not carried out. Most clinicians believe that the benefit of chemotherapy is minimal for patients with early T1N0 tumours and can be omitted. The majority of these cases are surveillance-detected adenocarcinomas on a background of Barrett's oesophagus.

Gastro-oesophageal cancer: peri-operative chemotherapy

MAGIC (**M**edical Research Council **A**djuvant **G**astric **I**nfusional **C**hemotherapy) trial: Peri-operative chemotherapy vs surgery alone for resectable gastro-oesophageal cancer.

AUTHORS: Cunningham D, Allum W, Stenning S et al.
REFERENCE: N Engl J Med (2006) 355, 11–20.
STUDY DESIGN: RCT
EVIDENCE LEVEL: 1b

Key message

First RCT to show that peri-operative chemotherapy is associated with significantly improved progression-free and overall survival in patients with resectable gastric cancer.

Impact

Although not previously favoured in the UK, peri-operative chemotherapy is now considered routinely for patients with operable (stage II and stage III) gastric or lower oesophageal adenocarcinoma.

Aims

Surgery for locally advanced gastric and lower oesophageal tumours has variable outcomes. The 'ECF' (epirubicin, cisplatin, and 5-fluorouracil (5-FU)) chemotherapy regime alone had been demonstrated to improve survival. This trial was designed to determine whether three cycles of ECF given before and after surgery, with curative intent, could improve outcomes.

Methods

Patients: 503 patients from 56 international centres (mainly UK).

Inclusion criteria:
- Histologically confirmed adenocarcinoma of stomach/lower oesophagus;
- ≥Stage II, with no evidence of distant metastases/locally advanced inoperable disease;
- World Health Organization performance status of 0 or 1;
- No previous chemotherapy/radiotherapy.

Groups: Surgery in both included oesophagogastrectomy, or total/distal gastrectomy depending on tumour site. Extent of lymphadenectomy decided by treating surgeon:
- S: Surgical resection alone (n=253);
- CSC: Peri-operative chemotherapy (3 pre- and 3 post-operative cycles of IV ECF) and surgery (n=250).

Primary endpoint: Overall survival.

Secondary endpoints: Progression-free survival, surgical and pathological assessments of downstaging, and quality of life.

Follow-up: Final analysis when either 320 patients (or approximately 90%) had died or had F/U for minimum of 2y. Median F/U=49 (CSC)/47 months (S).

Results

Endpoints	CSC group	S group	*p*
Overall survival (at 5y)	36.3%	23%	0.008
T1 and T2 tumours	51.7%	36.8%	0.002
Curative resection	79.3%	70.3%	0.03

- CSC group had significantly higher likelihood of disease-free (HR=0.66, 95% CI=0.53 to 0.81, *p*<0.001) and overall survival (HR=0.75, 95% CI=0.59 to 0.93, *p*=0.008). 13% increase 5y survival; 25% decrease in risk of death.
- Similar incidence of post-operative complications and 30d mortality.

Discussion

In patients with resectable tumours, peri-operative ECF reduced tumour size and stage, significantly improving disease-free and overall survival vs surgery alone. No increase in peri-operative morbidity or mortality was observed. The treatment effect was similar regardless of age, sex, performance status, and primary tumour site. In many centres, the treatment of metastatic gastric cancer now involves replacing infusional 5-FU with an oral alternative, capecitabine; this may make the regimen more attractive to patients and avoids the risks associated with Hickman lines. In addition, studies are being conducted replacing nephrotoxic cisplatin (given over several hours with high fluid loads) with non-nephrotoxic oxaliplatin (can be given quickly and may improve convenience and efficacy). A follow-on study (UK NCRI ST03) will randomise patients to either peri-operative chemotherapy with ECX (epirubicin, cisplatin, and capecitabine) or ECX plus vascular endothelial growth factor (VEGF) receptor inhibitor, bevacizumab, an antibody that has shown encouraging results in other tumour types, including colorectal and lung.

Problems

- Study was originally designed for patients with gastric cancer only. Due to lower than anticipated recruitment rates, eligibility criteria were extended to include patients with lower oesophageal adenocarcinomas.
- Several other studies using a variety of neoadjuvant or adjuvant regimens of chemotherapy with or without radiotherapy have failed to demonstrate such significant survival benefits.
- Reported 5y survival of 23% in the 'surgery only' group is relatively low compared with the results of non-randomised studies from specialist centres in Japan and the West. In most of these centres, extensive D2 lymphadenectomy is routinely performed for gastric cancer.
- Only 42% of those assigned to receive chemotherapy completed three post-operative cycles. The post-operative component of the regimen may be poorly tolerated, conferring no additional benefits; therefore, many clinicians are inclined to omit it.

Gastric cancer: D1 vs D2 resection

> Patient survival after D1 and D2 resections for gastric cancer: long-term results of the Medical Research Council (MRC) randomised surgical trial.
>
> **AUTHORS:** Cuschieri A, Weeden S, Fielding J et al.
> **REFERENCE:** Br J Cancer (1999) 79, 1522–30.
> **STUDY DESIGN:** RCT
> **EVIDENCE LEVEL:** 1b

Key message
This large RCT shows the classical Japanese D2 resection to offer no survival advantage over the less extensive D1 resection, in patients with gastric cancer.

Impact
Routine distal pancreatectomy and splenectomy, as an integral part of D2 resection for middle and upper third gastric tumours, has now been abandoned, even by the proponents of D2 surgery. The value of extended (D2) lymphadenectomy is still debated.

Aims
Despite low 5y survival rates, surgery is the only proven effective therapy for gastric carcinoma. Observational studies from Japan and selected specialist Western centres have reported impressive results following D2 resections for potentially curable gastric cancer. This MRC trial was designed to determine whether the apparent superiority of D2 surgery could be confirmed in an RCT.

Methods
Patients: 400 patients from 32 surgeons at multiple centres in Europe.

Inclusion criteria:
- Age >20y;
- Histologically proven and potentially curable gastric cancer;
- No contraindication to major surgery and no other malignancy.

Groups: Type of gastrectomy (total or subtotal) determined according to site of the primary tumour:
- D1 resection: included removal of lymph nodes within 3cm of tumour (n=200);
- D2 resection: included removal of the second tier of lymph nodes (N2) in all cases and pancreaticosplenectomy for middle and proximal third tumours (n=200).

Primary endpoint: Overall survival.

Secondary endpoints:
- Post-operative morbidity and mortality;
- Effect of lymphadenectomy on survival;
- Effect of pancreatectomy and splenectomy on survival.

Follow-up: At regular intervals until death or until study conclusion. Median F/U=6.5y. Intention-to-treat analysis was conducted.

Results

- Overall 5y survival rates similar in the 2 arms (35% for D1 and 33% for D2; p=0.4). Disease-specific survivals and survivals after exclusion of operative deaths also similar (p>0.05).
- Post-operative morbidity and mortality significantly higher in the D2 group compared with the D1 group (46% vs 28% for morbidity, p=0.001; and 13% vs 6.5% for mortality, p=0.04).
- Subgroup analysis showed that inclusion of distal pancreatectomy and perhaps splenectomy in the resection adversely affected the overall survival of the patients. Furthermore, it provided evidence that extended D2 lymphadenectomy without pancreatectomy or splenectomy may be superior to D1 resection in terms of long-term survival.

Discussion

This trial failed to reproduce the impressive results reported in case series from Japan for D2 resections, and its findings are very similar to those reported in a Dutch trial of similar design. It is noteworthy that although overall survival was similar in the 2 arms of the trial, further analysis of the data provided some evidence that D2 resection without pancreatectomy and splenectomy may be associated with improved long-term survival compared with the standard D1 resection.

Problems

- Deficient quality control: it is impossible to ascertain whether the operating surgeons were performing true 'Japanese style' D2 resections or not. In fact, there is evidence of significant 'non-compliance and contamination' in relation to the extent of lymphadenectomy, i.e. some patients assigned to D2 resection had less radical dissection and some patients assigned to D1 resection had more extensive dissection, making interpretation of the value of lymphadenectomy problematic.
- In accordance with the prescribed protocol, all patients with middle and proximal third tumours assigned to D2 group underwent distal pancreatectomy and splenectomy. This, and other studies, have shown that inclusion of these procedures is associated with increased post-operative mortality and reduced overall survival. They are no longer considered integral parts of D2 resections unless there is direct tumour invasion.
- In this study, the reported overall survival for D2 resections was much lower, and the reported post-operative mortality was much higher than the respective figures reported in retrospective studies from Japan and from specialist centres in the West.

Cholecystectomy: type of surgery

Laparoscopic vs mini-laparotomy cholecystectomy.

AUTHORS: McMahon A, Russell I, Baxter J *et al.*
REFERENCE: Lancet (1994) 343, 135–8.
STUDY DESIGN: RCT
EVIDENCE LEVEL: 1b

Key message
First RCT to show improved outcomes following elective laparoscopic cholecystectomy vs an open procedure, in patients with cholelithiasis.

Impact
Laparoscopic cholecystectomy is now the procedure of choice for patients with symptomatic gallstones requiring elective surgery.

Aims
Laparoscopic cholecystectomy rapidly became routine practice in the UK despite the lack of credible (level 1) evidence that it had advantages over the open procedure. This trial was designed to compare laparoscopic with open cholecystectomy, to ascertain whether the perceived advantages of laparoscopic surgery could be confirmed under controlled conditions.

Methods
Patients: 302 patients from 7 consultant surgeons at 5 hospitals in Scotland.

Inclusion criteria:
- Symptomatic cholelithiasis without common bile duct (CBD) stones;
- Elective surgery.

Exclusion criteria:
- Extensive previous upper abdominal surgery (e.g. gastrectomy);
- Abnormal liver function tests or dilated CBD (however, these patients were included if pre-operative cholangiogram was normal).

Groups:
- Laparoscopic cholecystectomy (n=151);
- Mini-laparotomy cholecystectomy (n=148).

Endpoints:
- Duration of operation;
- Post-operative hospital stay;
- Post-operative physical and social functioning (modified Short Form-36 (SF36) questionnaire and Hospital Anxiety and Depression Scale (HADS);
- Complication rate;
- Cost of hospital.

Follow-up: Intention-to-treat analysis. Outpatient review at 10d and 4wk; and postal questionnaires at 1, 4, and 12wk post-surgery.

Results

Endpoint	Laparoscopic	Open	p
Operation time (mean)	71min	57min	<0.001
Hospital stay (median)	2d	4d	<0.001
Return to paid work	5wk	6wk	>0.05
Complication rate	17%	20%	>0.05
Cost to hospital (mean)	£1,486	£1,090	<0.001

- 3 randomised patients did not undergo cholecystectomy (2 because of liver metastases; 1 because of severe cirrhosis).
- Laparoscopic cholecystectomy was associated with lower pain scores, lower morphine consumption, smaller reduction in post-operative pulmonary function, and better O_2 saturation up to 24h post-operatively (p<0.01 for all endpoints).
- Laparoscopic patients also returned more quickly to leisure and social activities and had significantly better physical and social functioning scores up to 4wk after surgery (p<0.05). No differences in physical and social functioning seen between the groups after 3 months.

Discussion

Laparoscopic cholecystectomy was introduced into routine surgical practice without prior confirmation that it had advantages over the open procedure. These data suggested, for the first time, that elective laparoscopic surgery reduced hospital stay and accelerated post-operative recovery without an increase in complication rates. Subsequent non-randomised studies have shown that the risk of injury to the common bile duct has increased since the introduction of laparoscopic cholecystectomy, compared with historical controls. However, this risk remains low and reduces further as the surgeon's experience of the procedure increases. Laparoscopic cholecystectomy is more expensive than its open counterpart; however, the savings from reduced hospital stay and earlier return to work can offset some of the additional costs.

Problems

- In this trial, neither the researchers nor the patients were blinded to the type of procedure performed. Therefore, introduction of bias cannot be excluded completely for some of the results. One subsequent study that used single-blind methodology failed to demonstrate any significant advantages in terms of hospital stay and post-operative recovery.
- This trial included elective cases only, although subsequent studies have also confirmed benefits over open cholecystectomy in subsets of patients with acute cholecystitis.

Cholecystectomy: timing of surgery

Prospective randomised study of early vs delayed laparoscopic chole-cystectomy for acute cholecystitis.

AUTHORS: Lo C, Liu C, Fan S *et al.*
REFERENCE: Ann Surg (1998) 227, 461–7.
STUDY DESIGN: RCT
EVIDENCE LEVEL: 1b

Key message
First RCT to show that early laparoscopic cholecystectomy for acute cholecystitis has significant medical and socioeconomic advantages compared with conservative initial management followed by interval chole-cystectomy.

Impact
In specialist centres, laparoscopic cholecystectomy within 72h of admission is now the preferred approach for the management of patients with acute cholecystitis.

Aims
In the pre-laparoscopic era, randomised studies had shown that early open cholecystectomy for acute cholecystitis was safe and associated with shorter total hospital stay and faster recovery. This trial was undertaken in order to determine whether the same advantages would apply following the introduction of laparoscopic techniques.

Methods
Patients: 99 patients at a single centre in Hong Kong.

Inclusion criteria:
- Clinical picture consistent with acute cholecystitis associated with leukocytosis and/or ultrasonic evidence of acute inflammation;
- Patients presenting within 7d from the onset of their symptoms and considered to be fit for laparoscopic surgery;
- No evidence of spreading peritonitis, no concomitant malignancy or pregnancy, and no previous upper abdominal surgery.

Groups:
- Early: Laparoscopic cholecystectomy within 72h of admission (n=45);
- Delayed: Initial conservative management followed by laparoscopic cholecystectomy within 8–12wk (n=41).

Endpoints:
- Conversion rate to open procedure (calculation of statistical power of study based upon this);
- Operative time;
- Failure of conservative management;
- Complication rate;
- Length of total hospital stay and recuperation time.

Follow-up: At 1wk post hospital discharge, and every 4wk thereafter.

Results

Endpoint	Early	Delayed	p
Conversion rate (to open)	11%	23%	0.2
Operative time (min)*	135 (75–220)	105 (50–290)	0.02
Complication rate	13%	29%	0.07
Total hospital stay (d)*	6 (2–16)	11 (5–33)	<0.001
Recuperation period (d)*	12 (3–30)	19 (5–59)	<0.001

* Values represent medians (range).

- 4 patients in the early group and 9 patients in the delayed group were excluded after randomisation, for a variety of reasons.
- 8 patients in the delayed group required urgent surgery. 7 of the remaining 33 were readmitted with recurrent symptoms (1 required urgent surgery).

Discussion

Previous non-randomised studies indicated that early laparoscopic cholecystectomy in patients with acute cholecystitis was associated with high conversion rates and increased morbidity. The data from this study suggested for the first time that early laparoscopic cholecystectomy (within 72h of admission) was not only feasible and safe, but was also associated with a significantly shortened total hospital stay and recuperation period.

Problems

- This trial was relatively small and a significant number of patients were withdrawn after randomisation. However, subsequent randomised studies have confirmed its main findings.
- The authors commented that laparoscopic cholecystectomy following acute cholecystitis was more difficult (regardless of the timing of the procedure), and a modification of the standard technique was often required. They suggested that these procedures should only be undertaken by experienced laparoscopic surgeons.
- Surgeons in the UK have been slow to adopt a policy of early surgery in patients with acute cholecystitis mainly because of the logistical problems that such a policy would pose. Elective lists are fully booked well in advance, access to the emergency list for semi-urgent cases can be problematic, and as mentioned previously, an experienced laparoscopic surgeon would have to be available at all times.

Acute gallstone pancreatitis: endoscopic treatment

Controlled trial of urgent endoscopic retrograde cholangiopancreatography and endoscopic sphincterotomy vs conservative treatment for acute pancreatitis due to gallstones.

AUTHORS: Neoptolemos J, London N, James D *et al.*
REFERENCE: Lancet (1988) 2, 979–83.
STUDY DESIGN: RCT
EVIDENCE LEVEL: 1b

Key message
First RCT to show improved outcome in patients with acute gallstone pancreatitis who undergo early endoscopic retrograde cholangio-pancreatography (ERCP) and sphincterotomy, compared with those who have conservative management.

Impact
ERCP ± sphincterotomy, within 48 to 72h of admission, is now included in the treatment algorithm for patients with predicted severe acute pancreatitis secondary to gallstones, particularly when there is evidence of persistent biliary obstruction.

Aims
Acute pancreatitis is a potentially lethal complication of gallstones. To date, very few treatments or interventions (other than supportive measures) have been shown to modify its natural history. This trial was designed to determine whether urgent ERCP and sphincterotomy could reduce the morbidity and mortality of acute gallstone pancreatitis.

Methods
Patients: 121 patients at a single centre in the UK.

Inclusion criteria:
• Age >18y;
• Serum amylase >1000 iu/L and compatible clinical picture;
• Suspected gallstones on ultrasound and biochemistry;
• No other identifiable cause of pancreatitis.

Groups:
• ERCP ± sphincterotomy within 72h of admission (n=59);
• Conservative management (n=62);

Patients in both groups were classified as having predicted 'mild' or 'severe' attack using modified Glasgow (Imrie) criteria. (*Gut* (1984) 25, 1340–6).

Endpoints:
• Morbidity and mortality;
• Length of hospital stay;
• Subgroup analysis according to the predicted severity of the attack.

Results

Endpoints	Early ERCP	No early ERCP	p
Mortality			
Overall	2%	8%	ns
Predicted mild	0	0	–
Predicted severe	4%	18%	ns
Complications			
Overall	17%	34%	0.03
Predicted mild	12%	12%	ns
Predicted severe	24%	61%	<0.01
Hospital stay (median)			
Predicted mild	9d	11d	ns
Predicted severe	9.5d	17d	0.03

• ERCP successfully completed in 88% of cases. Only 1 procedure-related complication occurred.

Discussion

This trial was the first to demonstrate that urgent ERCP and sphincterotomy during an attack of acute gallstone pancreatitis was not only feasible and safe, but also improved the outcome of patients with predicted severe attacks. Although the observed reduction in mortality did not reach statistical significance, there was a significant reduction in the overall incidence of complications and a significant reduction in the length of hospital stay for patients with predicted severe attacks of pancreatitis, who underwent early ERCP and sphincterotomy.

Problems

• 10 patients were excluded from analysis after randomisation because an alternative diagnosis was made (not by intention-to-treat analysis). 15 more patients that were included in the final analysis did not have the diagnosis of gallstones confirmed on subsequent investigations.

• Patients with predicted mild as well as predicted severe attacks were recruited. This and subsequent studies have demonstrated that only patients with predicted severe attacks benefit from early ERCP and sphincterotomy; patients with evidence of persistent biliary obstruction benefit the most.

• A treatment protocol that includes early ERCP and sphincterotomy would require an abdominal ultrasound scan being performed within 24h of admission in all cases, and an experienced endoscopist being available 7d a week. These facilities may not always be available in hospitals that treat patients with acute gallstone pancreatitis.

Acute pancreatitis: prophylactic antibiotics

Prophylactic antibiotic treatment in patients with predicted severe acute pancreatitis: a placebo-controlled, double-blind trial.

AUTHORS: Isenmann R, Runzi M, Kron M et al.
REFERENCE: Gastroenterology (2004) 126, 997–1004.
STUDY DESIGN: RCT
EVIDENCE LEVEL: 1b

Key message
To date, this is the only double-blind, placebo-controlled RCT to investigate the role of antibiotics in acute pancreatitis. It shows that prophylactic antibiotics do not improve outcomes in patients with predicted severe acute pancreatitis.

Impact
This well designed trial provided evidence against the routine use of prophylactic antibiotics in patients with predicted severe acute pancreatitis, a common practice in the UK.

Aims
Previous trials of antibiotic prophylaxis in the management of acute pancreatitis have been inconclusive due to inadequate power or poor design. This trial used, for the first time, double-blind methodology to determine whether a combination of prophylactic IV antibiotics could improve the outcome of patients with predicted severe acute pancreatitis compared with placebo.

Methods
Patients: 114 patients from 19 centres in Germany.

Inclusion criteria:
- Abdominal pain of <72h duration in combination with a 3-fold elevation of serum amylase or lipase and;
- CRP >150mg/L or evidence of pancreatic necrosis on CT.

Groups: Study medication changed to open antibiotic treatment when there was evidence of systemic clinical deterioration:
- Antibiotics: Ciprofloxacin (400mg bd IV) plus metronidazole (500mg bd IV) for up to 21d (n=58);
- Placebo: For up to 21d (n=56).

Primary endpoint: Incidence of infected pancreatic necrosis confirmed by operative smears or by fine needle aspiration.

Secondary endpoints:
- Mortality rate;
- Incidence of local and systemic complications. A Clinical Severity Score (CSS) was devised to assess the magnitude of systemic complications;

- Incidence of surgical intervention for pancreatic necrosis;
- Length of intensive care unit (ICU) and total hospital stay.

Results

Primary endpoint	Antibiotics	Placebo	p
Infected necrosis	12%	9%	ns
Secondary endpoints			
Mortality	5%	7%	ns
CSS, median points (range)	1 (0–4)	1 (0–4)	ns
Surgical intervention	17%	11%	ns
Hospital stay, median d (range)	21 (7–237)	18 (3–129)	ns

- Study medication switched to open antibiotic treatment due to clinical deterioration in 28% (antibiotic group) vs 46% (placebo group) (p=0.04).

Discussion

Although previous trials had reported conflicting results, surveys show that the majority of UK surgeons routinely use prophylactic antibiotics in the management of patients with predicted severe acute pancreatitis. This well designed, double-blind and placebo-controlled study did not detect any significant benefits in terms of overall morbidity and mortality, need for surgical intervention, ICU stay, and total hospital stay, in patients with predicted severe pancreatitis who received prophylactic ciprofloxacin and metronidazole, compared with those who did not. The authors concluded that antibiotics should be used 'on demand'.

Problems

- Significantly higher proportion of placebo group patients required switch to non-study medication due to clinical deterioration (46% vs 28%), suggesting that prophylactic antibiotics may have a protective effect against the development of systemic (extra-pancreatic) complications. Furthermore, the fact that antibiotics were started in nearly half the placebo group after a median of 5d introduces bias against the treatment effect, making interpretation of the results more difficult.
- Some meta-analyses have shown marginal effects in favour of antibiotic prophylaxis. However, published trials show significant heterogeneity in terms of the antibiotic regimens used, populations studied, and endpoints analysed, making the results of such meta-analyses less reliable.
- Recently published guidelines of the British Society of Gastroenterology conclude that there is insufficient evidence to make recommendations for or against the routine use of prophylactic antibiotics in patients with predicted severe acute pancreatitis.

Pancreatic cancer: adjuvant therapy

ESPAC-1 (European Study group for PAncreatic Cancer) trial: Randomised trial of chemoradiotherapy and chemotherapy after resection of pancreatic cancer.

AUTHORS: Neoptolemos J, Stocken D, Friess H *et al.*
REFERENCE: N Engl J Med (2004) 350, 1200–10.
STUDY DESIGN: RCT
EVIDENCE LEVEL: 1b

Key message
First RCT to show that adjuvant chemotherapy improves outcome in patients with resectable pancreatic cancer, whereas adjuvant chemoradiotherapy has an adverse effect on survival.

Impact
In the UK, adjuvant chemotherapy is now considered routinely following resection for potentially curable pancreatic cancer.

Aims
Pancreatic cancer has a very poor prognosis, with overall 5y survival rates of less than 4%. Although adjuvant chemotherapy has been proposed to offer survival advantages, previous trials on adjuvant chemotherapy and/ or radiotherapy had been inconclusive due to inadequate power or poor design. The ESPAC undertook this trial to determine whether adjuvant chemoradiotherapy and maintenance chemotherapy, after pancreatic resection with curative intent, offered a survival advantage in patients with localised pancreatic cancer.

Methods
Patients: 289 patients from 53 centres in 11 European countries.

Inclusion criteria: Randomisation done post-surgery and included patients with histologically confirmed ductal adenocarcinoma of the pancreas who underwent macroscopically complete (potentially curative) resection.

Exclusion criteria: Positive resection margins.

Groups (2x2 factorial design):
- Chemoradiotherapy alone (20Gy in 2wk) plus fluorouracil (n=73);
- Chemotherapy alone (6 cycles of fluorouracil) (n=75);
- Combination of chemoradiotherapy and chemotherapy (n=72);
- No adjuvant treatment (n=69);

Primary endpoint: 2y survival rate (survival=date of resection to death).

Secondary endpoints:
- Incidence of adverse effects;
- Incidence of recurrence;
- Quality of life measures.

Follow-up: Every 3 months until death. Median F/U=47 months for surviving patients. Results analysed on an intention-to-treat basis.

Results

	Chemoradiotherapy (n=145)	No chemoradiotherapy (n=144)	*p*
5y survival	10%	20%	0.05
	Chemotherapy (n=147)	No chemotherapy (n=142)	*p*
5y survival	21%	8%	0.009

- Deaths/adverse events: 2 treatment-related deaths and 29 serious adverse events reported. Majority occurred in the chemoradiotherapy groups. All but 12 of the 237 recorded deaths were disease-related.
- Quality of life: No significant differences in the quality of life measures between the treatment groups.

Discussion

In spite of recent advances in the diagnosis and management of patients with pancreatic cancer, the long-term results of surgical resection alone remain poor. These data suggested, for the first time, that the addition of post-operative chemotherapy significantly improved survival in patients with resectable pancreatic cancer, whereas adjuvant chemoradiotherapy had a deleterious effect.

Problems

- This trial was not designed to have sufficient statistical power to compare survival in the four treatment groups directly. However, it is not clear why survival in the chemotherapy alone group was so much better than survival in the chemoradiotherapy plus chemotherapy group (5y survival 29% and 11%, respectively), given that only two treatment-related deaths were observed.
- Since the inception of this trial, new chemotherapy agents have become available. Gemcitabine, for example, has been shown to be superior to fluorouracil in the management of advanced pancreatic cancer and is the subject of ongoing trials in the adjuvant setting.
- This study has been criticised for the complexity of its design which makes comparisons with other trials problematic. In North America, for example, adjuvant chemoradiotherapy has been adopted as standard for resectable pancreatic cancer based on the results of a relatively small USA-based trial, which demonstrated improved survival in the chemoradiation group compared with observation alone.

Colorectal cancer: screening

Effect of faecal occult blood screening on mortality from colorectal cancer.

AUTHORS: Scholefield J, Moss S, Sufi F et al.
REFERENCE: Gut (2002) 50, 840–4.
STUDY DESIGN: RCT
EVIDENCE LEVEL: 1b

Key message
UK-based RCT demonstrating a significant reduction in mortality from colorectal cancer (CRC) in a large population that was offered screening by faecal occult blood (FOB) testing.

Impact
A national screening programme for CRC is currently being rolled out across the UK and will include all individuals between the ages of 60 and 69y.

Aims
CRC is the second commonest cause of cancer deaths in the UK. This trial was designed to determine whether screening by FOB testing could reduce the mortality from CRC in the screened population vs controls. As concerns had been raised about possible adverse effects (such as colonoscopy-related complications and psychological harm) in the screened population, the authors also examined mortality from other causes in detail.

Methods
Patients: 152,850 patients living in the Nottingham area of the UK.

Inclusion criteria:
• Individuals aged 45–74y;
• No previous CRC or other serious illness within the last 5y.

Groups:
• FOB testing every 2y. Those with positive tests offered colonoscopy and then treated accordingly (n=76,466);
• No intervention (n=76,384).

Primary endpoint: CRC-related mortality.

Secondary endpoints
• Incidence of CRC;
• All-cause mortality;
• Cause specific mortality with special reference to ischaemic heart disease (IHD) and suicide.

Follow-up: Through local hospital records and flagging at the Office for National Statistics. Case notes reviewed for all certified and registered CRC cases. Median F/U=11.7y. Intention-to-treat analysis.

Results

Primary endpoint	Intervention	No intervention	*p*
CRC mortality	0.7	0.8	<0.01
Secondary endpoints			
Incidence of CRC	1.5	1.5	0.7
All-cause mortality	24.1	24.1	0.8
IHD mortality	5.9	5.9	ns
Suicide	0.07	0.07	ns

Values represent rates per 1,000 person-years.

Discussion

This large trial demonstrated a 13% reduction in mortality from CRC among individuals who were offered screening by FOB testing. A reduction of 27% was seen when only individuals who accepted the invitation for screening were included in the analysis. Furthermore, in contrast with some early reports, there was no evidence of increased mortality from IHD or suicide in the screened group. Based on the results of this and other studies, a national screening programme for colorectal cancer has now been established in the UK.

Problems

- In spite of the fact that only 57% of subjects in the intervention group accepted the invitation for screening, a significant reduction in mortality from CRC was observed in this study. With increasing public awareness, it is anticipated that compliance rate will be higher in the national screening programme and as a result, mortality from CRC will reduce even further in the screened population.
- One of the benefits expected of screening is an overall reduction in the incidence rate of CRC as more polyps are treated endoscopically before they turn malignant. Such reduction has not been observed in this study yet, but it is likely that will become apparent with longer F/U.
- Alternative screening strategies have been proposed for CRC, but they have not gained acceptance in the UK for a variety of reasons. Colonoscopy, for example, is associated with a low compliance rate and significant risk of complications. Virtual colonoscopy and faecal DNA tests are still being evaluated as screening tools.

Colorectal cancer: open vs laparoscopic surgery

> **Medical Research Council CLASICC** (<u>C</u>onventional vs <u>L</u>aparoscopic-<u>A</u>ssisted <u>S</u>urgery <u>I</u>n patients with <u>C</u>olorectal <u>C</u>ancer) **trial:** Short-term endpoints of conventional vs laparoscopic-assisted surgery in patients with colorectal cancer.
>
> **AUTHORS:** Guillou P, Quirke P, Thorpe H *et al.*
> **REFERENCE:** Lancet (2005) 365, 1718–26.
> **STUDY DESIGN:** RCT
> **EVIDENCE LEVEL:** 1b

Key message
First UK RCT to show that the short-term outcome of laparoscopically-assisted surgery for colon cancer is equivalent to open surgery.

Impact
Laparoscopic surgery is increasingly adopted by UK surgeons in the management of patients with colorectal cancer. It is now recommended by the UK's National Institute for Health and Clinical Excellence (NICE) as an alternative to open surgery.

Aims
Early non-randomised studies had raised concerns about the oncological safety of laparoscopic resections in the management of patients with colorectal cancer. This trial was designed to compare short-term clinical and pathological endpoints in patients randomly assigned to open or laparoscopic surgery. These endpoints had been used as predictors of the long-term outcome of patients with colorectal cancer, in terms of disease recurrence and overall survival.

Methods
Patients: 794 patients from 27 centres in the UK.

Inclusion criteria:
- Operable colorectal cancer (except for transverse colon malignancies);
- Suitable for right or left hemicolectomy, sigmoid colectomy, anterior resection, or abdominoperineal resection.

Exclusion criteria:
- Pregnancy or contraindications to pneumoperitoneum (chronic cardiac or pulmonary disease);
- Acute gastrointestinal (GI) obstruction *or* GI disease requiring surgery;
- Synchronous adenocarcinomas *or* malignant disease in past 5y.

Groups:
- Laparoscopically assisted resection (n=526);
- Conventional (open) resection (n=268).

Primary endpoints:
- Rate of positive resection margins;
- Proportion of Dukes' C2 tumours;
- In-hospital mortality.

Secondary endpoints:
- Complication rates during surgery (at 30d and at 3 months);
- Quality of life measures up to 3 months after surgery;
- Transfusion requirements.

Follow-up: At 1 and 3 months after surgery, then every 3 months for the first year, every 4 months the second year, and every 6 months thereafter. Analysis by intention-to-treat and by actual treatment received.

Results

- Intention-to-treat analysis: no significant differences seen between the groups in relation to any primary/secondary endpoints.
- Conversion rates and complications: 29% of laparoscopic group underwent conversion to open surgery (25% with colonic cancer and 34% with rectal cancer). Complication rates, transfusion requirements, and proportion of Dukes' C2 tumours significantly higher in the converted group than the other two.
- Resection margins: Among patients who underwent anterior resection, subgroup analysis revealed a 2-fold increase in the rate of positive resection margins in the laparoscopic group vs the open group (not statistically significant: 12% vs 6%, respectively; $p=0.2$).

Discussion

The results of this trial suggested that open and laparoscopic surgery for colorectal cancer were equivalent in terms of 'radicality' of local dissection, lymph node harvesting, and in-hospital morbidity and mortality. As these short-term endpoints are considered reliable surrogate markers of disease-free interval and overall survival, it is likely that the long-term outcome would also be equivalent in the two treatment groups.

Problems

- Although the endpoints examined in this trial are considered accurate predictors of long-term outcome, the final results should be awaited before final conclusions can be drawn. However, other trials of similar design (and longer F/U periods) have already reported no differences in disease-free and overall survival between treatments.
- Of some concern is the non-significant increase in the rate of positive resection margins in the subgroup of patients who underwent anterior resection for rectal cancer. More RCTs are needed to clarify this issue.
- About a third of patients assigned to the laparoscopic group underwent conversion to open surgery. More importantly, this subgroup of patients suffered significantly increased in-hospital morbidity and mortality. Although conversion rates fell (suggesting that some participating surgeons were relatively inexperienced with the laparoscopic procedure), it would be useful to identify patient-related risk factors for conversion so that unplanned open surgery and its associated morbidity can be minimised.

Colorectal cancer: anti-angiogenic treatment

Bevacizumab colon study: Bevacizumab plus Irinotecan, Fluorouracil, and Leucovorin for Metastatic Colorectal Cancer.

AUTHORS: Hurwitz H, Fehrenbacher L, Novotny W et al.
REFERENCE: N Engl J Med (2004) 350, 2335–42.
STUDY DESIGN: RCT
EVIDENCE LEVEL: 1b

Key message
This RCT confirms the benefit of an anti-angiogenic treatment (bevacizumab) in advanced colorectal cancer.

Impact
Tumour angiogenesis is established as a valid target for treatment of cancer. Bevacizumab can be clinically justified as an addition to standard drugs in patients with metastatic disease. It is an expensive addition that confronts publicly funded health systems with a challenge of affordability.

Aims
Angiogenesis is one of six molecular 'hallmarks of cancer', identified in the late 20th century. Vascular endothelial growth factor (VEGF) is one of its key biological regulators. Bevacizumab is a mouse-derived monoclonal antibody against VEGF. This trial aimed to determine whether bevacizumab could improve survival in metastatic colorectal cancer when added to standard chemotherapy with irinotecan, bolus fluorouracil, and leucovorin (IFL).

Methods
Patients: 313 patients from 164 sites in the USA, Australia, and New Zealand.

Eligibility criteria:
- Histologically confirmed metastatic colorectal carcinoma;
- Bidimensionally measurable disease;
- Good performance status (Eastern Cooperative Oncology Group, ECOG, 0 or 1);
- Life expectancy >3 months;
- No prior treatment for metastatic disease;
- Adequate organ function (kidney, liver, blood, heart, brain).

Groups: Bevacizumab could continue as maintenance after 96wk:
- 1: IFL (once weekly for 4wk, cycle repeated every 6wk) and bevacizumab (every 2wk) (n=103);
- 2: IFL (once weekly for 4wk, cycle repeated every 6wk) and placebo (every 2wk) (n=100);

- 3: Fluorouracil, leucovorin (once weekly for 6wk, cycle repeated every 8wk) and bevacizumab (every 2wk) (n=110).

Once safety of bevacizumab established, recruitment for this group stopped; results not reported.

Primary endpoint: Overall survival (OS).

Secondary endpoints:
- Progression-free survival (PFS);
- Objective response: complete response (CR) and partial response (PR);
- Duration of response;
- Hospitalisation.

Follow-up: Tumour assessment 6-weekly to 24wk, then 12-weekly until treatment end. All CR/PR subject to confirmatory assessment after 4wk.

Results

Primary endpoint	Placebo	Bevacizumab	HR	*p*
Median OS (months)	15.6	20.3	0.66	<0.001
Secondary endpoints				
Median PFS (months)	6.2	10.6	0.54	<0.001
Objective response	45%	35%	–	0.004
Duration (months)	10.4	7.1	0.62	0.001
Hospitalisation	39.6%	44.9%	–	ns

- There was a higher incidence of grade 3 and 4 adverse events with bevacizumab, mainly hypertension, treatable with standard oral drugs.

Discussion

Anti-angiogenic treatment for cancer was first proposed by Folkman in 1971 (*J Exp Med* (1971) 133, 275–88), but its development in the intervening three decades had been slow. This was the study that finally confirmed the paradigm. Bevacizumab was at least as effective as any other agent tested in phase III trials for colorectal cancer, and was comparably tolerated to placebo.

Problems

- Challenges remain to understand the role of bevacizumab in relation to oxaliplatin, a newer cytotoxic active in colorectal cancer. This illustrates the continually shifting goalposts in phase III trials. At the time this study was designed, IFL was at the leading edge of drug treatment for colorectal cancer. At the time of the study's reporting, oxaliplatin was starting to appear in standard drug combinations.
- Access to bevacizumab is limited in publicly funded health systems on account of its high cost. Selection of patients who will benefit could be improved by identifying surrogate markers of response.
- There is research interest in markers of response to anti-angiogenic treatment. Several image-based markers of vascular function are being developed, including dynamic contrast MRI, positron emission tomography with oxygen-15 water, dynamic perfusion CT, and Doppler ultrasound.

Rectal cancer: total mesorectal excision

Mesorectal excision for rectal cancer.
AUTHORS: MacFarlane J, Ryall R, Heald R et al.
REFERENCE: Lancet (1993) 341, 457–60.
STUDY DESIGN: Observational study
EVIDENCE LEVEL: 3

Key message
Meticulous surgical technique and surgical specialisation can improve the outcome of patients with operable rectal cancer.

Impact
In the UK, total mesorectal excision (TME) is now the procedure of choice for resectable rectal cancer and is almost exclusively carried out by specialist colorectal surgeons.

Aims
Local recurrence is a serious problem in the management of rectal cancer with an incidence ranging from 15% to 45% after conventional surgery. In an effort to determine the standards that would be acceptable for the surgical treatment of rectal cancer, the authors of this study reviewed the outcome of a large cohort of patients with resectable tumours who had been treated with TME alone (no adjuvant therapies).

Methods
Patients: Prospectively collected data from 281 consecutive TME resections for rectal cancer, over a 13y period.

Protocol:
• Data retrospectively analysed by an independent assessor;
• Subset of 135 'high risk' patients analysed separately and comparisons made with the results of a contemporaneous North American trial that investigated the effect of adjuvant chemotherapy and chemoradiotherapy in the outcome of resectable rectal cancer;
• In accordance with the inclusion criteria, the 'high risk' group only included patients with Dukes' B and C tumours up to 12cm from the anal verge, who underwent macroscopically complete resection.

Endpoints:
• Local and overall recurrence rate;
• Disease specific survival.

Follow-up: Every 3 months for the first 2y, every 6 months for the next 3y, and yearly thereafter. Median F/U=7.7y.

Results
• Recurrence rate:
  • 200 patients underwent anterior resections with curative intent.
  • Local recurrence rate (at 5y)=4%.
  • Overall recurrence rate (at 5y)=18%.

- High-risk group: Among the 135 'high risk' patients:
  - Local recurrence rate (at 5y)=5% (95% CI 0 to 11%).
  - Overall recurrence rate (at 5y)=22%.
  - Disease-specific 5y survival=78% (95% CI 68 to 88%).
- Surgery and radiotherapy group:
  - Local recurrence rate (at 5y)=25%.
  - Overall recurrence rate (at 5y)=62.7%.
- Surgery and radiotherapy and chemotherapy group:
  - Local recurrence rate (at 5y)=13.5%.
  - Overall recurrence rate (at 5y)=41.5%.

Discussion

Local recurrence after surgical resection for rectal cancer causes disabling symptoms and is difficult to treat. These data suggested that TME could significantly reduce the incidence of local recurrence, perhaps improving overall survival. Interestingly, recurrence rates in this study following resection alone were much lower than those previously reported following conventional surgery combined with adjuvant chemotherapy and radiotherapy. Subsequent studies from other units have confirmed the superiority of TME to conventional surgery. The technique has been adopted by colorectal surgeons worldwide.

Problems

- This was an observational study, and therefore introduction of some bias is almost inevitable. However, the presented data were collected prospectively and analysed by an independent assessor, thus minimising such bias as much as possible.
- The authors compared their results with those of a contemporaneous US trial that greatly influenced the management of colorectal cancer at the time. Although the reported differences in recurrence rates were impressive, such comparisons between studies are unreliable because they are based on diverse populations with distinct characteristics.
- Based on their excellent results, the authors questioned the need for adjuvant therapies after TME for rectal cancer. Subsequent studies have demonstrated that pre-operative radiotherapy combined with TME reduces the risk of local recurrence even further and adjuvant chemotherapy may improve overall survival in selected cases.

Rectal cancer: neoadjuvant radiotherapy

Pre-operative radiotherapy combined with total mesorectal excision for resectable rectal cancer.

AUTHORS: Kapiteijn E, Marijnen C, Nagtegaal I et al.
REFERENCE: N Engl J Med (2001) 345, 638–46.
STUDY DESIGN: RCT
EVIDENCE LEVEL: 1b

Key message

First RCT to show that a short course of neoadjuvant radiotherapy reduces the risk of local recurrence in patients with rectal cancer who undergo total mesorectal excision (TME).

Impact

In the UK, neoadjuvant radiotherapy is now recommended for the majority of patients with resectable rectal cancer.

Aims

Previous studies of pre-operative radiotherapy for rectal cancer have been criticised because surgery was not standardised to include TME, a procedure that has been shown to significantly reduce the risk of local recurrence. This trial was designed to determine whether addition of neoadjuvant radiotherapy increased the benefit of TME in terms of local control of disease and overall survival.

Methods

Patients: 1861 patients from 108 European and Canadian centres.

Inclusion criteria:
- Histologically confirmed rectal adenocarcinoma up to 15cm from the anal verge;
- No pelvic fixation of the tumour and no distant metastases;
- No previous or coexisting malignancy.

Groups:
- Short course of radiotherapy (5Gy on each of 5d) followed by TME resection (n=924);
- TME resection alone (n=937);

56 patients (27 in the radiotherapy group) were found to be ineligible for participation after randomisation and were excluded from analysis.

Endpoints:
- Local and overall recurrence (at 2y);
- Overall survival at 2y;
- Post-operative morbidity and mortality.

Follow-up: Clinical evaluation every 3 months for the first year, and yearly thereafter. Annual liver imaging and endoscopy. Median F/U=24.9 months.

Results

Endpoint	Radiotherapy	No radiotherapy	p
Local recurrence	2.4%	8.2%	<0.001
Overall recurrence	16.1%	20.9%	0.09
Overall survival	82%	81.8%	0.8

- There was no evidence that the treatment effect of radiotherapy varied in accordance with tumour location, TNM staging, or type of procedure.
- Overall post-operative mortality was 3% (no difference between the groups). Patients assigned to radiotherapy had higher blood loss during surgery (1000mL vs 900mL; $p<0.001$) and more perineal complications (26% vs 18%; $p=0.05$) compared with the surgery alone group.

Discussion

This trial demonstrated that a short course of pre-operative radiotherapy could further reduce the risk of local recurrence, when used in combination with TME; this was without a significant increase in post-operative morbidity and mortality. Furthermore, this study confirmed that the good results of TME could be reproduced on a larger scale provided the surgeons were adequately trained in performing the procedure.

Problems

- This study did not show an improvement in overall survival in the radiotherapy plus surgery group after a short median F/U period of 2y. It is expected that benefits in survival will become apparent with longer F/U.
- In this trial, only patients with mobile tumours were included. There is evidence that short courses of pre-operative radiotherapy do not result in downstaging of locally advanced tumours. Therefore, accurate pre-operative staging is important. More locally advanced, fixed tumours should be treated with longer courses of pre-operative radiotherapy.
- The protocol of this trial did not allow the use of adjuvant chemotherapy. There is now evidence that post-operative chemotherapy may also be beneficial in selected cases of rectal cancer.

Anal fissure: non-surgical management

A randomised, prospective, double-blind, placebo-controlled trial of glyceryl trinitrate ointment in treatment of anal fissure.

AUTHORS: Lund J, Scholefield J.
REFERENCE: Lancet (1997) 349, 11–4.
STUDY DESIGN: RCT
EVIDENCE LEVEL: 1b

Key message
First RCT to show that topical application of glyceryl trinitrate (GTN) is effective in over two thirds of patients with chronic anal fissure, thus obviating the need for surgery.

Impact
Medical management has now replaced surgery as the first-line treatment for chronic anal fissure.

Aims
The uncertain aetiology of anal fissures makes determining ideal treatment difficult. Lateral internal sphincterotomy is an effective treatment for chronic anal fissure, but can result in minor impairment of continence in up to 30% of patients. Conservative treatment with topical preparations has been reported to be of limited efficacy in chronic fissures. Nitric oxide (NO), released by organic nitrates, can reduce maximum anal resting pressure (MARP), amounting to a 'chemical' sphincterotomy. This randomised, double-blind, placebo-controlled trial was designed to determine the effectiveness of topical GTN in the management of patients with chronic anal fissure.

Methods
Patients: 80 patients from 2 hospitals in the UK.

Inclusion criteria: Consecutive patients attending outpatients:
• Clinical evidence of chronic anal fissure (primary or recurrent);
• Duration of symptoms more than 6wk with fibrosis at fissure base.

Groups:
• GTN ointment (0.2%): bd for up to 8wk (n=38);
• Placebo: bd for up to 8wk (n=39).

3 patients excluded after randomisation (2 did not have a chronic fissure and 1 was lost to F/U).

Primary endpoint: Healing of fissure after 8wk.

Secondary endpoints:
• Severity of anal pain measured by visual analogue pain score;
• Incidence of headache;
• MARP and anodermal blood flow measured before and after the first application of ointment (GTN or placebo).

Follow-up: Every 2wk for 8wk.

Results

Primary endpoint	GTN	Placebo	*p*
Healing of fissure	68%	8%	<0.001
Secondary endpoints			
Median pain score			
Pre-treatment	73	56	ns
At 4wk	22.5	44.5	<0.05
Headache	58%	12%	<0.05

- Significant reduction in MARP and significant increase in anodermal blood flow found after the first application of the ointment in the GTN group. No changes were seen in the placebo group.

Discussion

Previous studies had demonstrated that topical application of nitrates could achieve a reversible 'chemical sphincterotomy' by transiently reducing the resting anal pressure and increasing the blood flow to the sphincter. These data suggested for the first time that GTN ointment could become first-line treatment for chronic anal fissure, greatly reducing the need for surgery and its associated risks.

Problems

- In this trial, 58% of patients in the GTN group complained of headaches soon after the application of the ointment. However, this was transient in the majority of cases, lasting <30min. Only one patient had to discontinue the treatment because of side effects.
- This trial was not designed to investigate the long-term outcome of patients after successful initial treatment with GTN. However, this and other studies have shown that GTN is also effective in the management of patients with recurrent anal fissures.
- Since the publication of this study, other non-surgical treatments for anal fissure have become available. Topical application of diltiazem, for example, has been shown to be at least as effective as GTN and is associated with a significantly lower incidence of headache. Botulinum toxin injections have also shown promising results.

Hernia repair: type of surgery

Laparoscopic vs open repair of groin hernia: a randomised comparison.

AUTHORS: The MRC Laparoscopic Groin Hernia Trial Group.
REFERENCE: Lancet (1999) 354, 185–90.
STUDY DESIGN: RCT
EVIDENCE LEVEL: 1b

Key message

First large UK trial to show significant advantages for patients who undergo laparoscopic repair of groin hernia compared with those who have an open procedure.

Impact

Laparoscopic repair of groin hernia is increasingly gaining acceptance in the UK and is already the procedure of choice in many other countries. Laparoscopic surgery has now been approved in the UK as one of the treatment options for the repair of inguinal hernia.

Aims

Surgeons in the UK have been slow to adopt laparoscopic repair of inguinal hernia mainly because of early reports of rare serious complications during and after surgery. This trial was designed to compare laparoscopic with open repair of groin hernia in order to evaluate its safety, and to determine whether it was associated with any advantages for the patient.

Methods

Patients: 928 patients from 26 hospitals in the UK and Ireland.

Inclusion criteria:
- Primary or recurrent femoral or inguinal hernia (unilateral or bilateral) that was not incarcerated and not inguinoscrotal;
- Fit for anaesthesia.

Exclusion criteria:
- Previous midline or paramedian incision;
- Uncorrected coagulation disorder;
- Pregnancy.

Groups:
- Laparoscopic repair: either transabdominal preperitoneal (TAPP) or totally extraperitoneal (TEP) according to surgeon preference (n=468);
- Open repair (n=460).

Princple outcome measures:
- Complications;
- Return to usual social activities;
- Groin pain persisting 1y post-operatively;
- Cost to health services.

Follow-up: Clinical review at 1wk, postal questionnaire at 3 months, questionnaire and clinical review at 1y.

Results

Measure	Laparoscopic (n=468)	Open (n=460)	p
Intra-operative complications			
Major	3 (0.6%)	1 (0.2%)	ns
Overall	25 (5.6%)	6 (1.4%)	<0.001
Post-operative complications	108 (29.9%)	155 (43.6%)	<0.001
Return to social activities (d)	10 (7–21)	14 (7–28)	<0.01
Pain in the groin at 1y	113 (28.7%)	133 (36.7%)	0.02
Recurrence at 1y	7 (1.9%)	0	0.02

- Laparoscopic repair cost (UK) £314 more than open repair. The difference decreased to £129 when 100% reusable equipment was used.

Discussion

Early non-randomised studies had raised concerns regarding the safety of laparoscopic repair of inguinal hernia. In this trial, although more serious complications occurred in the laparoscopic group (3 vs 1), the numbers were too small for meaningful analysis. Furthermore, this study demonstrated clear advantages associated with laparoscopic repair in terms of wound-related complications, time for return to usual social activities, and persistent pain in the groin following the procedure (all three patients who reported severe pain after 1y were in the open repair group).

Problems

- All three serious intra-operative complications in this trial occurred in the TAPP group. A recent meta-analysis confirmed a small but statistically significant difference between the two types of laparoscopic repair in terms of major (visceral or vascular) complications. However, there is evidence that the incidence of these complications reduces with experience and is exceedingly low when the procedures (both TAPP and TEP) are performed by experienced surgeons.
- There was a higher incidence of recurrence in the laparoscopic vs the open group after 1y. However, subsequent trials and meta-analyses have not found significant differences between the two procedures.
- There is little direct evidence to support the view that one laparoscopic procedure (TAPP or TEP) is superior to the other. One small, randomised trial that compared the two procedures found no differences in any of the outcome measures it examined. The choice of procedure largely depends on the individual surgeon's experience.
- Laparoscopic hernia repair is more expensive than open repair, although the cost difference is significantly lower when reusable instruments are used.

Post-operative nutrition

> Post-operative enteral vs parenteral nutrition in malnourished patients with gastrointestinal cancer: a randomised multicentre trial.
>
> **AUTHORS:** Bozzetti F, Braga M, Gianotti L et al.
> **REFERENCE:** Lancet (2001) 358, 1487–92.
> **STUDY DESIGN:** RCT
> **EVIDENCE LEVEL:** 1b

Key message
Enteral feeding reduces post-operative complications of gastrointestinal (GI) surgery, but is associated with a greater incidence of GI side effects. Enteral feeding reduces overall lengths of hospital stay.

Impact
The initial aim should be to start enteral feeding. If this is not tolerated, a low threshold should be maintained for changing to a parenteral feed.

Aims
Malnutrition is associated with poorer post-operative outcomes. Enteral nutrition is physiologically more natural than parenteral nutrition and is often advocated after major GI surgery despite this assumption having only been validated by small trials. Other advantages include its lower costs. This study aimed to evaluate the efficacy and tolerability of enteral vs parenteral feeding in malnourished patients having surgery for GI malignancy.

Methods
Patients: 317 patients at 10 centres in Italy.

Inclusion criteria:
- Weight loss ≥10% of usual body weight in past 6 months;
- Histological proven GI cancer;
- Major planned elective surgery.

Exclusion criteria:
- Age <18y;
- Hepatic dysfunction (Child-Pugh >2);
- Renal dysfunction (serum creatinine >265.2micromol/L or haemodialysis);
- Cardiac dysfunction (New York Heart Association (NYHA) Class >3);
- History of stroke;
- Karnofsky performance status <60;
- Pregnant;
- Ongoing infection;
- Intestinal anastomosis without diverting stoma.

Groups:
- Enteral nutrition (jejunostomy catheter/nasojejunal feeding tube placed at surgery)(n=159);

- Parenteral nutrition (n=158).

Feeding regimes designed to be isocaloric and isonitrogenous for 1wk.

Primary endpoint: Occurrence of post-operative complications: 17 individual infections and non-infectious complications defined (wound infection, abdominal abscess, pulmonary tract infection, urinary tract infection, bacteraemia, wound dehiscence, bleeding, anastamotic leak, respiratory failure, circulatory insufficiency, renal dysfunction, renal failure, hepatic dysfunction, pancreatic fistula, delayed gastric emptying, multiple organ dysfunction syndrome).

Secondary endpoints:
- Length of post-operative stay;
- Adverse effects;
- Treatment crossover.

Results

	Enteral (n=159)	Parenteral (n=158)	*p*
Complications (all post-op)	54 (34%)	78 (49%)	0.005
Length of stay (d)	13.4 (SD 4.1)	15 (SD 5.6)	0.009
Adverse effects	56 (35%)	22 (14%)	<0.0001
Crossover	14 (9%)	0	<0.0001

Discussion

This study showed that enteral post-operative feeding in malnourished patients with GI cancer decreased post-operative complications, but was not always well tolerated. GI adverse events such as diarrhoea, vomiting, abdominal distension, and cramps, were more common with enteral feeding. However, these were generally mild and required crossover to parenteral feed in only 9%. Enteral nutrition also decreased length of post-operative hospital stay.

Problems

- Although several similar studies have been undertaken on this subject, none have been as rigorous or on a similar scale to this. However, this trial only discussed the merits of enteral feeding in malnourished GI cancer patients, rather than patients pre-operatively malnourished from other causes.

Intensive care

Introduction

'Anyone can give an anaesthetic and that is the problem' (paraphrased dialogue with Lord Nuffield when endowing the first chair in anaesthesia). The same sentiment could have easily been expressed for intensive care two decades ago when it was often considered, especially by those not practicing the specialty, as the 'part time hobby' for those from a range of specialties.

The phenomenal developments clinically, academically, organisationally, and professionally, over the last two decades, have all defined a specialty that has not only come of age, but has established a distinct distance from its parent specialties. It is a rapidly progressing field with ideas, concepts, and innovations driving clinical progress. As a relatively young speciality, Intensive Care strives to establish a solid evidence base. Through the papers considered in this chapter, various innovations are described that have had a direct impact on practice.

Many of the developments that now arise in Intensive Care are easily promulgated to other parts of the Hospital, as the selected trials help demonstrate. Even now it can be seen that some have, so far, stood the tests of both time and clinical trials, while others have not. Trials themselves are problematic. Few things seem to work. It may well be that trial methods and, in particular, endpoints (tried and tested in other specialties in relatively homogeneous populations to assess therapeutic interventions) may be inappropriate in heterogeneous populations testing the supportive interventions that are common in Intensive Care.

Young and dynamic, the evidence base is recognised to be fluid, not concrete. However, recognition of a shortfall in hard evidence is a potent driver for innovation and for testing existent concepts. None of the trials described here are the 'last word', but are merely interim reports, both a healthy and honest position for a young specialty.

ARDS: optimal tidal volume

> **ARDSNet** (**A**cute **R**espiratory **D**istress **S**yndrome **Net**work)
> **study:** Ventilation with lower tidal volumes as compared with tra-
> ditional tidal volumes for acute lung injury and the acute respiratory
> distress syndrome.
>
> **AUTHORS:** The Acute Respiratory Distress Syndrome Network.
> **REFERENCE:** N Engl J Med (2000) 342, 1301–08.
> **STUDY DESIGN:** RCT
> **EVIDENCE LEVEL:** 1b

Key message

In acute lung injury (ALI) or acute respiratory distress syndrome
(ARDS), a lower tidal volume strategy is associated with lower mortality
and fewer ventilator-dependent days. The trial was stopped early due to
lower mortality in the lower tidal volume group.

Impact

This paper has influenced practice across the globe. Arguably, there
was already a trend towards using lower tidal volumes in patients with
ALI/ARDS, but practice is often slow to change. This study encouraged
intensivists to modify their ventilation strategies in these patients.

Aims

Patients with ALI and ARDS have mortality rates of 40–50%. Traditional
mechanical ventilation strategies utilise tidal volumes of around 10mL/kg – larger
than the 7–8mL/kg volumes in resting normal subjects. With patients
prone to stretch-induced lung injury, release of inflammatory mediators,
and subsequent non-pulmonary organ failure, this study aimed to discover
whether a lower tidal volume approach would be protective and reduce
mortality.

Methods

Patients: 861 patients at 10 centres across the USA.

Inclusion criteria:
- Age >18y, not pregnant;
- Intubated and receiving mechanical ventilation (for <36h);
- Acute decrease in ratio P_aO_2:FiO_2 ≤300;
- Bilateral pulmonary infiltrates on CXR.

Key exclusion criteria:
- Evidence of left atrial hypertension or PCWP ≤18mmHg;
- Increased intracranial pressure (ICP)/neuromuscular disease impairing
  breathing/sickle cell/severe chronic respiratory disease/chronic liver
  disease/severe burns/any condition with 6 month mortality >50%;
- Previous bone marrow or lung transplant.

Groups:
- Traditional: Ventilated at 12mL/kg tidal volume (11.8±0.8) (n=432);

- Low-volume: Ventilated at 6mL/kg tidal volume (6.2±0.8) (n=432).

Primary endpoint: Mortality pre-discharge (independently breathing).

Secondary endpoints:
- Breathing without assistance by 28d;
- Ventilator-free days (d1–28 for >48h);
- Organ/organ system failure-free days;
- Barotrauma.

Follow-up: Daily monitoring for 28d. F/U to death, d180, or until patient breathing on their own at home.

Results

Primary endpoint	6mL/kg	12mL/kg	*p*
Mortality	31%	39.8%	0.007
Secondary endpoints			
Breathing without assistance by 28d	65.7%	55%	<0.001
Ventilator-free days	12±11	10±11	0.007
Barotrauma (d1–28)	10%	11%	0.4
Organ/organ system failure-free days	15±11	12±11	0.006

Discussion

The headline finding of decreased mortality has encouraged change in ventilation practice. However, many clinicians questioned why high tidal volumes were used in the control group. This raised the question of whether the findings were that lower tidal volumes improved survival rates or that higher volumes worsened them. Despite other supporting evidence, practice change has been slow, with many intensivists resistant to lower volume strategies for reasons that remain unclear.

Problems

- As above, the use of 12mL/kg tidal volume in the 'traditional' group outstrips standard practice (of approximately 10mL/kg).
- Only 16% of eligible patients were enrolled, limiting the ability to generalise the results.
- There was an early positive end expiratory pressure (PEEP) difference between the groups; although this was small, it may have led to the positive result (rather than the differences in tidal volume).

Ventilation: continuous IV sedation

The use of continuous IV sedation is associated with prolongation of mechanical ventilation.

AUTHORS: Kollef M, Levy N, Ahrens T *et al.*
REFERENCE: Chest (1998) 114, 541–8.
STUDY DESIGN: Observational, prospective, cohort
EVIDENCE LEVEL: 2a

Key message

Continuous IV sedation appears to lengthen the duration of mechanical ventilation. The study also suggests that actively reducing the use of sedation shortens ventilation time.

Impact

Prior to the publication of this paper, some specific sedative agents had been identified as worsening outcomes, but the practice of continuous sedation had never really been questioned. Oversedation was common. Many units now have a policy of regular sedation holds and patient assessment, which is tending to reduce the depth of sedation and reduce the cumulative effects. The issue of the potentially deleterious use of sedation has now been clearly identified.

Aims

An increased duration of ventilation is associated with increased morbidity and mortality. Amongst other reasons, the likelihood of ventilator-associated pneumonia (VAP) is directly related to the length of ventilation. This study aimed to discover whether the use of unbroken sedative regimes, compared with bolus or no sedative policies, had a significant impact on duration of ventilation.

Methods

Patients: 242 consecutive patients at 1 centre in the USA.

Inclusion criteria:
- Age >17y and requiring mechanical ventilation;
- Admission to intensive care unit (ICU) >24h.

Groups:
- Continuous IV sedation during mechanical ventilation;
- Bolus IV sedation or no sedation.

Primary endpoint: Duration of mechanical ventilation.

Secondary endpoints:
- ICU length of stay;
- Hospital length of stay;
- Hospital mortality;
- Acquired organ system derangements.

Results

Primary endpoint	Continuous sedation	Bolus/none	p
Duration of ventilation	185h	55.6h	<0.001
Secondary endpoints			
ICU stay (mean d)	13.5d	4.8d	<0.001
Hospital stay (mean d)	21d	12.8d	<0.001
Hospital mortality	30%	33.6%	0.6
Acquired organ system derangements (n.)	3.1	2.5	0.01

Discussion

Sedation without regular assessment resulted in prolonged ventilation as well as longer ICU and hospital stay, at least between the two groups studied, even when potential confounding variables were taken into account. Despite this, the study did not show an effect on hospital mortality. Common sense tells us that the longer a patient remains in ICU, the more likely they are to contract other infections, with inevitable effects on morbidity and mortality. This paper made it clear that continuous IV sedation is potentially harmful, and challenged intensivists to make the distinction between patients who require ventilation and those who require both ventilation and sedation.

Problems

- This was a prospective cohort study, not an RCT, so no direct causal relationship between continuous IV sedation and prolongation of mechanical ventilation could be confirmed.
- The agents used for continuous sedation were mainly lorazepam and fentanyl. Many ICUs use shorter-acting agents such as propofol (and now remifentanil); it remains unclear what effect other sedative techniques may have had.
- This study was confined to a single centre: approaches to sedation vary considerably between units and countries.

Goal-directed therapy: increasing peri-operative oxygen delivery

A randomised clinical trial of the effect of deliberate peri-operative increase of oxygen delivery on mortality in high-risk surgical patients.

AUTHORS: Boyd O, Grounds R, Bennett E.
REFERENCE: JAMA (1993) 270, 2699–707.
STUDY DESIGN: RCT
EVIDENCE LEVEL: 1b

Key message
In high-risk surgical patients, peri-operative treatment with dopexamine decreases mortality.

Impact
The findings of this trial suggest that a high level of monitoring and inotropic support could decrease mortality. This has had huge implications for peri-operative care. While its implementation has been patchy (for a range of reasons), the principles have gained increasing popularity.

Aims
Early studies had identified surviving high-risk surgical patients as having higher post-operative cardiac output and improved systemic oxygen delivery (DO_2). 'Goal-directed' therapy involves monitoring cardiac output and other parameters to guide fluid replacement and inotrope therapy in order to increase cardiac output. However, although studies had suggested improved outcomes after major surgery, this process leads to increased cardiac oxygen requirement, with the suggestion that patients are at increased risk of myocardial ischaemia. The β_2 agonist and dopamine analogue, dopexamine, can increase DO_2 without increasing demand. This trial aimed to assess the effects of deliberately increasing peri-operative DO_2 on mortality and morbidity in high-risk surgical patients.

Methods
Patients: 107 surgical patients at 1 centre in the UK.

Inclusion criteria: Patients undergoing surgery >1.5h, with/or any of:
- Age >70y;
- Chronic cardiovascular/respiratory disease;
- Extensive surgery;
- Massive blood loss;
- Septicaemia;
- Respiratory failure (P_aO_2 <8kPa/FiO_2 >0.4 or mechanical ventilation);
- Abdominal catastrophe and haemodynamic instability;
- Acute renal failure (urea >20, creatinine >260);
- Late-stage vascular disease involving aortic disease.

Groups:
- DO_2 increase group: to >600mL/min/m^2, using dopexamine (n=53);
- Control group (n=54).

Primary endpoint: 28d mortality.

Secondary endpoints:
- 28d mortality in abdominal surgery patients;
- 28d mortality in vascular surgery patients;
- Complication rates.

Follow-up: To hospital discharge *or* 28d.

Results

Primary endpoint	Dopexamine	Control	*p*
Hospital mortality	5.7%	22.2%	0.02
Secondary endpoints			
Mortality: abdominal surgery patients	0	25%	0.05
Mortality: vascular surgery patients	10%	21%	0.3
Number of complications	0.68(±0.16)	1.35 (±0.2)	0.008

Discussion

Surgical outcomes can be improved by physiological optimisation. How much of this is due to the choice of inotrope remains contentious. Dopexamine appeared to have significant mortality benefit, but improved outcomes in the protocol group may have been due to other factors such as increased fluid administration, the role of dopexamine as a splanchnic vasodilator, or just enhanced care. Therefore, the benefits may have been unrelated to any DO_2 increase. Whilst it is clear the treatment group did better, it is not entirely clear why. Although some recent studies (*Crit Care* (2005) 9, R687–93) have also shown post-operative goal-directed therapy with dopexamine to reduce complications and decrease length of hospital stay, the issue of using dopexamine to increase oxygen transport to supranormal levels remains contentious.

Problems

- Single-centre study.
- Extremely high mortality in vascular surgical control group does not correlate with recent national UK data.
- All patients had pulmonary artery catheters inserted; not applicable to current practice.
- Despite 'as expected' higher fluid requirements in the treatment group, this is not considered as a proposed mechanism in the conclusions.
- Dopexamine effects on other organs are not considered in the mortality data.

Intravenous resuscitation: choice of fluid

> **SAFE (Saline vs Albumin Fluid Evaluation) study:** A comparison of albumin and saline for fluid resuscitation in the intensive care unit.
>
> **AUTHORS:** The SAFE Study Investigators.
> **REFERENCE:** N Engl J Med (2004) 350, 2247–56.
> **STUDY DESIGN:** RCT
> **EVIDENCE LEVEL:** 1b

Key message

There are no differences in outcomes between saline and albumin when used for resuscitation in the intensive care unit (ICU) setting.

Impact

This study refuted the claims of a meta-analysis published by the Cochrane collaboration that purported to show an increased mortality in critically ill patients given albumin, which led clinicians to question their use of resuscitation fluids. There was no difference between normal saline and albumin, but the study led to increased interest in seeking real benefits between different fluid recipes.

Aims

There remains continued debate as to the optimal choice of fluid for IV fluid resuscitation. Although albumin-containing fluids had been proposed to improve outcomes, previous meta-analyses had shown mixed results in terms of mortality benefit over crystalloid solutions. This study aimed to address the uncertainty surrounding the effects of albumin on the survival of critically ill patients.

Methods

Patients: 6997 patients at 16 ICUs in Australia and New Zealand.

Inclusion criteria:
- ICU patients;
- Age >18y;
- Requiring fluid administration to maintain intravascular volume;
- No cardiac surgery, burns, or liver transplant patients.

Groups:
- Albumin: received 4% albumin (n=3410);
- Saline: received 0.9% normal saline (n=3418).

Primary endpoint: 28d mortality.

Secondary endpoints:
- Proportion of patients with new organ failure;
- Duration of mechanical ventilation;
- Duration of renal replacement therapy (RRT);
- Duration of ICU stay;
- Duration of hospital stay.

Follow-up: Until 28d or death.

Results

Primary endpoint	Albumin	Saline	*p*
28d mortality	20.9%	21.1%	0.9
Secondary endpoints			
% no new organ failure	52.7%	53.3%	0.9
Duration of mechanical ventilation: (d)	4.4±6.1	4.3±5.7	0.4
Duration of RRT (d)	0.48±2.28	0.39±2.0	0.4
Duration of ICU stay (d)	6.5±6.6	6.2±6.2	0.4
Duration of hospital stay (d)	15.3±9.6	15.6±9.6	0.3

Discussion

Conclusions from meta-analyses asking similar questions have shown conflicting results. A Cochrane Group analysis *(BMJ* (1998) 317, 235–40) showed an increased risk of death of 6%, whereas Wilkes *et al. (Ann Intern Med* (2001) 135, 149–64) showed no significant difference in outcome. This study has put the remaining concerns over the safety of albumin in the critically ill to rest. This study also served to highlight the inherent dangers of meta-analysis, and showed large, well-planned, multicentre clinical trials can be successfully performed in critical care medicine in order to answer specific questions; for example, if the calculated power of a study involved 7,000 patients, surely a similarly powered meta-analysis would need similar numbers? The Cochrane Collaboration had only 1,419 patients from 30 studies.

Problems

• Neither albumin nor normal saline (a crystalloid) are common resuscitation fluids in many UK ICUs, a point not addressed.
• Patients with traumatic brain injury seemed to have a worse outcome with albumin, suggesting that further studies are needed.
• The saline group had significantly more fluid administered; this could have led to 'unblinding' bias. Furthermore, normal saline is associated with hyperchloraemic acidosis, but the albumin group received albumin in saline.

Glycaemic control in critically ill patients

Intensive insulin therapy in critically ill patients.

AUTHORS: Van den Berghe G, Wouters P, Weekers F et al.
REFERENCE: N Engl J Med (2001) 345, 1359–67.
STUDY DESIGN: RCT
EVIDENCE LEVEL: 1b

Key message
Tight glycaemic control reduces morbidity and mortality in critically ill patients in the surgical intensive care unit (ICU).

Impact
Tight glycaemic control has been adopted across the board in ICU despite the difficulty in other units of repeating these results.

Aims
Previous studies in critically ill patients had noted a correlation between impaired hepatocyte response to insulin and an increased risk of death. However, there had been no controlled trials. This study hypothesised that either a relative deficiency of insulin or increased insulin resistance was present in critically ill patients. It aimed to discover whether correction of these imbalances had an effect on mortality and other complications.

Methods
Patients: 1548 patients at 1 ICU in Belgium.

Inclusion criteria: All invasively ventilated patients.

Groups:
- Conventional treatment: target blood glucose 10–11.1mmol/L (n=783);
- Intensive treatment: target blood glucose 4.4–6.1mmol/L (n=765).

Primary endpoint: ICU mortality.

Secondary endpoints:
- Mortality: patients in ICU >5d;
- Need for prolonged intensive care;
- Deaths in patients with multi-organ failure (MOF) and proven septic focus;
- Need for prolonged ventilation; or renal replacement therapy;
- Critical illness polyneuropathy;
- Bloodstream infection.

Follow-up: To death or discharge from hospital.

Results

Baseline features	Conventional treatment	Intensive treatment
Male	71%	71%
Age (mean)	62.2±13.9y	63.4±13.6y
Blood glucose >110mg/dL (>200mg/dL)	76% (13%)	73% (11%)

Reason for ICU admission = cardiac surgery in 63% (conventional group) and 62% (intensive group).

Primary endpoint	Conventional treatment	Intensive treatment	p
ICU mortality	8%	4.6%	<0.04
Secondary endpoints			
Mortality (ICU >5d)	20.2%	10.6%	0.005
Deaths: MOF and septic focus	33	8	Not reported
Need for prolonged ICU	15.7%	11.4%	0.01
Need for prolonged ventilation	11.9%	7.5%	0.003
Renal replacement therapy	8.2%	4.8%	0.007
Critical illness polyneuropathy	51.9%	28.7%	<0.001
Bloodstream infection	7.8%	4.2%	0.003

Discussion

This study clearly showed that tight glycaemic control improved both morbidity and mortality in the ICU population studied. It is concordant with observations in obstetrics, cardiology, and in everyday glucose control. The largest mortality reduction was in patients with MOF with a proven septic focus (33 vs 8), but the numbers were so small that no statistical analysis was performed. This raises the question of whether another study focusing on this subgroup should be undertaken. The fact that the study population was almost exclusively surgical with low APACHE (Acute Physiology And Chronic Health Evaluation) scores makes its application to UK ICUs somewhat difficult. However, the approach is logical and should be easy to adopt and monitor – perfect for a protocol. The concept has been incorporated into ICU practice the world over, although it has proved difficult for other studies to match these results.

Problems

- Single-centre study, with almost exclusively surgical patients;
- APACHE II scores averaged 9—very low in comparison to average UK ICU scores.
- Hypoglycaemic events significantly higher in control group, a serious concern in the critically ill. This side effect has been seen in everyday practice in many units incorporating tight glycaemic control.

Sepsis: role of steroids

Effect of treatment with low doses of hydrocortisone and fludrocortisone on mortality in patients with septic shock.

AUTHORS: Annane D, Sébille V, Charpentier C et al.
REFERENCE: JAMA (2002) 288, 862–71.
STUDY DESIGN: RCT
EVIDENCE LEVEL: 1b

Key message

Treatment of relatively adrenal-deficient septic shock patients with low dose hydrocortisone and fludrocortisone for 1wk reduces mortality in non-responders to the short Synacthen test (SST); however, overall evidence for steroid use in Addisonian patients is unequivocal, with or without critical illness.

Impact

The recommendations of this study were immediately and widely accepted into intensive care practice. Many intensivists routinely perform SSTs on patients with septic shock and continue steroids in those with relative adrenal insufficiency. Many more give empirical steroids pending results, with some not even bothering with the SST.

Aims

Severe sepsis has been proposed to be associated with adrenal insufficiency or systemic glucacorticoid resistance secondary to inflammation. Smaller studies had confirmed improved arterial BP response to inotropes following low doses of hydrocortisone, in patients with septic shock. Therefore, this study aimed to assess whether steroid replacement therapy by low doses of corticosteroids could improve 28d survival in patients with septic shock and relative adrenal insufficiency.

Methods

Patients: 300 patients at 19 intensive care units (ICUs) in France.

Inclusion criteria: Age ≥18y, fulfilling standardised septic shock criteria.

Groups:
- Hydrocortisone 50mg (qds) and 50mcg fludrocortisone (od) (n=151);
- Placebo (n=149).

Primary endpoint: 28d mortality in non-responders (NR).

Secondary endpoints:
- 28d mortality in responders (R) and all patients;
- ICU, hospital, and 1y mortality in both subgroups and all patients;
- Time to withdrawal of vasopressor in both groups and all patients.

Follow-up: To 28d, discharge from ICU and hospital, and at 1y.

Results

Primary endpoint	Placebo	Corticosteroids	p
NR 28d mortality	63%	53%	0.04
Secondary endpoints			
R 28d mortality	53%	61%	1.0
All patient 28d mortality	61%	55%	0.09
NR ICU mortality	70%	58%	0.02
R ICU mortality	59%	67%	1.0
All ICU mortality	68%	60%	0.08
NR hospital mortality	72%	61%	0.04
R hospital mortality	59%	69%	0.8
All hospital mortality	69%	63%	0.1
NR 1y mortality	77%	68%	0.07
R 1y mortality	71%	69%	0.6
All 1y mortality	75%	68%	0.08
NR time to vasopressor withdrawal	10d	7d	0.001
R time to vasopressor withdrawal	7d	9d	0.5
All time to vasopressor withdrawal	9d	7d	0.01

Discussion

Among the treated non-responders, there was a significant positive effect on mortality. However, there was a trend towards a deleterious effect on ICU and hospital mortality from treatment in the responders. There was no overall effect on mortality when all patients were considered. Steroids are used for sepsis in many institutions, but there remains inconsistency in implementation of the SST. The CORTICUS trial *(Crit Care Med* (2007) 35, 1012–8) aimed to clarify matters, but was underpowered and failed to show significant benefits from steroid use. It also showed a trend to higher hyperglycaemia rates in the treatment group. There may be a place for steroids in severe sepsis for those with adrenal insufficiency, but the evidence is, at best, equivocal.

Problems

- Patients (in the first half) who had received etomidate, a potent adrenal suppressant, were not excluded; this seriously compromised what could/should have been a truly landmark paper.
- The premise of using a relatively complex means of differentiating patients based on a test that takes time to provide results is intrinsically flawed and inevitably results in over-treatment.
- The single positive result produced an 'ethical' impediment to doing further trials to assess the trial's reliability, a new problem for evidence-based medicine.
- No patient demographics were specified, which would have been relevant to the interpretation of the results (e.g. medical vs surgical condition, etc.)

Sepsis: activated protein C

PROWESS (**P**rotein C **W**orldwide **E**valuation in **S**evere **S**epsis) **study:** Efficacy and safety of recombinant human activated protein C for severe sepsis.

AUTHORS: Bernard G, Vincent J, Laterre P *et al.*
REFERENCE: N Engl J Med (2001) 344, 699–709.
STUDY DESIGN: RCT
EVIDENCE LEVEL: 1b

Key message
Treatment with activated protein C (APC) decreases 28d mortality in patients with severe sepsis with no significant increase in serious bleeding events.

Impact
The first study of its kind with a positive outcome. While APC has been adopted in many units, controversy still rages about longer-term outcomes and major bleeding risk. It was associated with the development of the 'Surviving Sepsis' campaign and an international protocol.

Aims
Sepsis has been suggested to cause activation of the coagulation cascade, leading to multi-organ failure by microvascular sludging with microthrombi. Correspondingly, severe sepsis is associated with a high mortality rate, despite appropriate and timely antimicrobial therapy. It had previously been noted that patients with severe sepsis given APC had reduced inflammatory and coagulation cascade markers. This study aimed to ascertain whether increasing levels of protein C (noted to be low in patients with sepsis) decreased mortality.

Methods
Patients: 1690 patients at 164 centres across 11 countries.

Inclusion criteria:
- Age >18y;
- Met infection criteria (known or suspected infection), based upon standard accepted criteria (evidenced by ≥1 of: white cells in normally sterile body fluid, perforated viscus, radiographic evidence of pneumonia in association with production of purulent sputum, syndrome associated with high risk of infection, e.g. ascending cholangitis);
- 3 out of 4 of modified systemic inflammatory response syndrome (SIRS) criteria (included temperature, heart rate, white cell count, respiratory rate);
- ≥1 new organ failure <24h.

Exclusion criteria:
- Pregnancy or breastfeeding;
- Platelets <30,000/mm³ *or* conditions/drugs associated with increased bleeding risk (except prophylactic anticoagulation or low-dose aspirin) *or* known hypercoagulable condition/recent thromboembolic disease;

- Very poor performance status/aggressive treatment undesirable;
- Advanced HIV, end-stage renal failure, portal hypertension, organ transplant.

Groups:
- Treatment: drotrecogin alfa (recombinant human APC) 24mcg/kg/h, for 96h (n=871);
- Placebo: normal saline with or without 0.1% HAS (albumin) (n=857).

Primary endpoint: 28d all-cause mortality.

Secondary endpoints: Included: subgroup analysis according to plasma protein C level and serious adverse events (including bleeding).
Follow-up: Data collected for 28d or until death.

Results

Recruitment stopped after 1520 patients recruited (second interim analysis) due to significant differences in mortality rates between groups.

Primary endpoint	Placebo (n=758)	Treatment (n=792)	p
28d all-cause mortality	30.8%	24.7%	0.005
Secondary endpoints			
Protein C deficient patients	32.1%	25.7%	0.009
Non-protein C deficient patients	26.7%	15.6%	0.06
Serious bleeding events	2.0%	3.5%	0.06

Discussion

This appeared to be an exciting step forward in the battle to find effective treatments against sepsis. APC was associated with a reduction in the relative risk of death of 19.4%, and an absolute risk reduction of 6.1%, giving a number needed to treat (NNT) of 16. Serious bleeding occurred in more patients in the treatment arm, but no other adverse effects were associated with the drug. Biochemical evidence of a reduction in inflammation and coagulopathy was demonstrated. Subsequent trials have suggested that the improvement in mortality and the increase in major bleeding events may well be more evenly balanced than first thought. This, coupled with the high cost of APC (average UK £5000 per patient) has meant that after an initial flurry of treatment activity, many clinicians have become increasingly cautious about its use.

Problems

- Extensive exclusion criteria (including the further exclusion of moribund patients midway through the study) means evidence of APC's efficacy is unavailable for adults without multi-organ dysfunction and high disease severity scores.
- Change in APC-producing master cell bank during study; effect unclear.
- Only 28d mortality considered; recent studies suggest mortality benefit is lost after this period.
- The precise mechanism of action associated with benefit remains uncertain; a perceived benefit without a convincing mechanism.

Prevention of GI bleeding

A comparison of sucralfate and ranitidine for the prevention of upper gastrointestinal bleeding in patients requiring mechanical ventilation.

AUTHORS: Cook D, Guyatt G, Marshall J et al.
REFERENCE: N Engl J Med (1998) 338, 791–97.
STUDY DESIGN: RCT
EVIDENCE LEVEL: 1b

Key message

Mechanically ventilated patients receiving ranitidine have significantly lower gastrointestinal (GI) bleeding rates than those given sucralfate.

Impact

This paper effectively ended the use of sucralfate in intensive care units (ICU). Ranitidine became the mainstay of stress ulcer prophylaxis despite the trend towards higher ventilator-associated pneumonia (VAP) rates.

Aims

Patients with respiratory failure and coagulopathy and/or sepsis are common in ICU. It is these patients who have been shown to be at the highest risk of upper GI bleeding. This study aimed to evaluate the rates of GI bleeding, ventilator-associated pneumonia and mortality, in mechanically ventilated patients given either ranitidine or sucralfate as stress ulcer prophylaxis.

Methods

Patients: 1200 patients at 16 ICUs in Canada.

Inclusion criteria: Mechanically ventilated patients (>48h) with:
• No established gastrointestinal bleeding on admission;
• No pneumonia on admission;
• No prior stress ulcer prophylaxis.

Groups:
• Ranitidine (50mg IV tds) or placebo (n=596);
• Sucralfate (1g via nasogastric tube, bd) or placebo (n=604).

Primary endpoint: GI bleeding.

Secondary endpoints:
• Ventilator-associated pneumonia;
• Length of ICU stay;
• ICU mortality.

Follow-up: To death or ICU discharge.

Results

Primary endpoint	Ranitidine	Sucralfate	p
GI bleeding	1.7%	3.8%	0.02
Secondary endpoints			
Ventilator-associated pneumonia	19.1%	16.2%	0.2
Length of ICU stay (Mean d) (range)	9 (5–15)	9 (5–17)	0.3
ICU mortality	23.5%	22.8%	0.3

Discussion

This study showed a statistically significant benefit of H_2 antagonist use compared with placebo or sucralfate, for stress ulceration-related GI bleeding. It failed to show a significant increase in ventilator-associated pneumonia. The latter had been implied by a previous meta-analylsis *(Crit Care Med* (1991) 19, 942–9) and led to a swing away from H_2 antagonist use, for many years. The real clinical benefit of these agents still remains contentious. The cost-to-benefit ratio of prophylaxis increases dramatically in lower-risk patients. Thus, the clear benefit of administering H_2 antagonists to prevent GI bleeding among many patients in an ICU remains to be shown. More recent studies have not helped clarify the real role of H_2 antagonists, partly due to variations in the definition of either clinically significant bleeding or nosocomial pneumonia. Most ICU clinicians will prescribe an H_2 antagonist in non-enterally fed patients.

Problems

- There were very small numbers of patients with clinically important GI bleeding (ranitidine group: 10/596; sucralfate group: 23/604).
- A large number of patients (70%) were receiving concomitant enteral nutrition, believed to reduce the risk of GI bleeding.
- Unreported incidence of coagulopathy or duration of prophylaxis prior to GI bleeding.

Pulmonary artery catheterisation

The effectiveness of right heart catheterisation in the initial care of critically ill patients.

AUTHORS: Connors A, Speroff T, Dawson N et al.
REFERENCE: JAMA (1996) 276, 889–97.
STUDY DESIGN: Observational, prospective, cohort
EVIDENCE LEVEL: 2a

Key message
Inserting pulmonary arterial catheters (PACs) in critically ill patients
appears to increase mortality.

Impact
This paper caused huge controversy in the intensive care unit (ICU) community. Almost immediately, practice changed, with clinicians becoming
more reluctant to use PACs because of its findings. Most importantly, it
caused clinicians to critically review the true value of the data they were
measuring. Although there has been severe criticism of the paper in the
intervening years, there is no doubt that the everyday use of the PACs is
now a thing of the past.

Aims
Pulmonary artery catheterisation to measure cardiac function has long
been felt to improve management of critically ill patients. However, for
a variety of reasons, including difficulty in randomisation of patients, RCT
data had been lacking. This study examined the association between the
use of PAC in the first 24h of ICU admission and survival, length of stay,
and cost.

Methods
Patients: 5735 patients at 5 hospitals in the USA.

Inclusion criteria: Designed to identify patients with an aggregate 6 months
mortality of 50% in ≥1 of the following criteria:
- Acute respiratory failure;
- Chronic obstructive pulmonary disease (COPD);
- Congestive heart failure;
- Cirrhosis;
- Non-traumatic coma;
- Colon cancer (metastatic to liver);
- Non-small cell lung cancer (stage III or IV);
- Multi-organ failure with malignancy or sepsis.

Groups:
- PAC inserted in the first 24h of ICU stay (n= 2184);
- PAC not inserted in the first 24h of ICU stay (n= 3351).

Primary endpoint: 30d survival.

Secondary endpoints:
• 2 and 6 months survival;
• Total cost of hospital stay;
• Length of ICU stay.

Follow-up: To 6 months or death.

Results

Primary endpoint	No PAC	PAC	p
30d survival	69.4%	62%	<0.001
Secondary endpoints			
2 months survival	62.8%	54.5%	<0.001
6 months survival	53.7%	46.3%	0.001
Total cost of stay (x $1,000)	74.3	131.9	<0.001
Length of ICU stay (mean d)	10.3	15.5	<0.001

Discussion

Prior to this study, PACs were in widespread use in ICUs across the world. Though the methodology can be criticised, this study was a wake-up call that sparked a sea change in practice: many clinicians stopped using PACs and there was a clamour for RCTs in the field. The single-blinded, placebo-controlled PAC-Man study (*Lancet* (2005) 366, 472–7) showed that there was no overall advantage or disadvantage to using PACs in the ICU. Most importantly, few studies show any clear benefit. The decision remains with the clinician as to whether or not to use PACs; however, there is no doubt the clinical skills required to place them are becoming a rare commodity.

Problems

• The study was neither randomised nor controlled.
• Patients receiving PACs were appreciably sicker than those who did not, with higher both APACHE (Acute Physiology And Chronic Health Evalution) and TISS (therapeutic intervention scoring system) scores.
• The catheter was studied, not the use to which it was put, and there was no information as to specific areas in which it was useful.
• Similar measurements derived by newer devices are now being increasingly employed in an identical manner, begging the question 'is the problem the tool or how it is used?'

Central venous catheter: optimal frequency of changes

A controlled trial of scheduled replacement of central venous and pulmonary arterial catheters.

AUTHORS: Cobb D, High K, Sawyer R *et al.*
REFERENCE: N Engl J Med (1992) 327, 1062–8.
STUDY DESIGN: Controlled trial
EVIDENCE LEVEL: 2a

Key message
Routine catheter replacement after 3d does not prevent infection, with new site insertions causing more complications. 'Railroading' lines over guidewires increases bloodstream infections.

Impact
This, along with other studies conducted in the 1990s, persuaded most clinicians that regular (usually weekly) invasive line changes were unnecessary and caused more complications. It is now widely accepted in clinical practice that lines should be changed only if there is evidence of infection and they have been *in situ* for several days.

Aims
Central venous catheters (CVCs), commonly used in critically ill patients, can pose a hazard of serious infections and mechanical complications. Observational studies had linked catheter use for >3–4d with higher infection rates; however, although this led to a practice of scheduled CVC replacement among some centres, this practice was not evidence-based. This study aimed to evaluate the efficacy of scheduled CVC replacement every 3d, by the use of guidewire exchange, new puncture site, replacement when clinically indicated in a new site, or exchange over a guidewire.

Methods
Patients: 160 patients (523 catheters) at 1 intensive care unit (ICU) in the USA.

Inclusion criteria:
- Subclavian or internal jugular line for >72h;
- INR <1.85;
- Platelet count >50,000/mm^3.

Groups:
- Catheters replaced every 3d via new puncture site (n=35);
- Catheters exchanged over guidewire every 3d (n=40);
- Catheters replaced when clinically indicated via new puncture site (n=41);
- Catheters exchanged over guidewire as clinically indicated (n=44).

- *Primary endpoint:* Infectious complications (bloodstream, colonisation, catheter site).

Secondary endpoints: Various mechanical complications, including:
- Pneumothorax;
- Arrhythmia;
- Suspected thrombosis;
- Bleeding;
- Mortality.

Follow-up: To 60d or death.

Results
- Complications occurring in first 3d of catheterisation (numbers=catheters):

Primary endpoint	1	2	3	4
Bloodstream infection	1/109	4/220	1/94	2/100
Catheter colonisation	6/109	10/220	5/94	26/100
Catheter site infection	0/109	1/220	1/94	0/100
Secondary endpoints				
Pneumothorax	2/109	2/220	1/94	1/100
Arrhythmia	0/109	1/220	2/94	1/100
Suspected thrombosis	2/109	0/220	1/94	0/100
Bleeding	1/109	0/220	0/94	1/100

No statistically significant differences in complication rates among the four groups.

Discussion
This study clearly demonstrated that there was no patient benefit to third day CVC changes. Guidewire exchanges ('railroading') appeared to non-significantly increase infection rates. Rates of CVC infection had previously been quoted at 2.5–70%, with suggested reasons for this wide range including variations in local practice to detect infection. Previous reports had shown many risk factors for CVC-related infection, including type of catheter, insertion site and technique, apparatus, patient characteristics, and duration of catheterisation.

Problems
- Very small cohort of patients;
- Very small numbers of complications;
- No standardisation of insertion technique or person—technicians defined only as first or second year residents.

Chapter 24

Neurosurgery

Introduction

The Edwin Smith papyrus is a transcription of several Ancient Egyptian documents dating back to the 17th century BC. It contains the world's first descriptions of neuroanatomy and details the diagnosis and management of head and spinal trauma, which remain accurate to this day. Since these ancient times, not until the turn of the 20th century—heralded by the discovery of antisepsis by Lister and the development of anaesthesia—was the field of neurosurgery really born.

Initially, it was the general surgeons who undertook neurosurgery. Based on the studies of mapping neurological function to the brain by Hughlings Jackson and David Ferrier, Sir Rickman Godlee (1849–1925), nephew of Joseph Lister, and Sir William MacEwen (1848–1924), a Scotsman, were the first surgeons who were able to locate an intracranial tumour by clinical examination, and thereby able to resect it. The work of these pioneers opened the door to specialist neurosurgeons.

Sir Victor Horsley (1857–1916), godson to Queen Victoria and son of the man who invented the Christmas card, was the world's first appointed specialist neurosurgeon. Working from the then known National Hospital for the Paralysed and Epileptics, he pioneered a series of firsts: laminectomy for spinal neoplasm, carotid ligation for cerebral aneurysm, curved skin flap, transcranial approach to the pituitary gland, intradural division of the trigeminal nerve root for trigeminal neuralgia, and surface marking of the cerebral cortex. With wide-ranging ability, Horsley also influenced other fields of medicine, one example being his study of the innervation of the larynx with Sir Felix Semons, resulting in the law that now defines the movement of the larynx.

Harvey Cushing (1869–1939) was educated at Yale, then Harvard Medical School, and worked in a number of prestigious institutions, including Johns Hopkins where he met his mentors, Halsted and Osler. The first to extensively attempt the trans-sphenoid approach to the pituitary, his tireless study of his pituitary patients led to his descriptions of 'Cushing's disease' and 'Cushing's syndrome.' Furthermore, he pioneered surgery of skull base lesions and meningiomas. Amongst his many important scientific contributions is his discovery of the 'Cushing's response' and the development of the anaesthetic chart, which he devised whilst an intern anaesthetising patients at Massachusetts General Hospital.

Since the time of these innovators, neurosurgery has developed at a rapid pace alongside technological advances such as CT, MRI, stereotaxis, microscope, and neuroendoscopy. We look forward to an exciting century of development as neurosurgery continues to demand more from technology, and now biotechnology, and these disciplines rise to meet that challenge.

Surgery for temporal lobe epilepsy

An RCT of surgery for temporal lobe epilepsy.

AUTHORS: Wiebe S, Blume W, Girvin J *et al.*
REFERENCE: N Engl J Med (2001) 345, 311–8.
STUDY DESIGN: RCT
EVIDENCE LEVEL: 1b

Key message

First RCT to demonstrate the superiority of surgery over prolonged medical therapy in the treatment of temporal lobe epilepsy.

Impact

Patients in whom temporal lobe epilepsy is suspected should be referred for surgical assessment at an early stage of their management.

Aims

Epilepsy is a relatively common and debilitating condition affecting a young, working population. Medical therapy is limited by side effects, drug interactions, and the need for monitoring. Although advances in neuroimaging and surgical technique have made surgical treatment more feasible, little robust evidence exists to support its safety and efficacy. This study aimed to assess whether surgical management of temporal lobe epilepsy was both as efficacious and safe as medical therapy.

Methods

Patients: 80 patients at 1 university centre in Canada.

Inclusion criteria:
- Age ≥16y;
- Seizures with strong temporal lobe semiology for >1y: clinically assessed by an epileptologist, MRI, EEG, and neuropsychology;
- Poorly controlled seizures with medication: seizures occurring at least every 1 month despite ≥2 anticonvulsants (one being phenytoin, carbamazepine, or valproic acid).

Groups:
- Surgical (n=36; 4 subsequently did not undergo surgery);
- Medical (n=44; 4 crossed over from the surgery group).

Primary endpoint: Freedom from seizures impairing awareness (i.e. complex or partial seizures) at 1y.

Secondary endpoints/measurements:
- Free of all seizures, including auras;
- Quality of life score.

Follow-up: At 3, 6, and 12 months, by three epileptologists (two of whom were blinded to the patients' treatment group).

Results

	Surgical	Medical	p
Primary endpoint			
Free of seizures impairing awareness at 1y	58%	8%	<0.001
Secondary endpoints			
Free of all seizures, including auras	38%	3%	<0.001
Quality of life*	73.8	64.3	<0.001

* Adjusted mean global scores on the Quality of Life in Epilepsy Inventory-89.

Adverse events	Surgical	Medical
Other	1 (wound infection)	0
Neurological	25 (see discussion)	0
Deaths	0	1 (unexpected)

• No significant difference between groups in severity of seizures, numbers attending school/employed, and cases of depression.

Discussion

This was the first robust evidence supporting surgery for the treatment of temporal lobe epilepsy. Although surgery resulted in more neurological complications than medical treatment alone, these were relatively minor and the benefits outweighed the risks: one small thalamic infarct causing thigh sensory abnormalities, two cases of decline in verbal memory affecting occupation, and 22 asymptomatic superior subquadrantic visual field defects.

Problems

• The surgical group also received optimal medical therapy for the duration of F/U. It is unclear if this was reduced over this time period and it would have been of interest to see if patients could have been rendered medication-free.
• 1y F/U duration is short. However, there is evidence to suggest that seizure-related outcome at 1y following temporal lobectomy is a reasonable predictor of subsequent outcome, and F/U continues.
• No indication of optimal timing of surgery. Patients may benefit undergoing surgical intervention earlier than 1y into their management.

Parkinson's disease: deep brain stimulation

Neurosurgery at an earlier stage of Parkinson's disease.

AUTHORS: Schüpbach W, Maltête D, Houeto J *et al.*
REFERENCE: Neurology (2007) 68, 267–71.
STUDY DESIGN: RCT
EVIDENCE LEVEL: 1b

Key message
Bilateral subthalamic nucleus (STN) stimulation, early in the course of mild to moderate Parkinson's disease (PD), improves quality of life.

Impact
First RCT to show STN stimulation should be considered in younger patients with PD, who are still in employment and in whom the disability of this chronic and progressive disease may be postponed.

Aims
Strong evidence supports bilateral STN stimulation for advanced PD. However, data assessing the impact of neurostimulation earlier in the disease process is scant. This study aimed to determine whether early STN stimulation in young patients with more recent disease onset could improve quality of life and prevent the psychosocial degradation that negatively impacts on productivity.

Methods
Patients and groups: 20 patients at 1 centre in France.

Inclusion criteria:
- Age <55y, with normal brain MRI and PD for 5–10y;
- Mild to moderate motor symptoms;
- Motor fluctuations with 'off periods' for >25% of the day;
- A professional activity of any kind;
- Absence of severe psychiatric disease or dementia;
- Impaired social and occupational functioning due to PD.

Groups: Matched and randomised in pairs to:
- Bilateral STN stimulation (n=10);
- Best medical treatment, adapted to each patient (n=10).

Primary endpoint: Relative change in overall quality of life (based upon Parkinson's Disease Questionnaire, PDQ39).

Secondary endpoints:
- Impact on activities of daily living (Unified Parkinson's Disease Rating Scale, UPDRS II questionnaire);
- Severity of motor disability: examinations conducted, unblinded, both 'off' and 'on' medication (UPDRS III);
- Reduction in daily dose of levodopa equivalence;
- Levodopa-induced motor complications (UPDRS IV);

- Cognition, frontal lobe function, anxiety, and psychiatric morbidity (Comprehensive Psychiatric Rating Scale, CPRS; Mattis Dementia Rating Scale, MADRS; Brief Anxiety Scale, BAS).

Follow-up: At 6, 12, and 18 months.

Results

At 18 months	Surgical	Medical	p
Primary endpoint			
Improved quality of life	24%	0%	<0.05
Secondary endpoints			
Improved activities of daily living	−27%	28%	<0.05
Improved severity of motor disability 'off' medication	−29%	69%	<0.05
Reduction in daily dose of levodopa	−12%	57%	<0.05
Improved levodopa-induced motor complications	−15%	83%	<0.05

- Motor scores 'on' medication did not change for either group.
- Cognition and frontal lobe function remained stable in both groups.
- Anxiety and psychiatric morbidity improved significantly in the surgical group, with no change in the medical group.
- 5 patients had transient hypomania after surgery; 4 surgical vs 3 medical patients had transient depression during F/U.
- One surgical patient had the lead cable severed at implantation.

Discussion

Adverse effects of surgery were mostly mild and transient. Low complication rates may be due to the younger trial population. The marked benefit and relative safety of surgery over medical therapy makes STN stimulation an option in those with PD, before severe motor disability and levodopa-associated motor effects develop.

Problems

- This was an unblinded, open-label study, as sham surgery was considered unethical. However, it would be unlikely for any placebo effect of surgery to persist for 18 months.
- Although a very small trial, there were enough subjects to power the study; the results require validation in a larger, multicentre study.
- 18 months is a short F/U for a disease that can span decades. Long-term F/U is essential to assess the durability of STN stimulation and its effect on disease progression.

Degenerative disk disease: surgical procedure

A prospective, randomised, multicentre Food and Drug Administration (FDA) investigational device exemptions study of lumbar total disc replacement with the CHARITE™ artificial disc vs lumbar fusion.

AUTHORS: Blumenthal S, McAfee P, Guyer R et al.
REFERENCE: Spine (2005) 30, 1565–75.
STUDY DESIGN: RCT
EVIDENCE LEVEL: 1b

Key message
Artificial disc replacement is a safe and effective treatment option for lumbar degenerative disc disease (DDD).

Impact
Artificial disc replacement can be considered as an alternative to anterior fusion for lumbar DDD. However, it remains to be accepted as a routine treatment in the absence of long-term follow-up data.

Aims
Lumbar DDD and subsequently increased spine movement at that level is a cause of lower back pain. Lumbar fusion aims to eliminate this abnormal movement. Although previous trials had supported this practice, there was also evidence to show that fusion of one level created abnormal movement at adjacent levels, resulting in the need for further surgery. Artificial discs are designed with the aim of preserving normal movement and preventing subsequent adjacent level disease. The aim of this trial was to test this hypothesis.

Methods
Patients and groups: 304 patients at 14 centres in the USA.

Inclusion criteria:
- Age 18–60y with single level, symptomatic DDD at L4–L5 or L5–S1;
- Back and/or leg pain without nerve root compression;
- Pain with a visual analogue score (VAS) ≥40;
- Oswestry disability index (ODI) ≥30;
- Ability to tolerate an anterior abdominal surgical approach;
- Failure to respond to non-fusion treatment for at least 6 months.

Groups: Randomised (in a 2:1 ratio) to:
- Artificial disc (n=205);
- Control, anterior lumbar body fusion (n=99).

Primary endpoints:
- Level of back and/or leg pain (VAS);
- Quality of life (ODI);
- Clinical success (fulfillment of 4 criteria): ≥25% improvement in ODI at 2y, no device failure, no major complications, no neurological deterioration.

Secondary endpoints:
- Duration of hospital stay;
- Narcotic medication use;
- Work status following surgery.

Follow-up: At 6wk, 3 months, 1y, and 2y.

Results

At 2y	Test Group	Control	p
Primary endpoints			
Pain, VAS*	40.6%	34.1%	0.1
ODI*	48.5%	42.4%	0.3
Clinical success	63.6%	56.8%	0.0004
Secondary endpoints			
Mean hospital stay	3.7d	4.2d	0.004
Narcotic use	72.2%	85.9%	0.008
Work status	62.4%	65%	0.5

* Expressed as mean improvement from baseline.

- Both groups significantly improved from baseline following surgery.
- No statistically significant difference in complications (e.g. development of new neurological deficits or device failures requiring re-operation), and no deaths in either group.

Discussion

The artificial disc tested was a safe and effective option for DDD. Whether it is superior to traditional anterior lumbar body fusion remains unclear; the F/U period of 2y is too short to determine if the artificial disc will indeed prevent adjacent level disease, as previous studies assessing adjacent level disease with lumbar fusion had F/U of up to 15y.

Problems

- This trial was unblinded; this may have introduced bias.
- Anterior lumbar body fusion is an established surgical procedure, with which surgeons will have had substantial experience; those unfamiliar with the artificial disc were allowed only five non-randomised cases to ensure technical competence.
- This trial was limited to levels L4–L5 and L5–S1, and to the CHARITE™ disc (DePuy Spine). Subsequent results for other levels of disease and other available artificial discs should be extrapolated with caution.

Back pain: surgery and rehabilitation

Medical Research Council (MRC) spine stabilisation trial: RCT to compare surgical stabilisation of the lumbar spine with an intensive rehabilitation programme for patients with chronic low back pain.

AUTHORS: Fairbank J, Frost H, Wilson-MacDonald J et al.
REFERENCE: BMJ (2005) 330, 1233–39.
STUDY DESIGN: RCT
EVIDENCE LEVEL: 1b

Key message

This is the first RCT to address the relative efficacy of surgery compared to intensive rehabilitation for lower back pain. Although surgery improves back pain-associated quality of life (based upon a disability index scoring system), the overall results demonstrate no clear evidence in support of surgical intervention.

Impact

In patients suffering with lower back pain, a period of intensive rehabilitation should be considered before surgical intervention.

Aims

Chronic back pain is a common and debilitating condition. Although about 1,000 lumbar fusions are performed per year in the UK, no clear evidence exists to support this practice over conservative management. This trial was designed to compare the efficacy of surgical stabilisation with an intensive rehabilitation programme for symptom relief, in patients with chronic lower back pain.

Methods

Patients and groups: 349 patients at 15 centres in the UK.

Inclusion criteria:
- Age 18–55y;
- >1y history of lower back pain;
- Uncertainty principle: deemed suitable for spinal stabilisation, but clinician and patient uncertainty as to which treatment strategy would be best.

Exclusion criteria:
- Infection or other comorbidities making one of the trial interventions unsuitable (e.g. inflammatory disease, tumours, fractures);
- Pregnancy.

Groups:
- Surgical stabilisation (n=176; 4% crossed to rehabilitation);
- Intensive rehabilitation programme (n=173; 28% crossed to surgery).

Primary endpoint:
- Quality of life, Oswestry disability index (ODI);

- Shuttle walking test: standardised, progressive, maximal test of walking speed and endurance.

Secondary endpoints/measurements:
- Physical health (e.g. physical functioning, role limitation and Short Form-36 questionnaire (SF36)); Mental health (e.g. social functioning, energy and vitality, SF36)

Follow-up: At 6 months, 1y, and 2y. Overall, 20% lost to F/U.

Results

At 2y	Estimated difference between surgery and rehabilitation (95% CI)*	p*
Primary endpoint		
ODI	−4.1 (−8.1 to −0.1)	0.04
Shuttle walking test	34 (−8 to 77)	0.1
Secondary endpoints		
SF36 physical	2.0 (−1.2 to 5.3)	0.2
SF36 mental	−0.2 (−2.9 to 2.6)	0.9

* Difference in change=surgery group score–rehabilitation group score (hence *p* value relates to whether difference in surgical group was significant or not, as compared with rehabilitation).

- Complications: Intra-operative complications occurred in 19 surgical cases: 11 patients required further operative intervention during the F/U period. Rehabilitation was not associated with any specific complications.

Discussion

Surgery was significantly better at improving back pain than rehabilitation (based upon the ODI quality of life scoring system). However, the difference of 4.1 points represented only a very small clinical difference, with overall differences in reporting of pain as an isolated symptom being non-significant. Additionally, in the face of all other outcomes being non-significant, this result requires cautious interpretation. After consideration of the complications and costs associated with surgery, the overall evidence supporting spinal stabilisation for back pain is limited.

Problems

- Selection bias was potentially introduced by only randomising patients deemed suitable for spinal stabilisation.
- There is a lack of blinding in the F/U assessment, although overall scores from the questionnaires were calculated centrally.
- Significant numbers were lost to F/U (20%). This challenges the internal validity of the trial, although statistical analyses adjusting for this loss yielded similar results to above.
- A significant number of patients allocated to rehabilitation crossed over to surgery during the F/U period. As this was an intention-to-treat analysis, these patients were considered as part of the control group, with a potential impact on the overall result.

Head trauma: prophylactic phenytoin

A randomised, double-blind study of phenytoin for the prevention of post-traumatic seizures.

AUTHORS: Temkin N, Dikmen S, Wilensky A *et al.*
REFERENCE: N Engl J Med (1990) 323, 497–502.
STUDY DESIGN: RCT
EVIDENCE LEVEL: 1b

Key message
Phenytoin only provides effective seizure prophylaxis in the short term following severe head injury.

Impact
Phenytoin may be considered for seizure prophylaxis following severe head injury. But also considering the need for therapeutic monitoring and idiosyncratic reactions, if started, its use should be limited to 1wk.

Aims
Seizures are a relatively common complication of severe head injury and can be extremely debilitating. Phenytoin had therefore been used for many years for the prevention of seizures, despite the evidence base being inconclusive and limited by subtherapeutic levels of drug and limited statistical power. This study aimed to assess whether prophylactic phenytoin reduced the incidence of seizures following severe head trauma.

Methods
Patients: 404 patients at 1 centre in the USA.

Inclusion criteria: One of the following:
- Age ≥16y;
- Cortical contusion on CT scan;
- Subdural, epidural, or intracerebral haematoma;
- Depressed skull fracture;
- Penetrating head wound;
- Seizure within 24h of injury;
- Glasgow Coma Score (GCS) ≤10.

Groups:
- Phenytoin (n=208);
- Placebo (n=196; 15 patients crossed over).

Primary endpoint: Occurrence of seizures, either 'early' (occurring from time of drug loading to d7) or late (d8 or later).

Secondary endpoints: Adverse effects.

Follow-up: Over 2y.

Results

	Phenytoin	Placebo	p
Primary endpoint			
Occurrence of early seizures	3.6%	14.3%	0.001
Occurrence of late seizures	27.5%	21.1%	>0.2
Secondary endpoints			
Rash causing stopping of treatment	17	4	<0.01
Other drug reactions	12	8	Not stated

- Mortality rates of both treatment groups were similar: 14% (n=49, phenytoin group) and 15% (n=41, placebo group) died during the 1wk F/U period, and 24% and 21%, respectively, died by 2y.

Discussion

This trial provided robust evidence that phenytoin could prevent seizures up to 1wk following severe head injury. Benefits were not seen after this period. Admirably, the maintenance of therapeutic drug levels in this study, compared to those before, was achieved.

Problems

- Crossover of patients from the placebo group to the phenytoin group, and stopping of treatment due to idiosyncratic reactions in this intention-to-treat analysis, may have obscured results. However, secondary analysis considering these factors did not reveal a different result.
- With a lack of benefit seen beyond 1wk, there was some concern as to whether the study had sufficient power to detect a potentially beneficial effect. However, statistical analysis did confirm that the power was sufficient.

Spinal metastases: surgical decompression

Direct decompressive surgical resection in the treatment of spinal cord compression caused by metastatic cancer.

AUTHORS: Patchell R, Tibbs P, Regine W et al.
REFERENCE: Lancet (2005) 366, 643–8.
STUDY DESIGN: RCT
EVIDENCE LEVEL: 1b

Key message

Surgery followed by radiotherapy (RT) is markedly superior to RT alone for spinal cord compression secondary to spinal metastases.

Impact

Patients with a single spinal metastasis causing spinal cord compression should be referred to neurosurgery for consideration of spinal decompression rather than immediately to radiation oncology.

Aims

Spinal cord compression due to metastasis is a common and debilitating complication of cancer. Previous trials had not supported the role of decompressive laminectomy, demonstrating no benefit over RT alone. However, an alternative surgical procedure for tumour removal, resulting in immediate circumferential decompression, had shown benefits over RT in previous uncontrolled series' and meta-analyses. This trial aimed to test this technique in a randomised and controlled setting.

Methods

Patients: 101 patients at 7 centres in the USA.

Inclusion criteria:
- Age ≥18y, with general medical status acceptable for surgery;
- Tissue-proven cancer diagnosis (not of CNS or spinal column origin);
- ≥1 neurological symptom or sign;
- Not totally paraplegic for ≥48h prior to surgery;
- Single spinal metastasis causing spinal cord compression;
- Expected survival of ≥3 months.

Groups:
- Surgery and RT (n=50; 4 had no/incomplete RT);
- RT alone (n=51; 10 crossed over to surgery following substantial decline in motor strength during RT).

Primary endpoint: Maintenance of, or gaining the ability to walk after treatment (i.e. able to take ≥2 steps with each foot unassisted, even if a cane or walker is needed).

Secondary endpoints: See Results section.

Follow-up: Assessment every 4wk until the trial end *or* death. Median F/U=102d (surgery) and 93d (RT).

Results

	Surgery and RT	RT	p
Primary endpoint			
Ability to walk after treatment	84%	57%	<0.001
Secondary endpoints			
Duration continence was maintained	156d	17d	0.02
Improved or maintained function post-treatment	86%	60%	0.006
Improved or maintained muscle strength post-treatment	91%	61%	0.0008
Median dexamethasone equivalent dose	1.6mg	4.2mg	0.009
Median opioid equivalent dose	0.4mg	4.8mg	0.002
30d mortality rate	6%	14%	0.3
Median duration of hospital stay	10d	10d	0.9

Discussion

The clear superiority of surgery and RT over RT alone led to premature closure of the trial. Of note, pre-operative neurology between the two groups was similar, and subgroup analysis of those able and unable to walk at study entry also reflected the significant benefits of surgery (data not shown). Importantly, surgery did not lead to an increase in hospital stay. This is overwhelming evidence supporting decompressive surgery for those with single spinal metastases causing spinal cord compression.

Problems

- Strict inclusion and exclusion criteria led to a selection bias; only patients hypothesised to do well post-surgery were randomised.
- Neurological assessments were unblinded. However, the reasonable F/U period should have compensated for this.
- No standard surgical protocol was followed. However, there was a common aim: to provide direct circumferential decompression of the spinal cord and to provide spinal stabilisation where necessary.

Brain metastases: radiotherapy and surgery

Whole brain radiation therapy with or without stereotactic radiosurgery boost for patients with 1 to 3 brain metastases: phase III results of the Radiation Therapy Oncology Group (RTOG) 9508 randomised trial.

AUTHORS: Andrews D, Scott C, Sperduto P et al.
REFERENCE: Lancet (2004) 363, 1665–72.
STUDY DESIGN: RCT
EVIDENCE LEVEL: 1b

Key message
Stereotactic radiosurgery (SRS) boost treatment confers a survival advantage over whole brain radiation alone and improves functional autonomy in those with a single, unresectable brain metastasis.

Impact
Those with single unresectable brain metastasis should be considered for SRS boost treatment in addition to whole brain radiation therapy (WBRT).

Aims
Brain metastases are the commonest intracranial tumours. Prognosis is poor, with median survival of only 1–2 months. Survival can be extended to 6 months by WBRT, and may be improved further if WBRT is preceded by surgical resection. SRS had been proposed as a less invasive alternative to surgery in those surgically unfit, or with unresectable metastases in deep seated or eloquent parts of the brain. This trial aimed to assess the benefits conferred by SRS for those with 1–3 unresectable metastases receiving WBRT.

Methods
Patients: 331 patients from multiple RTOG institutions in the USA and Canada.

Inclusion criteria:
- Age ≥18y, with no previous cranial radiation;
- Contrast-enhanced MRI showing 1–3 unresectable brain metastases outside of the brain stem or ≥1cm from the optic apparatus, with maximum diameter 4cm (for the largest lesion), and additional lesions not exceeding 3cm in diameter;
- Treatment for systemic cancer completed >1 month ago;
- Karnofsky Performance Score (KPS) >70.

Groups:
- WBRT and SRS boost RSS within 1wk of completing WBRT (n=164);
- WBRT alone (n=167).

Primary endpoint: Overall survival (subgroup analysis: survival by number of brain metastases and analysis of potential prognostic factors).

Secondary endpoints:
• Overall time to tumour progression;
• Local control rate;
• Performance measures (KPS, steroid use, mental status).

Follow-up: At 3, 6, and 9 months; then at 1y.

Results

	WBRT and SRS	WBRT alone	*p*
Primary endpoint			
Overall survival	6.5 months	5.7 months	0.1
Survival (single brain metastasis)	6.5 months	4.9 months	0.04
Secondary endpoints			
Time to tumour progression	Not reported		0.1
Overall local control	82%	71%	0.01

• No difference between groups: early and late toxicities, rate of neurological death, mental status.
• Univariate and multivariate analysis:
  • Recursive partitioning analysis (RPA) class and tumour type were prognostic factors independent of metastasis number.
  • RPA class 1 and squamous/non-small cell carcinomas had significantly better outcomes with the addition of SRS.
  • SRS also conferred a statistically significant improvement in KPS and decreased steroid use at 6 months.

Discussion

Addition of SRS to WBRT improved survival, local control rates, and performance measures in those with single, unresectable brain metastasis. SRS should be considered for these patients, especially in those deemed RPA class 1 and with squamous/non-small cell tumours. As SRS improved performance measures in all patients, it may also still be considered for those with multiple brain metastases. Trials comparing surgery and SRS have failed to accrue enough patients due to strong biases of treating physicians and informed patients. However, there are ongoing trials comparing SRS alone with WBRT and SRS.

Problems

• 19% (n=31) of the SRS group did not receive SRS. As this was an intention-to-treat analysis, this group was still analysed as having had SRS, thus potentially affecting outcomes.
• A significant number of MRIs were not available for assessment at 3 months F/U, thereby affecting analysis of secondary outcomes.

Glioblastoma: adjuvant chemotherapy

Radiotherapy plus concomitant and adjuvant temozolomide for glioblastoma.

AUTHORS: Stupp R, Mason W, van den Bent M *et al.*
REFERENCE: N Engl J Med (2005) 352, 987–96.
STUDY DESIGN: RCT
EVIDENCE LEVEL: 1b

Key message
Addition of temozolomide to radiotherapy confers a significant survival advantage for patients with glioblastoma with minimal toxicity.

Impact
Temozolomide is now used as routine adjuvant therapy for those with glioblastoma.

Aims
Glioblastoma multiforme is the commonest adult primary brain tumour. Despite surgical resection and radiotherapy (RT), prognosis remains poor, with a median survival of 1y from diagnosis. Temozolomide, an alkylating agent that depletes the DNA repair enzyme, O^6-methylguanine DNA methyltransferase (MGMT), had been shown to potentially improve survival in phase II studies. This phase III trial aimed to substantiate this finding.

Methods
Patients: 573 patients at 85 centres in 15 countries.

Inclusion criteria:
- Age 18–70y;
- Histologically confirmed glioblastoma (World Health Organization (WHO) grade IV astrocytoma);
- WHO performance status of ≤2;
- Adequate haematological, renal, and hepatic function;
- Those receiving a stable or decreasing dose of corticosteroids.

Groups:
- RT and temozolomide (daily temozolomide during RT, followed by 6 cycles of adjuvant treatment) (n=287);
- RT (n=286).

Primary endpoint: Overall survival.

Secondary endpoints/measurements:
- Progression-free survival;
- Safety.

Follow-up: Maximum F/U=24 months. Median F/U=28 months.

Results

	RT and temozolomide (95% CI)	RT alone (95% CI)
Primary endpoint		
Median survival	14.6 months (13.2 to 16.8)	12.1 months (11.2 to 13.0)
2y survival rate	26.5% (21.2 to 31.7)	10.4% (6.8 to 14.1)
Secondary endpoints		
Median progression-free survival	6.9 months (5.8 to 8.2)	5 months (4.2 to 5.5)
Grade 3–4 haemotologic toxicity	Concomitant: 7% Adjuvant: 14%	0
Severe infections	Concomitant: 3% Adjuvant: 5%	2%

- At 28 months, 480 patients (84%) had died.
- Hazard ratio for death in the RT and temozolomide group vs RT alone was 0.63 (95% CI 0.52 to 0.75, $p<0.001$).

Discussion

The addition of the chemotherapeutic agent, temozolomide, to RT significantly prolonged the survival of patients with newly diagnosed glioblastoma. Median increase in survival was 2.5 months and the relative reduction in risk of death was 37%. Furthermore, chemotherapy was safe, with minimal toxicity. Interestingly, a translational study involving methylation of the MGMT promoter (resulting in gene silencing) was associated with a striking survival advantage in patients treated with RT and temozolomide. In the future, therapy may be tailored to the tumour's biological profile.

Problems

- It is not clear from this study whether temozolomide is required, both concomitantly and as an adjuvant to RT. Ongoing studies are assessing the optimum RT and temozolomide regime.
- 85% of the RT and temozolomide group and 94% of the RT alone group had disease progression. At this point, further treatment was at the physician's discretion, which included both surgery and salvage chemotherapy. Salvage therapies may have influenced overall outcomes in this intention-to-treat analysis.

Subarachnoid haemorrhage: nimodipine

BRANT (**BR**itish **A**neurysm **N**imodipine **T**rial): Effect of oral nimodipine on cerebral infarction and outcome after subarachnoid haemorrhage.

AUTHORS: Pickard J, Murray G, Illingworth R *et al.*
REFERENCE: BMJ (1989) 298, 636–42.
STUDY DESIGN: RCT
EVIDENCE LEVEL: 1b

Key message
Oral nimodipine reduces cerebral infarction, thereby improving outcomes following aneurysmal subarachnoid haemorrhage (SAH).

Impact
Oral nimodipine (at a dose of 60mg every 4h, for 21d) is given routinely to patients following aneurysmal SAH.

Aims
Cerebral ischaemia or infarction is a common, debilitating complication of aneurysmal SAH. Previous studies to investigate the effects of the calcium channel antagonist, nimodipine, on the incidence of these complications, had been inconclusive. This study aimed to establish the exact effects and outcomes of nimodipine after aneurysmal SAH.

Methods
Patients: 554 patients at 4 centres in the UK.

Inclusion criteria:
- Age ≥18y;
- Within 96h of onset of aneurysmal SAH;
- Proven SAH on lumbar puncture and/or CT;
- Presence of an aneurysm subsequently proven on angiography or necropsy, or (in 2 cases) typical appearance of a giant aneurysm on CT;
- Absence of major renal, pulmonary disease, pre-existing cardiac decompensation, or recent myocardial infarction.

Groups:
- Nimodipine (60mg PO every 4h, for 21d) (n=278);
- Placebo (n=276).

Protocol: Treatment initiated within 96h of ictus and routinely continued for 21d in survivors. CT performed within 24h of trial entry and repeated if clinically indicated.

Primary endpoint: Incidence of cerebral infarction.

Secondary endpoints/measurements:
- Outcome at 3 months: 'poor outcomes', i.e. 3 of the 5 Glasgow Outcome Scale (GOS) categories (death, vegetative state, and severe disability);
- Adverse reactions.

Follow-up: At 3 months.

Results

	Nimodipine	Placebo	p
Primary endpoint			
Incidence of cerebral infarction	22%	33%	0.03
Secondary endpoints			
Poor outcomes	20%	33%	< 0.001
Death	43	60	< 0.06
Adverse reactions	17	10	–
Withdrew due to adverse drug reactions	8	3	–

- Adjusting for prognostic factors (e.g. sex and loss of consciousness) did not change the significant reduction in cerebral infarction and poor outcome associated with nimodipine.
- Adverse events included cardiovascular (hypotension, flushing) and hepatic (impaired liver function) effects.

Discussion

Nimodipine significantly reduced the rate of cerebral infarction and improved outcomes following aneurysmal SAH. Although cerebral ischaemia classically occurs between 7–10d following SAH, the need for early and prolonged institution of nimodipine was reflected by only 37% of ischaemic events in this trial occurring within this time frame. Furthermore, this trial specifically analysed SAH secondary to aneurysmal rupture. The results should not be extrapolated to SAH of other causes, where evidence supporting the benefit of nimodipine is lacking.

Problems

- Treatment was discontinued in 130 patients (70 in the nimodipine group and 60 in the placebo group). The main reason was due to absence of an aneurysm on angiography. It does not seem that these patients were then excluded from statistical analysis, potentially affecting outcomes.

Intracerebral bleed: early surgery

STICH (International Surgical Trial in IntraCerebral Haemorrhage): Early surgery vs initial conservative treatment in patients with spontaneous supratentorial intracerebral haematomas.

AUTHORS: Mendelow A, Gregson B, Fernandes H et al.
REFERENCE: Lancet (2005) 365, 387–97.
STUDY DESIGN: RCT
EVIDENCE LEVEL: 1b

Key message

Early neurosurgical intervention confers no prognostic or survival benefit for patients with spontaneous supratentorial intracerebral haemorrhage (SSIH).

Impact

In patients with SSIH but no clear indication for immediate surgery, it would be reasonable to consider a period of conservative treatment first and only to proceed to surgery if the clinical indication arises.

Aims

SSIH has a reported mortality of >40%. Decompression of the haematoma, thereby reducing intracranial pressure and increasing cerebral perfusion to the penumbra around the haematoma, is believed to improve outcomes. However, early clinical trials had yielded conflicting results. This trial aimed to provide an up-to-date analysis of the potential benefits of early surgery in treating those with SSIH.

Methods

Patients: 1033 patients at 107 international centres.

Inclusion criteria:
- CT evidence of SSIH, with a minimum haematoma diameter of 2cm;
- Presenting within 72h of haemorrhage;
- Glasgow Coma Score of ≥5;
- No structural cause of haemorrhage e.g. aneurysms, arteriovenous malformation, tumour, trauma;
- Uncertainty regarding benefits of surgery or conservative management.

Groups:
- Surgery within 24h of randomisation (n=496; surgery delayed in 465);
- Conservative management (n=529; 140 crossed over).

Primary endpoint: Prognosis-based outcome, as indicated by the Glasgow Outcome Scale (GOS).

Secondary endpoints:
- Mortality;
- Barthel Index (score of 10 activities of daily living);
- Modified Rankin scale (6-point scale of degree of disability).

Follow-up: At 6 months.

Results

	Early surgery	Conservative therapy	p
Primary endpoint			
Favourable	26%	24%	0.4
Secondary endpoints			
Mortality	36.3%	37.4%	0.7
Favourable outcome: Barthel Index	27%	23%	0.1
Favourable outcome: Rankin Scale	33%	28%	0.1

- Subgroup analysis revealed a statistically significant outcome from early surgery if the haematoma was ≤1cm from the cortical surface (p=0.02).

Discussion

Early surgery was not shown to confer any prognostic or survival benefits compared with initial non-neurosurgical management. However, it would seem that in a pre-specified subgroup (those with a haematoma ≤1cm from the cortical surface), early surgery might be potentially beneficial. In a further attempt to establish whether certain populations would benefit from early surgery, *post hoc* analysis of STICH data has indicated that patients with intraventricular haemorrhage and/or hydrocephalus have a much poorer outcome with surgery than those who do not. Therefore, an ongoing randomised trial (STICH 2) aims to assess whether patients with lobar intracerebral haemorrhage without these complications would benefit from early surgery.

Problems

- Results of the subgroup analysis require caution in interpretation as the study was not powered to assess these subgroups.
- Substantial crossover from the conservative arm to the surgical arm occurred (26%). As this was an intention-to-treat analysis, this group was still considered in the conservative arm for statistical analysis, thereby potentially influencing the overall outcome.
- In 28 patients (6%), surgery was delayed beyond 24h after randomisation; the impact of this upon the overall result is unclear.

Intracranial aneurysm: treatment of rupture

> **ISAT (International Subarachnoid Aneurysm Trial):** of neuro-surgical clipping vs endovascular coiling in 2,143 patients with ruptured intracranial aneurysms: a randomised comparison of effects on survival, dependency, seizures, rebleeding, subgroups, and aneurysm occlusion.
>
> **AUTHORS:** Molyneux A, Kerr R, Yu L et al.
> **REFERENCE:** Lancet (2005) 366, 809–17.
> **STUDY DESIGN:** RCT
> **EVIDENCE LEVEL:** 1b

Key message

Endovascular coiling is associated with lower mortality and disability than surgical clipping at 1y after aneurysmal subarachnoid haemorrhage (SAH). This benefit appears to continue for at least 7y. However, coiling is associated with a higher risk of rebleeding.

Impact

In Europe, this has led to a shift in practice in favour of coiling. However, there are important study criticisms that need to be considered.

Aims

SAH and subsequent rebleeding are common and debilitating complications of ruptured cerebral aneurysm. There are two treatment options targeted at managing this: endovascular coiling and surgical clipping. Although some preliminary results have been published (*Lancet* (2002) 360, 1267–74), this was the first complete RCT that aimed to compare the safety and efficacy of these two approaches.

Methods

Patients: 2143 consecutive patients at 42 international neurosurgical centres.

Inclusion criteria:
- SAH secondary to ruptured intracranial aneurysm (CT or lumbar puncture proven) within 28d;
- Aneurysm treatable by either technique.

Groups:
- Surgical clipping (n=1070; 39 had coiling first, 19 died prior to procedure);
- Endovascular coiling (n=1073; 9 had clipping first, 7 died prior to procedure).

Primary endpoint: Death or dependence at 1y.

Secondary endpoints: Rate of seizures and rebleeding.

Follow-up: Range=1–7y. Questionnaire at 2 months, 1y, and annually to measure modified Rankin scale. Further admissions recorded. Endovascular group patients had F/U angiogram, as did some of the surgical group.

Results

At 1y	Surgical clipping (n=1055)	Endovascular coiling (n=1063)	p
Primary endpoint			
Death/dependent	30.9%	23.5%	0.0001
Secondary endpoints			**Relative risk (95% CI)**
Rebleeds (n)	39	45	1.15 (0.75 to 1.75)

- Treatment effect remained heterogeneous within predefined subgroups of age, World Federation of Neurosurgeons SAH grading, and aneurysm site. Advantage was maintained in those followed-up to 7y.
- Coiling associated with significant decrease in seizures after first procedure (relative risk=0.52, 95% CI=0.37 to 0.74).
- >4 times as many patients undergoing coiling needed additional procedures.

Discussion

One year F/U data suggest endovascular coiling to be superior to surgical clipping of ruptured aneurysms; the risk reduction equates to 74 patients avoiding death or dependency at 1y for every 1000 patients treated. However, coiling is more expensive and appeared to be associated with increased rebleeding rates. As rebleeds can occur for up to 30y, the absolute risk reduction of death and dependence may potentially fall with long-term analysis; data is awaited to elucidate the durability of the results. Although this trial has been widely criticised, particularly in the USA, it is the first of its kind and has led to a change in practice in Europe.

Problems

- 95% aneurysms located in the anterior circulation, 90% were smaller than 10mm, and 80% patients were of good clinical grade. Extrapolation of this data beyond these parameters requires caution.
- Potential selection bias: of 9278 eligible patients, only 2143 were randomised. Of the non-randomised remainder, more underwent clipping than coiling. Therefore, patients should perhaps still undergo clipping if this is the surgeon's preference: trial data is limited to patients in whom the best option is unclear.
- Most centres in Europe, Australia, and Canada. Only two patients from the USA, where the degree of neurovascular practitioner sub-specialisation is different locally. Practitioner expertise may limit applicability of results to different regions.

Obstetrics and gynaecology

Introduction

The history of obstetrics and gynaecology is as old as the history of child-birth, and according to some obstetricians, perhaps even older. Evidence of dedicated and skillful aid during labour appears in ancient Hindu, Egyptian, Grecian, and Roman cultures. There are also less accurate records and legends. One of them says that the great Roman emperor, Julius Caesar, was born by abdominal route, the procedure later named after him. This is unlikely to be true as his mother Aurelia died at the age of 76; the first accurate record of a mother surviving a caesarean dates from the 19th century, when lower segment sections and suturing of the incision became routine practice.

In the Middle Ages, childbirth and the practice of obstetrics were ripe with superstitions and secrecy. From the 14th to the 17th century, many midwives and female healers were accused of being witches, and were hunted and executed. Modern Clinical Governance processes tend to be less drastic.

In 16th century London, two obstetricians, the Chamberlen brothers, revolutionised the management of obstructed labour by inventing obstetric forceps. However, their contribution to the EBM of the time is questionable, as the brothers went to great length to keep their invention a secret within the family. When they arrived at the home of the labouring woman, their assistants would carry a large box with a pair of forceps in it. Everybody had to leave the room and the patient was blindfolded for the procedure. It was not until 130 years later that the secret finally leaked out for the benefit of many. Fortunately, the results of clinical trials now have more urgent time frames.

Modern obstetricians and gynaecologists are less shy and secretive and more generous with their inventions, sharing them with their peers and patients alike. EBM is now deeply rooted in obstetrics and gynaecology with many large, effective, often multinational trials providing evidence to improve practice and the care of women.

Tubal ectopic pregnancy: type of surgery

Management of unruptured ectopic gestation by linear salpingostomy: a prospective RCT of laparoscopy vs laparotomy.

AUTHORS: Vermesh M, Silva P, Rosen G et al.
REFERENCE: Obstet Gynaecol (1989) 73, 400–4.
STUDY DESIGN: RCT
EVIDENCE LEVEL: 1b

Key message
This is the first RCT to show similar efficacy and safety for laparoscopic linear salpingostomy, vs routine laparotomy. However, laparoscopic procedures result in shorter recovery times and are more cost-effective.

Impact
The UK's Royal College of Obstetricians and Gynaecologists 2004 'Green Top' Guidelines on the management of tubal pregnancy now quote a laparoscopic approach for the management of ectopic pregnancies as preferable to the open approach, in haemodynamically stable patients.

Aims
Prompt management of tubal ectopic pregnancy is key to preserving fertility and reducing morbidity. With ultrasound and β-hCG assays often allowing diagnosis prior to rupture, linear salpingostomy by laparotomy had become an established procedure. Although laparoscopic approaches had been suggested to confer acceptable rates of subsequent intrauterine pregnancy and lower morbidity, a direct comparison of these two surgical approaches had yet to be undertaken. This study aimed to compare factors including morbidity, fertility outcome, and cost, between laparoscopy and laparotomy for linear salpingostomy.

Methods
Patients: 60 women (80% Mexican-American, 10% White, 5% Black, 5% Asian) at 1 centre in the USA.

Inclusion criteria: Women with ectopic pregnancy:
- Age >18y with a desire for future fertility;
- Stable vital signs and haematrocrit >30%.

Exclusion criteria:
- Ruptured tube or diameter of tubal gestation >5cm;
- Location of ectopic other than isthmus or ampulla;
- Presence of pelvic adhesions limiting visualisation.

Groups:
- Laparoscopy (n=30);
- Laparotomy (open surgery) (n=30).

Primary endpoint: Safety-related complications (intra-operative and short-term).

Secondary endpoints:
- Efficacy-confirmed tubal patency at hysterosalpingography (HSG);
- Intra-operative blood loss;
- Cost and length of hospital stay;
- Pregnancy rates (in those seeking conception).

Follow-up: β-hCG levels every 3d until level ≤1.5miu/L. HSG at 12wk.

Results

	Laparoscopy	Laparotomy	*p*
Primary endpoint (complications)			
Intra-operative	2 cases*	0	–
Short-term	1 post-op fever	2 wound infections 1 post-op fever	–
Secondary endpoints			
Patent HSG	80% (16/20)	89% (17/19)	ns
Mean intra-operative blood loss	79mL (±18)	195mL (±24)	<0.001
Length of stay	1.4d (±0.1)	3.3d (±0.2)	<0.001
Pregnancy rates	56% (10/18)	58% (11/19)	ns

* The two cases requiring laparotomy (for haemostasis) both had gestations of 5cm diameter.

- All pregnancies conceived within 6 months of surgery.
- Cost savings=US$150/patient undergoing laparoscopy (vs laparotomy).

Discussion

Two subsequent RCTs have confirmed these findings (*Fertil Steril* (1992) 57, 998–1002, *and Fertil Steril* (1992) 57, 1180–5). In women who desired future fertility, the subsequent tubal patency and intrauterine pregnancy rates were similar between the open and laparoscopic groups. There was a trend towards lower repeat ectopic pregnancies if a laparoscopic approach was used, but also higher rates of persistent trophoblast.

Problems

- 60 patients were recruited to this trial, and only 228 women were studied in total between all three relevant trials. This may be insufficient to look at small differences between the two interventions.
- All authorities agree that in haemodynamically unstable situations, treatment should be by the most expedient route (e.g. salpingectomy rather than a conservative method) and probably an open approach.

Pre-eclampsia: preventing seizures

> **MAGPIE (MAGnesium sulphate for the Prevention of Eclampsia) trial:** Do women with pre-eclampsia and their babies benefit from magnesium sulphate?
>
> **AUTHORS:** Altman D, Carroli G, Duley F et al.
> **REFERENCE:** Lancet (2002) 359, 1877–90.
> **STUDY DESIGN:** RCT
> **EVIDENCE LEVEL:** 1b

Key message

Magnesium sulphate halves the risk of women with pre-eclampsia developing seizures and also reduces the risk of maternal death, with no associated substantive side effects to mother or baby.

Impact

This trial clearly showed the effectiveness and safety of magnesium sulphate in the treatment and prevention of this serious disorder of pregnancy. As such, it has now become established as the treatment of choice for this condition.

Aims

Hypertensive disorders of pregnancy are the second leading cause of maternal mortality. Pre-eclampsia is a multisystem disorder complicating 2–8% of pregnancies and can lead to eclampsia-superimposed convulsions. The mainstream treatment for severe pre-eclampsia has been the use of anticonvulsants (e.g. diazepam). Although magnesium sulphate has shown promising early results, its use has not been validated by robust clinical trials to prove its efficacy. This study aimed to confirm whether magnesium sulphate could reduce the risk of eclampsia and was safe for mother and baby.

Methods

Patients: 10,141 women at 33 international centres.

Inclusion criteria: Cases of pre-eclampsia in women who had not yet given birth or were ≤24h post-partum, with:
- BP ≥140/90mmHg;
- Proteinurea ≥1+.

Groups:
- Magnesium sulphate: (n=5071);
- Placebo (n=5070).

Protocol:
- IV: Loading dose of 8mL (4g of either magnesium sulphate or placebo) diluted with normal saline, given IV over 10–15min. Followed by IV maintenance infusion (over 24h) of 2mL/h (1g/h of either agent);
- IM: Alternatively, IM injection used, with same 8mL loading dose, and maintenance of 20mL trial treatment given as 10mL (5mg of either agent) into each buttock, followed by 10mL (5g of either agent) every 4h for 24h.

Primary outcome: Eclampsia and (for women randomised before delivery), neonatal mortality rate.

Secondary outcome: Maternal morbidity.

Follow-up: Until discharge from hospital post-delivery.

Results

	Magnesium sulphate (n=5055)	Placebo (n=5055)	Relative risk (95% CI)
Primary outcomes			
Eclampsia	40 (0.8%)	96 (1.9%)	0.42 (0.29 to 0.60)
Maternal death	11 (0.2%)	20 (0.4%)	0.55 (0.26 to 1.14)
Risk of baby dying	576 (12.7%)	558 (12.4%)	1.02 (99% CI 0.92 to 1.14)
Secondary outcomes			
Any serious morbidity	196 (3.9%)	183 (3.6%)	ns

Discussion

This was, by far, the largest and most robust clinical trial conducted on hypertensive disease of pregnancy. It was a multinational study across a diverse population, involving a wide range of clinical settings in both rich and poor countries. The trial design was robust, as were the results. Compared to placebo, magnesium sulphate reduced the risk of eclampsia by 58%. Maternal mortality was lower in the magnesium sulphate group, but there was no clear difference between the groups in the risk of baby dying. However, although maternal mortality was lower in the magnesium sulphate group, there was no clear difference between groups in any measure of serious maternal morbidity.

Problems

- Although the maternal mortality was lower in the magnesium group, the numbers were too small (11 vs 20) to draw firm conclusions. There were 9 more deaths in the placebo group, but they were in the renal failure, embolism, and infection categories, which are unlikely to be affected by the administration of magnesium sulphate.

Preterm rupture of membranes and spontaneous labour: antibiotics

ORACLE (Overview of the Role of Antibiotics in Curtailing Labour and Early delivery): Broad-spectrum antibiotics for preterm, prelabour rupture of foetal membranes (A1) and spontaneous preterm labour (A2).

AUTHORS: Kenyon S, Taylor D, Tarnow-Mordi W (ORACLE Group).
REFERENCE: Lancet (2001) 357, 979–88 (A1) and 989–94 (A2).
STUDY DESIGN: RCT
EVIDENCE LEVEL: 1b

Key message

<u>A1:</u> Routine erythromycin use in preterm, prelabour rupture of membranes (pPROM) is associated with improved neonatal outcome. Co-amoxiclav (either alone or in combination with erythromycin) should not be used in pPROM as it is associated with a higher incidence of neonatal necrotising enterocolitis. <u>A2:</u> Antibiotics should not be routinely prescribed in spontaneous preterm labour when there is no evidence of clinical infection.

Impact

The recommendations of this trial have, in particular, influenced the management of pPROM by introducing routine use of erythromycin. Any significant improvement in the management of this condition would have a large impact on neonatal survival rates and morbidity.

Aims

Preterm delivery accounts for 75–80% of all neonatal morbidity and mortality; 30–40% of cases involve pPROM. There is uncertainty about the role of infection (especially subclinical) in preterm labour and, although used, there had been uncertainty regarding the true efficacy of prophylactic antibiotics in both spontaneous preterm labour (SPL) with intact membranes, and pPROM. This study was designed to compare routine use of erythromycin, co-amoxiclav, or both, in women with pPROM (Arm 1, A1) and SPL with intact membranes (Arm 2, A2).

Methods

Patients: 4809 (A1)/6295 (A2) women at 161 international centres.

Inclusion criteria:
- A1: Patients with pPROM, <37wk gestation;
- A2: Suspected/definite SPL with intact membranes, <37wk gestation.

Exclusion criteria: Already on/predicted need for antibiotics.

Groups:
- Erythromycin (250mg) and co-amoxiclav (325mg) (n=1192 A1; 1565 A2);
- Erythromycin only (n=1197 A1; 1611 A2);
- Co-amoxiclav only (n=1212 A1; 1550 A2);
- Placebo (n=1225 A1; 1569 A2).

Primary outcome: Composite of death before discharge, O_2 need at 36wk postnatal gestational age, and major cerebral abnormality on ultrasonography.

Secondary outcomes:
- A1: Delivery <37wk; gestation and weight at birth; respiratory distress syndrome (RDS); surfactant use; neonatal infection/necrotising enterocolitis (NEC); time on O_2, the ventilator, and in hospital.
- A2: Delivery within 48h/1wk; mode of delivery; days in hospital; maternal antibiotic use post-delivery/pre-discharge; gestation and weight at birth; admission to neonatal intensive care unit or special care baby unit.

Follow-up: Up to discharge from hospital.

Results

- A1: Primary composite outcome

	Erythromycin	Placebo	*p*
All infants	151/1190 (12.7%)	186/1225 (15.2%)	0.08
Singletons	125/1111 (11.2%)	166/1149 (14.4%)	0.02

- A1 Secondary outcomes (erythromycin): No significant increase in delivery <37wk, multiple pregnancy, necrotising enterocolitis (NEC), respiratory distress syndrome (RDS), or time on O_2/ventilation. Significant decrease in surfactant use (12.8% vs 16.3%, $p=0.02$).
- A2: Primary composite outcome

Erythromycin	Co-amoxiclav	Both	Placebo
90 (5.6%)	76 (5.0%)	91 (5.9%)	78 (5.0%)

Discussion

A1: Significantly fewer patients in the erythromycin group (among singleton pregnancies) had primary composite outcomes vs placebo. Erythromycin was also associated with prolongation of pregnancy, reduction in surfactant use, and other positive secondary outcomes. Although co-amoxiclav was associated with prolongation of pregnancy, it was also associated with a significant rise in the incidence of neonatal necrotising enterocolitis (NEC).

A2: None of the antibiotics were associated with lower rates of primary composite outcome vs placebo, and none prolonged pregnancy, influenced mode of delivery, or length of hospital stay. Rate of maternal infection was lower with antibiotics, but at a greater risk of neonatal supplementary O_2 need at 36wk of age with erythromycin.

Problems

- A1: Primary composite outcome included somewhat diverse phenomena, although separate analyses did look at each sub-component. Analysis of the subgroup in which significant decrease in the risk of primary outcome was found (pPROM and singleton pregnancy) was neither pre-specified in the methods nor tested for interaction between treatment group and pregnancy type; this poses a slight risk of the finding being due to chance.
- A2: As antibiotics did not decrease the rates of primary composite outcome, the authors concluded that the role of subclinical infection in premature birth might have been overestimated. However, as the trial did not report assessments of amniotic fluid/placenta microbiology or indicators of an inflammatory response, this conclusion may be inappropriate.

Prelabour rupture of membranes: management at term

TERMPROM trial: Induction of labour compared with expectant management for prelabour rupture of the membranes at term.

AUTHORS: Hannah M, Ohlsson A, Farine D *et al.*
REFERENCE: N Engl J Med (1996) 334, 1005–10.
STUDY DESIGN: RCT
EVIDENCE LEVEL: 1b

Key message

Women with prelabour rupture of membranes (PROM) at term have similar outcomes with both active (induction of labour) and expectant management. Neonatal infection and caesarean section rates are comparable in both groups. IV oxytocin is associated with lower maternal infection rates, and women prefer induction of labour.

Impact

With comparable outcomes between groups for this common condition, this trial has reassured clinicians and patients alike that they can together decide on a management option best suited to their needs and the capabilities of local service provisions. The results of this trial have been incorporated in protocols and guidelines worldwide.

Aims

PROM affects approximately 8–10% of all pregnancies. 90% of these women will spontaneously start labour within 24h. The risk of neonatal infection is a major concern with prolonged rupture of membranes. Although the risk is thought to be small in the first 24h, it increases thereafter. On the other hand, a premature intervention may increase the risk of unnecessary caesarean section. Therefore, there remained no agreement as to whether early induction of labour or expectant management should be used. This trial was designed to assess and compare the available management options.

Methods

Patients: 5,041 women at 72 international centres.

Inclusion criteria:
- Women with prelabour rupture of membranes at term;
- ≥37wk gestation;
- Single foetus in cephalic presentation.

Groups:
- Labour induced immediately with:
  - IV oxytocin (n=1258);
  - Prostaglandin E2 gel (n=1259);
- Expectant management for up to 4d (in absence of complications). Labour induced with either:
  - Oxytocin (n=1263) *or*
  - Prostaglandin E2 gel (n=1261).

Primary outcome: Neonatal infection.

Secondary outcomes:
- The need for caesarean section;
- Other measures of maternal, foetal, and neonatal health;
- Patient evaluation of the care they received.

Results

	Induction		Expectant	
	Oxytocin (n=1258)	**Prostaglandin (n=1263)**	**Oxytocin (n=1259)**	**Prostaglandin (n=1261)**
Rate of neonatal infection	2%	3%	2.8% OR 0.7; 95% CI 0.4 to 1.2	2.7% OR 1.7; 95% CI 0.1 to 1.8
Rate of caesarean section	10.1%	9.6%	9.7% OR 1.0; 95% CI 0.8 to 1.4	10.9% OR 0.9; 95% CI 0.7 to 1.1

OR=odds ratio; OR/95% CI=vs same group who underwent induction.

Discussion

Both immediate induction of labour with syntocinon (oxytocin) or prosta-glandins, and expectant management of up to 96h with induction of labour in the presence of any complications (signs of foetal or maternal infection), had similar outcomes. Caesarean section rates were not significantly different in any of the groups and were not raised in the early intervention group. Maternal wishes should be taken into account when managing PROM. In this trial, immediate induction of labour with syntocinon was considered the 'best' option by the authors, with comparable caesarean section rates and the lowest rates of clinical chorioamnionitis. This was also the patients' preferred choice.

Problems

- Although the authors concluded that oxytocin led to fewer infections and was preferred by patients, in practice, the difference in service provisions and resources between different countries and hospitals should be taken into account in the decision making process; this was not discussed by the authors.

Breech presentation: mode of delivery

Term breech trial: Planned caesarean section vs planned vaginal birth for breech presentation at term: a randomised multicentre trial.

AUTHORS: Hannah M, Hannah W, Hewson S *et al.*
REFERENCE: Lancet (2000) 356, 1375–83.
STUDY DESIGN: RCT
EVIDENCE LEVEL: 1b

Key message
For breech presentation at term, planned caesarean section (CS) is safer for the foetus than planned vaginal delivery. Maternal complications are similar in both groups.

Impact
This trial has finally tipped the balance in favour of caesarean section, having provided evidence that it is the safer option.

Aims
Breech presentation affects 3–4% of pregnancies at term. In recent years, vaginal breech deliveries in the Western world have been dramatically falling, mainly due to the fear of litigation. The evidence to date has been inconclusive, supporting neither planned CS nor vaginal birth as a method of choice. However, previous trials were small and possibly skewed due to poor outcomes in premature babies in whom breech is more prevalent. Some studies were also biased because women were not randomly allocated to different groups. This large RCT for breech at term aimed to resolve this contentious issue.

Methods
Patients: 2088 women at 121 international centres (26 countries).

Inclusion criteria: Women with a singleton live foetus in a frank or complete breech presentation at term.

Exclusion criteria:
- Evidence of foeto-pelvic disproportion;
- Foetus clinically large or estimated weight of ≥4000g;
- Presence of hyperextension of the foetal head;
- Contraindication to either labour or vaginal delivery.

Groups:
- Planned CS (section scheduled for ≥38wk gestation) (n=1043);
- Planned vaginal birth (attended by experienced clinicians) (n=1045).

Primary outcome: Perinatal or neonatal mortality at ≤28d of age and serious neonatal morbidity.

Secondary outcomes: Maternal mortality or serious maternal morbidity during the first 6wk postpartum.

Follow-up: Mothers and babies had F/U to 6wk postpartum. 3 months and 2y F/U performed in selected centres.

Results

	Caesarean (n=1039)	Vaginal birth (n=1039)	Relative risk (RR) and *p*
Primary outcome			
Perinatal and neonatal mortality, and serious neonatal morbidity	17/1039 (1.6%)	52/1039 (5.0%)	RR 0.33 *p*<0.0001
Secondary outcome			
Maternal mortality or serious maternal morbidity	41/1041 (3.9%)	33/1042 (3.2%)	RR 1.24 *p*<0.4

Discussion

The ideal management of breech foetus at term had previously been controversial. In the absence of robust RCT data, clinicians had been guided by medico-legal concerns, data from non-randomised trials and personal preferences. This trial showed that the perinatal and neonatal mortality, as well as serious neonatal morbidity, was three times lower if delivery was by elective caesarean section, as compared with vaginal delivery.

Problems

Numerous criticisms of the study design, methods, and conclusions:
- Inclusion criteria were not always strictly adhered to and some candidates enrolled in the study were not suitable for vaginal breech delivery (e.g. a foetus with a large meningomyelocoele).
- Some centres lacked adequate diagnostic resources. Hyperextension of the foetal neck is a contraindication for vaginal breech delivery, but in one third of cases assigned to the vaginal delivery group, an ultrasound scan was not performed to check for this condition.
- A subsequent 2y F/U of toddlers (in selected centres) did not show significant differences in outcome between the two techniques.
- A number of cases with neonatal mortality or morbidity were attended during labour by a practitioner with inadequate experience in vaginal breech delivery. Although this may indicate flaws in executing the trial methodology, it also represents the reality in most hospitals today: clinicians skilled in the art of vaginal breech delivery have become a rarity.

Hormone replacement therapy

WHI (Women's Health Initiative) study: Risks and benefits of oestrogen plus progesterone in healthy post-menopausal women.

AUTHORS: Rossouw J, Anderson G, Prentice R et al.
REFERENCE: JAMA (2002) 288, 321–33.
STUDY DESIGN: RCT
EVIDENCE LEVEL: 1b

Key message

First trial to directly demonstrate that hormone replacement therapy (HRT) carries an increased risk of coronary heart disease, stroke, breast cancer, and venous thrombosis.

Impact

In conjunction with the observational Million Women Study (MWS) the WHI results have shaped the 2004 guidelines issued by the Committee of Safety of Medicine (CSM) to prescribe HRT 'in the lowest dose for the shortest possible time' in women with severe menopausal symptoms (after fully informing them of the added risks). This has also been the subject of several Consensus Statements, published by the British (BMS), European (EMAS), and International (IMS) Menopause Societies.

Aims

The WHI study included both RCT and observational elements. While the latter looked at the impact of lifestyle factors on health outcomes, the RCT component was divided into three arms. This arm aimed to evaluate the benefits and risks associated with HRT in post-menopausal women with an intact uterus. The other two arms evaluated (i) the effects of dietary modification on breast/colorectal cancer and cardiovascular risk and (ii) the effect of calcium and vitamin D supplementation on osteoporotic fracture and colorectal cancer risk.

Methods

Patients: 16,608 women from 40 centres in the USA.

Inclusion criteria:
- Age 50–79y;
- Post-menopausal (defined as no vaginal bleeding for 6 months (12 months if age 50–54y), or a history of previous post-menopausal hormone therapy use);
- Uterus still present.

Exclusion criteria:
- Any medical condition likely to cause predicted survival <3y;
- Prior breast/other cancer (in past 10y), except non-melanoma skin cancer;
- Low haematocrit or platelet count;
- Medical conditions causing poor compliance.

Groups:
- Oestrogen (conjugated equine oestrogen 0.625mg/d) and progesterone (medroxyprogesterone acetate 2.5mg/d) (n=8506);
- Placebo (n=8102).

Primary endpoints:
- Coronary heart disease (CHD), includes non-fatal myocardial infarction and CHD deaths, and need for coronary artery bypass graft (CABG) or percutaneous transluminal coronary angioplasty (PTCA);
- Invasive breast cancer.

Secondary endpoints: Included:
- Fractures;
- Other cardiovascular disease not in primary endpoint;
- Endometrial, colorectal, and other cancers.

Follow-up: Symptom review at 6wk, then every 6 months thereafter. F/U stopped after 5.2y (intended to be 8.5y).

Results

Primary endpoint	HRT (n=8506)	Placebo (n=8102)	Hazard ratio	Nominal 95% CI
CHD	164	122	1.29	1.02 to 1.63
Invasive breast cancer	166	124	1.26	1.00 to 1.59
CABG/PTCA	183	171	1.04	0.84 to 1.28
Secondary endpoint				
Stroke	127	85	1.41	1.07 to 1.85
Venous thromboembolic disease	151	67	2.11	1.58 to 2.82
Endometrial cancer	22	25	0.83	0.47 to 1.47
Colorectal cancer	45	67	0.63	0.43 to 0.92
Hip fractures	44	62	0.66	0.45 to 0.98
Vertebral fractures	41	60	0.66	0.44 to 0.98
Total fractures	650	788	0.76	0.69 to 0.85
Death	231	218	0.98	0.82 to 1.18

Discussion

This trial was stopped early as women with a uterus who were taking the combined oestrogen and progesterone HRT were found to have an excessive risk of breast cancer. Therefore, it was felt the health risks associated with treatment exceeded the health benefits. At the time of stopping, the risks of CHD, stroke, pulmonary embolism, and invasive breast cancer were significantly increased in the HRT group. There were smaller reductions in the numbers of hip fractures and colorectal cancers.

Problems

- Only one dose of oral oestrogen and progesterone was investigated, hence the risks may not apply to HRT with lower hormone doses or to other routes of HRT administration. It is also unclear whether the excess risks were due to the oestrogen or progesterone component.
- This trial did not include patients who had prior hysterectomy.
- The reduction in fracture risk or incidence of colorectal cancer may have been underestimated due to early trial termination.

PCOS: metformin treatment

Ovarian function and metabolic factors in women with oligomenor-rhoea treated with metformin in a randomised, double-blind, placebo-controlled trial.

AUTHORS: Fleming R, Hopkinson Z, Wallace A *et al.*
REFERENCE: J Clin Endocrinol Metab (2002) 87, 569–74.
STUDY DESIGN: RCT
EVIDENCE LEVEL: 1b

Key message
Metformin therapy improves ovulation in oligomenorrhoeic women with polycystic ovaries.

Impact
Metformin treatment is routinely used in women with polycystic ovarian syndrome (PCOS).

Aims
The role of insulin resistance in the aetiology of PCOS is well recognised, as is the link with the metabolic syndrome. This RCT aimed to confirm anecdotal evidence for the benefit of oral hypoglycaemics in PCOS.

Methods
Patients: 94 patients (2 withdrew before treatment) at 1 centre in the UK.

Inclusion criteria:
- Aged <35y;
- Women with oligomenorrhoea (cycle length >41d; <8 cycles/y) or amenorrhoea and polycystic ovaries.

Exclusion criteria:
- Significant hyperprolactinaemia;
- Abnormal thyroid function tests;
- Congenital adrenal hyperplasia.

Groups:
- Metformin (n=45);
- Placebo (n=47).

Endpoints:
- Ovarian function;
- Anthropometric criteria;
- Glycaemic indices;
- Leptin;
- Lipid profile.

Follow-up: At 14wk after treatment (between 12–16wk).

Results

Ovarian function and dropout rate:

Endpoint	Metformin (n=45)	Placebo (n=47)	p
Ovulation frequency	23%	13%	<0.01
Day to first ovulation (d)	23.6	41.8	0.02
Failed to ovulate	8	17	0.04
Luteal ratio	23%	13%	<0.001
Luteal phases with progesterone concentration <7ng/mL	2 (8%)	5 (13%)	ns
Dropout rate	15%	5%	<0.05

Metabolic parameters:

Change from baseline	Metformin	Placebo
BMI (SD)	−0.6*	0.3*
Waist/hip ratio	0	0
Leptin (ng/mL)	−3.8	−2.1
Fasting insulin (miu/L)	−0.4	−0.9
Fasting glucose (nmol/L)	0	0.1
Total cholesterol (nmol/L)	−0.11	−0.03
Triglycerides (mmol/L)	0.01	0.04
VLDL (mmol/L)	0.02	0.12
LDL (mmol/L)	−0.2	−0.14
HDL (mmol/L)	0.06*	0

*$p<0.05$; all other values=ns.

Discussion

This study showed a significant, but modest, benefit of metformin treatment on ovarian function, as well as anthropometric and HDL lipid measurements, in patients with PCOS. The increase in the ovulation rate occurred much more rapidly with metformin. However, there were no changes in androgen concentrations, glucose, insulin, triglyceride, or VLDL levels. Subgroup analysis suggested that the least androgenic patients were more likely to respond to metformin treatment.

Problems

- There was a high (significant) dropout rate in the metformin group (more than 30%) mainly due to gastrointestinal side effects; this compliance issue has important clinical relevance.
- The effect of different metformin doses on ovarian and metabolic function was not analysed.

PCOS: infertility treatment

Clomiphene, metformin, or both for infertility in the Polycystic Ovary Syndrome.

AUTHORS: Legro R, Barnhart H, Schlaff W et al.
REFERENCE: N Engl J Med (2007) 356, 551–66.
STUDY DESIGN: RCT
EVIDENCE LEVEL: 1b

Key message
Clomiphene is more effective than metformin for the treatment of polycystic ovarian syndrome (PCOS)-related infertility.

Impact
Clomiphene is considered the best first-line treatment for infertility in patients with PCOS.

Aims
PCOS is the commonest reproductive endocrinopathy and represents a major cause of subfertility. This study aimed to determine whether clomiphene, metformin, or a combination of the two therapies would result in the highest birth rate in patients with PCOS-related infertility.

Methods
Patients: 626 patients from multiple centres in the USA.

Inclusion criteria:
- History of oligomenorrhoea (no more than 8 menses/y);
- Hyperandrogenaemia.

Exclusion criteria:
- Hyperprolactinaemia;
- Congenital adrenal hyperplasia;
- Thyroid disease;
- Amenorrhoea not related to PCOS;
- Clinically suspected Cushing's syndrome;
- Androgen-secreting neoplasm.

Groups:
- CL: Clomiphene (n=209);
- M: Metformin (n=208);
- C: Combination of Metformin and Clomiphene (n=209).

Primary endpoints: Rate of live births.

Secondary endpoints:
- Rate of pregnancy loss;
- Singleton birth;
- Ovulation;
- Adverse events.

Follow-up: Up to 6 months.

Results

Endpoint (% of patients)	CL	M	C	*P* C vs M	C vs CL	CL vs M
Live births	22.5	7.2	26.8	<0.001	0.3	<0.001
Ovulation	49.0	29.0	60.4	<0.001	0.003	<0.001
Singleton pregnancies	94.0	100	96.9	1.0	0.5	1.0
First trimester pregnancy loss	22.6	40	25	0.2	0.7	0.1
Conception rate in those who ovulated	39.5	21.7	46	<0.001	0.2	0.002
Serious adverse events	3.3	1.0	5.3	0.02	>0.05	0.1

CL: Clomiphene M: Metformin C: Combination.

Discussion

PCOS is a major cause of infertility. Metformin had been used in recent years as first-line therapy, though data for its use had mainly been derived from small studies. This study demonstrated that conception, pregnancy, live births, and multiple births were significantly more likely to occur with clomiphene rather than metformin therapy. Despite clomiphene being more effective than metformin, only just over 20% of women gave birth. Compared with single agent treatment, females treated with combination therapy had higher ovulation rates, but this did not translate into higher pregnancy or live birth rates. Pregnancy-related adverse events were more common in the clomiphene and combination groups.

Problems

- There was a high dropout rate of 23.4–34.6% in the three groups, with the metformin group having a significantly higher dropout rate.
- Extended slow-release metformin was used instead of the more common immediate-release metformin. This may have contributed to the lower efficacy of metformin seen in this study.

Uterine fibroids: embolisation vs surgery

> **REST (Randomised trial of Embolisation vs Surgical Treatment):** Uterine artery embolisation vs surgery for symptomatic uterine fibroids.
>
> **AUTHORS:** Edwards R, Moss J, Lumsden M *et al.* (Committee of the randomised trial of embolisation vs surgical treatment for fibroids).
> **REFERENCE:** N Engl J Med (2007) 356, 360–70.
> **STUDY DESIGN:** RCT
> **EVIDENCE LEVEL:** 1b

Key message

In women with symptomatic fibroids, the lower cost and faster recovery after embolisation must be weighed against the need for further treatment in a minority. Surgery offered better long-term symptom control, but quality of life was similar at 1y.

Impact

These findings have helped clarify the treatment options for uterine fibroids.

Aims

Uterine fibroids are the commonest female reproductive tract tumour, associated with menstrual disorders, subfertility, miscarriage, and pressure effects. Uterine artery embolisation, a uterus sparing and less invasive procedure, has become increasingly popular *(Radiology* (2003) 226, 425–31). This study aimed to compare uterine artery embolisation with surgery (hysterectomy/myomectomy).

Methods

Patients: 157 patients at 27 centres in the UK.

Inclusion criteria:
- Age >18y with ≥1 fibroid (>2cm diameter) visible on MRI;
- Symptoms (menorrhagia/pelvic pain/pressure) warranting surgery.

Exclusion criteria:
- Pregnancy/severe contrast allergy/other contraindication to MRI/surgery;
- Subserosal pedunculated fibroids;
- Recent or ongoing pelvic inflammatory disease.

Groups: Randomised in a 2:1 ratio:
- Embolisation (n=106);
- Surgery (n=51).

Primary endpoint: Quality of life at 1y assessed using Medical Outcomes Study Short-Form 36 item general health questionnaire (SF36) .

Secondary endpoint: EuroQol-5D questionnaire to measure preferences for certain health outcomes, time until resumption of usual activities, recommendation to friend, 24h pain score, complications, and treatment failure (i.e needed later hysterectomy/repeat embolisation).

Follow-up: Outcomes at 1, 6, 12, and 21 months; then annual F/U.

Results

	Embolisation (n=95)	Surgery (n=45)	*p*
Symptom score (1 month)	1.5 (±2.4)	2.8 (±2.6)	0.004
Symptom score (12 months)	3.6 (±2.0)	4.3 (±11.7)	0.03
Pain score (24h)	3.0 (±2.1)	4.6 (±2.3)	<0.001
Hospital stay	1d	5d	<0.001
Minor complications	36 (34%) [mostly post-embolisation syndrome]	10 (20%) [mostly minor infections]	0.06
Major adverse events (at 1y)	13 (12%)	10 (20%)	0.2
Treatment failures (required additional procedure)	21 (20%) [10 (9%) during 1st year]	1 (2%) [myomectomy to hysterectomy]	Not stated
Mean cost saving	UK £951 (at 1y)	–	–

- **Symptoms:** No significant differences in quality of life at 1y. Embolisation group had less time before resuming all usual activities ($p < 0.001$).

Discussion

Neither treatment was perfect, both having pros and cons. Although quality of life at 1y was equal, symptom control was better with surgery. However, embolisation was cheaper with faster recovery and resumption of usual activities. The rate of complications did not differ significantly, but timing did: the surgical group's occurred largely during the hospital stay, while the embolisation group's occurred post-discharge. The major disadvantage of embolisation was that 20% required further treatment for recurrence or persistence of symptoms, half within the first year.

Problems

- No standardisation of technique for either procedure (2 types were used).
- Primary outcome (SF36) related to quality of life, and was not related to fibroid-specific symptoms.
- 'Time until resumption of usual activities' is open to bias, as patients may expect to take longer to recover from surgery.

Ophthalmology

Introduction

The commonest cause of treatable visual disability in the world is cataract. Historically, cataracts were removed (if they were removed at all) by an extremely unsatisfactory procedure called 'couching', an operation entailing puncture of the eye with a needle and an attempt to push the cloudy lens out of its normal location with the needle tip. The ultimate goal was to dislodge the lens and remove it away from the patient's visual axis. Not only was this procedure excruciatingly painful, but the visual results were often disastrous. These days, small incisional surgery is undertaken using phacoemulsification and implantation of an intraocular lens under local anaesthesia, resulting in a rapid and often spectacular improvement in vision. Justifiably, the operation is considered one of the most rewarding in all of medicine. However, it took many years of slow progress to develop the technique that is now used. The first intraocular lens implant was inserted by Sir Harold Ridley in 1949 and was met with opposition from the medical community. It took three decades of struggle before the procedure was undertaken routinely. Dr Charles Kelman first undertook small incisional surgery using phacoemulsification and aspiration of the cataract in 1967. Once again, it took almost two decades for this technique to be adopted. It could be argued that the reason for the slow progress in this field was the fact that randomised studies comparing these new techniques with established practice were not undertaken at an early stage. In recent years ophthalmologists have realised the importance of evidence-based studies of therapy in the other common causes of visual disability: diabetic retinopathy, chronic glaucoma, age-related macular degeneration, and the surgical treatment of myopia. The rapid acceptance of new therapy for these conditions has been a direct consequence of prospective RCTs. In this chapter, the most important studies in these fields will be considered.

Glaucoma: control of intraocular pressure

AGIS-7 (Advanced Glaucoma Intervention Study): The relationship between control of intraocular pressure and visual field deterioration.

AUTHORS: The AGIS Investigators.
REFERENCE: Am J Ophthalmol (2000) 130, 429–40.
STUDY DESIGN: RCT
EVIDENCE LEVEL: 1b

Key message

Consistently low intraocular pressure (IOP) measurements are associated with reduced progression of visual field defects in patients with advanced glaucoma.

Impact

Both a low average IOP (of <14mmHg) and an IOP consistently below 18mmHg lead to a dramatic slowing of visual field loss in patients with glaucoma. This study gives clinicians a target IOP to aim for in the management of glaucoma.

Aims

Previous studies had suggested a correlation between low IOP and reduced glaucoma progression. This study compared two regimens of surgical intervention in patients with glaucoma and poorly controlled IOP on maximally tolerated medical therapy. By aiming to keep IOP <18mmHg, this study aimed to assess the effect of both a low average IOP and an IOP consistently <18mmHg on the progression of visual field defects. This study was one of a series designed to provide a comprehensive overview of interventions for glaucoma.

Methods

Patients: 591 patients (789 eyes) at 11 centres across the USA.

Inclusion criteria:
- Age 35–80y;
- Open angle glaucoma (defined by raised IOP, glaucomatous visual field defect, and optic disc rim changes, uncontrolled by maximal topical medication);
- Phakic (eye containing a natural lens);
- Visual acuity (VA) better than 20/80;
- Both eyes enrolled only if simultaneously eligible.

Groups: Randomised to receive 1 of 2 sequences of surgical intervention:
- 1: Argon laser trabeculoplasty, trabeculectomy, trabeculectomy;
- 2: Trabeculectomy, argon laser trabeculoplasty, trabeculectomy;

Topical medication used as required after each intervention (up to a maximum combination) aiming for an IOP <18mmHg.

Primary endpoint: Visual field deterioration (measured by change in visual field score, with a positive score indicating deterioration).

Analysis: Two methods used: predictive analysis (PA) and associative analysis (AA). PA patients divided into 3 groups depending on IOP level during the first 18 months. AA patients divided into 4 groups based on the percentage of visits with IOPs <18mmHg.

Follow-up: Initial F/U at 3 months, then every 6 months for the duration of the study (range 4–7y).

Results (at 8 months):

IOP over first 18 months	Change in visual field score compared to lowest IOP group	p
<14mmHg (group A)	–	–
14–17.5mmHg (group B)	0.76	0.01
>17mmHg (group C)	1.89	<0.001

Percentage of visits IOP<18mmHg	Change in visual field score compared to group A	p
100% (group A)	–	–
75% (group B)	1.11	0.02
50% (group C)	1.97	<0.001
25% (group D)	2.42	<0.001

Discussion

Both methods of analysis concluded that consistently low IOP slowed glaucoma progression (as measured by visual field changes). IOP lowering effects were greatest in Group 1. Afro-American patients did better with initial laser trabeculoplasty, whereas Caucasians did better with initial trabeculectomy. Overall risk of cataract was 78%, with increased risk after the first trabeculectomy. In the lowest pressure group, some patients continued to progress despite low IOP.

Problems

- Only one visual field used as a baseline for each patient.
- Despite the title, the study included some patients with early glaucoma and excluded very advanced glaucoma.
- Disease staging was not attempted.

Glaucoma: medical vs surgical treatment

CIGTS (Collaborative Initial Glaucoma Treatment Study): Interim clinical outcomes in the collaborative initial glaucoma treatment study comparing initial treatment randomised to medications or surgery.

AUTHORS: Lichter P, Musch D, Gillespie B *et al.*
REFERENCE: Ophthalmology (2001) 108, 1943–53.
STUDY DESIGN: RCT
EVIDENCE LEVEL: 1b

Key message

Either medical or surgical treatment of newly diagnosed glaucoma result in a similar degree of visual field loss and a similar visual acuity after 5y. The intraocular pressure (IOP)-lowering effect of surgery is greater.

Impact

Initial medical therapy, which carries fewer risks than surgery, is a valid option for primary treatment of newly diagnosed glaucoma.

Aims

Visual field loss, and the subsequent blindness associated with open angle glaucoma, is often preventable if treated early. Initial studies had suggested that filtration surgery might be more efficacious than medical management (topical drops) for newly diagnosed disease. This study aimed to compare the outcome of primary surgical treatment with that of medical treatment, in patients with newly diagnosed glaucoma.

Methods

Patients: 607 patients at 14 clinical centres across the USA.

Inclusion criteria:
- Age 25–75y;
- Best corrected visual acuity (VA) better than 20/40 in both eyes;
- Newly diagnosed open angle glaucoma (including primary, pigmentary, and pseudoexfoliative).
- One of:
  - IOP ≥ 20mmHg and loss of 3 contiguous points on Humphrey visual field (HVF) and glaucomatous disc;
  - IOP 20–26mmHg and loss of 2 contiguous points on HVF;
  - IOP ≥27mmHg and suspected glaucomatous disc.
- No prior ocular surgery and no or limited prior topical treatment.

Groups: Both groups treated aggressively with a stepwise progression of treatments for pressure above target:
- Primary trabeculectomy (initially immediate procedure, proceeding to argon laser procedure if failure; with or without 5-fluorouracil at the surgeon's discretion) (n=300).
- Topical medication (usually commencing with a β-blocker) (n=307).

Primary endpoint: Visual field loss.

Secondary endpoints:
- Visual acuity;
- IOP;
- Cataract.

Follow-up: 4–5y.

Results

	Surgical group	Medical group	*p*
Primary endpoint			
Clinically significant visual field loss	13.5%	10.7%	Not stated
Secondary endpoints			
Clinically substantial VA loss at some point over 5y	7.2%	3.9%	Not stated
Average IOP	14–15mmHg	17–18mmHg	0.0001
Cataract surgery	17.3%	6.2%	0.0001

Discussion

Both baseline visual field score and initial post-operative visual acuity were worse in the surgical group than the medical group, but this difference was not sustained at 5y. The surgical group maintained a lower IOP (by about 3mmHg) throughout the study, but had a higher rate of cataract formation.

Problems

- Inclusion criteria may have allowed recruitment of some patients with ocular hypertension who had less risk of progression than those with early glaucoma.
- In the surgical group, initial trabeculectomy was sometimes augmented with 5-fluorouracil, which may affect outcomes.
- F/U was relatively short for a chronic condition such as glaucoma; longer-term data are needed before firm treatment recommendations can be made.

Glaucoma: topical medication

OHTS (<u>O</u>cular <u>H</u>ypertension <u>T</u>reatment <u>S</u>tudy): A randomised trial determines that topical ocular hypotensive medication delays or prevents the onset of primary open angle glaucoma.

AUTHORS: Kass M, Heuer D, Higginbotham E *et al.*
REFERENCE: Arch Ophthalmol (2002) 120, 701–13.
STUDY DESIGN: RCT
EVIDENCE LEVEL: 1b

Key message

Decreased risk of progression to primary open angle glaucoma (POAG) is observed with topical pressure-lowering treatment (vs no treatment) in individuals with ocular hypertension (OHT).

Impact

After clinical assessment of co-existent risk factors to identify appropriate patients, topical ocular anti-hypertensive treatment can be used to successfully decrease the likelihood of development of POAG.

Aims

Patients with OHT are at risk of developing POAG. African-American populations have an incidence five times that of Caucasians. This study was designed to compare risk of progression to POAG with and without topical ocular antihypertensive treatment.

Methods

Patients: 1636 patients at 22 centres across the USA.

Inclusion criteria:
- Age 40–80y;
- IOP between 24–32mmHg in the first eye and between 21–32mmHg in the second eye;
- Open angles;
- Normal optic discs and visual fields.

Groups:
- Topical medication: Investigators free to choose any commercially available agent to lower intraocular pressure (IOP) to ≤24mmHg with a minimum 20% reduction from baseline (n=817);
- No medication (n=819).

Primary endpoint: Development of POAG in one or both eyes (defined as reproducible visual field abnormality or reproducible optic disc deterioration attributed to POAG).

Secondary endpoints: Adverse events and side effects related to the topical medication.

Follow-up: Every 6 months for the duration of the study (median F/U=78 months).

Results (at 60 months)

	Treatment	No treatment	p
Primary endpoint			
Progression to POAG	4.4%	10.9%	<0.0001
Visual field change	1.8%	3.5%	0.002
Optic disc change	2.2%	6.2%	<0.001
Both field and disc changes	0.4%	1.1%	Not stated
Secondary endpoints			
Serious adverse events related to medication	None	None	–
Side effects: ocular	57%	47%	<0.001
Side effects: skin/hair/nails	23%	18%	<0.001
Side effects: iris colour (patients on prostaglandin analogues)	17%	7.6%	<0.001

Discussion

Reducing IOP in patients with OHT reduced the risk of progression to POAG. Topical treatment was generally safe, although patients should be made aware of the potential side effects. Analysis of the African-American patient subgroup showed treatment to be less protective with a higher incidence of progression to glaucoma. A sister publication (*Arch Ophthalmol* (2002) 120, 714–20) identified baseline factors that predict POAG onset in individual subjects.

Problems

- The population consisted of healthy volunteers with a mean age <60y. This may not represent patients with this condition in the general population, either in terms of outcome or medication side effects.
- The F/U of the African-American subgroup was 6 months less than that for the remainder of the patients, which may have affected the results.

Glaucoma: early treatment

EMGT (Early Manifest Glaucoma Trial): Factors for glaucoma progression and the effect of treatment.

AUTHORS: Leske M, Heijl A, Hussein M *et al.*
REFERENCE: Arch Ophthalmol (2003) 121, 48–56.
STUDY DESIGN: RCT
EVIDENCE LEVEL: 1b

Key message
Intraocular pressure (IOP)-lowering treatment reduces the rate of progression in some patients with early open angle glaucoma.

Impact
This is the first large RCT to demonstrate a benefit of treatment (vs no treatment) in Caucasian patients with early glaucoma. It identifies a number of baseline characteristics that can be related to the likelihood of disease progression.

Aims
Although various factors affecting the progression of glaucoma have been studied, opinions on their relative importance and the indications for therapy vary. This prospective RCT was designed to assess the effect of IOP reduction on disease progression in early glaucoma. It also aimed to identify the other baseline factors associated with a risk of disease progression.

Methods
Patients: 255 patients at 2 centres in Sweden.

Inclusion criteria:
- Age 50–80y;
- Newly diagnosed, untreated open angle glaucoma (based on presence of repeatable glaucomatous visual field defects in at least one eye, not attributable to any other cause).

Exclusion criteria:
- Advanced visual field defects;
- Visual acuity (VA) <0.5 (logMAR);
- Mean IOP >30mmHg *or* any IOP >35mmHg in at least one eye;
- Lens or media opacities.

Groups:
- IOP-lowering treatment with argon laser trabeculoplasty followed by topical betaxolol (n=129);
- No treatment (n=126).

Primary endpoint: Progression of glaucoma (defined by significant change from baseline in at least 3 points on 3 consecutive visual field (VF) tests *or* change in photographic optic disc appearance). Progression of glaucoma was compared for the treatment vs no treatment group, and then assessed to determine the effect of different baseline characteristics.

Follow-up: 4 pre-randomisation visits, then F/U every 3 months (median 6y).

Results

	Progression	*p*
Treatment group	45%	0.003
Control group	62%	
Age ≥68	57%	0.05
Age <68	49%	
IOP ≥21mmHg	63%	0.003
IOP <21mmHg	45%	
Mean deviation on VF ≤ −4db	59%	0.03
Mean deviation on VF > −4db	47%	

- Other baseline characteristics significantly (*p*<0.001) affecting progression were: presence of pseudoexfoliation, and both eyes eligible for study, i.e. bilateral disease (progression in 72% vs 47% of those with only one eye eligible).
- Factors having no significant effect were: sex, central corneal thickness, presence of disc haemorrhage, refractive error, or personal/family medical history.

Discussion

Reducing IOP by 25% from baseline reduced the risk of progression by 50%. The presence of certain risk factors made progression more likely. Some patients did not progress despite receiving no treatment, and some patients progressed despite receiving pressure-lowering treatment.

Problems

- This study excluded patients with advanced glaucoma or very high IOP, so results may not be applicable to these groups.
- Only Caucasian patients were included, which may limit application of the results to other ethnic groups.
- Treatment options were limited.

Age-related macular degeneration: laser photocoagulation

> **MPS (Macular Photocoagulation Study):** Argon laser photocoagulation for neovascular maculopathy: 5year results from RCTs.
>
> **AUTHORS:** The Macular Photocoagulation Study Group.
> **REFERENCE:** Arch Ophthalmol (1991) 109, 1109–14.
> **STUDY DESIGN:** RCT
> **EVIDENCE LEVEL:** 1b

Key message
Argon laser photocoagulation reduces severe visual loss in patients with extrafoveal choroidal neovascular membranes (CNVM). Despite this, recurrences are common and carry a poor prognosis.

Impact
Patients with extrafoveal CNVM can benefit from argon laser photocoagulation to stabilise vision and reduce the risk of severe visual loss. This standard UK practice is now being replaced in some centres by anti-VEGF (vascular endothelial growth factor) treatment. However, laser treatment is cheaper and retains a role for the time being.

Aims
Age-related macular degeneration (AMD) is one of the most common causes of visual loss in the Western world. Ocular histoplasmosis (OHS) is another factor implicated in some regions. This study aimed to investigate the efficacy and safety of argon laser photocoagulation treatment in patients with extrafoveal CNVM. Since CNVM causes visual loss in both AMD and OHS, this study aimed to compare 5y F/U results in patients with CNVM secondary to AMD, OHS, and with no known cause (idiopathic).

Methods
Patients: 565 patients (236 with AMD, 262 with OHS, and 67 with idiopathic CNVM) at multiple centres in the USA.

Inclusion criteria:
- Extrafoveal CNVM (defined as 200–2500micrometres from the centre of the foveal avascular zone on fluorescein angiography);
- Visual acuity (VA) >20/100;
- Visual symptoms related to CNVM;
- For AMD group: presence of drusen (accumulation of extracellular material in innermost layer of the choroid).

Exclusion criteria: Prior laser photocoagulation or coexisting ocular disease potentially affecting VA.

Groups:
- Argon laser photocoagulation treatment (n=119 in AMD group; 132 in OHS group; 33 in idiopathic group);

- No treatment (n=117 in AMD group; 130 in OHS group; 34 in idiopathic group).

Primary endpoint: Severe visual loss (loss of ≥6 lines from baseline).

Secondary endpoints/measurements:
- Level of visual acuity;
- Recurrence of CNVM (defined as visible leakage along the border of a treated lesion on fluorescein angiography ≥3 months after treatment).

Follow-up: At 3 and 6 months, then every 6 months for 5y.

Results

Outcome	Treatment	No treatment	p
Mean VA after 5y			
AMD group	20/125	20/200	0.002
OHS group	20/40	20/50	0.001
Idiopathic group	20/64	20/80	0.2
Mean change in VA			
AMD group	Loss 5 lines	Loss 7 lines	0.01
OHS group	Loss 1 line	Loss 4 lines	0.001
Idiopathic group	Loss 3 lines	Loss 4 lines	0.2
Proportion of eyes with severe visual loss			
AMD group	0.46	0.64	0.001
OHS group	0.12	0.42	<0.0001
Idiopathic group	0.23	0.48	0.04

- Similar reduction in visual loss 6 months post-treatment and up to the 5y figures shown here.
- Recurrence of CNVM occurred in 54% (AMD group), 26% (OHS group), and 34% (idiopathic group).

Discussion

Argon laser photocoagulation reduced the incidence of severe visual loss in eyes with CNVM secondary to a variety of causes, and was most effective for CNVM secondary to OHS. Despite this, visual prognosis for these patients was poor overall, with frequent recurrence of CNVM. Sister studies looked at treatment of juxtafoveal CNVM by krypton laser, and subfoveal CNVM by krypton or argon laser. In both studies, a reduction in severe visual loss was seen in the treated groups, but with high rates of recurrence. Despite the eventual benefit of laser in the subfoveal group, an initial immediate decrease in visual acuity was always seen.

Problems

- Some of the eyes originally assigned to 'no treatment' were later treated after intervention of the Data and Safety Monitoring Committee. The authors commented that this had little effect on comparisons made between treatment and control groups.

Age-related macular degeneration: VEGF antagonists

MARINA (Minimally classic/occult trial of the Anti-VEGF antibody Ranibizumab In the treatment of Neovascular Age-related macular degeneration study).

AUTHORS: Rosenfeld P, Brown D, Heier J et al. (MARINA group).
REFERENCE: N Engl J Med (2006) 355, 1419–31.
STUDY DESIGN: RCT
EVIDENCE LEVEL: 1b

Key message

Intravitreal injection of ranibizumab stabilises or improves vision in patients with minimally classic or occult choroidal neovascularisation due to age-related macular degeneration (AMD), with few serious side effects.

Impact

Given the high incidence of AMD, ranibizumab has the potential to have a significant impact on visual outcomes and is increasingly being used in this group of patients.

Aims

In the developed world, age-related macular degeneration (AMD) is a leading cause of blindness in patients aged >50y of age. Patients with neovascular AMD and minimally classic or occult lesions have poor visual prognosis, previously available treatments having shown limited success in stabilising vision. This phase III trial aimed to assess the efficacy of ranibizumab (a recombinant humanised monoclonal antibody that neutralises active vascular endothelial growth factor, VEGF) in stabilising vision.

Methods

Patients: 716 patients at 96 centres in the USA.

Inclusion criteria:
- Age ≥50y;
- Best corrected visual acuity (VA) equivalent to between 20/40 and 20/320;
- Primary or recurrent minimally classic or occult choroidal neovascularisation associated with AMD, involving the fovea and ≤12 optic disc areas;
- Recent disease progression (determined by fresh haemorrhage, change in vision, or observed increase in lesion size).

NB. 'Classic' and 'occult' are descriptions of appearance on fluorescein angiography.

Exclusion criteria: Previous subfoveal laser treatment, or verteporfin photodynamic therapy, or experimental treatments for wet AMD.

Groups: All patients received intravitreal injections every 1 month for 2y in one eye. Photodynamic therapy with visudyne was allowed if the lesion became predominantly classic.

- Ranibizumab 0.3mg (n=238);
- Ranibizumab 0.5mg (n=240);
- Sham injection (n=238).

Primary endpoint: Loss of <15 letters on Early Treatment of Diabetic Retinopathy Study (ETDRS) chart.

Secondary endpoints: Other adverse events (including endophthalmitis, uveitis, retinal detachment or tear, vitreous haemorrhage, and lens damage), change in VA from baseline.

Follow-up: Every 1 month for 2y.

Results

Primary endpoint	Ranibizumab 0.3mg (n=238)	Ranibizumab 0.5mg (n=240)	Sham (n=238)	*p*
Loss of <15 letters	94.5%	94.6%	62.2%	<0.001
Gain of ≥15 letters	24.8%	33.8%	5.0%	<0.001
Mean change in VA	+6.5 letters	+7.2 letters	−10.4 letters	<0.001
Adverse events (total)	1.2%	3.8%	5.0%	Not stated

Discussion

Clear benefits in stabilising or improving vision were observed in patients treated with ranibizumab as compared with control. The rate of serious adverse events was low (comparable to earlier studies), with an average rate of 1% (or 0.05% per injection) of endophthalmitis. The lower dose of ranibizumab provided as much benefit as the higher dose with a lower rate of side effects.

Problems

- The numbers in the trial may have been insufficient to detect less common adverse effects of the treatment.
- The study did not look at the effect of stopping treatment on visual acuity.

Age-related macular degeneration: VEGF antagonists vs photodynamic therapy

ANCHOR (ANti-VEGF antibody for the treatment of predominantly classic CHORoidal neovascularisation in age-related macular degeneration study): ranibizumab vs verteporfin for neovascular age-related macular degeneration.

AUTHORS: Brown D, Kaiser P, Michels M et al.
REFERENCE: N Engl J Med (2006) 355, 1432–44.
STUDY DESIGN: RCT
EVIDENCE LEVEL: 1b

Key message

Ranibizumab (a monoclonal anti-vascular endothelial growth factor (VEGF) antibody) is more effective than photodynamic therapy (PDT) in stabilising vision in patients with predominantly classic choroidal neovascularisation due to age-related macular degeneration (AMD).

Impact

This trial showed a marked improvement in visual outcome in patients with a particular type of neovascular AMD, with few serious side effects. This could have a huge impact on outcomes in this condition given the number of patients affected.

Aims

In the developed world, AMD is a leading cause of blindness in patients aged over 50. Previously available treatments had little success in stabilising vision. This study aimed to compare two different treatments of ranibizumab (a recombinant monoclonal anti-VEGF antibody) with verteporfin-based PDT in the treatment of predominantly classic choroidal neovascularisation associated with AMD.

Methods

Patients: 423 patients from multiple international centres.

Inclusion criteria:
- Age ≥50y;
- Predominantly classic choroidal neovascular membrane (CNVM) measuring ≤5400micrometres;
- Best corrected visual acuity (VA) between 20/40 and 20/320 Snellen equivalent;
- No previous treatment or structural damage to the foveal area.

Groups: Intravitreal injections carried out monthly. PDT carried out every 3 months according to angiographic findings.
- Intravitreal ranibizumab 0.3mg + sham PDT (n=140);
- Intravitreal ranibizumab 0.5mg + sham PDT (n=140);
- Sham intravitreal injection + PDT with verteporfin (n=143).

Primary endpoint: Loss of <15 letters on Early Treatment of Diabetic Retinopathy Study (ETDRS) chart.

Secondary endpoint:
- Morphological characteristics of choroidal neovascular lesion (CNVM);
- Adverse events including endophthalmitis, uveitis, retinal detachment or tear, vitreous haemorrhage, and lens damage.

Follow-up: Monthly for 24 months.

Primary endpoint	Ranibizumab 0.3mg + sham PDT	Ranibizumab 0.5mg + sham PDT	Sham injection + active PDT	p
Loss of <15 letters	94.3%	96.4%	64.3%	<0.001
Secondary endpoints				
Gain of ≥15 letters	35.7%	40.3%	5.6%	<0.001
Severe loss of vision (>30 letters)	0%	0%	13.3%	<0.001
Mean change in VA at 12 months	+8.5 letters	+11.3 letters	−9.5 letters	<0.001
Change in size of classic CNV (optic disc areas)*	−0.52	−0.67	0.54	<0.001
Change in size of whole lesion (optic disc areas)*	0.36	0.28	2.56	<0.001
Adverse events (total)	1.4%	3.5%	0.7%	Not stated

*One optic disc area = 2.54 mm^2 on the basis of one optic disc diameter of 1.8 mm.

Discussion

This study showed that intravitreal injection of ranibizumab was more effective than PDT (at both doses trialled) for stabilising or improving vision in patients with classic choroidal neovascularisation due to AMD.

_____ low rate of serious adverse events in all groups.

al may have been insufficient to detect less
ts of the treatment.
k at the effect of stopping treatment on visual

Diabetic retinopathy: laser photocoagulation

DRS (Diabetic Retinopathy Study): Photocoagulation treatment of proliferative diabetic retinopathy.

AUTHORS: The Diabetic Retinopathy Study Research Group.
REFERENCE: Am J Ophthalmol (1976) 81, 383–96 *and* Ophthalmology (1978) 85, 82–106.
STUDY DESIGN: RCT
EVIDENCE LEVEL: 1b

Key message

Scatter argon laser photocoagulation reduces the rate of development of severe visual loss in patients with proliferative diabetic retinopathy. Side effects of treatment, including loss of visual acuity and constriction of peripheral visual fields, are considered acceptable in eyes with moderate to severe retinopathy.

Impact

This was the first RCT to show the benefits of scatter laser photocoagulation in patients with proliferative diabetic retinopathy. The technique is now established worldwide as the prime treatment for this common and increasingly prevalent condition.

Aims

Patients with diabetes mellitus (DM) are at risk of developing proliferative retinopathy and subsequent visual impairment. Although photocoagulation had become a routinely used treatment, evidence for its efficacy and safety was limited. This study aimed to determine whether scatter photocoagulation was of benefit in preserving vision in these patients and whether there were differences in efficacy and safety of argon vs xenon photocoagulation.

Methods

Patients: 1758 patients at 15 centres in the USA.

Inclusion criteria:
- Age <70y;
- Proliferative diabetic retinopathy in at least one eye or s~~~~
  proliferative diabetic retinopathy in both eyes;
- Visual acuity (VA) of 20/100 or better in each eye.

Exclusion criteria: Previous photocoagulation.

Groups: One eye of each patient was randomly as~~~~
tocoagulation with argon (n=867) or xenon (n=8~~~~
acted as an untreated control.

Primary endpoint: VA worse than 5/200.

Secondary endpoints:
- Loss of VA due to treatment;
- Loss of visual field;
- Development or progression of proliferative retinopathy.

Follow-up: Every 4 months for up to 3y.

Results

Outcome	Laser groups	No laser group	Statistical significance*
Primary endpoint			
VA worse than 5/200 at 2y	6.4%	15.9%	Z=4.1
VA worse than 5/200 at 3y	10.5%	26.4%	Z=3.5
Secondary endpoints			
≥5 line decrease in VA at 6wk	4.2%	2.2%	Not stated
≥5 line decrease in VA at 4 months	6.8%	6.1%	Not stated
≥5 line decrease in VA at 1y	10.0%	15.9%	Not stated
≥5 line decrease in VA at 2y	13.7%	27.1%	Not stated

* Z value=difference between proportions of events observed in untreated and treated eyes divided by the SE of the difference. Positive Z value indicates a lower event rate in the treated group than in the untreated group.

- Reduction in severe visual loss was greater in the xenon group compared with the argon group.
- Xenon treatment carried a greater risk of loss of ≥5 lines of VA than treatment with argon or no treatment.
- There was substantial loss of peripheral visual field in the xenon group (only 48% retained ≥500° of field compared to 90% in the other groups).
- There was a statistically significant reduction in progression of all stages of retinopathy seen in the treatment groups (vs no treatment).

Discussion

The DRS study commenced in 1971. It showed photocoagulation to be effective in reducing severe visual loss (by >50%) in eyes with proliferative diabetic retinopathy and the development of high-risk characteristics across all stages of diabetic retinopathy. Xenon treatment led to a marked impairment of peripheral visual field, more so than argon treatment. Persistent decreases in visual acuity were twice as common in xenon-treated eyes than those treated with argon.

Problems

- Eyes in which severe macular oedema or ischaemia reduced VA to worse than 20/100 were excluded from this study.
- As this study was a comparison of immediate treatment vs no treatment, the possibility of deferred treatment in eyes with severe non-proliferative or mild proliferative retinopathy was not considered.

Diabetic retinopathy: photocoagulation for macular oedema

ETDRS (Early Treatment of Diabetic Retinopathy Study): Report number 1. Photocoagulation for diabetic macular oedema.

AUTHORS: Early Treatment Diabetic Retinopathy Study Group.
REFERENCE: Arch Ophthalmol (1985) 103, 1796–806.
STUDY DESIGN: RCT
EVIDENCE LEVEL: 1b

Key message

Eyes with clinically significant macular oedema associated with mild to moderate non-proliferative diabetic retinopathy benefit from treatment with focal argon laser treatment.

Impact

This trial defined a subtype of macular oedema in patients with mild to moderate non-proliferative diabetic retinopathy that benefits from focal argon laser treatment and is now normally treated. Macular oedema outside this classification carries a low risk of visual loss and need not be treated. Another arm of this study concluded aspirin therapy to have no ocular contraindications in patients with diabetes, hence not requiring it to be withheld when required for other indications.

Aims

Diabetic retinopathy causes visual loss through macular oedema, ischaemia, or proliferative disease. The ETDRS was designed to evaluate photocoagulation and aspirin treatment in the management of non-proliferative and early proliferative diabetic retinopathy. This first report looked at the question of whether argon laser photocoagulation was effective in the treatment of diabetic macular oedema. The study also considered when pan-retinal photocoagulation (PRP) treatment was most effective and whether aspirin treatment could alter the course of disease.

Methods

Patients: 1876 patients (2998 eyes) at 23 centres across the USA.

Inclusion criteria:
- Age 18–70y;
- Presence of mild to moderate diabetic retinopathy with clinically significant macular oedema (CSMO). Defined as ≥1 of:
  - Retinal thickening at or within 500micrometres of centre of macula;
  - Hard exudates at or within 500micrometres of the centre of the macula associated with retinal thickening;
  - Retinal thickening one disc area or larger, any part of which is within one disc diameter of the centre of the macula;
- Visual acuity of 20/200 or better (with macular oedema).

Exclusion criteria: Other significant ocular disease.

Groups:
- Immediate focal argon laser photocoagulation (repeated if clinically significant macular oedema persisted or developed during F/U) (n=1508 eyes);
- No treatment (n=1490 eyes).

Primary endpoint: Loss of ≥15 letters of visual acuity.

Secondary endpoints:
- Visual field loss;
- Change in colour vision score (Farnsworth–Munsell 100 hue test).

Follow-up: At 6 months, then every 4 months for 3y.

Results

% eyes with VA loss ≥15 letters	Laser group	No laser group	*p*
At 1y	5%	8%	0.01
At 2y	7%	16%	0.01
At 3y	12%	24%	0.01

- Similar differences between groups for final VA <50 letters (=20/100).
- For eyes with CSMO at time of recruitment, 35% had persistent CSMO at 1y in the laser group, compared to 63% in the no laser group.
- No significant differences seen between groups for visual fields or colour vision.

Discussion

This study showed, that for eyes with macular oedema associated with mild to moderate diabetic retinopathy, immediate laser photocoagulation reduced the proportion of eyes with significant visual loss. Visual prognosis was worse for eyes with a poorer VA at baseline. For eyes without CSMO, the rate of visual loss was low, with no benefit of laser treatment. The authors recommended that all eyes with CSMO associated with mild to moderate non-proliferative diabetic retinopathy be treated, and that treatment also be considered in eyes with CSMO associated with severe non-proliferative or proliferative disease. Further reports from the same study group showed that the benefit of PRP treatment outweighed the risks when carried out early in eyes exhibiting high-risk features. Eyes with mild to moderate non-proliferative retinopathy carried low risk of progression, and deferral of treatment was recommended. Another arm of this study (which randomised patients to 650mg od aspirin vs placebo) found no effect of aspirin on the progression of diabetic retinopathy, or development of preretinal or vitreous haemorrhage. Its use at a lower dose was associated with a 17% decrease in morbidity and mortality.

Problems

- Only a few patients with severe non-proliferative or proliferative diabetic retinopathy were included in the macular oedema part of the trial, so it is difficult to be certain about the magnitude of the treatment effect in these patients.

Myopia: surgical correction

> Evidence for superior efficacy and safety of LASIK over photorefractive keratectomy for correction of myopia.
>
> **AUTHORS:** Shortt A, Bunce C, Allan B.
> **REFERENCE:** Ophthalmology (2006) 113, 1897–908.
> **STUDY DESIGN:** Meta-analysis
> **EVIDENCE LEVEL:** 1a

Key message

Laser-assisted *in situ* keratomileusis (LASIK) is safer and more effective than photorefractive keratectomy (PRK) for the correction of myopia.

Impact

This meta-analysis of trials conducted in the 1990s revealed LASIK to be a safer and more effective method of refractive surgery to correct myopia than PRK. However, it did not consider other procedures for myopia (such as Epi-LASIK or LASEK), which may be preferred in certain clinical scenarios.

Aims

Two of the most common surgical treatments for correction of myopia are LASIK and PRK. LASIK involves creation of a thin corneal flap that is folded back while laser is used to reshape the corneal stroma, and is then replaced at the end of the procedure. With PRK, the epithelium is removed surgically before an excimer laser is used to reshape the anterior stroma. The epithelium regrows over a few days. This meta-analysis of prospective RCTs compared the safety and efficacy of these two types of refractive surgery in the correction of myopia.

Methods

Patients: 7 trials with a total of 683 eyes undergoing PRK, and 403 undergoing LASIK.

Inclusion criteria:
- Prospective RCT comparing LASIK and PRK;
- Correction of any myopia or ≤3 dioptres astigmatism;
- Age 18–60y;
- No ocular co-pathology or previous surgery;
- No systemic condition that could be associated with impaired wound healing.

Outcome measures:
- Efficacy:
  - Uncorrected visual acuity (UCVA) ≥20/20;
  - Post-operative spherical equivalent (SE) within ±0.50 dioptres from target.

Safety:
- Loss of ≥2 lines best spectacle-corrected visual acuity (BSCVA);
- Final BSCVA <20/40;
- Final BSCVA <20/25 when initial BSCVA ≥20/20.

Results

Outcome measure	No. of trials	Procedure	Odds ratio	*p*
UCVA better than 20/20 at 6 months	7	LASIK	1.72	0.009
UCVA better than 20/20 at 12 months	5	LASIK	1.78	0.01
Post-op SE±0.5D at 6 months	4	No significant difference	0.83	Not stated
Post-op SE±0.5D at 12 months	5	Trend towards LASIK but no significant difference	1.38	0.1
Loss ≥2 lines BSCVA	5	PRK	2.69	0.05
Final VA <20/40	4	Trend towards PRK but no significant difference	2.92	0.4
Final VA <20/25 when initial VA >20/20	4	No significant difference	0.93	Not stated

- Subgroup analysis of patients with correction of low myopia (<−6.0 dioptres) showed similar results.

Discussion

Analysis of the trials considered in this paper demonstrated the efficacy and safety of LASIK to be superior to that of PRK. This was supported by parallel analysis of a number of prospective case series', as described within the paper.

Problems

- Data collated and examined for this study related to trials conducted 5 or more years ago, which may not have included new techniques and modifications to existing techniques.
- A 1y F/U period may be insufficient to allow complete recovery from the procedure.
- Outcome measures between the trials were not standardised, making comparison more difficult.

Optic neuritis: steroids

ONTT (Optic Neuritis Treatment Trial): An RCT of corticosteroids in the treatment of acute optic neuritis.

AUTHORS: Beck R, Cleary P, Anderson M *et al.*
REFERENCE: N Engl J Med (1992) 326, 581–8.
STUDY DESIGN: RCT
EVIDENCE LEVEL: 1b

Key message
Intravenous (IV) steroid increases the rate of visual recovery in patients with optic neuritis, but with little effect on final visual outcome.

Impact
Treatment with IV steroid can be offered to patients developing optic neuritis, with the aim of speeding up visual recovery. Patients should be informed that treatment will make little difference to final visual outcome.

Aims
Optic neuritis is a cause of acute loss of vision that may be idiopathic or associated with multiple sclerosis (MS). Although steroids had been reported to improve outcomes, no consensus existed as to optimal treatment. This trial aimed to determine whether corticosteroid treatment changed the rate of recovery or visual outcome in patients with this condition.

Methods
Patients: 457 patients at 15 clinical centres across the USA.

Inclusion criteria:
- Age 18–46y;
- History consistent with acute optic neuritis, with visual symptoms for ≤8d;
- Presence of a relative afferent pupillary defect and visual field defect in the affected eye.

Exclusion criteria:
- Previous episode of optic neuritis in the same eye;
- Systemic disease (other than MS) that may cause optic neuritis.

Groups:
- IV group: IV methylprednisolone 250mg/6h for 6d followed by oral prednisolone 1mg/kg/d for 10d (n=151);
- Oral group: oral prednisolone 1mg/kg/d for 2wk (n=156);
- Placebo (n=150);

In both IV and oral groups, the dose of oral prednisolone was tapered over a further 4d.

Primary endpoint: Rate of recovery of visual field and contrast sensitivity.

Secondary endpoints: Rate of recovery of visual acuity and colour vision.

Follow-up: Initially at 4, 15, and 30d; 7, 13, and 19wk; then at 6 months, 1y, and 2y.

Results

Adjusted recovery rate for parameter measured	IV group	p (compared to placebo)	Oral group	p (compared to placebo)
Visual acuity	2.93	0.09	0.06	0.4
Visual field	16.27	0.00001	3.16	0.08
Contrast sensitivity	5.91	0.02	0.75	0.4

- Recurrent optic neuritis occurred significantly more frequently in the oral group compared to placebo ($p=0.02$), but not in the IV group.
- Rates of development of clinically definite MS were similar in all three groups.
- Incidence of minor side effects was higher in both steroid groups compared to placebo.
- Serious adverse effects occurred in two patients in the IV group (acute depression and pancreatitis), both of whom recovered completely.

Discussion

Increased rates of recovery from optic neuritis were found in patients treated with a regimen of IV methylprednisolone followed by oral prednisolone, as compared to placebo. This effect was not seen with oral prednisolone alone. There was little difference in final visual outcome. Rates of recurrence of optic neuritis were significantly higher in patients treated with oral steroid alone.

Problems

- Patients in the group receiving IV methylprednisolone were not mashed to treatment whereas those in the other two groups were.
- The oral and IV doses of steroid were very different. No group received a very high initial dose of oral steroid.

Ocular herpes simplex: antiviral treatment

> **HEDS-APT (Herpetic Eye Disease Study - Aciclovir Prevention Trial):** Aciclovir for the prevention of recurrent herpes simplex virus eye disease.
>
> **AUTHORS:** The Herpetic Eye Disease Study Group.
> **REFERENCE:** N Engl J Med (1998) 339, 300–6.
> **STUDY DESIGN:** RCT
> **EVIDENCE LEVEL:** 1b

Key message
Use of oral aciclovir over a 1y period reduces the risk of recurrence of ocular herpes simplex eye disease.

Impact
Ocular herpes simplex is a recurrent condition. Stromal keratitis and uveitis can cause a decrease in vision due to scarring. Use of oral aciclovir over a 12 month period reduces the risk of recurrent disease.

Aims
Ocular herpes simplex is a recurrent condition that can affect different parts of the eye. Complications, including stromal keratitis and uveitis, can cause visual loss due to scarring. Although aciclovir had been previously used in this condition, there was no consensus as to its role in treatment and prevention. This study aimed to evaluate the effect of treatment with oral aciclovir in reducing the recurrence rate of ocular herpes simplex virus (HSV) disease.

Methods
Patients: 703 patients at 74 clinical centres in the USA.

Inclusion criteria:
- Age ≥12y;
- Episode of ocular HSV in one or both eyes within the last 1y, but not within the last 30d;
- Immunocompetent, on no antiviral or topical treatment;
- No previous corneal surgery;
- No contraindication to treatment with aciclovir.

Groups:
- Oral aciclovir (400mg bd for 1y) (n=357);
- Placebo (n=346);

Both groups then stopped treatment, but remained under observation for a further 6 months.

Primary endpoint: One episode of recurrence of ocular HSV disease.

Secondary endpoints:
- Multiple episodes of recurrence of ocular HSV disease;
- Side effects or serious adverse events related to medication.

Follow-up: Examinations at 1, 3, 6, 9, and 12 months during treatment. Post-treatment observation at 13, 15, and 18 months. Recurrence=ocular surface infections, stromal keratitis, or iritis.

Results

	Aciclovir	Placebo	*p*
Primary endpoint			
Recurrence of ocular HSV disease during treatment period	19%	32%	<0.001
Recurrence of ocular HSV disease after treatment period	13%	14%	ns
Secondary endpoints			
>1 episode of recurrence	4%	9%	Not stated
Medication discontinued due to side effects	4%	5%	Not stated
Serious adverse events	0	0	—

Discussion

The HEDS-II study comprises two RCTs evaluating the role of oral aciclovir in the management of HSV eye disease. This study showed a significant reduction in the number of recurrences of ocular HSV disease in patients treated with long-term oral aciclovir. This effect did not persist after stopping medication but no rebound effect was seen. There was no difference in the rate of side effects between the groups and no adverse events in either group. Patients with stromal keratitis and uveitis are at greatest risk of long-term visual loss, particularly if disease is recurrent. The sister trial (HEDS-EKT 'epithelial keratitis trial') evaluated the benefits of oral aciclovir treatment for acute HSV keratitis, finding no benefit from the addition of oral aciclovir to topical trifluridine in preventing stromal keratitis or iridocyclitis. A study evaluating the effect of other factors (psychological, environmental, and biological) on recurrences of HSV eye disease is currently underway (HEDS-RFS 'recurrence factor study').

Problems

- This study considered immunocompetent patients only; it is impossible to say with certainty whether the result would also apply to immunocompromised patients.
- These results may not be relevant to patients who have undergone corneal grafting, as they were excluded from this study.

Otorhinolaryngology

Introduction

Unfortunately, otorhinolaryngology remains a specialty to which little time is devoted during medical school. However, symptoms from the ear, nose, or throat are among the most commonly encountered in non-specialist practice. Otorhinolaryngology patients constitute a large proportion of a primary care practitioner's workload. Many find considerable challenge in unravelling the problem of headache, facial pain, dizziness, persistent sore throat, hearing loss, or dysphagia.

The present inadequate training in the management of ear, nose, and throat disorders is regrettable. Much can be diagnosed from the history and clinical examination—especially, of course, with the additional benefits of flexible endoscopy of the upper aerodigestive tract. It is with these facts in mind that many of the trials highlighted in this chapter have been chosen. It is hoped that they will prove useful in managing patients in the primary care setting.

As with many specialties, carrying out randomised controlled surgical trials in otorhinolaryngology remains challenging. For many pathologies, the treatment outcome is patient's quality of life. Although otorhinolaryngologists have worked hard to develop validated measures of subjective outcomes, trial evaluation is much more complex than a convenient binary all-or-nothing scenario—or indeed a change in a unidimensional scale. Much pathology remains relatively rare to individual practitioners in the specialty, and hence, multicentre collaboration is becoming more popular. The pharmaceutical industry also has a relatively low profile in the specialty: traditionally, most industrial sponsorship supports nasal therapy or device development.

Despite these challenges to gathering evidence, otorhinolaryngologists have continued to embrace the RCT and to support a very active Cochrane Group, while also adopting the current trend for clinical databases and their ability to provide large scale audit data.

Otitis externa: topical drops

Clinical efficacy of three common treatments in acute otitis externa in primary care.

AUTHORS: van Balen F, Smit W, Zuithoff N *et al.*
REFERENCE: BMJ (2003) 327, 1201–5.
STUDY DESIGN: RCT
EVIDENCE LEVEL: 1b

Key message

Eardrops containing corticosteroids are more effective than acetic acid for the treatment of acute otitis externa (OE). Drops containing steroid and acetic acid are just as effective as steroid and antibiotic.

Impact

Steroid/antibiotic drops remain otolaryngologists' first-line treatment for acute OE. For continued symptoms (beyond 1wk) or for those in whom the small risk of ototoxicity is a concern with topical antibiotics, the use of steroid/acetic acid should be recommended.

Aims

Acute OE is a common condition, often predisposed to by persistently moist environments. Control of itching symptoms is improved by over-the-counter medications containing acetic acid. In primary care, antibiotic drops (with and without steroid) are commonly prescribed. With no consensus as to which treatment was optimal, this study aimed to compare the clinical efficacy of acetic acid, steroid/acetic acid combination, and steroid/antibiotic combination-containing eardrops in the treatment of acute OE in primary care.

Methods

Patients: 213 patients from 47 primary care centres in the Netherlands.

Inclusion criteria:
- Acute OE (defined as: redness/swelling of ear canal or debris in canal, with pain, itchiness, discharge, hearing loss for <3wk);
- Age >17y.

Exclusion criteria:
- Chronic OE;
- A furuncle;
- Acute otitis media;
- Perforated eardrum;
- Recent treatment for acute OE.

Groups:
- Acetic acid (7.2mg per g; 3 drops tds) (n=71);
- 0.1% triamcinolone and acetic acid (3 drops tds) (n=63);
- 0.66mg dexamethasone, 5mg neomycin and 10,000iu polymyxin B (3 drops tds) (n=79).

Any patient whose eardrum could not be visualised had a dry wick placed in the ear canal for 24h, with the drops applied to it.

Primary outcomes: Duration of symptoms as measured by a standardised daily diary kept by the patient.

Secondary outcomes: Cure rates at days 6–8, 13–15, and 20–22.

Follow-up: At baseline, then 7, 14, and 21d.

Results

- Significant difference in duration of symptoms (p=0.0005). Median duration to recovery=8d with acetic acid (95% CI 7.0 to 9.0), 7d with steroid/acetic acid (95% CI 5.8 to 8.3), and 6d with steroid/antibiotic (95% CI 5.1 to 6.9).

Cure rates	After 7d	After 14d	After 21d
Acetic acid	19/65	37/65	40/65
Steroid/acetic acid	29/61	46/61*	54/61*
Steroid/antibiotic	31/73	60/73*	63/73*

* Denotes a significant difference when compared to acetic acid (p=0.001).

Discussion

In the presence of acute OE, acetic acid drops were not as effective as either steroid/acetic acid or steroid/antibiotic; therefore, there is an option as to which to use as first-line treatment. Addition of antibiotic appeared to reduce the duration of symptoms. However, there remains a concern that many of the topical antibiotic drops may produce local hypersensitivity reactions and also contain ototoxic aminoglycosides, although risk of hearing loss with their use is low. For patients with continued symptoms and ear canal debris, aural toilet was very useful. For many in primary care, this option will not be available and should prompt referral. Combination of aural toilet and wick insertion did not affect outcomes between groups. 58% of patients had contact hypersensitivity on patch testing. Neomycin was the commonest sensitising agent. *(See also: Clin Otolaryngol (1990) 15, 155–8.)*

Glue ear: grommets

Grommets in otitis media with effusion: an individual patient data meta-analysis.

AUTHORS: Rovers M, Black N, Browning G *et al.*
REFERENCE: Arch Dis Childhood (2005) 90, 480–5.
STUDY DESIGN: Meta-analysis
EVIDENCE LEVEL: 1a

Key message

Watchful waiting is an appropriate management option for most children with otitis media with effusion (OME); this analysis suggests a period of observation of 12wk. Of those with persistent bilateral effusions, children ≥4y old with hearing loss ≥25dB in both ears persisting for ≥12wk, and children ≤3y in environments with a high infection load (e.g. attending day care) benefit most from grommets.

Impact

A period of watchful waiting for ≥3 months is now recommended for all children with glue ear before considering grommet insertion.

Aims

Persistent OME resulting in conductive hearing loss is commonly treated by the use of conventional ventilation tubes (grommets). Although smaller studies have proposed greater benefits in certain patient subgroups, this has not been substantiated by larger trials. This paper aimed to assess the effectiveness of grommets through an individual patient data (IPD) meta-analysis, thus providing suitable power to perform analysis on individual subgroups of patients.

Methods

- Literature search of all suitable RCTs using PubMed, proceedings of the international symposium on OME, and the Cochrane Library. Primary investigators of each trial asked to provide raw data for re-analysis.

Inclusion criteria:
- Trials randomised to a high standard;
- Children of age 0–12y;
- Persistent bilateral OME confirmed on tympanogram/otoscopy;
- Treatment arms=grommets vs watchful waiting.

Primary outcomes:
- Mean time spent with effusion (on tympanogram);
- Mean hearing loss (pure tone audiogram *or* age-related assessment);
- Language development (Reynell test);
- Effect modifiers included in the IPD: baseline hearing, acute otitis media, upper respiratory tract infections, day care attendance, gender, socio-economic status, siblings, season, breastfeeding, and parental smoking.

Results
- 7 of 10 RCTs deemed suitable to provide raw data for analysis;
- 801 patients received either grommets *or* watchful waiting;
- 433 randomised to treatment in 1 ear, with contralateral ear as control;
- In 1y F/U period, children receiving grommets had mean 19.7wk with effusion vs 37wk in watchful waiting group ($p<0.01$);
- No significant differences in mean language development at either F/U period of 6–9 months *or* 12–18 months.

Mean hearing levels during follow-up in trials:

F/U period (months)	Treatment group	n	Mean hearing (dB)	p
Baseline	Gr	296	40.1	0.4
	WW	278	39.3	
6	Gr	192	26.6	0.001
	WW	189	31.1	
12	Gr	198	27.3	0.8
	WW	181	27.6	
18	Gr	148	20.7	0.7
	WW	135	20.2	

Gr=grommets; WW=watchful waiting.

Discussion
Previous trials had only demonstrated marginal effects on hearing and language development post-grommet insertion. The most frequently cited, Paradise *et al.* (*N Engl J Med* (2001) 344, 1179–87; not included in this meta-analysis) did not demonstrate benefit in terms of developmental outcomes at 3y between early insertion of grommets only and watchful waiting with grommets, for persistent effusions. This meta-analysis added to this message: most children with OME can be observed for a period. IPD allowed appropriate subgroup analysis. The only factor associated with hearing differences was day care attendance; it was unclear as to whether this resulted from a presumed increase in the frequency of acute otitis media with secondary effusions. Interestingly, it was also found that hearing level at baseline was not necessarily a clear selection criterion, as previously thought. Hearing improvement with grommets appeared to provide a short-term benefit.

Problems
- There were patients in the watchful waiting group that went on to receive grommets. In one of the included trials, 85% of these children had received grommets by 18 months, but were analysed as part of the conservative group according to the 'intention-to-treat' analysis.

Otitis media: antibiotics

Primary care-based, randomised, double-blind trial of amoxicillin vs placebo for acute otitis media in children under 2y.

AUTHORS: Damoiseaux R, van Balen F, Hoes A *et al.*
REFERENCE: BMJ (2000) 320, 350–4.
STUDY DESIGN: RCT
EVIDENCE LEVEL: 1b

Key message
For children with acute otitis media (AOM) aged 6 months to 2y, the number needed to treat is 7–8 in order to improve symptomatic outcome at 4d.

Impact
Although most clinicians would advocate not prescribing antibiotics for AOM, practice remains varied due to parental pressure. This study justified an approach of analgesia as first-line treatment, with antibiotics reserved for clinical deterioration.

Aims
Antibiotics are routinely used to treat AOM despite debate as to their clinical effectiveness *(BMJ* (1997) 314, 1526–9). With issues such as antibiotic resistance and adverse effects to consider, some have advocated restricting prescribing for certain patients. This study aimed to determine the effect of antibiotic treatment for acute otitis media in children between 6 months to 2y of age.

Methods
Patients: 240 patients at primary care centres in the Netherlands.

Inclusion criteria:
- Acute middle ear infection, characterised by appearances of injection along handle of malleus and the annulus of the tympanic membrane, or acute otorrhoea.
- ≥1 symptom of: fever, recent earache, general malaise, or recent irritability.

Groups: Patients randomised into:
- Amoxicillin suspension (40mg/kg/d in 3 divided doses, for 10d) (n=117);
- Placebo suspension (same course) (n=123);

Both groups received oxymetazoline 0.0025% decongestant nasal drops (1 drop in each nostril tds for 7d).

Primary outcomes: Persistent symptoms at 4d (defined as earache, pyrexia ≥38°C, crying, or being irritable).

Secondary outcomes: Treatment failure at 11d (defined as above, or with no improvement in appearance of tympanic membrane).

Follow-up: Baseline GP visit. Day clinic on d4. Parents kept diary for 10d.

Results

Outcome	Amoxicillin (n=117)	Placebo (n=123)	Difference in % (95% CI)	p
Persistent symptoms at 4d	59%	72%	13% (1 to 25)	0.03
Unchanged eardrum at 4d	77%	83%	6% (−4 to 16)	0.3
Clinical treatment failure at 11d	64%	70%	6% (−6 to 18)	0.4
Median days of fever	2d	3d	1%	0.004
Median days of pain/crying	8d	9d	1%	0.4
Mean doses of analgesia in first 10d	2.3	4.1	1.8%	0.004

Discussion

Compared with placebo, amoxicillin improved symptoms at 4d. However, no differences were found between the groups at 11d in terms of symptoms or otoscopy findings. To improve symptoms at 4d in one child, 7–8 children would need to be treated (number needed to treat); the authors concluded that this was not sufficiently clinically important to warrant the prescription of antibiotics for every child aged between 6 months to 2y. The risk of intracranial complications secondary to AOM appeared low; only one patient of 123 treated with placebo developed meningitis and antibiotics were commenced on d2 due to a clinical deterioration. A retrospective study noted one case of meningitis in 3,000 cases of treated AOM (*Anales de Pediatria* (2004) 60, 125–32).

Problems

- Of the 362 patients eligible, 122 were not randomised for various reasons. Amongst these were 27 patients for whom antibiotics were deemed necessary. It is not stated why, but it is possible that these were clinically more severe cases.
- This study was not large enough to show whether antibiotics reduced the risk of meningitis.

Dizziness: exercise therapy

A RCT of exercise therapy for dizziness and vertigo in primary care.

AUTHORS: Yardley L, Beech S, Zander L et al.
REFERENCE: B J Gen Pract (1998) 48, 1136–40.
STUDY DESIGN: RCT
EVIDENCE LEVEL: 1b

Key message

Exercise therapy in the form of directed 'vestibular rehabilitation' (VR) is effective in improving symptoms of chronic dizziness and its secondary effects. This study demonstrates a benefit to patients with VR taught in a primary care setting, rather than at a specialist unit. However, patient motivation is important for VR to be effective.

Impact

This RCT highlights the role that directed exercise therapy, with supportive advice to help with secondary effects, has on a heterogeneous group of patients with dizziness. It also raises awareness of what can be achieved in the primary care setting.

Aims

Persistent and disabling dizziness/vertigo has multiple potential aetiologies and is commonly encountered in the primary care setting. For those cases caused by vestibular dysfunction, VR or 'balance retraining' through a series of graded exercises has been shown in uncontrolled studies to improve both dizziness and associated secondary symptoms of anxiety, neck pain, and situational phobias. This study aimed to compare VR with normal medical care, for a heterogeneous sample of dizzy patients in order to establish whether treatment could feasibly be provided in primary care.

Methods

Patients: 143 patients at 10 UK general (primary care) practices.

Inclusion criteria:
- Age >18y;
- Symptoms of dizziness or vertigo.

Exclusion criteria:
- Vigorous head/body movements contraindicated;
- Established non-vestibular cause of symptoms;
- Multiple life-threatening/progressive central disorders.

Groups:
- Control: received 'normal medical care' (n=76);
- VR: single session at baseline and 6wk. Therapist explained normal physiology and causes of dizziness. 8 sets of head and body movements taught, to be performed twice daily by the patient. Training in relaxation, slow breathing, and resumption of activity also given (n=67).

Primary outcomes: Validated questionnaires completed at baseline, 6wk, and 6 months for: symptoms of vertigo, anxiety/depression, and handicap. Testing with provocative movements and Romberg's test also carried out at the same intervals.

Follow-up: All patients had vestibular system assessments (nystagmus, Romberg's, and Unterberger's tests) at baseline and 6wk post-treatment.

Results

Outcome scores		VR	Control	*p*
Symptoms	Baseline	10.9	13.0	
	6 months	7.7	12.5	0.005
Anxiety/depression	Baseline	11.8	13.7	
	6 months	9.3	13.6	<0.001
Handicap	Baseline	17.0	19.1	
	6 months	14.8	18.4	ns
Provocative movements	Baseline	2.8	3.5	
	6 months	1.7	3.9	<0.001
Romberg positive	Baseline	48.6	46.2	
	6 months	55.0	43.3	0.01

Discussion

Basic VR, delivered at the primary care level, appeared to be effective for the group with moderate symptom outcome scores, as shown by an improvement in all but the vertigo handicap outcome scores. With the prevalence of dizziness (of any cause: diagnosed or non-specific) being high and the demand on formal VR programmes outweighing resources, exercise therapy administered in primary care may be cost-effective. Motivation by patients to perform the exercises and to continue on the programme was lacking, as demonstrated by a 1 in 4 dropout rate.

Problems

- The authors did state that the improvements noted were relatively modest and that further work needs to be done to optimise the treatment package.

Benign paroxysmal positional vertigo: Epley's manoeuvre

Short-term efficacy of Epley's manoeuvre: a double-blind, randomised trial.

AUTHORS: von Brevern M, Seelig T, Radtke A *et al.*
REFERENCE: J Neurol Neurosurg Psychiatry (2006) 77, 980–2.
STUDY DESIGN: RCT
EVIDENCE LEVEL: 1b

Key message
Epley's manoeuvre (EM) is shown to resolve posterior canal benign paroxysmal positional vertigo (PC-BPPV), both effectively and rapidly.

Impact
Well designed RCT for this common condition, confirming the efficacy of EM for PC-BPPV.

Aims
Abnormal endolymph flow in the semicircular canals caused by misplaced otoconia can lead to PC-BPPV, a condition associated with position dependent vertigo and nystagmus. EM, a technique involving five successive head positions, has been a well-known treatment. However, as BPPV can resolve spontaneously, rigorous evidence for the extent of its efficacy is limited, with some suggestions that the longer-term impact of treatment may be overestimated. This study aimed to evaluate the efficacy of EM for treatment of PC-BPPV, 24h after applying the manoeuvre.

Methods
Patients: 66 patients at 1 centre in Germany.

Inclusion criteria:
- Short-lasting vertigo (<1min) precipitated by head position changes;
- Nystagmus beating toward undermost ear in one of the lateral head-hanging positions of Dix–Hallpike (DHP) manoeuvre, lasting <30s;
- Brief latency between head positioning and onset of nystagmus.

Exclusion criteria:
- Bilateral BPPV;
- Previous treatment with EM;
- Involvement of the horizontal or anterior semicircular labyrinthine canals (both much rarer).

Groups:
- EM on the affected side (n=35);
- Sham procedure: EM on the normal side (n=31);

After the EM was performed once, it was repeated up to 3x until there was no nystagmus demonstrable on the DHP test. Sham procedure repeated as many times as the previous patient had received the EM.

Primary outcome: Successful treatment at 24h (defined by absence of positional vertigo and nystagmus on DHP performed twice).

Secondary outcomes: Successful treatment of controls when the EM was performed correctly after the initial 24h assessment.

Follow-up: Assessment after 24h by investigator blinded to previous treatment. DHP test performed. Telephone interview at 1wk and 1 month.

Results

	EM (n=35)	Sham (n=31)	*p*
Free of nystagmus at 24h	28 (80%)	3 (10%)	<0.001
Free of BPPV at 24h	28 (80%)	4 (13%)	<0.001
Free of BPPV at 1wk	33/35 (94%)	22/27 (82%)	ns
Free of BPPV at 1 month	30/35 (86%)	22/26 (85%)	ns
Required only 1 EM	15 (43%)	15 (48%)	ns

- 26/28 (93%) of EM group that were successfully treated by the EM to the affected side remained BPPV-free when seen after a further 24h (telephone interview).
- 5 patients in sham group lost to F/U.

Discussion

This study showed treatment of PC-BPPV with the EM (*Otolaryngol Head Neck Surg* (1992) 107, 399–404) to be more effective than a sham procedure at short-term F/U, thus demonstrating the real impact of the intervention. Longer interval studies with higher success rates may be confounded by spontaneous resolution of the condition. For such a common condition, there is a notable lack of high quality evidence. The results of this study support the conclusions of an earlier Cochrane review *(The Epley manoeuvre for BPPV. Cochrane Database Systematic Reviews 2004, Issue 2)*.

Problems

- The authors accept that this study did not actually answer the question of whether repeated EMs on the first session were more beneficial than one EM alone.

Epistaxis: first-line treatment

Management of epistaxis in children.

AUTHORS: Ruddy J, Proops D, Pearman K *et al.*
REFERENCE: Int J Pediatr Otorhinolaryngol (1991) 21, 139–42.
STUDY DESIGN: RCT
EVIDENCE LEVEL: 1b

Key message
First RCT to show that an antiseptic nasal barrier cream (Naseptin®) is as effective as silver nitrate cautery in reducing recurrent epistaxis in children, and as such, should be the first-line treatment option.

Impact
Most clinicians would now advocate an antiseptic nasal barrier cream as first-line treatment. Peanut allergy should be enquired about before prescribing Naseptin® cream as it does contain peanut oil.

Aims
Epistaxis is a common childhood condition and a frequent cause of otorhinolaryngology clinic referral. It is often treated with antiseptic creams (e.g. Naseptin®, containing chlorhexidine and neomycin) or silver nitrate cautery. This study aimed to compare Naseptin® cream with cautery in reducing childhood epistaxis.

Methods
Patients: 48 patients at 1 centre in the UK.

Inclusion criteria:
- Age 3–14y;
- ≥1 nose bleed in the previous 4wk;
- History of recurrent epistaxis.

Groups:
- Naseptin® cream, administered by parents to both nostrils bd for 4wk (n=24);
- Silver nitrate cautery to prominent vessels after local anaesthetic application (n=24);

Patients asked to record the number of nose bleeds in a 4wk period prior to F/U at 8wk.

Primary outcome: Number of nosebleeds in the preceding 4wk to F/U. 'Complete success' defined as no bleeds, 'partial success' as a 50% reduction in bleeds, 'failure' as <50% reduction.

Follow-up: At 8wk.

Results

Treatment	Complete success	Partial success	Failure	Lost to F/U
Naseptin®	12	4	7	1
Silver nitrate	13	3	6	2

No statistically significant differences between groups.

Discussion

Naseptin® was as effective as silver nitrate cautery as a first-line treatment. It should therefore be prescribed in primary care, being cost-effective with few side effects and certainly lacking the risk of septal perforation associated with recurrent cauterisation. More recent randomised studies have confirmed these findings and suggested Naseptin® to be an effective first-line treatment for adults too *(Clin Otolaryngol* (1999) 24, 228–31). As the authors highlight, there may be instances when one treatment is more suitable than the other; for example, Naseptin® was particularly good for septal crusting and vestibulitis, whereas point cauterisation may be more appropriate for obvious telangiectatic vessels. However, this study was too small to allow such stratification into subgroups.

Problems

- Calculating the power of identifying a % difference between the 'complete resolution' groups shows the power to be 6%. Hence, this is a low-powered study and there is a real chance (94%) that a true difference between treatments may have been missed. However, one could argue that any small benefit that one treatment may offer may still not merit a change to the study's main conclusion of first-line primary care treatment with the safer Naseptin®. As the power is so small, we cannot necessarily say that a treatment option is superior. It seems wise to recommend Naseptin® as the first-line treatment in primary care, but not be too dismissive of silver nitrate cautery in the specialist setting.

Treatment of chronic rhinosinusitis

Evaluation of the medical and surgical treatment of chronic rhinosinusitis.

AUTHORS: Ragab S, Lund V, Scadding G.
REFERENCE: Laryngoscope (2004) 114, 923–30.
STUDY DESIGN: RCT
EVIDENCE LEVEL: 1b

Key message

Both the medical and surgical treatment of chronic rhinosinusitis (CRS) significantly improve symptoms over 1y, with no differences found between the two groups other than total nasal volume, which is better following surgical management.

Impact

First prospective study of medical vs surgical treatment of CRS.

Aims

Although a common condition, there is a limited evidence base comparing the relative efficacy of treatments for CRS. This study aimed to conduct the first prospective RCT, evaluating the available medical treatments vs endoscopic sinus surgery (ESS) for both polypoid and non-polypoid CRS.

Methods

Patients: 90 patients at 1 centre in the UK.

Inclusion criteria:

- 8wk of persistent symptoms. At least 2 major, or 1 major and 2 minor symptoms (major: nasal congestion/obstruction, nasal discharge, facial pain/pressure, headache, olfactory disturbance; minor: fever, halitosis); *or*
- 4 episodes of recurrent acute rhinosinusitis lasting ≥10d.

Groups:

- Medical group: Initial 6wk nasal steroid spray treatment (Dexa-Rhinaspray® 2 puffs bd) and nasal douche. Then 12wk erythromycin (500mg bd for 2wk; then 250mg bd for 10wk), nasal douche, and intranasal steroids (spray for non-polyposis group, drops for polyposis group; 9 patients with polyposis received a tapering regime of oral steroids) (n=45);
- Surgical group (19 with polyposis, 23 with asthma, 2 with aspirin sensitivity, 25 with positive skin prick tests): Initial 6wk treatment of nasal steroid spray and nasal douche. Patients then underwent ESS (n=45).

Endpoints: Changes in pre- and post-operative status:
- Subjective assessments: Major symptom Visual Analogue Scales (VAS);
- Quality of life instruments: Sinonasal Outcome Test-20 (SNOT 20) and Short Form 36 Health Survey (SF36);
- Examination of the nose;

- Objective measurements of nasal physiology: Nitric oxide (NO), acoustic rhinometry, saccharine clearance test (SCT), minimum cross-sectional area (MCA).

Follow-up: At 6 months and 1y.

Results

| | % change from baseline for each group | | | |
| | Medical group | | Surgical group | |
Outcome	6 months	1y	6 months	1y
VAS of major symptoms	45.3	50.4	49.7	51.6
SCT	26.8	30.6	30.1	32.2
Total nasal NO	80.1	92.7	117.0	129.4
Total nasal volume	17.3	20.0	37.9*	37.5*
Total nasal MCA	25.4	29.8	43.7	42.4
Total endoscopic score	56.2	60.7	58.7	62.6

* Denotes a significant difference between groups ($p < 0.01$).

Discussion

This study showed the medical regimen of low-dose erythromycin, nasal douche, topical nasal steroids, and short courses of oral steroids (where indicated) was an effective therapy for CRS. Other than total nasal volume, there were no significant differences in outcomes between the medical and surgical groups. This study concluded that CRS should be treated medically for 3 months before assessing non-responders for surgery.

Problems

- Study was by its nature unblinded, a potential source of bias.

Snoring: surgical treatment

Palatoplasty for snoring: an RCT of 3 surgical methods.

AUTHORS: Clarke R, Yardley M, Davies C et al.
REFERENCE: Otolaryngol Head Neck Surg (1998) 119, 288–92.
STUDY DESIGN: RCT
EVIDENCE LEVEL: 1b

Key message
Uvulopalatopharyngoplasty (UVPP), laser palatoplasty, and diathermy palatoplasty are equally efficacious in the short term.

Impact
This was the first RCT to compare different palatal surgical techniques with an emphasis on post-operative morbidity and outcomes. The choice of optimal first-line procedure remains a subject of debate.

Aims
Snoring can be treated in many patients by simple measures, (e.g. dietary changes), and treatment of underlying conditions, e.g. (rhinitis). However in some patients, symptoms warrant palatal surgery. A variety of techniques are available, with limited long-term data as to their efficacy. This study aimed to compare the various palatal surgical options in an attempt to provide evidence for their use and appropriate selection.

Methods
Patients: 62 patients at 1 centre in the UK.

Inclusion criteria:
• Antisocial snoring;
• Failure to respond to conservative treatment;
• No significant nasal pathology.

Exclusion criteria: Sleep apnoea (as detected on overnight pulse oximetry).

Groups:
• UVPP, tonsillectomy, and uvulectomy (n=13);
• Laser (uvulectomy and soft palate mucosa midline strip excised) (n=18);
• Diathermy (excision as with the Laser) (n=16).

Primary outcomes: 100mm Visual Analogue Scores (VAS) at:
• 24 and 48h: nasal regurgitation, pain, and dysphagia;
• 1wk: taste/voice change, nasal regurgitation, pain, and dysphagia;
• 3 and 6 months: snoring (partner measured), nasal regurgitation, dysphagia, pain, and taste change. Alcohol/tobacco consumption and weight measured.

Follow-up: Review at 24h, 48h, 1wk, then 1, 3, and 6 months.

Results

- No significant differences noted pre-operatively between groups in terms of age, weight, collar size, alcohol/tobacco intake, snoring levels (measured on VAS and assessed by partners), pain, and dysphagia.
- No significant differences in pain or dysphagia between groups in first 48h post-operatively.
- Nasal regurgitation was worse with the UVPP up to 1 month, improving after this stage.
- The snoring level (on 100mm VAS scale) improved equally over the 6 months with each technique, as shown below:

Snoring level:	Diathermy	Laser	UVPP
Pre-operatively	90.5	89.3	81.7
1 month	21.3	39.1	12.4
3 months	19.9	27.7	21.7
6 months	23.9	30.4	36.3

Discussion

All three treatments were efficacious in reducing snoring levels in the short term. The study was carried out, in part, to establish the role of the newer palatal techniques, as compared to traditional treatment with UVPP. The authors concluded that this study could not recommend substituting the UVPP technique with the newer procedures. Diathermy could be as efficacious as the laser, avoiding the need for the expense associated with laser techniques. An interesting finding was that patients did not gain any weight after 6 months. As the authors commented, it was suggested by some that snoring could improve following surgery due to the loss of weight in the recovery period, and that snoring may deteriorate again as this weight was regained.

Problems

- The study lacked longer-term results. Benefits of surgery may decrease with time, e.g. whether the palatal stiffening procedures are as comparable with UVPP in the longer term.
- The use of VAS as the sole method of measuring outcomes could be criticised. Measures of general health, cognition, and sleepiness may have added further weight to the claim that surgery was highly efficacious.
- Although the aims were clearly stated, it may have been interesting to include a more conservative treatment group such as ear plugs for partners or mandibular repositioning splints.
- The study lacked a sample size/power calculation.

Sleep apnoea: treatments

Randomised crossover trial of two treatments for sleep apnoea/hypopnoea syndrome: continuous positive airway pressure and mandibular repositioning splint.

AUTHORS: Engleman H, McDonald J, Graham D *et al.*
REFERENCE: Am J Respir Crit Care Med (2002) 166, 855–9.
STUDY DESIGN: RCT
EVIDENCE LEVEL: 1b

Key message

Although mandibular repositioning splints (MRSs) and continuous positive airway pressure (CPAP) both improve outcomes in sleep apnoea/hypopnoea syndrome (SAHS), CPAP is more effective, with no difference in patient satisfaction between treatments.

Impact

Whereas previous studies have suggested patients prefer MRS, this study demonstrates no such preference. Both treatments are similar in terms of costs over 10y. The materially greater effectiveness of CPAP makes this the treatment of choice.

Aims

Evidence from systematic reviews had demonstrated the efficacy of two treatments in SAHS: CPAP and MRS. Although CPAP is often considered the treatment of choice, both this and MRS are not always well tolerated. This study aimed to compare the clinical effectiveness of long-term home treatment with CPAP and MRS on an intention-to-treat basis in a group of mixed severity SAHS with a crossover RCT.

Methods

Patients: 48 patients at 1 centre in the UK.

Inclusion criteria:
- Age 18–70y;
- Apnoea/Hypopnoea Index (AHI) ≥5/h;
- ≥2 symptoms of sleepiness, including Epworth Score ≥8, or reported sleepiness while driving.

Exclusion criteria:
- Fewer than 4 teeth remaining in either arch;
- Narcolepsy or significant periodic limb movements;
- Major medical illnesses;
- Shift work.

Groups:
- CPAP for 2 months followed by MRS for 2 months (n=24);
- MRS for 2 months followed by CPAP for 2 months (n=24).

Primary outcomes:
- Treatment use and effectiveness;
- Symptoms and sleepiness;
- General well-being;
- Cognitive performance.

Secondary outcomes: Subgroup analysis of patients with mild SAHS (AHI 5–15).

Follow-up: Outcomes measured by a limited home sleep study in the final 10d of each treatment, after at least 6wk of use.

Results

Outcome	Baseline measure (mean±SD)	After CPAP (mean±SD)	Effect size of CPAP compared to baseline	After MRS (mean±SD)	Effect size of MRS compared to baseline
AHI (per h)	31±26	8±6	0.9	15±16	0.6
Epworth Sleepiness Score	14±4	8±5	1.5	12±5	0.5

Discussion

This RCT compared two treatments rather than one treatment vs placebo. The authors justifiably mentioned this as a reason for the small to moderate effect sizes noted for the significant differences between the groups.

Problems

- The effect size of an intervention is an important concept to understand. It is a measure of the magnitude of the treatment effect. This study compared the effect size between the two groups. In our analysis, we calculated and presented the effect size of both treatments compared to baseline by dividing the clinical effect observed by the SD (e.g. for CPAP: 23/26); we felt that this better represented the clinical effect of the two treatments. Effect sizes were grouped roughly by Cohen into 0.2=small, 0.5=medium, and 0.8=large (*Psychol Bull* (1992) 112, 155–9). This does help to put these results into perspective: CPAP offered a 'large' effect for both outcomes, and MRS a 'medium' effect.

Surgery for recurrent throat infection in children

Tonsillectomy and adenotonsillectomy for recurrent throat infection in moderately affected children.

AUTHORS: Paradise J, Bluestone C, Colborn D *et al.*
REFERENCE: Pediatrics (2002) 110, 7–15.
STUDY DESIGN: RCT
EVIDENCE LEVEL: 1b

Key message
In moderate to severe cases, surgery reduces the number of subsequent throat infections.

Impact
This research group's findings have been used as evidence for the current UK guidelines for tonsillectomy in recurrent tonsillitis, with a threshold of ≥5 episodes per year, for at least 1y.

Aims
Tonsillectomy is one of the most commonly performed operations in children. Previous trials by the same group had stringent entry criteria, e.g. with 'recurrent' throat infection being defined as ≥7 episodes in the preceding year (*N Engl J Med* (1984) 310, 674–83). These studies had concluded tonsillectomy to be efficacious at reducing infection frequency and severity for at least 2y. This study aimed to address the efficacy of tonsillectomy in children less severely affected than in the previous trials.

Methods
Patients: 328 children at 1 centre in the USA.

Inclusion criteria:
- History of recurrent tonsillitis, pharyngitis, or tonsillopharyngitis;
- Meeting one of the following age-dependent criteria:
  - 3–6y: 5–6 episodes in past year *or* 4 episodes in each of past 2y;
  - 7–15y: 4–6 episodes in past year *or* 3 episodes in each of past 2y.

Exclusion criteria:
- Severe symptoms;
- Requiring adenotonsillectomy (obstructive sleep apnoea due to obstructing adenoids or persistent otitis media).

Groups: Three age groups: 3 and 4y; 5 and 6y; 7–15y. Two parallel RCTs:
- 3-way trial for patients with no apparent indication for adenoidectomy: tonsillectomy (n=58) *or* adenotonsillectomy (n=59) *or* control (n=60) groups;
- 2-way trial for those with ≥1 indication for adenoidectomy: adenotonsillectomy (n=73) *or* control (n=78).

Primary outcome: Number of throat infection episodes post-operatively or during control F/U. 'Episodes' based on 5 criteria score (degree of sore throat, maximum oral temperature, degree of malaise/reduced activity, degree of tonsillar/pharyngeal erythema, degree of anterior cervical lymphadenopthy) and rated mild (≤2), moderate (3–5), or severe (≥6).

Follow-up: 3y total F/U period. Biweekly assessment of day-to-day status. Clinical assessment at 6-weekly intervals and at time of acute illness.

Results

	Tonsillectomy	Adeno-tonsillectomy	Control
3-way trial			
Mean episodes of throat infection/ year	1.55	1.63	2.77
Mean episodes/y rated moderate to severe	0.09	0.08	0.33
2-way trial			
Mean episodes of throat infection/y	–	1.74	2.93
Mean episodes/year rated moderate-severe	–	0.07	0.28

- Surgical group outcomes significantly more favourable (both trials).
- However, illness rate in control groups was modest; over the 3y, proportion of moderate/severe episodes was 11.3% and 10.5%, respectively, with the number of such episodes ranging from 0.16–0.43/y.
- Adenotonsillectomy was no more efficacious than tonsillectomy alone in those children without an indication for adenoidectomy.
- Surgical complications occurred in 7.9% of children: 3 had primary haemorrhage, 7 had secondary haemorrhage.

Discussion

For children with moderate to severe symptoms of recurrent tonsillitis, surgery offered a modest benefit in terms of reducing the number of subsequent throat infections. However, after considering the risks involved in surgery and the relatively modest number of moderate to severe infections suffered by patients in the control groups, the benefits of surgery may have become less apparent. Other studies have demonstrated no benefit of surgery over watchful waiting for children with mild symptoms *(BMJ* (2004) 329, 651–4).

Problems

- This study concluded that the chosen criteria for tonsillectomy were not stringent enough to ensure that those children undergoing surgery truly benefited. Conversely, the fact that 20% of the controls in the 3-way trial and 24% of controls in the 2-way trial underwent surgery must have reduced the effect size of operating.

Acute sore throats in children: penicillin

Penicillin for acute sore throat in children.

AUTHORS: Zwart S, Rovers M, de Melker R *et al.*
REFERENCE: BMJ (2003) 327, 1324–7.
STUDY DESIGN: RCT
EVIDENCE LEVEL: 1b

Key message
Penicillin treatment has no benefit in reducing the average duration of symptoms, but may reduce streptococcal sequelae. Seven eligible children need to be treated to prevent a worsening illness in one child.

Impact
Confirms recommendations that most children with sore throats do not benefit from antibiotic treatment. Their prescription can be delayed for worsening symptoms or for signs of peritonsillar abscess formation.

Aims
15–30% of cases of pharyngitis are associated with group A streptococcus. Although penicillin had been demonstrated to be effective in adults, there was limited evidence for its efficacy in children. This double-blind study aimed to assess the effectiveness of penicillin treatment for 3d and 1wk, as compared with placebo, in resolving symptoms in children with sore throat.

Methods
Patients: 156 patients at primary care centres in the Netherlands.

Inclusion criteria:
- Children aged 4–15y;
- ≥2 of the 4 Centor criteria (fever, absence of cough, swollen and tender anterior cervical lymph nodes, tonsillar exudates);
- Excluded were those with an imminent peritonsillar abscess, intercurrent illnesses requiring antibiotics, and penicillin intolerance.

Groups:
- Penicillin V for 1wk (250mg tds for 4–10y olds/500mg tds for 10–15y olds) (n=46);
- Penicillin V for 3d followed by placebo for 4d (n=54);
- Placebo for 1wk (n=56).

Primary outcomes: Number of days until symptoms resolved permanently.

Secondary outcomes: Mean consumption of analgesia, absence from school, development of peritonsillar abscess, eradication of pathogen after 2wk, and recurrent episodes of sore throat over the next 6 months.

Follow-up: Diary kept nightly for 2wk to record extent of throat complaints, temperature, analgesia requirements. Patients then examined at 2wk by GP. Telephone interviews at 2, 4, and 6 months.

Results

	Placebo	Penicillin for 3d	Penicillin for 1wk
Mean duration of sore throat (d, 95% CI)	3.8 (3.3 to 4.3)	4.6 (4.0 to 5.2)	3.8 (3.2 to 4.4)
Mean absence from school (d, 95% CI)	2.4 (1.8 to 3.0)	2.3 (1.7 to 2.9)	2.8 (2.2 to 3.5)
Mean consumption of analgesia (d, 95% CI)	1.4 (1.0 to 1.8)	1.4 (1.0 to 1.9)	1.1 (0.7 to 1.6)

Discussion

This study demonstrated no significant benefit of prescribing penicillin over placebo in children with sore throat. The findings were similar for those children with proven group A streptococcal infections on throat swabs. One child (1wk penicillin group), two children (3d penicillin group), and 8 children (placebo group) suffered with streptococcal sequelae, usually in the form of a peritonsillar abscess. This study may have suggested that such effects were reduced by antibiotic treatment, but it lacked the power to provide any firmer conclusions. All patients with these sequelae subsequently improved with penicillin, suggesting it would be appropriate to adopt a 'watch and wait' strategy for those children whose symptoms do not resolve or deteriorate. A useful commentary followed this paper and calculated the number needed to treat as 7 children. *BMJ* (2003) 327, 1327–8.

Problems

- Limited power to confirm whether incidence of sequelae was reduced by antibiotic treatment.

Reflux laryngitis: proton pump inhibitors

Evaluation of omeprazole in the treatment of reflux laryngitis.

AUTHORS: Noordzij J, Khidr A, Evans B et al.
REFERENCE: Laryngoscope (2001) 111, 2147–51.
STUDY DESIGN: RCT
EVIDENCE LEVEL: 1b

Key message

Although there may be a placebo effect in the treatment of reflux laryngitis, with a lack of a 'no treatment' group, natural resolution of symptoms cannot be discounted. This study does show a benefit from proton pump inhibitors (PPIs) for mild hoarseness and throat-clearing symptoms.

Impact

Treatment of non-specific, subjective throat symptoms with PPIs (usually bd for long durations) remains commonplace, but still lacks a real evidence base; this RCT has become one of the most frequently cited from the limited literature.

Aims

Suppression of gastric acid with PPIs has been proposed by numerous studies to reduce laryngeal inflammation, and subsequently, the symptoms of reflux laryngitis. Although pH probe testing is the only accepted diagnostic technique, many previous studies have not utilised this. Therefore, this prospective, placebo-controlled, randomised, double-blind trial aimed to determine the efficacy of gastric acid suppression in the treatment of pH-proven reflux laryngitis.

Methods

Patients: 30 patients at 1 centre in the USA.

Inclusion criteria:
- >3 months history of ≥1 symptom (hoarseness, excessive phlegm, throat clearing, throat pain, lump in the throat, or chronic cough);
- Positive finding of laryngopharyngeal reflux noted on 24h dual probe pH monitoring.

Exclusion criteria: Other causes of symptoms found on laryngoscopy.

Groups:
- Oral omeprazole: 40mg bd for 2 months (n=15);
- Placebo: in an identical fashion (n=15).

Primary outcomes: Symptoms measured on a severity questionnaire, recorded individually and as a composite score.

Secondary outcomes: Laryngeal appearances, scored in a blind fashion from videostrobolaryngoscopy recordings.

Follow-up: At baseline, then 1 and 2 months.

Results

Mean symptom scores*	Omeprazole		Placebo	
Symptom	Initial	At 2 months	Initial	At 2 months
Hoarseness	331	254*	188	262
Throat pain	359	85	424	182
Lump in throat	238	121	281	179
Cough	347	234	308	328
Throat clearing	473	276*	712	632
Excessive phlegm	306	108	486	360
Dysphagia	129	18	314	119
Painful swallow	128	23	139	8
Heartburn	588	129	751	381
Composite score	2055	1079*	2399	1945

* Denotes significant difference vs placebo ($p=0.02$ hoarseness; $p=0.04$ throat clearing; $p=0.04$ composite score).

- No laryngeal signs changed significantly over treatment course (either group).

Discussion

There have been many observational studies lacking comparison groups, claiming PPIs to be effective in managing the throat symptoms presumed caused by reflux laryngitis. The benefits have not been reproduced in the few RCTs that compare PPI with placebo. Although this study showed benefit for mild hoarseness, throat clearing, and composite symptom score, it is the only RCT to do so. The overriding message from this and other RCTs is that there may be a significant placebo effect in treating what are predominantly subjective throat symptoms, but natural resolution over time cannot be excluded without a 'no treatment' group.

Problems

- Sample sizes were small and there appeared to be a significant difference between the two groups' baseline scores for certain symptoms. A larger RCT with the power to detect true differences in treatments is required.

Globus: speech therapy

The use of speech therapy in the treatment of globus pharyngeus patients.

AUTHORS: Khalil H, Bridger M, Hilton-Pierce M et al.
REFERENCE: Rev Laryngol Otol Rhinol (2003) 124, 187–90.
STUDY DESIGN: RCT
EVIDENCE LEVEL: 1b

Key message
Speech therapy significantly improves the sensation of a lump in the throat when compared to reassurance alone.

Impact
This study demonstrates the improvements that can be made in this common and often chronic condition, if time is taken to explain the underlying process to the patient and improve general throat hygiene. The study is of only a small sample size, but is one of only a few RCTs looking at treatment strategies for globus pharyngeus. Rather than advocate speech therapy for all patients, the study perhaps provides some evidence of how to successfully treat patients. Adopting this policy could improve the currently widespread practice of investigating patients with a lump in the throat (usually with a barium swallow or rigid oesophagoscopy) in order to provide reassurance that a malignancy does not exist.

Aims
Globus pharyngeus, a sensation of a lump in the throat, is a condition with an uncertain aetiology and a limited evidence base for treatments. This study aimed to investigate results from previous uncontrolled studies suggesting that speech therapy techniques improve outcomes in patients with globus pharyngeus.

Methods
Patients: 40 patients at 1 centre in the UK.

Inclusion criteria:
- Normal fibreoptic laryngoscopy;
- Normal full blood count;
- Normal barium swallow.

Exclusion criteria:
- Children;
- Pregnant females;
- History of upper aero-digestive tract malignancy.

Groups:
- Speech and language therapy: single 45–60min consultation covering an explanation of the condition, the role of stress in exacerbating symptoms, reassurance about the benign nature of the condition, elimination of throat clearing, adequate hydration, avoidance of smoking and excessive coffee or tea, exercises to relieve pharyngeal and laryngeal tension. Patients then told to practice these at home (n=20);

- Reassurance: by a nurse practitioner, with a standardised verbal format (including reassurance of benign nature of condition and its ability to spontaneously resolve) lasting 20–30min (n=20).

Primary endpoint: Measurement of globus symptoms on a 10-point visual analogue score (VAS) pre- and post-intervention.

Follow-up: At 3 months.

Results

Intervention	Median pre-intervention VAS	Median post-intervention VAS	*p*
Speech therapy	7.5	2	0.001
Reassurance	5	5	0.6

- 4 patients dropped out following randomisation.

Discussion

Symptoms of globus pharyngeus may be long-lasting and recurrent; the true measure of a treatment is whether it can control symptoms on a long-term basis, irrespective of whether repeat treatment sessions are required. Despite some limitations, this is an otherwise well-designed study that demonstrated the benefit of speech therapy. Simply providing reassurance did not improve symptoms.

Problems

- Short F/U period of only 3 months.
- The sample size was small and there appeared to be a difference in the baseline levels of symptoms between the two groups.
- 20–30min sessions of reassurance are far longer than most patients are likely to receive in a busy hospital clinic
- Globus pharyngeus is a complicated phenomenon and to measure its effects with VAS may be somewhat simplistic. The study would be improved with more detailed outcome measures, possibly to include general health and well-being questionnaires

Plastic and reconstructive surgery

Introduction

The current misinterpretation that the term 'plastic surgery' arose from making people look plastic or filling their breasts with plastic could not be further from the truth. The term 'plastic' was used in relation to plastic surgery long before the hydrocarbon-based material plastics were ever created. Derived from the Greek 'plastikos', the word means 'fit for moulding'—an apt description of plastic surgery's aim in using the body (or parts of it) to mould and reconstruct in the most functional and aesthetic way possible. Honorably, the parts utilised are often considered discardable and worthless from often overlooked bits of the body; this has permitted the specialty to gain in prominence and importance.

In plastic and reconstructive surgery, innovation and creativity has been foremost, with (occasionally) science and evidence following. Unlike for a number of other specialties, the advances in plastic surgery have largely come from imagination, innovations, and trial and error rather than from scientific trials. Somewhat more than for the rest of surgery, in plastics (where the art and craft of each particular surgeon counts immeasurably), RCTs of technique have failed to be generated, as requesting plastic surgeons to strictly follow a particular technique is akin to asking an artist to paint by numbers. Furthermore, assessing the outcome of surgery, particularly of aesthetic procedures, is practically impossible given that 'beauty is in the eye of the beholder'.

Fortunately, plastic surgeons are by nature critical of their own and others' results (especially of others), and seek constant perfection and reassurance. As is proven by this chapter, the era of evidence is finally among us, and scientific trials are now being performed in plastic surgery, albeit to answer the relatively minor—but no less important—questions.

Malignant melanoma: excision margins

Thin, stage I, primary cutaneous malignant melanoma: comparison of excision with margins of 1 or 3cm.

AUTHORS: Veronesi U, Cascinelli N, Adamus J et al.
REFERENCE: N Engl J Med (1988) 318, 1159–62.
STUDY DESIGN: RCT
EVIDENCE LEVEL: 1b

Key message
Narrow surgical lateral excision margins (1cm) are as effective as wide excision margins (3cm) in patients with melanomas of up to 1mm in thickness.

Impact
Current guidelines based on this RCT suggest that for patients with thin melanomas (<1mm thick), a surgical margin of 1cm is appropriate. This has resulted in a significant decrease in the number of cutaneous malignant melanoma patients requiring skin grafts as a result of the excision of their thin tumour. Subsequent studies have led guidelines to recommend >1cm excision in melanomas ≥2mm in depth.

Aims
Wide excision, with margins of 3–5cm, had been common practice for decades, despite this not being an evidence-based approach. Case reports had suggested that narrower margins were satisfactory in thin melanomas; however, consensus had not been reached as to the optimal size of the margin or the thickness of tumours that were amenable to such conservative approaches. This study aimed to compare outcomes following excision of thin, stage I, primary cutaneous malignant melanomas using margins of either 1 or 3cm.

Methods
Patients: 612 patients at multiple international centres.

Inclusion criteria: Clinical stage I melanoma ≤2mm thickness.

Exclusion criteria:
- Melanomas on the face, fingers, or toes;
- Multiple primary lesions or satellite lesions;
- Age >65y.

Groups:
- Narrow (1cm) excision margins (n=305);
- Wide (3cm) excision margins (n=307).

Evaluations: F/U every 2 months for 2y, then every 3 months from 3rd to 5th year.

Primary endpoints: Disease-free and overall survival.

Secondary endpoints: Local and regional recurrence, and distant metastases, according to site of first relapse.

Results

Primary endpoint	Narrow	Wide	p
Disease-free survival (at 55 months)	96.8%	96%	0.7

Discussion

For patients with thin melanomas (up to 1mm thickness), a narrow excision margin of 1cm was as effective a treatment as a wider margin of 3cm, at body sites excluding the face, fingers, and toes. Prior to this study, it was standard clinical practice to take wider margins of 3cm in patients with thin melanomas. This study did not satisfactorily clarify the optimal excision margin for melanomas of thickness between 1–2mm. A more recent multicentre RCT of 900 patients by Thomas *et al.* *(N Eng J Med* (2004) 350, 757–67) found a 1cm excision margin to have a greater risk of loco-regional recurrence than a 3cm margin in malignant melanomas of ≥2mm depth; however, there was no significant difference in survival at 60 months. There remains no clear evidence for choosing between 2–3cm excision margins.

Problems

- The results of this study suggested that narrow surgical margins (1cm) were as effective as wider margins (3cm) in patients with cutaneous melanoma no thicker than 2mm. However, the first sign of recurrent disease in three individuals within the study was local recurrence; all three patients had melanomas at least 1mm thick and had been treated with a narrow surgical margin of 1cm. Thus, the current British Association of Dermatologists' guidelines recommend that for melanomas between 1–2mm thick, the margin should be a minimum of 1cm, with a discussion of the case in a multidisciplinary team meeting and appropriate counselling of the patient. Many clinicians will take a wider margin with melanomas greater than 1mm thick.
- The F/U for this study was over a 5y period. It is not clear whether outcomes between the two treatment groups would differ beyond this time.
- Although surgical treatment is often a curative intervention for thin cutaneous malignant melanoma, adjuvant therapies for more advanced disease are currently ineffective.

Melanoma: lymph node status

MSLT (<u>M</u>ulticentre <u>S</u>elective <u>L</u>ymphadenectomy <u>T</u>rial): sentinel node biopsy or nodal observation in melanoma.

AUTHORS: Morton D, Thompson J, Cochran A *et al.*
REFERENCE: N Engl J Med (2006) 355, 1307–18.
STUDY DESIGN: RCT
EVIDENCE LEVEL: 1b

Key message
Large randomised trial showing that sentinel node biopsy may confer a survival benefit by permitting earlier lymphadenectomy. This trial also shows the staging reliability of sentinel node biopsy.

Impact
This trial reinforces the role of sentinel node biopsy in the management of melanoma, and the need for lymphadenectomy when the biopsy is positive.

Aims
Although resection is usually curative in most patients with clinically localised melanoma of intermediate thickness, metastasis to regional nodes occurs in 15–20%. Regional node metastasis is the most important prognostic factor in early-stage disease; for this reason, some have advocated immediate lymphaedenectomy. However, this is not without morbidity, and an overall survival advantage has not been demonstrated in the majority. Sentinel node biopsy is a technique that can be used to help accurately stage melanoma in order to determine whether more major lymph node resection is necessary. This study aimed to determine the value of sentinel node biopsy and the effects of completion lymphadenectomy on positive biopsies on survival and recurrence.

Methods
Patients: 1269 patients from multiple centres in the USA, Australia, and Europe.

Inclusion criteria: Primary melanoma (1.2–3.5mm deep) with:
• Clark level 3, with Breslow thickness >1mm;
• Clark level 4–5, with any Breslow thickness.

Groups: Randomised in 60:40 ratio to treatment groups. Both groups had wide excision of the primary melanoma:
• Observation of lymph nodes, with lymphadenectomy if they became palpable (n=500);
• Sentinel node biopsy, with lymphadenectomy if biopsy was positive (n=769).

Primary endpoint: Survival until death from melanoma.

Secondary endpoints:
• Survival without evidence of recurrence or metastasis (disease-free survival);
• Incidence of nodal metastases and survival once detected.

Follow-up: Every 3 months with examination, Chest X-ray, and bloods for first 2y; then every 4 months in y3; then every 6 months in y4–5; then annually until y10. Median F/U=59.8 months.

Results

Primary endpoint	Sentinel node	Observation	*p*
Melanoma-specific death	12.5%	13.8%	ns
Secondary endpoints			
Disease-free survival	78.3%	73.1%	0.009
5y survival once lymph basin treated	72.3%	52.4%	<0.001
Incidence of nodal metastases	19.4%	18.5%	ns

Discussion

This study confirmed the ability of sentinel node biopsy to accurately stage and provide prognostic evaluation of intermediate level melanomas. Positive sentinel node biopsy and immediate lymphadenectomy increased the 5y survival rate from 52.4% to 72.3%, compared with delayed lymphadenectomy for palpable lymph nodes, and reduced the death rate from 48.7% to 26.2%; it also reduced recurrence. This confirmed the findings of other smaller studies. In those without nodal disease, sentinel node biopsy did not affect survival or recurrence.

Problems

- Statistically, the results are only valid if the assumption that a positive sentinel node would progress to nodal disease is true.
- The median time to detection of nodal relapse in the observation group was 1.33y.
- This is an interim result; the final results of this study are still pending.

Facial basal cell carcinoma: type of resection

Surgical excision vs Mohs' micrographic surgery for basal cell carcinoma of the face.

AUTHORS: Smeets N, Krekels G, Osterag J et al.
REFERENCE: Lancet (2004) 364, 1766–72.
STUDY DESIGN: RCT
EVIDENCE LEVEL: 1b

Key message
There is no difference in the recurrence rates of primary or recurrent basal cell carcinoma (BCC), when treated with either surgical excision or Mohs' micrographic surgery (MMS).

Impact
MMS, which is more costly and time-consuming, can now safely be reserved for those multiply recurrent BCCs, morphoiec BCCs, or indistinct BCCs, in particularly anatomically sensitive areas.

Aims
BCC is the commonest skin cancer in Caucasians, with a rising incidence. It rarely metastasises, but the morbidity (and mortality) from some, particularly if large or incompletely treated, can be significant. There had been a widely held belief that recurrence rates of BCCs were lower when treated by MMS (utilising a systematic microscopic examination of the tumour site), compared with more commonly used surgical excision. However, MMS is a more time-consuming, hence more expensive, procedure. This study aimed to identify whether there were subsets of facial BCC in which MMS would be more effective than surgical excision.

Methods
Patients: 565 patients (612 BCCs) from 2 European centres.

Inclusion criteria: Facial BCC:
- Histologically confirmed BCC;
- At least 1cm in diameter if non-aggressive type *or* any size if aggressive type (morphoiec, micronodular, squamous differentiation, infiltrative, trabecular: these account for approximately 50% of cases);
- Recurrence must be biopsy-proven, any size.

Exclusion criteria: Life expectancy <3y.

Groups: Classified by primary or recurrent BCC status. 3mm resection margin used for both groups:
- Surgical excision (n=204 primary; 102 recurrent);
- MMS (n=204 primary; 102 recurrent).

Primary endpoint: Recurrence of the BCC.

Secondary endpoints:
- Incomplete excision;
- Suboptimal aesthetic results;
- Costs of treatment.

Follow-up: At 6 months and 18 months by researcher for photographs and aesthetic assessment, in addition to normal cancer F/U for recurrence. Mean F/U=2.66y.

Results

Primary endpoint	Surgical excision	MMS	p
Recurrence	8 cases	2 cases	ns
Secondary endpoints			
Incomplete excision	18% of primary and 32% of recurrences	No cases	<0.001
Defect size: primary/recurrent (cm²)	4.64/7.78	4.06/7.50	0.4/0.6
Suboptimal aesthetic	No difference		ns*
Cost (primary tumour)	€216.86	€405.79	<0.001

* But primary tumours had significantly better aesthetic outcome than recurrent (*p*=0.04).

Discussion

With 50% of BCCs comprising the aggressive type, the average primary size treated was 6–8mm, with recurrences 10–12mm. Excisions were performed by dermatologists, with an incomplete excision rate of 18% in primary tumours and 32% in recurrent tumours. Incomplete excisions were more likely in aggressive tumours, and those around the eyes and ears; most were re-excised. The study showed no significant difference in recurrence rates at a mean of 2y.

Problems

- The incomplete excision rate seemed very high.
- Followed an intention-to-treat protocol, so even though four patients were randomised to excision and had their results counted in that group, they had MMS.
- The study's conclusion (that MMS be used for tumours bigger than 1cm in diameter and recurrent tumours) is not consistent with the results presented.
- Unclear if costs represented each procedure or total cost per patient to treat initial disease, including treatment of incomplete excision.
- The BCCs undergoing MMS were curetted initially, but those in the surgical excision group were not.

Hypertrophic burn scars

Hypertrophic burn scars: analysis of variables.

AUTHORS: Deitch E, Wheelahan T, Rose M et al.
REFERENCE: J Trauma (1983) 10, 895–8.
STUDY DESIGN: Prospective, cohort
EVIDENCE LEVEL: 3

Key message
Burn healing period correlates with the risk of hypertrophic scarring. If the burn takes 14–21d to heal, there is a 33% risk of hypertrophic scarring. A healing period greater than 10d in Afro-Caribbean patients is associated with a higher risk of hypertrophic scarring.

Impact
This evidence gave additional impetus to the push for early excision/ debridement of burns. Burns assessed to take longer than 14d to heal should be excised. Those of uncertain potential can be observed, and if they remain unhealed at 10–14d, they should then be excised and grafted. Burns that are treated conservatively and take longer than 10–14d to heal should be treated with prophylactic compression garments.

Aims
Hypertrophic scarring is a major complication in patients experiencing thermal injury. This study aimed to determine the factors associated with an increased risk of development of hypertrophic burns scars.

Methods
Patients: 100 patients (245 burns) at 1 centre in the USA.

Inclusion criteria:
- Burns (superficial or moderate partial thickness) judged likely to heal within 3wk;
- Deeper burns in patients who refuse surgery.

Primary endpoint: Hypertrophic scars (increased thickness/elevation >2cm in diameter).

Secondary endpoint: Wound problems.

Follow-up: 9–24 months; assessed for hypertrophic scars.

Results
Baseline: 59 children, mean age=3y, total burn surface area (TBSA) average=14%; and 41 adults, mean age=37y, TBSA average=21%.

Would problems:
- 38% of patients developed wound problems;
- 26% (63 of 245 wound sites) became elevated or hypertrophic.

Risk of hypertrophic scarring:
- 78% if the burn took longer than 21d to heal;
- 33% if healing occurred in 14–21d;

- If healing occurred in a shorter period than 14d, the risk of hypertrophic scar was markedly lower, except in Afro-Caribbean patients in whom the overall incidence of wound problems was 2x that of other populations. In this group, healing had to occur within 10d to reduce the risk of hypertrophic scar formation.

Discussion

This study showed the strong correlation between time to heal a burn and the formation of hypertrophic scars. It also showed the racial differences in hypertrophic scar formation. Furthermore, there was a difference in site, with the chest, upper limb, and foot found to be sites most likely to develop hypertrophic scarring. Compression or pressure garment use made no difference to the development of wound problems.

Problems

- This was an observational study, though it is unlikely that a prospective RCT could be performed given the non-uniform mechanism of injury and the lack of equipoise, amongst other reasons. There was no statistical analysis of the significance of the results.
- The F/U period could have probably been longer, though by 9 months the tendency to hypertrophy would already be present.
- The inference that a less hypertrophic scar would result by surgically healing a burn that would take longer to heal if treated conservatively, remains unproven.

Vacuum-assisted closure

Comparing conventional gauze therapy to vacuum-assisted closure wound therapy.

AUTHORS: Mouës C, van den Bemd G, Heule F *et al.*
REFERENCE: J Plast Reconstr Aesthet Surg (2007) 60, 672–81.
STUDY DESIGN: RCT
EVIDENCE LEVEL: 1b

Key message
First randomised trial to show vacuum-assisted closure (VAC) to be at least as good as gauze dressings.

Impact
Although the evidence base is limited, VAC is used by some as the panacea to all wounds. This study showed that, in carefully selected patients, VAC decreased contracture compared to gauze-dressed wounds.

Aims
In patients requiring reconstructive surgery, wounds are often large, with extensive soft tissue loss. In many cases, immediate closure is not possible, with the first stage of management involving optimisation of the wound condition through aggressive debridement in order to remove necrotic tissue, bacteria, and foreign material. This is conventionally followed by application of topical dressings. Drainage of wounds is important, with suction drainage combined with foam dressings having been an established surgical practice. VAC had recently been proposed as demonstrating efficacy in promoting wound healing. This study aimed to compare the use of VAC with gauze dressings in the treatment of acute (early-treated) and chronic (late-treated) surgically debrided full-thickness wounds awaiting surgical closure.

Methods
Patients: 54 wounds (29 vacuum and 25 gauze) at 1 centre in The Netherlands.

Inclusion criteria:
• Full thickness wounds unable to be closed immediately due to crush, chronicity, or infection;
• Initial aggressive surgical debridement.

Exclusion criteria:
• Malignant disease;
• Exposed vessels, bleeding, or deep fistulas;
• Necrotic tissue or unstable skin around the wound;
• Osteomyelitis, uncontrolled diabetes, or psychiatric disorders.

Groups: Classified by early-treated wounds (≤4wk) vs late-treated wounds (>4wk):
• Vacuum (n=29; 12 early-treated, 17 late-treated);
• Conventional wet gauze dressings (n=25; 8 early-treated, 17 late-treated).

Primary endpoint: Period until wound 'ready' for surgery (i.e. healthy granulations and good wound scores).

Secondary endpoints:
- Wound scores: inflammation, slough, exudates;
- Wound surface area;
- Bacterial count;
- Complications.

Follow-up: All wound measurements taken at the point when the wounds were considered ready for surgical closure. Bacterial count biopsies were performed every 2–3d. Wound scores at every dressing change (every 12h gauze and 48h vacuum).

Results

Primary endpoint	Vacuum	Gauze	p
Period to wound readiness	6d	7d	ns
Secondary endpoints			
Wound scores='good'	69% in 1wk; 86% in 2wk	56% in 1wk; 84% in 2wk	ns
Wound area reduction	100% patients	77% patients	<0.05
Bacterial count	No change	No change	ns
Complications (pre-op)	4/29	2/25	ns
Treatment terminated	2 (sepsis, necrosis)	0	ns
Large complications (post-op)	4/25	3/21	ns
Osteomyelitis	4/29	1/25	ns

Discussion

The authors felt that VAC showed greatest difference in the 'late' group, though this was not statistically significant. Statistically, the significant differences were seen in the degree of wound contracture (with both techniques, but greater with VAC) and the daily relative wound score (significantly lower with VAC on d3, 6, and 8 ($p<0.05$), but not significant overall). Despite this, the trial concluded that vacuum therapy resulted in improved wound healing compared with gauze therapy.

Problems

- The manufacturers of VAC supported the trial; unclear impact.
- Despite randomisation by closed envelope assignment, unequal sample sizes occurred. Distribution of early and late wound types, and mechanisms, was unequal. Not all treatments were the same (e.g. 44% of the conventional group received topical antibacterial, whereas no patients in the vacuum group did.

Breast augmentation: type of implant

Textured or smooth implants for breast augmentation?
AUTHORS: Coleman D, Foo I, Sharpe D.
REFERENCE: Br J Plast Surg (1997) 50, 99–105.
STUDY DESIGN: RCT
EVIDENCE LEVEL: 1b

Key message
Textured implants lead to greatly reduced capsular contracture, compared with smooth implants.

Impact
Textured implants have become the silicon breast implant shell of choice.

Aims
The incidence of adverse capsular contracture following breast augmentation is high (approximately 30%), and many implant modifications have occurred to reduce this rate. Previous studies had largely been retrospective, leading to incomplete follow-up and unequal comparison of implants. This trial was designed to compare textured silicon implants with smooth implants, to ascertain whether there was a difference in adverse capsular contracture rates.

Methods
Patients: 53 consecutive women (100 breasts) at 1 centre in the UK.

Inclusion criteria:
• Primary bilateral breast augmentation;
• Already on the waiting list for surgery.

Groups: Randomised in theatre after pocket dissection and sizing to:
• Smooth implant (48 breasts);
• Textured implant (52 breasts);

Textured or smooth implants were otherwise identical in shape and bleed characteristics and were from the same manufacturer. All patients received intra-operative antibiotics and the pocket was washed with 5% povidine iodine.

Primary endpoint: Baker grade of capsular contracture. Grade 1–2=if patient said they could not feel the implant (i.e. normal appearance). Grade 3=firm breast and abnormal appearance. Grade 4=hard, painful breast with abnormal appearance.

Follow-up: At 1y, with questionnaires and clinical examination by one or more surgeons.

Results

Implant	Baker 1 and 2 (without contracture)	Baker 3 and 4 (with contracture)	Total (n)
Smooth	20	28	48
Textured	48	4	52
Total	68	32	100

$\chi^2 = 27.14$; $p < 0.0001$.

Discussion

This prospective RCT suggested that textured implants had markedly lower adverse capsular contraction rates. The reason for this is unknown. Subsequent studies have confirmed this finding, leading to textured implants becoming the shell of choice for bilateral augmentation.

Problems

- The only criterion used for capsular contracture was Baker's scale. This scale is a peculiar mixture of symptoms and signs, and is not objective.
- Not all patients were assessed by all three surgeons. Only one surgeon assessed some patients, although inter-rater reliability was rated as high.
- This trial confirmed benefit in using textured implants in both breasts. Subsequent studies have confirmed benefits in patients randomised to receive textured or smooth implants in either breast.

Breast reduction: drainage

Routine drainage is not required in reduction mammoplasty.

AUTHORS: Wyre S, Banducci D, Mackay D *et al.*
REFERENCE: Plast Reconstr Surg (2003) 111, 113–7.
STUDY DESIGN: RCT
EVIDENCE LEVEL: 1b

Key message
First randomised trial to show that drains are unnecessary in routine breast reduction surgery.

Impact
This trial inspired a larger (n=150) UK study that confirmed the findings. However, most surgeons still persist in draining breast reductions.

Aims
The use of closed suction drainage in reduction mammoplasty is standard practice in many centres; however, this is not evidence-based. Although it is believed that drainage reduces fluid accumulation, consequently leading to improved healing and cosmetic outcome, drainage itself is not without complication; in particular, drains cause discomfort to the patient, with some sources claiming that they can potentially increase post-operative infection rates. This study sought to clarify the situation.

Methods
Patients: 49 consecutive women at 1 centre in the USA.

Inclusion criteria: Routine breast reduction candidates:
• Bilateral breast reduction by the inferior pedicle technique.

Groups: Self-controlled—one breast each randomised to be:
• Drained;
• Undrained.

Primary endpoint: Complications (especially haematoma).

Secondary endpoints:
• Patient satisfaction (post-operative questionnaire to determine comfort level and overall satisfaction);
• Surgeons aesthetic outcome assessment.

Follow-up: Drains removed on post-operative d1. Average F/U=9 months (range 5–17 months).

Results

Primary endpoint	Drained (n=49)	Undrained (n=49)	p
Complications	6 (12%)	5 (10%)	ns
Haematoma	1 (2%)	1 (2%)	ns

- Secondary endpoints: 17 of 19 patients reported that the undrained breast was more comfortable; 2 of 19 reported little/no difference between either breast.
- Mean weight reduction: Drained breast=675g (360–1,090g); undrained breast=620g (380–1,011g).
- Surgeons' subjective observations: undrained breast observed to be slightly more swollen and weepy (serous fluid) from suture line in first 24h. Differences were not appreciable after 48h.

Discussion

Routine drainage is commonplace, despite studies suggesting that reduction mammoplasty can be conducted safely without the need for post-operative suction drainage. To date, there had never been a prospective study to address this issue. Although small, this trial was the first such prospective RCT to demonstrate that breast reductions could be safely left undrained with comparable outcomes between groups. The patients served as their own controls, and the volumes excised were similar between drained and undrained breasts.

Problems

- Small numbers. F/U intervals were not recorded, and only 63% of patient questionnaires were returned.
- Randomisation details were missing; it is unclear whether randomisation was performed at the end of the operation (after all haemostasis had been completed) or at the beginning (allowing some bias to occur in technique).
- Average excision volumes were smaller than in other studies on reduction mammoplasty. Furthermore, as the authors reported, there were no reductions >1,100g, hence applicability of these findings to large volume reductions is not possible.
- All but one patient underwent reduction using the inferior pedicle technique; correspondingly, the results are also not directly applicable to other reduction techniques.
- Different centres remove drains on different post-operative days; the authors of this study removed drains on the first post-operative day, hence the effect of longer drainage was not observed.

Flexor tendon rehabilitation

Digital function following flexor tendon repair in zone II: A comparison of immobilisation and controlled passive motion techniques.

AUTHORS: Strickland J, Glogovac S.
REFERENCE: J Hand Surg [Am.] (1980) 5, 537–43.
STUDY DESIGN: Controlled trial
EVIDENCE LEVEL: 2a

Key message

This is the first comparative study of rehabilitation techniques in flexor tendon repairs. It demonstrates the value of early mobilisation.

Impact

Along with the non-comparative reports on the topic, this study changed the treatment of flexor tendon injuries to one of primary repair and immediate mobilisation.

Aims

Flexor tendon injuries in zone II (flexor tendon lacerations that lie within the flexor synovial sheath from the A1 pulley in the palm to the level of the insertion of the flexor digitorum superficialis (FDS) tendon on the middle phalanx) were considered as lying within 'no man's land', and surgeons were advised not to attempt primary repair in this zone due to complications of failure and stiffness. With a delayed approach being advocated (even though this required FDS excision, a tendon graft, and only average results after prolonged therapy), it was not until the first reports of Verdan (J Bone Joint Surg (1960) 42, 647–57) and others that successful primary repair was demonstrated. These studies encouraged primary repair in acute injuries, but used immobilisation as the rehabilitation protocol. Despite improved results over delayed repair, further improvements were sought; Kleinert subsequently published his technique of 'passive dynamic mobilisation' (J Hand Surg [Am]. (1977) 2, 441–51), involving rehabilitation with passive flexion and active extension following tendon repair. This study aimed to compare the outcomes of immobilisation, with the early use of the Duran and Houser (1975, Mosby) technique of passive mobilisation (passive flexion and passive extension).

Methods

Patients: 37 patients with 50 consecutive flexor tendon injuries at 1 centre in the USA.

Inclusion criteria:
- Zone II flexor tendon injuries;
- Isolated injuries ± digital nerve injury.

Groups: Consecutively recruited:
- Immobilisation for 3.5wk, then gradual motion (n=3 had flexor digitorum profundus (FDP) tendon alone severed; n=22 had FDP and FDS severed);

- Mobilisation immediately with passive flexion, commencing active flexion at week 4.5 with rubber band (n=8 had FDP tendon alone severed; n=17 had FDP and FDS severed).

Primary endpoint: Range of motion of interphalangeal joints–'extensor lag'.

Secondary endpoint: Tendon rupture.

Follow-up: Average F/U=13 months.

Results

Primary endpoint	Immobilisation	Mobilisation	*p*
Range of motion	0% excellent	36% excellent	<0.005* and
	12% good	20% good	<0.05†
	28% fair	16% fair	
	11% poor	24% poor	
Secondary endpoint			
Rupture	4	1	Not stated

*=for 'excellent' and 'good' groups; †=for 'excellent', 'good', and 'fair' groups.

Discussion

Verdan first reported that primary repair of flexor tendons in 'no man's land' was a valid operation in fresh, cleanly cut wounds, which gave equal or better results than tendon grafts. However, he utilised a period of immobilisation following repair. This study demonstrated an advantage, in terms of range of motion and rupture rate, when mobilisation rather than immobilisation was used as the rehabilitation method following primary flexor tendon repair.

Problems

- Patients were not randomised.
- Increasing surgeon experience with primary tendon repair and rehabilitation may have biased the results.

Transplantation

Introduction

Organ transplantation is now a well-established therapy for selected patients with end-stage organ failure, for whom it is a life saving or life-enhancing experience. In the UK alone over 3,000 organ transplants are carried out each year, and this figure would be much higher were it not for the severe shortage of available organs. The majority of those fortunate enough to receive an organ transplant can now expect a good outcome, with average graft survival rates for kidney, liver, and heart transplantation in excess of 75% at five years. Because transplantation is now regarded as an almost routine event in modern medical practice, it is easy to lose sight of how, not so long ago and certainly within the professional careers of the authors of this chapter, organ transplantation was a very hazardous procedure with a high chance of failure.

The first successful human kidney transplant was carried out between genetically identical twins in 1954 at the Peter Bent Brigham hospital in Boston. This was a major advance but had little immediate impact on patient care, since the number of patients with kidney failure fortunate enough to have a healthy identical twin who wanted to give them a kidney was extremely small. Then when the antiproliferative drug azathioprine was developed in the late 1960s and used together with steroids to prevent graft rejection, successful transplantation of kidney allografts from cadaveric donors became possible and was performed increasingly during the 1970s. The world's first successful liver transplant was performed by Tom Starzl at the University of Colorado in 1967 and the first heart transplant was carried out in the same year by Christiaan Barnard at the Groot Schuur Hospital in Cape Town, although the scientific foundations for heart transplantation had already been established by Norman Shumway in the USA. In these early days, randomised clinical trials were not needed to establish the benefits of organ replacement surgery, since the alternative was either certain death or life long dialysis.

The modern era of organ transplantation only really became firmly established in the 1980s, with the introduction of powerful new immunosuppressive agents, notably ciclosporin and subsequently tacrolimus. These new agents not only improved the results of renal transplantation, but also allowed the widespread development of liver and thoracic organ transplantation, which prior to this had been limited to very few centres worldwide. Along too came the first of many large multicentre clinical trials to determine how best to immunosuppress patients undergoing organ transplantation—a question still very much under investigation today.

Over the last twenty years the results of transplantation have improved incrementally for a variety of reasons, including better recipient selection, improved anaesthetic and surgical techniques, the introduction of more effective anti-viral agents, and better post-transplant immunosuppressive management. Although new immunosuppressive agents have become available, ciclosporin and tacrolimus still remain the mainstay of most immunosuppressive regimens, despite their side effects, which ironically include nephrotoxicity. The problem of early graft loss from acute rejection is now uncommon and the main challenges today are chronic allograft rejection and the side effects of non-specific suppression of the immune response, namely infection and malignancy. Randomised clinical trials continue to inform and further improve clinical practice. Because transplantation today is such a success story, however, the traditional endpoints of one-year patient and graft survival are no longer sufficient and new and more sophisticated endpoints are needed that reflect graft function and quality of life after transplantation.

Cardiac transplantation: patient selection

> **COCPIT** (**C**omparative **O**utcomes and **C**linical **P**rofiles **I**n **T**ransplantation): An observational study comparing mortality among patients who underwent a heart transplant vs patients who did not, on a national heart transplant waiting list.
>
> **AUTHORS:** Deng M, De Meester J, Smits J et al.
> **REFERENCE:** BMJ (2000) 321, 540–5.
> **STUDY DESIGN:** Observational cohort study
> **EVIDENCE LEVEL:** 3

Key message
Patients who undergo cardiac transplantation do not have an overall survival benefit at 1y, compared with patients who do not. However, there is a survival benefit of up to 8 months in patients with severe heart failure stratified by the Heart Failure Survival Score (HFSS).

Impact
Patients placed on the waiting list for cardiac transplantation should be prioritised according to medical urgency.

Aims
This study aimed to investigate whether undergoing a heart transplant was actually associated with a survival benefit in patients on a cardiac transplant waiting list. These patients were stratified into high, medium, and low risk according to the heart failure survival score.

Methods
Patients: 889 patients in Germany in 1997.

Inclusion criteria:
- Listed for first time heart transplant between 1st Jan to 31st Dec 1997;
- Age >16y.

Exclusion criteria:
- Previous heart transplant.

Groups:
- High risk (HFSS <7.2) (n=107);
- Medium risk (HFSS 7.2 to 8.09) (n=360);
- Low risk (HFSS >8.09) (n=422).

Primary endpoint: Survival stratified by HFSS.

Follow-up: Minimum of 2y.

Results

	High risk	Me	780
Overall mortality at 1y	51%		
Mortality at 1y without transplant	32%	20%/18%	
Mortality at 1y after transplant	36%	24%/25%	0.2

* For high risk vs medium/low risk

Discussion

There have been considerable advances in medical and organ-saving management in patients with heart failure. Therefore, cardiac transplantation
in patients with less severe heart failure might not be as beneficial in the
present era. In this study, cardiac transplantation was not associated with
an overall improvement in survival within a year. However, high risk patients who underwent cardiac transplantation had a relative risk reduction
of death of up to 8 months. Efforts must be directed to refine the selection
of patients who might benefit from cardiac transplant.

Problems

- This study does not address the issue of improvements in quality of
  life, symptoms, or cost-effectiveness to society that cardiac transplantation might confer.
- Although the minimum follow-up in this study was 2y, results were
  only reported to 1y. It may be that medium- to long-term survival of
  patients with severe heart failure is improved by cardiac transplantation.

…ransplantation: single vs
…ung transplant

…ilateral lung transplantation for emphysema: A retro-
…tudy comparing outcomes among emphysema patients who
…ent either single or bilateral lung transplantation.

…HORS: Sundaresan R, Shiraishi Y, Trulock E et al.
…FERENCE: J Thorac Cardiovasc Surg (1996) 112, 1485–94.
STUDY DESIGN: Retrospective, cohort
EVIDENCE LEVEL: 3

Key message

Patients with emphysema who undergo bilateral lung transplantation demonstrate improved breathing mechanics, gas exchange, and functional status over patients who have a single lung transplant. There is also a trend towards better survival at 5y.

Impact

Patients with end-stage emphysema should ideally be offered bilateral lung transplant where feasible.

Aims

This study aimed to investigate whether there was a benefit for patients with emphysema who were being considered for transplantation to undergo bilateral rather than single lung transplant.

Methods

Patients: 119 patients at 1 centre in the USA.

Inclusion criteria:
- Underwent single or bilateral lung transplantation;
- All consecutive patients operated on between 1st July 1999 to 31st December 1994.

Exclusion criteria:
- Patients who underwent en bloc bilateral lung transplantation.

Groups:
- Single lung (n=50);
- Bilateral lung (n=69).

Primary endpoint: Survival at 5y.

Follow-up: 7 to 64 months.

Results

	Bilateral lung (n=69)	Single lung (n=50)	p
90d mortality	7.2%	10%	0.7
5y actuarial survival	53%	41%	0.3
Actual or predicted FEV_1 at 4y post-transplant	75%	50%	<0.05

Discussion

Lung transplantation was associated with an overall improvement in spirometry, functional capacity, and gas exchange over all pre-operative values. These improvements were even more significant in those receiving bilateral lung transplants. However, in light of severe organ shortages, it might be more beneficial to society to have two patients benefit with single lung transplantation rather than a single patient with bilateral lung transplantation.

Problems

• The bilateral lung transplant group were significantly younger than the single lung transplant group and so would naturally have an intrinsic survival advantage.
• Patients with α1-antitrypsin deficiency were included together with patients with chronic obstructive pulmonary disease (COPD) in this study on lung transplantation for end-stage emphysema. This could confound the outcomes as it combines two potentially different subgroups. In addition, the proportion of patients with COPD was significantly higher in the single lung transplant group.

Liver transplant: hepatitis C recurrence

Efficacy of antiviral therapy on hepatitis C recurrence after liver transplantation.

AUTHORS: Carrion J, Navasa M, Garcia-Retortillo M et al.
REFERENCE: Gastroenterology (2007) 132, 1746–56.
STUDY DESIGN: RCT
EVIDENCE LEVEL: 1b

Key message
Antiviral therapy with interferon plus ribavirin reduces disease progression in hepatitis C virus (HCV)-infected liver transplant recipients.

Impact
These findings suggest the importance of regular assessment with biopsy and portal pressure gradient measurement in HCV-positive recipients, with early antiviral therapy if there is evidence of disease recurrence.

Aims
HCV-related liver disease is the most common indication for liver transplantation. Patients undergoing liver transplantation for HCV always acquire HCV in their graft, often leading to chronic hepatitis and cirrhosis. Most centres start antiviral therapy if biopsy confirms liver damage, but the evidence that it prevents disease progression is limited. This study aimed to determine the effect of antiviral therapy (interferon plus ribavirin) on disease progression, compared to no treatment.

Methods
Patients: 81 patients at 1 centre in Spain.

Inclusion criteria:
- Age 18–70y with first liver transplant;
- Diagnosis of HCV recurrence (supported by positive HCV test, serum HCV-RNA, and liver biopsy).

Exclusion criteria:
- Medical: HBV or HIV infection, renal failure;
- Previous organ transplant.

Groups:
- A: mild HCV recurrence; no treatment (n=27);
- B: mild HCV recurrence: antiviral treatment (n=27);
- C: severe HCV recurrence: antiviral therapy (n=27).

Antiviral therapy=pegylated interferon α-2b (1.5 mcg/kg/wk) and ribavirin (dose adjusted for creatinine clearance) for 48wk.

Primary endpoint: Stable or improved histological response (fibrosis) on liver biopsy.

Secondary endpoints:
- HCV clearance (early/sustained);
- Hepatic venous pressure gradient (in around 50% randomised patients).

Follow-up: Every 2–4wk during treatment and every 8wk during 6 month F/U period. Liver biopsy performed at baseline and 6wk after completion of treatment. Paired measurements of hepatic venous pressure gradient performed on some patients.

Results

Histology	No treatment			Antiviral treatment			*p*
	Stable	Improved	TOTAL	Stable	Improved	TOTAL	
Mild HCV	7	1	8 (30%)	13	7	20 (74%)	0.001
Severe HCV	–	–	–	9	4	13 (46%)	–

- **Viral clearance:** 0% (control group) cleared HCV spontaneously vs 48% (treated patients with mild recurrence) and 19% (treated patients with severe recurrence) who showed a sustained virological response (undetectable HCV-RNA for >6 months) after completing treatment.
- **Portal pressures:** slight increase (control patients) and decrease (treated patients, especially in those with baseline portal hypertension) (*p*=0.05).

Discussion

This study suggested that early treatment of HCV recurrence with pegylated interferon α-2b and ribavirin slowed disease progression and, in around half of all patients, led to long-term viral clearance. As therapy is less effective for advanced recurrent HCV, particularly in recipients with cholestasis, there appears to be a good case for regular assessment (liver biopsy and hepatic venous portal gradient measurement) of HCV-positive transplant recipients and treatment with antivirals if recurrent disease is detected.

Problems

- Dose adjustments of antiviral therapy were commonly required, and treatment was interrupted in 22% of those with mild disease and 56% of those with severe disease, most often due to disease progression.
- Study design limitations (single centre, relatively small patient numbers, and limited F/U period).

Liver transplant: immunosuppression

> **TMC (Tacrolimus vs Microemulsified Ciclosporin) study:** Tacrolimus vs microemulsified ciclosporin in liver transplantation.
>
> **AUTHORS:** O'Grady J, Burroughs A, Hardy P et al. (with the UK and Republic of Ireland Liver Transplant Study Group).
> **REFERENCE:** Lancet (2002) 360, 1119–25.
> **STUDY DESIGN:** RCT
> **EVIDENCE LEVEL:** 1b

Key message
First RCT to show that outcomes after liver transplantation are better with tacrolimus compared with ciclosporin-based immunosuppression.

Impact
Tacrolimus-based immunosuppression is now the preferred treatment for most adults undergoing liver transplantation in the UK and in most liver transplant centres worldwide.

Aims
Calcineurin inhibitors are the mainstay of immunosuppressive protocols after liver transplantation, with the choice of agent being between tacrolimus and ciclosporin. These agents have the same mode of action, but differ in structure, side effect profile, and potential efficacy. This investigator-led trial compared tacrolimus with ciclosporin-based immunosuppression in adults undergoing liver transplantation.

Methods
Patients: 606 adults at 8 liver transplant centres in the UK and Republic of Ireland.

Inclusion criteria: Undergoing orthotopic liver transplantation:
- Age >18y;
- All indications for liver transplantation;
- First liver transplant (emergency and elective cases).

Exclusion criteria:
- Multi-organ or re-transplantation;
- Auxilliary transplant and incompatible donor blood group.

Groups: Both groups received similar concomitant immunosuppression (steroids and azathioprine) in this open-label, concentration-controlled study:
- Tacrolimus (n=301);
- Ciclosporin (n=305).

Primary endpoint: Cumulative endpoint comprising occurrence (whichever occurred earliest) of death, re-transplantation, or treatment failure for immunological reasons.

Secondary endpoints: Death, re-transplantation, treatment failure, graft rejection (acute or chronic), and change from protocol immunosuppression.

Follow-up: At 1 and 2wk; then at 1, 2, 3, 6, 9, and 12 months.

Results

A+12 months	Tacrolimus n=301	Ciclosporin n=305	p
Primary endpoint			
Death/re-transplantation/treatment failure for immunological reasons	62 (21%)	99 (33%)	0.001
Secondary endpoints			
Death	50 (17%)	72 (24%)	0.04
Re-transplantation	11 (4%)	31 (10%)	ns
Treatment failure (immunological reason)	6 (2%)	12 (4%)	ns

Discussion

This head-to-head comparison of tacrolimus and ciclosporin, with a carefully standardised protocol and involving a large number of patients, showed that tacrolimus gave a better clinical outcome 12 months after transplantation. Tacrolimus was superior for the composite primary endpoint of death, re-transplantation, and treatment failure, as well as for patient and graft survival.

Problems

• Relatively short F/U (1y), although the authors recently reported outcomes at 3y, confirming the early advantage of tacrolimus for the primary endpoint was maintained (*Am J Transplant* (2007) 7, 137–41).
• The trial included all indications for transplantation, but the proportion of patients with hepatitis C cirrhosis (10%) was very low compared to current clinical practice.
• Target trough blood concentrations of the treatment drugs were achieved during the first 6 months (when most primary endpoints occurred), but after 6 months, not all patents on ciclosporin had achieved their target drug concentration range.

Renal transplant: immunosuppression

A blinded, randomised clinical trial of mycophenolate mofetil for the prevention of acute rejection in cadaveric renal transplantation.

AUTHORS: Tricontinental Mycophenolate Mofetil Renal Transplantation Study Group.
REFERENCE: Transplantation (1996) 61, 1029–37.
STUDY DESIGN: RCT
EVIDENCE LEVEL: 1b

Key message
One of the first large randomised trials to show mycophenolate mofetil (MMF) to be associated with a lower rate of treatment failure after renal transplantation when compared to azathioprine (AZA).

Impact
MMF is now the anti-proliferative agent of choice in immunosuppressive regimens at most international renal transplant units.

Aims
Prophylactic immunosuppression after renal transplantation usually includes a calcineurin inhibitor (CNI), steroids, and an anti-proliferative agent, historically AZA. This trial was designed to evaluate AZA replacement (in a ciclosporin-based regimen) with the newer MMF, a more selective inhibitor of lymphocyte proliferation.

Methods
Patients: 503 patients at 21 European, Canadian, and Australian centres.

Inclusion criteria:
- Age >18y;
- First or second cadaveric renal transplant recipients;
- No severe gastrointestinal disorder.

Groups:
- MMF (1.5g bd) (n=164);
- MMF (1g bd) (n=173);
- AZA (100–150mg od, according to body weight) (n=166);

Drugs given according to blinded, double capsule protocol. Analysis of efficacy based on intention-to-treat. All groups received same concomitant immunosuppression (ciclosporin and corticosteroids).

Primary endpoint: Treatment failure within first 6 months (defined as biopsy confirmed graft rejection, graft loss, patient death, or discontinuation of study drug).

Secondary endpoints: Acute rejection not confirmed by histology. Safety analysis.

Follow-up: At 12 months.

Results

	AZA (n=166)	MMF (2g) (n=173)	MMF (3g) (n=164)
Primary endpoint			
Treatment failure	83 (50%)	66 (38%)	57 (35%)
Secondary endpoints			
Graft rejection (biopsy)	59 (36%)	34 (20%)	26 (16%)
Graft rejection (clinical/biopsy)	80 (48%)	55 (32%)	44 (27%)
Graft loss/death	7 (4%)	8 (5%)	6 (4%)

[*] For primary endpoint: AZA vs MMF (2g), $p=0.03$; AZA vs MMF (3g), $p=0.005$; MMF (2g) vs MMF (3g), $p=$ns.

Discussion

This study showed convincingly that substituting AZA with MMF (both 2g and 3g) was associated with reduced treatment failure at 6 months, with the difference remaining significant at 1y. MMF reduced the incidence and severity of acute rejection: the incidence of graft loss and patient death was not different between groups. The drugs were all relatively well tolerated although MMF 3g was associated with a numerically higher rate of gastrointestinal side effects and invasive cytomegalovirus (CMV) infections, leading the authors to suggest that the MMF dose should be adjusted according to clinical need. The finding that MMF reduces the incidence of acute rejection in ciclosporin-based regimens has been confirmed by other studies (*Transplantation* (1997) 63, 39–47—pooled data). The UK's National Institute for Health and Clinical Excellence (NICE) recognised the benefit of MMF in reducing the incidence of acute rejection, but stated that it was unlikely to be cost-effective compared to AZA and therefore, did not recommend it for routine use after renal transplantation. However, they did recommend MMF for cases of intolerance to CNI or a very high risk of nephrotoxicity requiring reduced exposure to CNI.

Problems

- AZA is about 50 times less expensive than MMF, and MMF has not been shown to improve graft survival in this setting.
- MMF was dosed irrespective of body weight or metabolism; concentration-controlled dosing may be more appropriate, but is unproven.
- The ciclosporin formulation used was not the better absorbed microemulsion formulation. This may explain why rejection rates were higher than currently seen.

Renal transplant: chimeric antibodies

Randomised trial of basiliximab vs placebo for control of acute cellular rejection in renal allograft recipients.

AUTHORS: Nashan B, Moore R, Amlot P et al.
REFERENCE: Lancet (1997) 350, 1193–8.
STUDY DESIGN: RCT
EVIDENCE LEVEL: 1b

Key message
First randomised trial to show prophylaxis with a chimeric antibody (basiliximab) directed against the interleukin-2 receptor (IL-2R) prevents acute rejection in recipients of kidney transplants.

Impact
Chimeric (basiliximab) or humanised (daclizumab) monoclonal antibodies to the IL-2R are now widely used as prophylaxis against acute rejection in renal transplant recipients.

Aims
Interleukin-2 (IL-2) induces T cell proliferation and plays a key role in the early immunological response to a kidney allograft. Immunosuppression via chimeric antibodies directed against IL-2R has been indicated in early studies to be well tolerated. This study aimed to determine whether administration of basiliximab at the time of renal transplantation was effective in reducing the incidence of acute allograft rejection.

Methods
Patients: 380 adult renal allograft recipients at 21 European and Canadian centres.

Inclusion criteria:
- First cadaveric renal transplant;
- Not highly sensitised to HLA antigens (<80% panel reactive antibodies);
- At least 1 HLA class I or II mismatch.

Groups:
- A: basiliximab (20mg infusion) (n=193);
- B: placebo (n=187).

Basiliximab/placebo administered on d0 (day of transplant) and 4. Both groups received dual immunosuppression (ciclosporin and steroids).

Primary endpoint: Acute rejection episode during the first 6 months.

Secondary endpoints:
- Histological severity of acute rejection;
- Biopsy proven rejection;
- Steroid-resistant rejection;
- Patient and graft survival;
- Safety and toxicity of basiliximab.

Follow-up: Up to 12 months.

Results *(376 eligible patients, on an intention-to-treat basis)*

	Placebo (n=186)	Basiliximab (n=190)	p
Primary endpoint			
Rejection during first 6 months	52%	34%	<0.001
Secondary endpoints			
Histologically severe rejection	15%	10%	ns
Biopsy-proven rejection	44%	30%	0.012
Steroid resistant rejection	23%	10%	<0.001
Graft survival (at 12 months)	87%	88%	ns
Patient survival (at 12 months)	97%	95%	ns

Discussion

This study demonstrated that basiliximab reduced the incidence of acute rejection following renal transplantation. No significant adverse events associated with the treatment drug were identified, and there was no evidence that infections were more common in patients receiving basiliximab. On the basis of this and similar studies using the humanised IL-2R antibody, daclizumab, IL-2R antibodies are now widely used (in conjunction with ciclosporin or tacrolimus, steroids, and an anti-proliferative agent) as induction therapy for the prevention of acute rejection after renal transplantation.

Problems

• The rate of acute rejection observed in the control group was higher than might now be expected.
• Only recipients considered to be at low to moderate risk of rejection were recruited.
• While IL-2R antibodies reduce the incidence of acute rejection, there is no evidence that they prolong graft survival.

Renal transplant: acute rejection

Efficacy and safety of tacrolimus compared with ciclosporin microemulsion in renal transplantation.

AUTHORS: Margreiter R (European Tacrolimus vs Ciclosporin Microemulsion Renal Transplantation Study Group).
REFERENCE: Lancet (2002) 359, 741–6.
STUDY DESIGN: RCT
EVIDENCE LEVEL: 1b

Key message

Tacrolimus is more effective than ciclosporin for preventing acute rejection after renal transplantation. However, graft survival rates are equivalent and choice of agent may be influenced by the differing side effect profiles.

Impact

Although both tacrolimus and ciclosporin are widely used as primary immunosuppression after kidney transplantation, tacrolimus is now used more frequently by most transplant centres. The UK's National Institute for Health and Clinical Excellence (NICE) guidelines state that the initial choice of calcineurin blocker for an individual should be based on the relative importance of the differing side effect profiles.

Aims

Calcineurin inhibitors (CNI) are the mainstay of immunosuppression for renal transplantation. This open-label trial was designed to determine which of the two primarily available agents (tacrolimus or ciclosporin) was most effective in terms of efficacy and side effects.

Methods

Patients: 560 kidney transplant recipients at 50 European centres.

Inclusion criteria:
- Age 18–60y;
- Primary or subsequent renal transplant (from cadaveric and living donors aged 5–60y).

Exclusions:
- High risk of immunological rejection (>50% panel reactive antibodies);
- Previous non-renal allograft.

Groups: Tacrolimus and ciclosporin both given to achieve target blood concentrations. Both groups received corticosteroids and azathioprine:
- Ciclosporin (n=273);
- Tacrolimus (n=287).

Primary endpoint: First biopsy-proven acute rejection episode within 6 months of transplant and time to first rejection episode.

Secondary endpoints:
• Patient and graft survival;
• Severity of acute rejection, overall rate of rejection (including non-biopsy proven), and rate of steroid resistant rejection;
• Safety and tolerability.

Follow-up: At 6 months.

Results

	Ciclosporin (n=273)	Tacrolimus (n=287)	p
Primary endpoint			
Biopsy-proven rejection	101 (37%)	56 (20%)	<0.0001
Secondary endpoints			
Severe rejection	18 (7%)	4 (1%)	ns
All acute rejection	139 (51%)	93 (33%)	<0.0001
Steroid resistant rejection	57 (21%)	27 (9%)	<0.0001
Recipient survival	267 (99%)	284 (99%)	ns
Graft survival	249 (92%)	271 (95%)	ns

Discussion

These results showed that tacrolimus was more effective than ciclosporin for preventing acute rejection after renal transplantation, however, no difference in graft or patient survival was apparent. For both agents, the drug blood target levels achieved were satisfactory and within the therapeutic target range. The overall frequency of side effects was similar for the two agents. As expected from the well-known side effect profiles, ciclosporin was associated with more cosmetic side effects (hirsutism and gum hyperplasia) whereas tacrolimus produced more neurotoxicity (tremor).

A well-recognised long-term complication of both agents is non-reversible nephrotoxicity, leading to deteriorating graft function. Some success has been achieved by withdrawal of CNI in the post-transplant period. Recent studies (*Am J Transplant* (2005) 5, 2496–503) have found switching patients with suboptimal graft function to sirolimus-based immunosuppression improves GFR, an option recommended by NICE for adults with proven intolerance (including nephrotoxicity) to CNI. Sirolimus is associated with common side effects of its own (such as skin rash and mouth ulcers); however, these usually respond to dose reduction. Optimal timing of this switch is not yet established, and it is unclear whether switching patients with satisfactory renal function is desirable.

Problems

• Potential variability between centres in diagnosing acute rejection and undertaking biopsy, although this would have affected both groups.
• Histological assessment of biopsies was undertaken locally rather than centrally, although all centres used Banff criteria to assess rejection.
• It cannot be assumed that differences in the incidence of acute rejection necessarily translate into reduced graft survival in the longer term.

Renal transplant: surgical approach in donors

> Comparison of laparoscopic and mini-incision, open-donor nephrectomy: single-blind RCT.
>
> **AUTHORS:** Kok N, Lind M, Hansson B *et al.*
> **REFERENCE:** BMJ (2006) 333, 221.
> **STUDY DESIGN:** RCT
> **EVIDENCE LEVEL:** 1b

Key message

Compared to mini-incision open-donor nephrectomy, laparoscopic donor nephrectomy allows faster recovery, produces less physical fatigue, and results in better quality of life.

Impact

This trial confirms the benefits of the laparoscopic approach in minimising donor discomfort and recovery, supporting widespread adaptation of this approach.

Aims

Kidney donation by living donors is increasing, and many centres undertake nephrectomy using a laparoscopic approach rather than by the traditional open flank incision. Laparoscopic nephrectomy had been shown to be safe and effective. This two-centre, prospective, single-blind RCT aimed to determine the best surgical approach (laparoscopic or mini-incision open surgery) for minimising donor fatigue and improving post-operative recovery.

Methods

Patients: 105 living kidney donors at 2 Dutch transplant centres. 5 operations cancelled.

Inclusion/exclusion criteria: Donors were not excluded on the grounds of obesity or multiple renal arteries.

Groups: Randomisation undertaken <12h before surgery:
- Laparoscopic donor nephrectomy (n=50);
- Mini-incision, open-donor nephrectomy (10–12cm muscle splitting incision anterior to 11th rib and a retroperitoneal approach) (n=50).

Right nephrectomy undertaken if both kidneys suitable for transplantation. Post-operatively, all donors received patient controlled analgesia (IV morphine) and were offered paracetamol (1g qds) until discharge.

Blinding: Patients and medical staff blinded during early post-operative period: only the surgical team were aware of the randomisation group. Post-operatively, wounds were covered with a standard dressing.

Primary endpoint: Physical fatigue (assessed by the multidimensional fatigue inventory) at 1, 3, 6, and 12 months short-term.

Secondary endpoints: Physical functioning score (Short Form 36 (SF36)), length of hospital stay, pain, duration of surgery, and graft function/survival.

Follow-up: Up to 1y. Day of discharge determined by the donor.

Results

	Laparoscopic	Open mini-incision	*p*
Primary endpoint			
Mean physical fatigue at 1 month (SD)	8.7 (3.9)	11.1 (4.5)	0.02
Secondary endpoints			
Median total morphine requirement (range)	16mg (0–93)	25mg (1–107)	0.005
Median length of stay (range)	3d (1–6)	4d (2–8)	0.003
Mean physical functioning score at 1 month (range)	80 (19)	70 (17)	0.02
Graft survival at 1y	100%	98%	ns

Discussion

Although laparoscopic nephrectomy appeared safe and efficacious, and had become the standard surgical approach in many transplant centres, there were few prospective RCTs assessing the safety benefits of this technique. This study showed that even when open nephrectomy was modified to reduce morbidity, laparoscopic donor nephrectomy remained superior and was associated with reduced post-operative pain, earlier discharge from hospital, and a better recovery from surgery. The advantages (in terms of reduced physical fatigue and improved physical functioning) were still apparent 1y after surgery.

Problems

- The study did not avoid potential bias caused by attitudes of health care staff after discharge.
- Differences in the incidence of serious adverse events after donor nephrectomy were too infrequent to be detected in a trial of this size.
- Laparoscopic nephrectomy is a technically challenging operation and requires extensive laparoscopic surgery experience. This may limit its universal use.

Combined kidney-pancreas transplantation

Improved survival in patients with insulin-dependent diabetes mellitus and end-stage diabetic nephropathy 10y after combined pancreas and kidney transplantation.

AUTHORS: Tydén G, Bolinder J, Solders G et al.
REFERENCE: Transplantation (1999) 67, 645–8.
STUDY DESIGN: Retrospective, cohort
EVIDENCE LEVEL: 3

Key message
Compared to kidney transplantation alone, successful combined kidney-pancreas transplantation has a beneficial effect on the late complications of diabetes and reduces long-term mortality.

Impact
Combined kidney-pancreas transplantation is the treatment of choice for carefully selected patients with insulin-dependent diabetes mellitus (IDDM) and end-stage kidney disease.

Aims
In patients with IDDM, pancreatic transplantation aims to restore normo-glycaemia, thereby preventing the secondary complications of diabetes. This study aimed to determine whether combined kidney-pancreas transplantation improved the long-term complications of diabetes and reduced mortality.

Methods
Patients: 29 patients at 1 centre in Sweden.

Inclusion criteria:
- Long-standing IDDM;
- End-stage diabetic nephropathy;
- Evaluated and deemed suitable for combined kidney-pancreas transplantation.

Groups:
- 1: Patients with kidney-pancreas transplants whose pancreas graft had survived >2y (n=14);
- 2 (Controls): 15 patients with kidney-pancreas transplants who had lost their pancreas graft through technical complications (n=9) or rejection (n=1) within 1y of transplantation or who had elected for kidney transplantation alone (n=5).

Evaluation:
- Glycated haemoglobin;
- Nerve conduction studies;
- RR-variations in ECG (autonomic function);
- Mortality.

Follow-up: At least annually for 10y after transplantation.

Results

- In contrast to the control group, recipients of kidney-pancreas grafts maintained normal levels of glycated haemoglobin and showed significantly improved nerve conduction and RR-variations after 4 and 8y.
- At 10y, 3/14 patients with kidney-pancreas grafts had died (all from cardiovascular complications) vs 12/15 control patients (10 from cardiovascular complications, 1 from uraemia, and 1 unknown cause).
- The difference in mortality was statistically significant at 6y ($p<0.05$) and remained significant at 10y ($p<0.01$).

Discussion

Patients with IDDM and end-stage diabetic nephropathy are well known to have a very high mortality from cardiovascular disease, irrespective of whether they undergo kidney transplantation. Pancreatic transplantation restores normoglycaemia and might be expected to reduce the cardiovascular complications. This single centre study compared patients with a successful kidney-pancreas transplant with those also accepted for combined transplantation but whose pancreas graft had failed or had not taken place. It showed convincingly that a successful pancreas graft provided protection from death from cardiovascular complications in this high-risk patient group.

Problems

- The main limitation of the study was the small number of patients followed up.
- The patients in this study underwent segmental pancreas transplantation whereas most centres now undertake whole organ transplantation (pancreas plus a segment of duodenum). This is unlikely to have influenced the results.

Pancreatic islet transplantation

International trial of the Edmonton protocol for islet transplantation.

AUTHORS: Shapiro J, Ricordi C, Hering B et al.
REFERENCE: N Engl J Med (2006) 355, 1318–30.
STUDY DESIGN: Prospective, cohort
EVIDENCE LEVEL: 2b

Key message

Islet transplantation may be beneficial in selected patients with type 1 diabetes mellitus (DM) and unstable glycaemic control but rarely results in long-term independence from insulin therapy.

Impact

Interest in transplantation of isolated pancreatic islets as a treatment for patients with type 1 DM and refractory hypoglycaemia increased following early success in Edmonton. This multicentre study confirmed the benefits but also highlighted the limitations of the Edmonton protocol. If long-term independence from insulin treatment is the goal, whole organ pancreas transplantation is currently the better option.

Aims

Despite advances in treatment, a proportion of patients with type 1 DM remain disabled by refractory hypoglycaemia. Islet cell transplantation by the Edmonton protocol (glucocorticoid-free immunosuppressive therapy combined with infusion of fresh islets from ≥2 pancreases from diseased donors) has, in small studies, been shown to achieve high rates of sustainable insulin independence. This international multicentre, phase I/II, single group study aimed to determine the feasibility and reproducibility of the Edmonton protocol for pancreatic islet transplantation in the treatment of patients with type 1 DM and poor glycaemic control.

Methods

Patients: 36 adult patients at 9 international centres (6 in North America and 3 in Europe).

Inclusion criteria:
- Age 18–65y with type 1 DM for >5y;
- Severe hypoglycaemic lability or hypoglycaemic unawareness.

Islet transplantation: Islets isolated from deceased donor pancreases using Liberase and transplanted by percutaneous transhepatic portal embolisation. Patients received 1–3 islet infusions.

Immunosuppression: Comprised daclizumab induction therapy followed by steroid-free maintenance regimen of sirolimus and tacrolimus.

Primary endpoint: Insulin independence (freedom from need for exogenous insulin) with adequate glycaemic control, 1y from final transplant.

Secondary endpoints: Included insulin independence with adequate glycaemic control during F/U, improved glycaemic control, and reduced need for exogenous insulin compared to pre-transplantation.

Follow-up: All except one patient were followed up for 2y. 21 patients were followed for ≥3y after transplantation.

Results

- 16/36 (44%) satisfied the primary endpoint.
- 10/36 (28%) partial graft function and markedly improved glycaemic control.
- 10/36 (28%) complete graft failure.
- Although 21/36 became insulin-independent during F/U, 16/21 (76%) were insulin-dependent again by 2y, and only 5/16 patients who were insulin independent at 1y remained independent at 2y.
- Adverse events associated with transplant procedure included 2 patients who required laparotomy (1 intraperitoneal haemorrhage and 1 bile leak). No reported deaths.

Discussion

This study demonstrated that islet transplantation (according to the Edmonton protocol) in carefully selected patients with type 1 DM resulted in insulin independence, but that this was not sustained over time. However, patients may still benefit from improved glycaemic control. The major downside was the need for long-term immunosuppression.

Problems

- Islet isolation is problematic and requires considerable experience. It is also expensive and wasteful of pancreases. In this study, only 45% of islet isolations undertaken were used for transplantation.
- Many recipients require islets obtained from ≥2 donor pancreases; the availability of donors falls far short of the anticipated demand for islets.
- The side effects from immunosuppressive therapy, including nephrotoxicity, remain problematic.
- Calcineurin inhibitor (CNI) exacerbated renal impairment is a complication.
- Failed islet transplantation results in sensitisation to HLA, which has implications for future islet and kidney transplantation.

CMV infection: antivirals

> **VICTOR study:** Oral valganciclovir is non-inferior to IV ganciclovir for the treatment of cytomegalovirus disease in solid organ transplant recipients.
>
> **AUTHORS:** Asberg A, Humar A, Rollag H et al. (Victor study group).
> **REFERENCE:** Am J Transplant (2007) 7, 2106–13.
> **STUDY DESIGN:** RCT
> **EVIDENCE LEVEL:** 1b

Key message
This large, multicentre, randomised, open-label study provides the best evidence to date that oral valganciclovir is as safe and effective as IV ganciclovir for the treatment of non-life-threatening (mild to moderate) cytomegalovirus (CMV) infection (including tissue-invasive disease) in recipients of sold organ transplants.

Impact
All patients can be given oral valganciclovir, with the advantage that treatment can be continued on an outpatient basis as it does not require intravenous (IV) administration.

Aims
Despite preventative strategies, CMV disease remains a major problem following solid organ transplantation, responsible for considerable morbidity. Although IV ganciclovir is usually an effective treatment, it requires long-term IV access and frequent hospital admission, which is expensive and inconvenient for patients. Oral valganciclovir has been proposed to provide a simpler and more convenient alternative. This open-label, active, drug-controlled, non-inferiority study aimed to determine whether oral valganciclovir (an oral pro-drug of ganciclovir, providing improved bioavailability) was as safe and effective as IV ganciclovir for treating CMV infection.

Methods
Patients: 321 adult recipients of solid organ transplants at 42 international centres. 74%=renal, 7%=liver, and 6%=heart transplantation.

Inclusion criteria: Virological and clinical evidence of CMV disease.

Exclusion criteria: Life-threatening CMV disease (as defined by local investigators).

Groups:
- Valganciclovir (900mg bd) (n=164);
- Ganciclovir (5mg/kg IV bd) (n=157);

Trial drugs were for 21d and doses adjusted according to renal function. After 21d, all patients transferred to valganciclovir (900mg od) for 28d.

Primary endpoint: Successful treatment (defined as eradication of CMV viraemia at d21, i.e. <600 viral copies/mL plasma).

Secondary endpoints:
- Clinical assessment of CMV disease;
- Time to undetectable viraemia (<200 copies/mL);
- Viral load kinetics;
- Safety and tolerability.

Follow-up: At d21 and 49.

Results

	IV Ganciclovir	Valganciclovir	*p*
Primary endpoint			
Viraemia eradication (d21)	48%	45%	ns
Secondary endpoints			
Treatment success (d21)	80%	77%	ns
Treatment success (d49)	84%	85%	ns
Time to viraemia eradication	19d	21d	ns
Viral load half life	10d	12d	ns
Adverse events	64%	70%	ns

- 46% had invasive CMV disease (49% of ganciclovir group; 43% valganciclovir group).

Discussion

Oral valganciclovir was as effective as IV ganciclovir for the treatment of non-threatening (mild to moderate) CMV infection, with no significant differences in outcomes.

Problems

- Treatment was not blinded.
- The trial size was relatively small for a non-inferiority study.
- The majority of patients were kidney transplant recipients, limiting the general applicability of the conclusions for non-renal transplants.
- Overall, the percentage of patients clearing their viraemia (<50%) was less than expected (65%). This raises questions about the optimal length of treatment. Longer-term F/U on CMV recurrence and resistance would be informative.
- The conclusions cannot be extrapolated to include paediatric recipients of organ transplants.

Trauma and orthopaedics

Introduction

The earliest evidence of orthopaedic principles in practice comes from the ancient Egyptian civilisation. Egyptian mummies have been found with splints on broken bones, and wall paintings depicting crutches are known to be 5,000 years old. Hippocrates (the Father of Medicine) wrote extensively on the treatment of fractures and dislocations, with detailed descriptions of reduction and splinting methodology, much of which is still valid today.

The word 'orthopaedics' derives from the Greek for 'straight child', and this reflects the origins of the specialty: addressing deformities in children. It was coined by Nicholas Andry with his text *Orthopaedia* of 1741. The Tree of Andry remains the symbol of orthopaedics throughout the world.

Jean Andre Venel is considered by many to be the father of orthopaedics, having opened the first orthopaedic hospital in 1780. Since then, the specialty has expanded to include trauma, joint disease, deformity correction, tumours, and conditions of the soft tissues of the musculoskeletal system.

The pioneering work of Sir John Charnley in the 1960s developed low friction arthroplasty of the hip, revolutionising the treatment of arthritis to the point where it seems that there are few joints left that cannot be replaced!

The recent advances in biomechanics and biomaterials are resulting in new and improved procedures, often with more reliance on high tech solutions. While such techniques as arthroscopy and arthroplasty have improved over the years, it is only with high quality research that true advances can be demonstrated (and failures averted) at the earliest stage. The principles of orthopaedics must remain to alleviate pain, correct deformity, and restore function, whatever technique is used.

Developmental dysplasia of the hip: ultrasound screening

> Universal or selective screening of the neonatal hip using ultrasound. A prospective, randomised trial of 15,529 newborn infants.
>
> **AUTHORS:** Holen K, Tegnander A, Bredland T *et al.*
> **REFERENCE:** J Bone Joint Surg (2002) 84(B), 886–90.
> **STUDY DESIGN:** RCT
> **EVIDENCE LEVEL:** 1b

Key message

This is the largest randomised trial to show that universal ultrasound (US) screening for neonatal hip dysplasia is unnecessary. It demonstrates the importance of proper screening for high-risk neonates and effective clinical examination of the hips postpartum in reducing cases of late presentation.

Impact

The use of US only for those neonates at high risk of dysplasia or with abnormal clinical examination remains an established and accepted standard.

Aims

This study was designed to assess whether universal screening of all neonates with hip US postpartum conferred a clear advantage over existing systems of only screening those neonates at high risk of having developmental dysplasia of the hip (DDH). The aim was to establish whether the additional time and expense of screening would reduce the rate of late diagnosis of DDH, which was 3 per 1,000 prior to the study.

Methods

Patients: 15,529 neonates at 1 European centre.

Inclusion criteria: All babies born between 1988–92.

Groups:
- Universal screening group: clinically examined on the first day of life and all had hip US on around the third day after birth (n=7840);
- Selective screening group: clinically examined and only those at high risk were examined with US (n=7689).

High-risk: Defined as having hip instability/doubtful stability on examination, family history of hip dysplasia, breech position, or foot deformities.

Clinical examination: Performed by a senior paediatrician and included Ortolani and Barlow tests. Repeated by orthopaedic surgeons at time of US.

Primary endpoint: Late detection, defined as the diagnosis of hip dysplasia, subluxation, or dislocation, in a baby >1 month of age.

Follow up: Range=6–11y. Mean F/U=8.5y.

Results

	Examination and universal US (n = 7840)	Examination and selective US (n = 7689)
Had US	7489 (95.5%)	872 (11.3%)
Late detection of DDH	1 (0.13 per 1000) (due to protocol failure)	5 (0.65 per 1000)
Rate of treatment (with Frejka pillow*)	0.96%	0.86% (ns)

* Abducts and flexes hip

- No significant differences between groups for gender, birth rank, mean birth weight, or risk factors (e.g. breech position, family history, foot deformities, etc.).
- Universal group:
  - Those who did not have US were either premature and transferred to intensive care, or died perinatally.
  - The relative risk of late diagnosis of DDH was 0.21 for the universal group (not statistically different, $p=0.2$).

Discussion

Previous trials had shown similar results, but were not as large or as well designed. This study emphasised the importance of careful attention to the identification of those neonates at risk for DDH, and the need for thorough clinical examination.

Problems

- Although this study had a large number of participants, there were only five positive results in one group and one in the other; this makes type 2 error possible.
- The study showed a dramatic reduction in late DDH presentation in both groups, suggesting that the study protocol itself improved diagnosis rate significantly. Therefore, it could be suggested that the control group (selective screening) was not representative of current screening programme outcomes.

Dynamic hipscrew: tip-apex distance in predicting failure

The value of the tip-apex distance in predicting failure of fixation of peritrochanteric fractures of the hip.

AUTHORS: Baumgaertner M, Curtin S, Lindskog D et al.
REFERENCE: J Bone Joint Surg (Am) (1995) 77, 1058–64.
STUDY DESIGN: Retrospective review
EVIDENCE LEVEL: 3

Key message
First trial to describe the concept of tip-apex distance (TAD). This study shows greatly reduced failure rates with dynamic hip screw fixation using a tip-apex distance of <25mm.

Impact
All dynamic hip screws are now performed with the aim of placing the screw in the centre of the head (in the anteroposterior and lateral planes) and minimising the tip-apex distance.

Aims
The main mechanism of failure in dynamic hip screw fixation of intertro-chanteric hip fractures is so-called 'cutout' of the screw. This is the collapse of the neck-shaft angle into varus with subsequent extrusion of the hip screw, and is related to the position of the hip screw. The authors of this study proposed the TAD, the sum of the distance from the tip of the screw to the apex of the femoral head on an anteroposterior radiograph and the same distance on a lateral radiograph, as a description of the screw position. The aim of this study was to assess the value of the TAD in predicting cutout of the lag screw.

Methods
Patients: 193 patients with 198 dynamic hip screws *in situ* at 1 centre in the USA.

Inclusion criteria: All patients with dynamic hip screw fixation of a peritro-chanteric hip fracture:
- >3 months F/U;
- Either definitive union of the fracture or failure of fixation (which applied to all patients studied).

Groups: Broadly classified into following groups for analysis:
- TAD of ≤24mm;
- TAD of ≥25mm.

Primary endpoint: Screw cutout.

Follow-up: Minimum of 3 months (mean F/U=13 months).

Results

Primary endpoint	TAD <25mm	TAD >25mm	p
Cutout	No occurrence	20.5% of patients	<0.0001

- 0% of screws with a TAD <25mm cutout (n=0/120).
- 2% of screws with a TAD <30mm cutout (n = 3/150).
- 27% of screws with a TAD >30mm cutout (n=13/48).

Cutout:
- Average age of patients 9y older than those with intact fixation (p=0.02);
- More common when unstable fractures were fixed (p=0.03);
- Significantly higher when a 150° side plate was used (p=0.005).

Failure:
- Non-significant trend to failure in hips with a poor reduction of the fracture (p=0.06).

Discussion

Previous trials had shown failure rates for dynamic hip screw fixation of intertrochanteric hip fractures to be as high as 23%. This had been attributed to malposition, with the position having been defined by a complex division of the femoral head into zones. This was the first study to link cutout to a specific measurement. This study showed cutout rates of only 8%, showing the technique to be more reliable than previously thought.

Problems

- This was a retrospective study (studying this phenomenon as a prospective study with deliberate malpositioning would be highly unethical).
- There was only a short F/U period and a high rate of exclusion due to incomplete data collection.

Hip fractures: hemiarthroplasty vs internal fixation

Hemiarthroplasty vs internal fixation for displaced intracapsular hip fractures in the elderly.

AUTHORS: Parker M, Khan R, Crawford J et al.
REFERENCE: J Bone Joint Surg (2002) 84(B), 1150–5.
STUDY DESIGN: RCT
EVIDENCE LEVEL: 1b

Key message

This study provides definitive evidence for the benefits of hemiarthroplasty over internal fixation in patients 70–90y of age, with displaced intracapsular hip fractures.

Impact

Hemiarthroplasty is now confirmed as the operation of choice in displaced, intracapsular hip fractures in all but the most elderly and frail patients. This has greatly reduced the need for revision surgery in this vulnerable group of patients.

Aims

Although previous studies had suggested arthroplasty to be associated with fewer of the later complications noted with internal fixation (such as displacement, non-union, or avascular necrosis), numbers were either small or the trials were not randomised. The study was designed to compare the intra-operative, post-operative, and delayed outcomes of reduction and screw fixation of subcapital hip fractures with those of hemiarthroplasty. With the early post-operative period being associated with complications dependent on blood loss and operative time, these factors were considered for each group. Long-term success was defined by avoidance of the need for further procedures and by survival.

Methods

Patients: 455 patients at 1 UK centre.

Inclusion criteria: All patients with displaced, intracapsular hip fracture:
- Age >70y old;
- Fit for either surgical procedure;
- No rheumatoid arthritis or significant osteoarthritis of the hip;
- No chronic renal failure, Paget's disease of bone, fracture through a tumour, or other metabolic bone disease;
- Surgery within 48h of the fracture, performed by the first author.

Groups:
- Internal fixation: closed reduction and internal fixation with 3 parallel, cancellous screws (n=226);
- Uncemented hemiarthroplasty (n=229).

Primary endpoint: Death.

Secondary endpoints:
- Requirement for further surgical procedure of the hip;
- Deep infection;
- Avascular necrosis of the hip (only applicable to the fixation group);
- Pain and function of the hip;
- Limb shortening.

Follow-up: At 1, 2, and 3y after surgery, with hip scores, residential status, and range of motion noted.

Results

	Internal fixation (n=223)	Hemiarthroplasty (n=223)	*p*
Primary endpoint			
Cumulative survival	0.74	0.73	ns
Secondary endpoints			
Re-operation	90 (56%)	12 (5.4%)	Not stated
Deep infection	No Cases	2.6%	0.03
Avascular necrosis	11 (4.9%)	0	ns

Discussion

Fixation was associated with a shorter intra-operative time and less blood loss, compared with hemiarthroplasty. This did not translate to a difference in mortality. Over one third of the fixation patients had evidence of fracture displacement or non-union at F/U. For patients between 70–90y of age, hemiarthroplasty had clear benefits in terms of fewer complications and lower overall hospital stay (when readmissions for further surgery were considered). The lower complication rates with hemiarthroplasty in this elderly population were in keeping with the results of other studies and meta-analyses.

Problems

- The study F/U period was only up to 3y (although there is continued follow-up of the cohort).
- The outcome of reoperation in the internal fixation group is not described in detail.

Hip arthroplasty: femoral head size and joint wear

The effect of femoral head size on wear of the polyethylene acetabular component.

AUTHORS: Livermore J, Ilstrup D, Morrey B.
REFERENCE: J Bone Joint Surg (Am) (1990) 72, 518–28.
STUDY DESIGN: Prospective, observational study
EVIDENCE LEVEL: 2b

Key message

First clinical trial to reliably establish the relationship between femoral head size and different patterns of wear, in total hip replacement.

Impact

The use of an intermediate femoral head size (28mm) is associated with the best wear characteristics in total hip replacement, and has become the standard for conventional bearings.

Aims

Acetabular component wear is associated with the formation of debris and subsequent activation of macrophages. This leads to bone resorption and failure of the arthroplasty. This study followed patients with three sizes of femoral head (22mm, 28mm, and 32mm) articulating with corresponding acetabular components, to assess the impact of head size on linear wear and volumetric wear.

Methods

Patients: 385 patients at 1 centre in the USA.

Inclusion criteria:
- Primary hip arthroplasty with acetabulum from a single manufacturer;
- Plain radiograph available from just after the arthroplasty and at least 9.5y later.

Groups:
- 22mm head with 22mm internal diameter socket (n=227);
- 28mm head with 28mm internal diameter socket (n=98);
- 32mm head with 32mm internal diameter socket (n=60).

Follow-up: Immediately post-operative and annual radiographs for a minimum of 9.5y. Linear wear and volumetric wear measured on radiographs by a single observer and validated by multiple measurements. Patients' weight was also recorded for correlation with wear.

Results

Head Size	Mean linear wear (mm/y)	Mean volumetric wear (mm³/y)
22mm	0.13	47.4
28mm	0.08	48.4
32mm	0.10	84.1

- 28mm heads had the lowest linear wear ($p<0.001$);
- 32mm heads had the highest volumetric wear ($p<0.001$);
- 22mm heads had the highest linear wear (ns);
- High patient weight increased volumetric wear ($p=<0.05$).

Discussion

These findings validated previous theoretical and laboratory work that suggested lower head diameters increased linear wear and higher diameters increased volumetric wear. The use of a 28mm head also had benefits in terms of increased stability of the hip, when compared with a smaller 22mm head diameter. The study also correlated increased wear with proximal femoral resorption and osteolysis of the proximal femur—important features associated with the failure of hip replacements. Since this study, the use of a 28mm head has quickly become the recommended standard.

Problems

- This was a non-randomised trial. Head size was based upon the surgeons' preferences for individual patients.
- During the study period, 1,964 patients had hip arthroplasty at the unit; the reasons for only including a small number of them are not clear.
- The study does not address the rates of wear in very large head diameters (>32mm) or with alternative bearing surfaces such as metal on metal, ceramic on ceramic/polyethylene, or metal on highly cross-linked polyethylene.

Femoral fracture: timing of surgery

Early vs delayed stabilisation of femoral fractures. A prospective randomised study.

AUTHORS: Bone L, Johnson K, Weigelt J *et al.*
REFERENCE: J Bone Joint Surg (Am) (1989) 71, 336–40.
STUDY DESIGN: RCT
EVIDENCE LEVEL: 1b

Key message

First prospective study to show increased complications with delayed fixation of femoral fractures.

Impact

Early fixation of femoral fractures is now the standard throughout the Western world. Delays beyond 24h are avoided, if at all possible. The use of traction as initial treatment is no longer considered useful, even in multiply injured patients. This has greatly reduced the incidence of adult respiratory distress syndrome (ARDS) in trauma patients.

Aims

Fat embolism syndrome, leading to ARDS, is associated with a high mortality rate. Previous studies had noted lower rates in those fixed early; however, these were very prone to bias. This study aimed to assess whether time of fixation was independently associated with complication rates.

Methods

Patients: 178 patients at 1 centre in the USA.

Inclusion criteria: All cases of femoral shaft fracture:
- Age 16–75y;
- Seen within 24h of injury.

Exclusion criteria: Low-energy trauma and age >65y.

Groups: Injury severity score (ISS) calculated using the Hospital Trauma Index. Randomly assigned to early stabilisation (ES, surgery within 24h) or late stabilisation (LS, initial treatment with traction, then stabilised >48h post-injury). Randomised into:
- ES of isolated fracture femur (ISS <18) (n=42);
- ES and multiple injuries (ISS >18) (n=46);
- LS of isolated femoral fracture (ISS <18) (n=53);
- LS and multiple injuries (ISS >18) (n=37).

All associated injuries were treated as normal. Open fractures were washed out early, then either fixed (ES) or put back onto traction (LS).

Follow-up: Daily arterial blood gas (ABG) measurements until P_aO_2 >75mmHg (on room air).

Results

	n	Mean ISS	Mean hospital stay	Respiratory complications (abnormal ABG)	ARDS	PE/FE
Early isolated	42	11.3	7.3d	5 (4)	0	1/0
Early multiple	46	31.8	17.3d	16 (15)	1	0/0
Late isolated	53	11.5	10.4d	14 (12)	0	2/0
Late multiple	37	31.3	26.6d	50 (33)	6	1/2

ABG= arterial blood gas; PE=pulmonary embolus; FE=fat embolus.

• Other respiratory complications: 7 cases of pneumonia and 2 cases of pulmonary dysfunction.

Discussion

The lack of specific and successful treatments for ARDS results in death in up to 50% of patients; therefore, prevention is a priority. This study was important as it compensated for the non-randomised nature of previous trials, which had been flawed in their methodology (there was a tendency for the less severely injured to have early stabilisation). This study showed an improvement in the respiratory health of those fixed early. This also helped to reduce inpatient stay costs.

Problems

• Unfortunately, there was no statistical analysis to determine the significance of the results.
• This study is now a little dated and showed the results of only one centre with the availability of all trauma services. In practice, it can be difficult to access general, orthopaedic, neurological, and plastic surgery services urgently; this makes it difficult to maintain this standard of approach.

MRI assessment of knee injuries

Effectiveness of MR imaging in selection of patients for arthroscopy of the knee.

AUTHORS: Vincken P, ter Braak B, van Erkell A *et al.*
REFERENCE: Radiology (2002) 223, 739–46.
STUDY DESIGN: Prospective, multicentre, partially randomised
EVIDENCE LEVEL: 2b

Key message

In a general population, a combination of clinical examination and magnetic resonance imaging (MRI) is effective in the selection of patients for arthroscopy, thus reducing unnecessary invasive investigations.

Impact

These findings have increased the evidence base towards supporting non-invasive investigation of knee injuries.

Aims

MRI of the knee has a high degree of sensitivity and specificity for injury to individual intra-articular structures. More relevant to patient management is the correct selection of those patients who require arthroscopy, based on the overall appearance of the knee (composite diagnosis). This study aimed to evaluate MRI in patients with a high clinical suspicion of internal derangements, in order to identify those who required arthroscopic therapy.

Methods

Patients: 430 consecutively referred patients at 3 centres in The Netherlands.

Inclusion criteria:
- Age between 16–45y;
- ≥4wk of pain, swelling, instability, and/or locking of the knee;
- High chance of internal derangement (based on physical examination).

Exclusion criteria:
- Known joint disease, history of locked knee, or previous knee surgery;
- Clinical diagnosis of retropatellar chondromalacia;
- Prior MRI or arthrographic diagnosis or contraindication to either;
- Fracture.

Protocol: All patients underwent MRI within 2wk and were divided into:
- Normal;
- Abnormal but arthroscopic treatment not required;
- Abnormal with arthroscopic treatment required;

Composite diagnosis based on the combination of the degree of individual structure damage. Half of the negative patients (normal and no treatment) underwent arthroscopy and the other half were treated conservatively.

Results

- Patient demographics: mean age=30.6y; 69.5%=male.
- Arthroscopy: indicated in 221 patients (undertaken in 200). Remaining patients randomised as: 105 for arthroscopy (93 undertaken) and 104 for conservative treatment.

Correlation between positive (needed treatment) and negative MRI, and arthroscopy:

		Arthroscopy	
		+	**−**
MRI	+	179	21
	−	13	80

Accuracy for composite diagnosis (needing arthroscopy) and individual injuries:

Injury	Composite diagnosis	Medial meniscus	Lateral meniscus	Anterior cruciate ligament rupture
Sensitivity	87	84	70	70
Specificity	88	94	95	95
PPV	89	90	81	60
NPV	86	91	91	97

Discussion

This paper looked at the usefulness of knee MRI in guiding management rather than detecting structural damage. The higher sensitivity of composite diagnosis was explained by the fact that injuries to more than one individual structure led to a positive MRI result, and that injuries were often not isolated. This helped compensate for the relatively low sensitivity of MRI for individual structures. This study differs to previous ones in that it defines both its patient selection and the need for arthroscopy criteria.

Problems

- Only half the negative group underwent arthroscopy, introducing a verification bias. The authors compensated for this by doubling the figures from this group.
- The radiologist reporting the MRI was not blind to the clinical findings. The authors claimed this represented real practice more closely.

Anterior cruciate ligament reconstruction: choice of graft

A 10y comparison of anterior cruciate ligament reconstructions with hamstring tendon and patellar tendon autograft.

AUTHORS: Pinczewski L, Lyman J, Salmon L et al.
REFERENCE: Am J Sports Med (2007) 35, 564–74.
STUDY DESIGN: RCT
EVIDENCE LEVEL: 1b

Key message

This is the first randomised, prospective study into the 10y results of hamstring tendon and patellar tendon autograft for anterior cruciate ligament (ACL) reconstruction. The use of both autografts is supported, with no clear benefit of using either one over the other.

Impact

The reduction in donor site symptoms in the hamstring tendon donors has led to a trend towards using hamstring graft, but both techniques remain popular. The positive results at 10y support the use of operative techniques to reconstruct the unstable knee.

Aims

There had been no previous prospective studies comparing long-term outcomes of the different types of ACL repair. Large numbers of papers had supported the use of either hamstring tendons or patellar tendon as graft. Previous comparative work had failed to separate the benefits and drawbacks of each technique. This study aimed to compare the functional results, re-rupture rate, and complication rates of the two common methods of ACL reconstruction.

Methods

Patients: 180 patients at 1 centre in Australia.

Inclusion criteria:
• Isolated, unilateral ACL injury;
• Symptomatic instability of the knee.

Exclusion criteria: History of previous cruciate ligament surgery.

Groups: Single surgeon operating on both groups:
• PT group: Bone patellar tendon bone autograft (n=90);
• HT group: Ipsilateral, four-strand hamstring tendon autograft (n=90).

Both groups were entered into a standardised, accelerated rehabilitation programme after surgery.

Results

- Both groups showed normal or near normal knee function in 97% of patients.
- Pain on strenuous activity was more common in the PT group ($p=0.05$).
- Rates of graft rupture were equivalent in each group, with all ruptures associated with graft laxity at 2y after surgery.
- Kneeling pain ($p=0.01$) and harvest site symptoms ($p=0.001$) were more common in the PT group.
- Radiographic evidence of osteoarthritis was more common in the PT group ($p=0.05$).

Discussion

It was possible to get excellent results with hamstring or patellar tendon reconstruction of the ACL. The authors recommended the use of hamstring autograft because of the reduction in donor site morbidity and radiographic signs of osteoarthritis. It may be of significance to avoid the use of patella tendon in patients whose work involves kneeling down. It is of particular note that the hamstring graft group did not suffer noticeable ill effects associated with the loss of strength in deep flexion of the knee, first noted in 1996 (*J Jap Clin Sports Med Assoc* (1996) 6, 681-6), and again shown in the intervening years.

Problems

- The study was not blinded for the outcome measures; this would be very difficult because of the differences in scars in each group.
- This study represented the results of a very experienced surgeon in a specialist centre, and did not include the 'learning curve' for the change to hamstring graft that other surgeons would have to go through.
- Frank osteoarthritis takes many years to develop, and yet longer F/U is required to establish if the increase in radiographic signs of osteoarthritis in the patella tendon group lead to increased risk of painful arthritis.

External fixation of long bones: coated pins

Hydroxyapatite-coated Schanz pins in external fixators used for distraction osteogenesis.

AUTHORS: Pommer A, Muhr G, David A.
REFERENCE: J Bone Joint Surg (Am) (2002) 84, 1162–6.
STUDY DESIGN: RCT
EVIDENCE LEVEL: 1b

Key message
Coating of external fixator pins significantly reduces the rates of loosening and infection. These should be the implants of choice in distraction osteogenesis and for other procedures requiring prolonged fixation.

Impact
Hydroxyapatite (HA)-coated pins are now used in limb reconstruction to improve fixation to bone.

Aims
One of the commonest complications of external stabilisation during limb reconstruction is loosening of the fixator pins. This dramatically increases the chances of infection, which can have devastating consequences. HA had been shown to improve fixation of bone to a variety of other implants in human and animal models. This study aimed to compare the pullout strength, loosening rates, and infection rates of uncoated titanium pins, with HA-coated pins.

Methods
Patients: 46 patients at 1 centre in Germany.

Inclusion criteria: All patients with distraction osteogenesis in the 2y study period.

Groups:
- Control group: AO/ASIF 3.8mm diameter titanium Schanz pins (n=23);
- Experiment group: identically shaped steel pins coated with a 50 micrometer HA layer (n=23).

Primary endpoint: Need to replace external fixator pin.

Secondary endpoints:
- Radiological loosening: presence of a continuous radiolucent line on both sides of the screw on the near cortex;
- Clinical loosening: pain, erythema, warmth, swelling, or discharge at the pin site;
- Pin site infection: assay from secretions swabbed from the pin site;
- Significant infection: acute bone marrow infection;
- Extraction torque at the time of removal.

Results

- Total of 334 pins inserted;
- Average age=39y (±14.1, range 18–61y).

	Uncoated pins (23 patients, 169 pins)	HA-coated pins (23 patients, 165 pins)	p
Primary endpoint			
Pins needing replacing	22	0	<0.001
Secondary endpoints			
Loosening	22	0	<0.001
Pin site infection	20	0	<0.001
Significant infection	1	0	ns
Pullout torque	0.10 N-m	0.43 N-m	<0.001

Key: N-m = Newton meter

Discussion

Earlier trials had attempted to reduce the micromotion of pins in the bone by pre-stressing the pins or using different pin designs; these had not been successful. This study used HA-coated pins (HA was integrated into the cortices around the whole diameter of the pins), allowing for more effective dissipation of all forces, thus reducing the peak force per unit area. The significant differences observed in this study showed that HA-coated pins reduced both morbidity and hospital stay for patients.

Problems

- Limited numbers.
- The control group used titanium pins and the experimental group used stainless steel. These materials have different stiffnesses that could affect the strength of anchoring.
- The pins were not standardised for depth of insertion and contact area with cortical bone.
- The study did not address whether this was a cost-effective improvement.

Fracture stabilisation: type of nails

Reamed or unreamed nailing for closed tibial fractures. A prospective study in Tscherne C1 fractures.

AUTHORS: Court-Brown C, Will E, Christie J *et al.*
REFERENCE: J Bone Joint Surg (1996) 78, 580–3.
STUDY DESIGN: RCT
EVIDENCE LEVEL: 1b

Key message
First RCT to demonstrate the significantly improved fracture union with the use of reamed nails, compared with unreamed nails.

Impact
Reamed intramedullary nailing has become the treatment of choice for closed, lower limb, long bone diaphyseal fractures.

Aims
Intramedullary reaming is associated with damage to the endosteal vascularity of long bones. Previous animal studies had conflicting results, with one showing delayed blood supply return with reamed nail insertion and another showing a 6-fold increase in periosteal blood supply following reaming. This study randomised patients with closed tibial fractures and minimal soft tissue damage (the commonest subtype of tibial fracture) to receive either reamed or unreamed intramedullary nailing, in order to determine the outcomes of either type of nail.

Methods
Patients: 50 patients at 1 UK centre.

Inclusion criteria: Unilateral diaphyseal tibial fracture:
- Skeletally mature;
- Tscherne 1 soft tissue injury pattern.

Groups:
- Grosse–Kempf reamed intramedullary nail (n=25);
- AO UTN, (n=25).

Primary endpoint: Union of fracture.

Secondary endpoints:
- Need for revision surgery (exchange intramedullary nailing);
- Malunion (>5° angular or rotational malalignment, or >1cm of leg length discrepancy);
- Metalwork breakage;
- Return to work.

Follow-up: Radiography and functional assessment at 3, 6, and 12 months.

Results

	Reamed nail	Unreamed nail	p
Primary endpoint			
Mean time to union	15.4wk	22.8wk	<0.01
Secondary endpoints			
Needed reoperation	0	20%	0.05
Malunion	0	16%	ns
Metalwork break	4%	52%	ns
Mean time to return to work	10.9wk	9.3wk	ns

Discussion

The insertion of unreamed nails was slightly quicker and less technically challenging than for reamed nails. However, there was a significant
cost in terms of time to union and need for exchange nailing. Because
of this, the authors recommended that all simple fractures of the tibial
diaphysis be treated with a statically locked, reamed intramedullary nail.
This has subsequently become the gold standard in treating long bone
diaphyseal fractures.

Problems

- There were only 50 patients, making the study prone to type 1 errors.
- The manufacturers of the unreamed nail did not recommend full
  weightbearing in the early post-operative period, but the surgeons
  allowed this, potentially leading to the high rate of metalwork fracture.

Preventing sepsis: ultraclean air theatres

Effect of ultraclean air in operating rooms on deep sepsis in the joint after total hip or knee replacement: a randomised study.

AUTHORS: Lidwell O, Lowbury E, Whyte W et al.
REFERENCE: BMJ (1982) 285, 10–4.
STUDY DESIGN: RCT
EVIDENCE LEVEL: 1b

Key message
First RCT to show a significant reduction in sepsis in total hip and total knee arthroplasties performed in ultraclean air theatres, compared with conventionally ventilated 'plenum' theatres. It also links the use of parenteral antibiotics to a reduction in infection rates.

Impact
Ultraclean air systems are now the standard in joint replacement practice. The British Orthopaedic Association recommends that all joint replacements should be carried out in ultraclean air theatres.

Aims
Deep sepsis is a significant cause of failure in total joint replacement and usually requires two-stage revision surgery to resolve the infection. This study was designed to elucidate the relationship between deep sepsis and theatre design. It sought to relate the numbers of deep infections to bacterial counts in air samples and to further relate the bacterial counts to the use of plenum theatres, ultraclean air theatres, and ultraclean air theatres in which the surgeons wore body exhaust suits.

Methods
Patients: 8136 operations at 15 British and 4 Swedish Orthopaedic units.

Inclusion criteria: Primary hip or knee arthroplasty:
- Control theatres ventilated by a positive pressure air supply (plenum theatre);
- Each surgeon operated in both conventional and ultraclean theatres;
- Air samples taken during the operations in each theatre type.

Groups: Divided in a 2:1:1 ratio (for logistical reasons):
- Plenum theatre (control) (n=4133):
- Ultraclean air theatre with surgeons wearing conventional gowns (n=1789);
- Ultraclean air theatre with surgeons wearing exhaust suits (n=2133).

Primary endpoint: Bacterial infection within the joint associated with clinically apparent tissue damage.

Secondary endpoints: Possible sepsis based on the following criteria:
- Isolation of potentially pathogenic micro-organisms from the joint;
- Raised erythrocyte sedimentation rate (ESR) in patients who had previously normal rates;

- Suggestive histological findings;
- Abnormal X-ray;
- Abnormal pain;
- Fever at the time of repeat operation.

Follow-up: Up to 1y after the last patient had entered the trial in each centre (mean F/U=2–2.5y).

Results

	Conventional	Ultraclean	p
Primary endpoint			
Sepsis or probable sepsis	1.5%	0.6%	<0.001
Secondary endpoint			
Possible sepsis	0.5%	0.5%	ns

	No antibiotics		Antibiotics		p
	Operations (n)	Septic (n)	Operations (n)	Septic (n)	
Control	1,161	39	2,969	24	<0.001
Ultraclean	1,060	13	2,863	10	<0.01

Discussion

Previous trials had demonstrated infection rates in primary hip and knee arthroplasty of up to 10%. This study revealed a 2.6-fold decrease in deep sepsis in patients operated on in ultraclean theatres. This was further broken down into a 2-fold decrease in ultraclean theatres alone and a 4-fold decrease in ultraclean theatres combined with exhaust suits. This supports the theory that airborne bacteria are a significant cause of infection in arthroplasty surgery. The study also revealed a 3-fold reduction in infection rates amongst those patients receiving parenteral antibiotics.

Problems

- There were a multitude of different theatre designs used to obtain appropriate numbers rather than a standard design for one conventional and one ultraclean theatre type.
- The study did not control for the use of parenteral antibiotic prophylaxis or the use of antibiotic laden cement. There was an association found between reduced infection risk and receipt of antibiotics, but this was not randomised, so could not be properly assessed.
- The actual rate of use of exhaust suits remains low because of comfort problems experienced by operating surgeons.

Urology

Introduction

Urology has become a sub-specialty of surgery relatively recently. However, its roots in EBM are deep. The removal of stones from the urinary bladder is an ancient art based upon a single piece of evidence: that pain from the bladder is only cured by removal of the stone. The devices used to remove stones bear testimony to the ingenuity of those who designed and improved them, based upon simple evidence of the newer versions working better. From the early days of ureteric tongs to crush stones, 1824 saw the first successful lithotripsy with the 'trilabium'—a device with three claws to hold a stone, and a drill to fragment it. Such innovations were refined based upon improved clinical outcomes; as rod lenses eventually entered mainstream urological practice, blind stone fragmentation was replaced by safer visual stone identification and removal.

Modern Urology has been at the forefront of EBM. The extracorporeal lithotripter is a prime example of the development of a new technique from laboratory to patient. Evolution through *in vitro* followed by *in vivo* animal and human experiments has led to the development of the newer generations of machines, capable of being used without anaesthesia. These are very different from the prototype HM-3 (human-model-3 machine) that required both an anaesthetised patient and a ready water bath. Evidence-based innovations in Urology are not confined to minimally invasive surgery. Radical prostatectomy is considered a gold standard curative option for early prostate cancer. Doyens, like Patrick Walsh, have refined the technical aspects of this highly complex operation by documenting each step precisely and objectively analysing outcomes. As a result, today's Urologists have the benefit of extensive anatomical knowledge of the pelvis, urinary sphincter, and the neurovascular bundles. The emergence of exciting technological innovations such as laser and robotic surgery continues to attest to the role of evidence-based practice in Urology.

Continuing changes in medical practice are inevitable. With the need to ensure that the patient remains the focal point in the minds of those who bring about such changes, EBM has become the safety net. When appropriately interpreted, the use of evidence will hopefully ensure that these remain changes for the benefit of patients rather than passing changes in fashion.

Acute pyelonephritis: antibiotic treatment

Comparison of ciprofloxacin (7 days) and trimethoprim-sulfamethoxazole (14 days) for acute uncomplicated pyelonephritis in women.

AUTHORS: Talan D, Stamm W, Hooton T *et al.*
REFERENCE: JAMA (2000) 283, 1583–90.
STUDY DESIGN: RCT
EVIDENCE LEVEL: 1b

Key message
When treating acute uncomplicated pyelonephritis in women, 7d of ciprofloxacin produces 91% clinical cure rates at 3–7wk, and achieves higher bacteriological and clinical cure rates than 14d trimethoprim-sulfamethoxazole.

Impact
This study demonstrates the effectiveness of an oral fluoroquinolone for uncomplicated pyelonephritis in women, where the uropathogen is fluoroquinolone-susceptible.

Aims
At the time of this study, the optimum duration of antibiotic therapy for acute uncomplicated pyelonephritis remained unclear, with the choice of appropriate empirical antimicrobial being necessarily dependent on local susceptibility data. This study was designed to compare bacteriological and clinical outcomes in women treated as outpatients for pyelonephritis, with either 7d ciprofloxacin or 14d trimethoprim-sulfamethoxazole.

Methods
Patients: 378 patients (255 fulfilled criteria for analysis of efficacy) at 25 outpatient centres in the USA.

Inclusion criteria:
- Premenopausal women, age >18y;
- Clinical diagnosis of acute uncomplicated pyelonephritis (loin tenderness, pyuria, and oral temperature >38°C);
- Evaluable for efficacy analysis if >10^4 bacterial colony forming units (cfu)/mL in pre-therapy midstream urine (MSU) or >10^3 cfu/mL in catheter sampled urine (CSU) and study antibiotic received for at least 5d (or bacteriological or clinical failure required an alternative antimicrobial).

Exclusion criteria:
- Severe sepsis;
- Diabetes mellitus or other immunocompromise;
- Urological abnormality or severe renal impairment;
- Persistent vomiting or pregnancy;
- Antimicrobial within previous 72h or sulphonamide/fluoroquinolone allergy.

Groups:
- Ciprofloxacin (500mg bd PO for 7d, with or without initial 400mg IV dose), then placebo (for 7d) (n=191; 66 received initial dose IV; 111 evaluable for bacteriological outcome at 22–48d);
- Trimethoprim-sulfamethoxazole (160/800mg bd PO for 14d, with or without initial IV ceftriaxone 1g dose) (n=187; 61 received initial dose IV ceftriaxone; 108 evaluable for bacteriological outcome at 22–48d).

Primary endpoint: Bacteriological and clinical cure rates 4–11d post-treatment.

Secondary endpoints included:
- Bacteriological and clinical cure rates 22–48d post-treatment;
- Adverse drug events assessed by questionnaire.

Follow-up: Between d4–11 and 22–48 post-treatment.

Results

Primary endpoint	7d ciprofloxacin	14d trim-sulf	p
Bacteriological cure	112/113 (99%)	90/101 (89%)	0.004
Clinical cure	109/133 (96%)	92/111 (83%)	0.002
Secondary endpoints			
Bacteriological cure	94/111 (85%)	80/108 (74%)	0.08
Clinical cure	96/106 (91%)	82/106 (77%)	0.02
Adverse drug events	46/191 (24%)	62/187 (33%)	ns

Trim-sulf: trimethoprim-sulfamethoxazole.

Discussion

Escherichia coli was isolated in the pre-treatment urine specimens in >90% subjects in the efficacy evaluated group; overall 18.4% of urinary isolates (n=47) were resistant to trimethoprim-sulfamethoxazole vs 0.4% (n=1) resistant to ciprofloxacin. The superior cure rates in the ciprofloxacin group are likely, in great part, to reflect these resistance rates. The study emphasises the importance of up-to-date susceptibility data for uropathogens in the population in question when determining initial empirical therapy.

Problems

- Trimethoprim-sulfamethoxazole is now not the usually recommended first-line agent for uncomplicated pyelonephritis due to unacceptably high resistance rates and a relatively high incidence of adverse drug events.
- The trial does not reflect clinical practice, in which the antimicrobial agent is changed at the earliest opportunity if indicated by bacteriological susceptibility data.
- Assessment of clinical cure may have been biased by physicians having access to bacteriological culture and susceptibility results.
- The optimal duration of antimicrobial therapy is not answered by this study; it is possible that a longer course of fluoroquinolone may have resulted in greater cure rates at 22–48d.

Vesicoureteral reflux in children: surgical vs medical management

> **IRS (International Reflux Study):** Ten-year results of randomised treatment of children with severe vesicoureteral reflux. Final report of IRS in children.
>
> **AUTHORS:** Jodal U, Smellie J, Lax H et al.
> **REFERENCE:** Pediatr Nephrol (2006) 21, 785–92.
> **STUDY DESIGN:** RCT
> **EVIDENCE LEVEL:** 1b

Key message

Treatment of children with vesicoureteral reflux (VUR) using antimicrobial prophylaxis or surgical reimplantation of the ureter has similar effects on renal scarring and renal growth.

Impact

The management of VUR is controversial, but this study has shown that the differences between various treatment options are not as significant as some suggest.

Aims

Severe VUR presents a difficult management problem in children, with no consensus as to whether medical or surgical management is best. It had been unclear whether the benefits of reimplanting the ureter (and therefore reducing the reflux) were great enough to warrant the risks of surgery, or whether simply preventing or treating urinary tract infections (UTIs) was all that was required to prevent the development of progressive reflux nephropathy. This 10y study aimed to clarify optimal management.

Methods

Patients: 306 patients at 16 centres in the USA and 8 in Europe.

Inclusion criteria: Severe (grade III or IV) VUR:
- Age <11y (infants <1y only eligible if reflux grade IV);
- Normal BP;
- Glomerular filtration rate (GFR) ≥70mL/min per 1.73m^2.

Groups:
- Medical (continuous low-dose co-trimoxazole, trimethoprim or nitrofurantoin) (n=155);
- Surgical (ureteral reimplantation procedure of surgeon's choice) (n=151).

Primary endpoint: Development of new renal scars and impairment of renal growth.

Secondary endpoints:
- Recurrence of UTI;
- Renal function (measured by EDTA clearance);

- New hypertension;
- Somatic growth.

Follow-up: Voiding cystourethrogram at 6, 18, 30, 42, and 54 months, and at 6, 8, and 10y. Intravenous urogram (IVU) and dimercaptosuccinic acid (DMSA) study done at 6, 18, 54 months, and 10y.

Results

- 252 children completed 10y F/U.

Primary endpoint	Surgical (n=127)	Medical (n=125)	p
New renal scarring	22	20	ns
Secondary endpoints			
UTI	50	48	ns
Febrile UTI	17	32	<0.03
Renal function GFR(9SD)	115 mL/min (±27)	119 mL/min (±16)	ns

Discussion

This trial demonstrated comparable results with either strategy. However, all the children in this trial had well preserved renal function, in contrast with other studies of children with more advanced kidney disease (in which outcomes such as new hypertension and end-stage kidney disease are more common). Extended F/U to detect any difference in adult chronic kidney disease (and subsequent requirement for renal replacement therapy) would be desirable, but is not planned.

Problems

- Minimally invasive endoscopic injection procedures are now available to treat VUR; this study does not help decide when they should be used.
- Unsatisfying surgical results were reported in 17%, which is higher than most series in the literature (94–99% success rate).
- There is little evidence to suggest that continuous low-dose antimicrobial prophylaxis is any better than placebo at preventing scarring, so this might not be an appropriate control group.

Renal cell cancer: laparoscopic nephrectomy

> Laparoscopic nephrectomy for renal cell cancer: evaluation of efficacy and safety: a multicentre experience.
>
> **AUTHORS:** Cadeddu J, Ono Y, Clayman R et al.
> **REFERENCE:** Urology (1998) 52, 773–7.
> **STUDY DESIGN:** Retrospective, cohort
> **EVIDENCE LEVEL:** 3

Key message

Laparoscopic surgery is safe and feasible for localised renal cell cancers, and is not associated with an increased risk of port site or retroperitoneal recurrence. 5y mortality comparable to open surgery.

Impact

This, and other studies have led to a greater acceptance of laparoscopic surgery for renal cancers. Laparoscopy is now the first-line approach.

Aims

Treatment of renal cell carcinoma (RCC) depends upon clinical stage and grade. Radical nephrectomy had formerly been the first-line procedure for resectable localised tumours. However, subsequent studies had concluded laparoscopy nephrectomy to be a safer and minimally invasive procedure for the treatment of RCC. This study aimed to evaluate the long-term outcomes of radical laparoscopic nephrectomy.

Methods

Patients: 157 patients, retrospectively identified from 5 international centres: USA (2), Canada (1), Japan (1), and Australia (1).

Inclusion criteria: Patients that had undergone radical laparoscopic nephrectomy for clinically localised, pathologically confirmed RCC (between 1991–7), $T_{1-2} N_0 M_0$.

Identifiable outcomes: Morbidity, disease-free status, and cancer-specific survival.

Follow-up: All patients had F/U physical examination and CXR; 75% had CT scans. 25 patients who did not have CT scans were from Canada where the standard protocol did not include a CT assessment. Mean F/U=19.2 months (range 1–72 months). 51 patients had F/U ≥2y.

Results

- Age: Mean age at surgery=61y (range 27–92).
- Surgical approach: 139 transperitoneal and 18 retroperitoneal. 6 (3.8%) converted to open procedures (laparotomy).
- Complications: In 15 patients (9.6%). Included ileus (4), UTI (2), pulmonary embolus (2).
- Mortality: No cancer-specific mortalities at F/U.

- Recurrence: No laparoscopic port site or renal fossa recurrences. 4 patients developed metastatic disease and 1 developed local recurrence.
- Survival: 5y actuarial survival=91% (94.8).

Discussion

Other studies have shown laparoscopic radical nephrectomy to be associated with shorter inpatient stay, less post-operative pain, and a quicker return to normal activity (*J Urol* (1996) 155, 1180–5). The main aim of this study was to exclude an increased risk of local and port site recurrences associated with laparoscopy. No cases were reported. Methods to prevent recurrence include the use of an endoscopic bag, ensuring sufficient excision margins and morcellating the kidney within a bag. In addition, 5y survival rates were comparable to open surgery, which range between 60–93% for localised disease.

Problems

- A retrospective study; with more clearly defined risks and benefits for laparoscopic surgery, an RCT comparison with open surgery would be neither warranted or justifiable. This study is an example of much of 'surgical technique' literature, which, by its inherent nature, and reliance upon individual operator skill, is difficult to assess in higher-level studies.
- Long-term F/U is necessary to determine and compare 10y survival rates with open surgery.
- 25 patients did not receive F/U CT scans. This may have led to an underestimation of recurrences.

Renal cell cancer: anti-angiogenic therapy

Sunitinib vs interferon alpha in metastatic renal cell carcinoma.

AUTHORS: Motzer R, Hutson T, Tomczak P *et al.*
REFERENCE: N Engl J Med (2007) 356, 115–24.
STUDY DESIGN: RCT
EVIDENCE LEVEL: 1b

Key message

Sunitinib has higher response rates and longer progression-free survival than interferon-alpha (IFN-α) in patients with metastatic renal cell carcinoma (RCC).

Impact

This study is still ongoing, although promising results so far are leading to a increased use of sunitinib.

Aims

RCC is highly resistant to chemotherapy, and cytokines such as interleukin-2 (IL-2) or (IFN-α) are often used as first-line treatment. Higher dose IL-2 had been shown to confer survival advantage over lower dose regimens (e.g. *J Clin Oncol* (2003) 21, 3127–32), however, overall response rates remained poor (<20%). The anti-angiogenic agent, sunitinib, an inhibitor of the tyrosine kinases thought to be upregulated in clear cell carcinoma (including vascular endothelial and platelet-derived growth factors) had shown promising results (*JAMA* (2006) 295, 2516–24). This phase III study aimed to compare outcomes of sunitinib with IFN-α in the treatment of RCC.

Methods

Patients: 750 patients at 101 international centres.

Inclusion criteria:
- Age ≥18y with untreated metastatic clear cell type RCC;
- Eastern Cooperative Oncology Group (ECOG): performance status 0/1.

Exclusion criteria:
- Comorbidities: significant coronary artery disease (past 1y); uncontrolled hypertension, hepatic/renal/haematological impairment;
- Brain metastases;
- Previous systemic therapy for RCC.

Groups: Doses reduced if adverse events. Randomisation stratified by lactate dehydrogenase (LDH) levels, performance status, and previous nephrectomy.
- Sunitinib (50mg od PO for 4wk, followed by a 2wk break) (n=375);
- IFN-α (3–9MU SC 3x/wk) (n=375).

Primary endpoint: Progression-free survival.

Secondary endpoints: Objective response rate, overall survival, patient-reported outcomes and safety.

Follow-up: Imaging assessment (at baseline, d28 of cycles 1–4, and then every two cycles until treatment end). Images reviewed by blinded third party. Quality of life (QoL)/adverse event assessments (at baseline; d1 and d28 of each cycle; treatment end). Regular examinations and laboratory investigations. Median F/U=6 months (sunitinib) and 4 months (IFN-α).

Results

	Sunitinib (n=375)	IFN-α (n=360)	p
Median treatment duration	6 months (1–15)	4 months (1–13)	–
Discontinued treatment (total)	127 (34%)	234 (62%)	Significant (p not stated)
Discont. (adverse events)	30 (8%)	47 (13%)	0.05
Discont. (disease progression)	92 (25%)	170 (45%)	<0.001
Discont. (withdrew consent)	5 (1%)	17 (8%)	<0.001
Adverse events requiring dose interruption/reduction	38%/32%	32%/21%	ns
Objective response rate	103/335 (31%) 95% CI 26 to 36	20/327 (6%) 95% CI 4 to 9	<0.001
Median progression-free survival	11 months (95% CI 10 to 12)	5 months (95% CI 4 to 6)	<0.001
Death	13%	17%	0.02 (HR=0.65)
Ongoing treatment at study end	248 (66%)	126 (34%)	Significant (p not stated)

- Baseline: Comparable demographic/disease characteristics.
- Crossover: After interim analysis, patients in the IFN-α group with progressive disease crossed over into the sunitinib arm.
- Side effects: Significantly higher in sunitinib group (despite lower discontinuation rates): diarrhoea, hypertension, vomiting, hand foot syndrome, and haematological (leukopaenia, neutropaenia, thrombocytopaenia) ($p<0.05$). IFN-α group=more grade 3/4 fatigue ($p=0.05$, ns).
- QoL: significantly better scores in sunitinib group ($p<0.001$).

Discussion

Previous studies had reported objective response rates of about 42% when sunitinib was given to patients failing cytokine therapy (IFN-α/IL-2). This was the second interim analysis of an ongoing study, with promising initial results of longer progression-free survival and response rates to sunitinib.

Problems

- Early results are promising, but more long-term data is required.
- Study sponsored by Pfizer, but blinded and independently reviewed.

Renal colic: imaging

Diagnosis of acute flank pain: value of unenhanced helical CT.

AUTHORS: Smith R, Verga M, McCarthy S *et al.*
REFERENCE: Am J Roentgenol (1996) 166, 97–101.
STUDY DESIGN: Prospective, cohort
EVIDENCE LEVEL: 2b

Key message
Unenhanced spiral computed tomography (CT) has a high sensitivity and specificity in providing rapid diagnosis of renal colic.

Impact
The usefulness of CT as an adjunct for stone diagnosis is undisputed, particularly in patients with renal impairment, indeterminate cases, and for suspected pathologies other than stones. However its use as the primary investigation for renal colic is still debated. Some centres now use CT as their first-line investigation.

Aims
Intravenous urography (IVU) had been the gold standard for investigating renal colic pain and urinary tract calculi since its introduction in the 1920s. The previous assumption that 90% of urinary tract calculi were radio-opaque on plan X-ray, was refuted by studies comparing helical CT with radiography, which reduced this figure to about 50%. Initial pilot studies by the same team had suggested unenhanced spiral CT to have the advantage of increased speed and lack of need for contrast. With a number of conditions presenting with similar symptoms and leading to diagnostic uncertainty, this study aimed to evaluate the diagnostic abilities of unenhanced helical CT in the assessment of patients with acute flank pain and uncertain clinical diagnosis.

Methods
Patients: 210 patients (98 men, 112 women) at 1 centre in the USA.

Inclusion criteria: Patients between 18–85y of age with acute flank pain referred for imaging evaluation.

Protocol: All patients underwent an unenhanced CT. Scans were reviewed blindly and jointly by two investigations. Ureteric stone disease considered if a calcified density was identified within the ureteric lumen, at the anatomic location of the ureterovesical junction, or within the bladder, *or* if there was ureteral dilatation and standing of the perinephric fat on the symptomatic side without a stone being evident.

Follow-up: Recruitment over 18 months.

Results
- Ureteral stones:
  - In 99 patients, CT scans showed urolithiasis. Of these, 57 had confirmatory imaging studies (16 excretory urography; 16 retrograde pyelography or nephrostography; 16 serial plain

radiography or evidence of stone passage; 4 ultrasonography; 2 contrast-enhanced CT; 2 F/U unenhanced CT; 1 F/U enhanced CT);
- 25 of 29 patients without confirmatory imaging studies recovered stones from urine. Small (2–3mm scans) stones were retrospectively identified on CT from the remaining 4 (symptoms resolved);
- 5 patients had stones that showed unilateral ureteral dilatation (all 5 recovered stones from the urine).

Comparison of actual to CT diagnosis:

Actual diagnosis	CT diagnosis		
	Stone +ve	Stone –ve	Total
Stone +ve	100	3	103
Stone –ve	4	103	107
Total	104	106	–

- Unenhanced CT:
  - Negative predictive value=97%; positive predictive value=96%.
  - Sensitivity=97%; specificity=96%; accuracy=97%.

Discussion

Unenhanced CT provided accurate detection of stones in patients with acute flank pain. CT was also able to diagnose a range of other conditions, including appendicitis, diverticulitis, and ovarian pathology. An advantage of CT was its speed; the entire examination could be completed in about 5min. Furthermore, the lack of need for contrast agents avoided the potential complications of contrast allergy and nephropathy. Other studies have since confirmed that an unenhanced CT provides enhanced detection of radiolucent stones compared to an IVU and can also detect alternative pathologies in patients with pain not caused by urolithiasis (*B J Urol Int* (2000) 85, 632–6). Radiation dose has been reported to be about three times higher with CT, with the literature quoting the additional lifetime risk of developing radiation-induced cancer from CT as 1 in 4000 vs 1 in 43,000 for IVU. However, some authors consider the risk of increased radiation can be somewhat balanced by that of fatal anaphylactic reactions to low osmolality contrast media (*LOCM, BM J Roentgool* (1991) 156, 825–32). LOCM is used in the UK for IVU and carries a risk of death of 1 in 111,000.

Problems

- Limited information specified about the inclusion criteria.
- This study did not consider the various practical issues associated with CT use, such as metal implants (that can limit views), availability of a CT scanner and a radiologist, and the types of CT scanners available in the UK. Furthermore, CT provides no detail regarding functional drainage or urothelial abnormalities. A CT scan is potentially more expensive, and is variably available outside the 9–5 working day, particularly in smaller centres, with possible diagnostic delays due to a lack of prompt reporting capabilities.

Ureteroscopy for upper urinary tract calculi

Management of upper urinary tract calculi with ureteroscopic techniques.

AUTHORS: Tawfiek E and Bagley D.
REFERENCE: Urology (1999) 53, 25–31.
STUDY DESIGN: Prospective, cohort
EVIDENCE LEVEL: 2b

Key message

In experienced hands, ureteroscopy and laser lithotripsy are safe and reliable methods for the management of ureteric and intrarenal calculi.

Impact

Application of ureterorenoscopy and laser has become the norm for the management of such cases.

Aims

Flexible ureteroscopy had been reported to provide improved access over rigid scopes for the treatment of upper ureteric and renal calculi. This study aimed to review outcomes in patients with ureteric and renal calculi treated by fibreoptic ureteroscopy and laser/electrohydraulic energy-techniques that, alongside extracorporeal shock wave lithotripsy (ESWL), have virtually replaced open surgery. Patients failing ESWL, having impacted or large stones, or distal obstruction, require treatment with ureteroscopic techniques. This study aimed to assess stone clearance and upper tract function during F/U.

Methods

Patients: 155 patients (73 male, 82 female) at 1 centre in the USA.

Inclusion criteria: All patients with ureteric or renal (upper urinary tract) calculi.

Techniques: All endoscopic manipulations were retrograde with the help of semi-rigid or fibreoptic ureteroscopes. Holmium YAG laser was used in 92.6% (n=113) of cases. Electrohydraulic lithotripsy was used in the remainder.

Follow-up: 1995 to 1997. Pre-operative clinical evaluation with imaging kidney, ureter, and bladder (KUB) X-ray, intravenous urogram (IVU) ± ultrasound (US) scan. 3 months F/U to assess stone clearance and upper tract function.

Results

- Mean age=49y (range 14–88).
- Site: Calculi=renal (n=59) and ureteric (n=82) (29 proximal, 19 mid and 34 distal ureter).

- Size: Stone size ranged from 3–40 mm. 78.7% (n=122) were 3–10mm. 56.8% (n=88) of the patients had single stones, 43.2% (n=67) had multiple calculi.
- Clearance: All patients with ureteric calculi were cleared of stones, regardless of location, with a single procedure. The success rate for clearance of renal stones (less than 3mm fragment) was 87.6%. 21% (n=33) stones retrieved intact; 79% (n=122) required lithotripsy.
- Operating time: Median 90min (range 20–240).
- Complications: Nil from ureteroscopy and no recurrent strictures at 3 months.

Site of stone	Stone-free at 3 months
Renal	64/73 (87.6%)
Lower pole	20/23 (87%)
Calyceal diverticula	4/5 (80%)
Proximal ureter	28/29 (96.5%)
Mid-ureter	19/19 (100%)
Distal ureter	34/34 (100%)

Discussion

This was the first large-scale study to demonstrate a high success rate with this technique in clearing upper urinary tract calculi. Stone fragmentation and subsequent clearance of renal calculi was also demonstrated as satisfactory. Therefore, laser fragmentation is a reliable, safe, and effective method of treatment for calculi in the upper ureter and the renal pelvis.

Problems

- Cohort study, and this technique was not compared with any other endoscopic method of stone fragmentation. Consequently, this limits the ability to determine the relative statistical significance of the results.

Stress urinary incontinence: tension-free vaginal tape

A multicentre study of tension-free vaginal tape (TVT) for surgical treatment of stress urinary incontinence.

AUTHORS: Ulmsten U, Falconer C, Johnson P *et al.*
REFERENCE: Int Urogynaecol J (1998) 9, 210–3.
STUDY DESIGN: Prospective, open, cohort
EVIDENCE LEVEL: 2b

Key message
First prospective RCT to show tension-free vaginal tape (TVT) insertion to be a safe and effective surgical procedure for the treatment of stress urinary incontinence.

Impact
TVT has become a standard procedure for the management of these patients.

Aims
Some studies have reported urinary continence rates in women to be as high as 52%. Stress incontinence is thought to be due to laxity of the vagina or its supporting ligaments. Colposuspension (surgically elevating the bladder neck) was a commonly used treatment, with 1y cure rates of up to 95%. TVT is a form of low-tension urethropexy, involving the use of a plastic sheath-covered polypropylene mesh. Early studies had proposed TVT sling insertion to be a quick and simple procedure for the treatment of stress urinary incontinence. This multicentre study aimed to further assess the safety and efficacy of this procedure.

Methods
Patients: 131 women at 6 centres in Scandanavia.

Inclusion criteria:
- Demonstrable genuine stress urinary incontinence (at least grade II on Ingelman–Sundberg scale);
- Symptoms for several years (mean=3y);
- No previous surgery for incontinence;
- Included irrespective of high or low urethral pressure.

Follow-up:
- At 2, 6, and 12 months. Post-operative F/U was standardised and included urodynamic assessment whenever possible;
- '*Significant improvement*' defined by negative stress test (repeated cough provocation with a filled bladder), >90% improvement in modified quality of life (QoL) assessment, >75% improvement in visual analogue score, and <10g leakage on 24h pad test;
- '*Cure*' defined as no post-operative urine leakage;

- All procedures performed using standardised technique, under local anaesthesia, with plastic sheath covered with prolene/ethicon TVT. 90% day cases.

Results

Baseline:
- Mean age=53y (35–88); mean parity=2(0–5).
- No women showed signs/symptoms of prolapse.
- All postmenopausal women were on systemic or local therapy.
- Mean operating time: 28min (range 19–41).
- Cure: 119 patients (91%; pad testing confirming 90% continence).
- Significant improvement: 9 patients (7%). Remainder did not have full bladder control, but did demonstrate reduced leakage.
- Complications: 1x bladder perforation, 1x wound infection, 3x acute urinary retention requiring short-term catheterisation, and 1x retro-pubic haematoma (spontaneously resolved). No tape rejection.

Discussion

This multicentre study confirmed the safety and efficacy of TVT as a minimally invasive surgical treatment method for stress urinary incontinence. It also confirmed that the procedure could be performed safely as a day case under local anaesthesia, with low complication rate even with less experienced operators.

Problems

- Short F/U period, although the authors' earlier data had suggested high 'cure' rates at 3y. Definitive long-term outcome data is required.
- The aim of this study was to determine safety and efficacy rather than to compare TVT with other surgical techniques; therefore, more comparative data with other techniques is needed (e.g. with Burch colposuspension).

Bladder cancer: neoadjuvant chemotherapy

> Neoadjuvant chemotherapy plus cystectomy compared with cystectomy alone for locally advanced bladder cancer.
>
> **AUTHORS:** Grossmaan B, Natale R, Tangen C *et al.*
> **REFERENCE:** N Engl J Med (2003) 349, 859–66.
> **STUDY DESIGN:** RCT
> **EVIDENCE LEVEL:** 1b

Key message
Neoadjuvant chemotherapy reduces the likelihood of residual disease, correspondingly improving survival.

Impact
As a result of this study, Urologists and Oncologists are increasingly using neoadjuvant chemotherapy in appropriate patients with locally advanced disease.

Aims
Patients with locally advanced bladder cancer have a high risk of tumour recurrence and metastases despite radical cystectomy, consequently leading to a poor prognosis. Previous studies had shown no improvement in survival from pre-operative radiotherapy; however, high rates of response had been noted from chemotherapy. This phase III study was designed to evaluate the impact of neoadjuvant chemotherapy in addition to cystectomy.

Methods
Patients: 317 patients at 126 centres in the USA.

Inclusion criteria:
- Patients suitable for radical cystectomy;
- Muscle invasive ($T_2 N_0 M0$ to $T_{4a} N_0 M_0$) transitional cell carcinoma;
- Adequate renal, hepatic, and haematological function;
- Southwest Oncology Group (SWOG) performance criteria 0–1.

Exclusion criteria: Previous pelvic irradiation.

Groups: Divided by age (>65 vs <65y) and stage (superficial muscle invasion vs more extensive disease):
- Cystectomy alone (n=154);
- Combination chemotherapy (3x 28d cycles) prior to cystectomy (n=153).

Chemotherapy regime: M-VAC (methotrexate, vinblastine, doxorubicin, cisplatin).

Primary endpoint: Survival after cystectomy.

Secondary endpoints: To quantify the effect of neoadjuvant M-VAC chemotherapy on tumour downstaging.

Follow-up: Mean F/U=8.7y (combination), 8.4y (cystectomy).

Results

	Cystectomy alone (n=154)	Cystectomy and neoadjuvant chemotherapy (n=153)	p
Median survival (all)	46 months	77 months	0.05
Median survival (<65y)	67 months	104 months	0.05
Median survival (≥65y)	30 months	61 months	
Median survival (T2)	75 months	105 months	0.05
Median survival (T3/T4a)	24 months	65 months	
No residual disease seen at cystectomy	15%	38%	<0.001
Bladder cancer deaths	n=77	n=54	0.002
5y overall survival	43%	57%	0.06

Discussion

Neoadjuvant chemotherapy prior to cystectomy improved survival in locally advanced bladder cancer. Combination chemotherapy appeared to confer an advantage over single agent therapy in these carefully selected patients and did not appear to increase surgical complication rates. A more recent study (*B J Urol Int* (2006) 97, 42–7) has also suggested benefit for adjuvant cisplatin-based regimens, with significant improvement in progression-free and overall survival.

Problems

- Only 87% patients in the chemotherapy arm received one complete chemotherapy course, with 33% having life-threatening granulocytopaenia and 72% experiencing side effects defined as moderate to severe. Therefore, survival advantages need to be balanced against the toxicity of treatment and delay in cystectomy in the cohort who fail to respond (studies have shown fewer patients receive adjuvant chemotherapy, compared with neoadjuvant).
- Other large trials have not shown such positive results, although differing chemotherapy regimes have been used, with some also combined with radiotherapy.

Benign prostatic hyperplasia: medical treatment

MTOPS (**M**edical **T**herapy **O**f **P**rostatic **S**ymptoms): The long-term effect of doxazosin, finasteride and combination therapy on the clinical progression of benign prostatic hyperplasia.

AUTHORS: McConnell J, Roehrborn C, Bautista O et al.
REFERENCE: N Engl J Med (2003) 349, 2387–98.
STUDY DESIGN: RCT
EVIDENCE LEVEL: 1b

Key message
A combination of doxazosin and finasteride is better than either drug alone in preventing the progression of obstructive (lower tract) urinary symptoms in benign prostatic hyperplasia (BPH).

Impact
Combination therapy has become part of the first-line treatment protocol for BPH, especially for prostate volumes >40mL.

Aims
Previous studies had shown the effectiveness of α-blockers and finasteride in relieving the lower urinary tract symptoms (LUTS) of BPH, with no benefits seen from combined treatment. As BPH is progressive, this study aimed to determine whether doxazosin and finasteride, either alone or in combination, could also delay or prevent BPH clinical disease progression.

Methods
Patients and groups: 3047 men (116 for a pilot study, 2931 for the full study) at 17 centres in the USA.

Inclusion criteria:
- Age >50y, with no prior medical/surgical treatment;
- American Urological Association (AUA) symptom score: 8–30;
- Max. urinary flow rate (Qmax): 4–15mL/s and voided volume >125mL.

Exclusion criteria:
- Prostate Specific Antigen (PSA) >10ng/mL;
- Supine BP <90/70mmHg.

Groups:
- Placebo (n=737);
- Doxazosin (n=756);
- Finasteride (n=768);
- Combination therapy (n=786).

Primary endpoints:
- Overall clinical disease progression;
- Increase in AUA score >4 (commonest recorded);
- Acute urinary retention (AUR);
- Renal insufficiency (secondary BPH): creatinine increase >50% baseline;
- Recurrent urinary tract infections (>2/y) or hygienically unacceptable incontinence.

Secondary endpoints:
• Changes over time in AUA score, Qmax, PSA, and prostate volume;
• Need for surgical intervention (e.g. TURP, laser, open prostatectomy).

Follow-up: Recruitment from 1993–1998. Mean F/U=4.5y.

Results

	Primary outcome events	NNT	NNT (PSA >4.0ng/mL) [20% men]	NNT (prostate vol. >40mL) [30% men]	RR of developing increase in AUA>4
Placebo	128	–	–	–	–
Doxazosin	85	13.7	–	–	45% decrease (p<0.001)
Finasteride	89	15.0	7.2	7.2	30% decrease (p=0.02)
Combination	49	8.4	4.7	4.9	64% decrease (p<0.001)

NNT=number needed to treat to prevent one instance of disease progression.

• AUR events: 18 (placebo) vs 6 (finasteride, p=0.009) and 4 (combination, p<0.001). Doxazosin delayed time to AUR, but did not decrease incidence (p<0.2).
• Need for invasive treatment: Finasteride and combination decreased need by 64%. No change with doxazosin.
• Symptom score: 4y mean decrease in score=4.9 (placebo) vs 6.6 (doxazosin, p<0.001), 5.6 (finasteride, p<0.001) and 7.4 (combination, p<0.001).
• Median prostate volume change: 24% decrease (placebo and doxazosin), 19% decrease (finasteride and combination).
• Major side effects: Doxazosin (dizziness, postural hypotension, asthenia), finasteride (erectile dysfunction, decreased libido, abnormal ejaculation).
• Clinical progression: Compared with placebo, doxazosin decreased risk by 39% (p<0.001), finasteride by 34% (p=0.002) and combination by 66% (p<0.001).

Discussion

Although both drugs alone showed a significant decrease in clinical progression, combination treatment was significantly better than monotherapy in reducing the incidence of AUR and need for invasive treatments.

Problems

• Large numbers discontinued, primarily due to adverse side effects: 18% (combination), 24% (doxazosin) and 27% (finasteride).
• Breast cancer diagnosed in four men using finasteride/combination treatment; this is a higher figure than reported by other trials (e.g. PCPT).
• Two previous 1y trials had shown no benefit of combination over monotherapy (Veterans Affairs (*N Engl J Med* (1996) 335, 533–9); PREDICT (*Curr Urol Rep* (2003) 4, 267–8)). Difference likely to be due to consideration of larger prostate volumes.

Benign prostatic hyperplasia: surgical treatment

Photo selective vaporisation (PVP) vs transurethral resection of the prostate (TURP): a prospective bi-centre study of peri-operative morbidity and early functional outcome.

AUTHORS: Bachmann A, Schurch L, Ruszat R *et al.*
REFERENCE: Eur Urol (2005) 48, 965–71.
STUDY DESIGN: Prospective, non-randomised, controlled
EVIDENCE LEVEL: 2b

Key message

PVP is a safe alternative to TURP, with comparable outcomes at 6 months.

Impact

PVP is increasingly being used as an alternative to TURP in patients requiring surgical intervention.

Aims

TURP has been the gold standard surgical treatment for the management of the lower urinary tract symptoms (LUTS) of benign prostatic hyperplasia (BPH). TURP is not without morbidity and less invasive techniques such as PVP had been proposed. The PVP laser is designed to be maximally absorbed by only the superficial tissue layers, potentially leading to less damage of structures. This study aimed to compare the early outcomes of PVP with TURP.

Methods

Patients: 101 patients at 2 centres in Switzerland.

Inclusion criteria:
- Patients with BPH, associated LUTS and max. flow rate (Qmax) <15mL/s;
- Transvesically measured post-void residual (Vres) >100mL and <400mL;
- International Prostate Symptom Score (IPSS) >7.

Exclusion criteria:
- Symptomatic response to α-blockers (mild LUTS);
- Definitive surgical indications (recurrent UTI, chronic renal impairment, recurrent prostatic bleeding), so unsuitable for α-blockers;
- Neurogenic bladder disorders (e.g. detrusor instability/hyperreflexia);
- Urethral strictures;
- Acute/repeated urinary retention or need for indwelling catheter.

Groups:
- Standard protocol TURP (n=37);
- PVP with GreenLight PV laser (n=64);

All patients initially received 6wk of α-blockers (to exclude those with mild LUTS). Patients with abnormal digital rectal examination or PSA >3ng/dL also underwent transrectal ultrasound-guided biopsies. All patients post-operatively catheterised.

Endpoints and follow-up: Qmax, Vres, IPSS, and quality of life 'Bother-score' recorded at discharge and 1, 3, and 6 months post-surgery. Secondary parameters recorded included intra- and peri-operative/post-discharge morbidity.

Results

	TURP	**PVP**	**p**
Qmax (at 6 months)	19.1mL/s	18.1mL/s	ns*
Vres (at 6 months)	14.4mL	12.9mL	ns*
IPSS at 6 months (% improvement)	4.8 (72%)	5.2 (71%)	ns*
Operating time (min)	49.4 (±16.0)	59.6 (±24.4)	0.047
Irrigation solution use	21.1L	8.8L	<0.001
Intra-operative severe bleeds	4	0	0.02
Serum Hb (1h post-op)	12.9g/dL	13.7g/dL	0.03
Serum Na$^+$ (1h post-op)	135.3mmol/L	137.9mmol/L	0.01
Serum Hb <10g/dL (discharge)	8 (21.6%)	4 (6.3%)	0.03
Mean post-op catheterisation	3.0d	1.8d	<0.001
UTI (post-discharge)	4 (10.8%)	7 (10.9%)	ns
Total complications	16 (42.2%)	25 (39.1%)	ns
Discharged with catheter (secondary to retention)	1 (2.7%)	5 (7.8%)	ns
Mean inpatient stay (d)	7.1 (±1.8)	5.5 (±2.7)	<0.001

* PVP only: comparison to previous control $p=0.01$ (Qmax); $p=0.03$ (Vres); $p=<0.001$ (IPSS).
Key: Na$^+$=sodium; Hb=haemoglobin

Discussion

PVP is a useful alternative to TURP, with comparable outcomes in terms of relief of LUTS. It may confer an advantage for certain groups of patients (such as those on anticoagulation) and can reduce inpatient stay. The quoted average stay of 7.1d for TURP could be debated as excessive. A disadvantage of PVP is that no tissue can be retained for histological examination. Interestingly, despite a larger dimension of prostate volume reduction post-TURP, prostate volume in the PVP group appeared to rise after an initial fall (not discussed by the authors).

Problems

- Not a randomised trial. Disproportionate group sizes, with limited numbers and no long-term data beyond 6 months.
- Different surgeons operated on each group.
- Debatable clinical significance of 1h post-procedure Hb/Na$^+$ measurements, with no documented cases of transfusion or transurethral resection (TUR) syndrome in either group.
- Morbidity associated with prostatic biopsy was not recorded.

Prostate cancer prevention: finasteride

PCPT (Prostate Cancer Prevention Trial): The influence of finasteride on the development of prostate cancer.

AUTHORS: Thompson I, Goodman P, Tangen C et al.
REFERENCE: N Engl J Med (2003) 349, 215–24.
STUDY DESIGN: RCT
EVIDENCE LEVEL: 1b

Key message
Long-term therapy with finasteride decreases the incidence of prostate cancer, although there is a small increase in high-risk cancers and sexual side effects.

Impact
The outcomes were greeted with a mixed reception due to concerns regarding the higher incidence of high-grade tumours with finasteride.

Aims
Most approaches to prostate cancer focus on treatment rather than prevention. Androgens are known to influence the development of prostate cancer. Finasteride (a 5-α reductase inhibitor) inhibits the conversion of testosterone to dihydrotestosterone, the primary prostatic androgen. This study aimed to determine whether finasteride could prevent prostate cancer in men aged $\geq$55y.

Methods
Patients: 18,882 men from 221 centres in the USA. 92% white, 4% African-American, 4% other ethnicity.

Inclusion criteria:
- Age $\geq$55y, no significant comorbidities or evidence of prostate cancer;
- Normal digital rectal examination (DRE);
- Prostate Specific Antigen (PSA) $\leq$3.0ng/mL;
- American Urological Association (AUA) symptom score <20.

Groups:
- 5mg finasteride (n=9423);
- Placebo (n=9459).

Primary endpoint: Development of prostate cancer (histologically proven).

Other factors assessed:
- Changes over time of PSA and prostate volume;
- Effect of finasteride on stage/grade of any developing prostate cancer;
- Accuracy of DRE and PSA in detecting prostate cancer.

Follow-up: Recruitment from 1993–1997. Stopped in 2003 (significantly lower incidence of prostate cancer in those taking finasteride). Mean F/U=7y. Annual PSA and DRE measurements. Prostate biopsy if PSA >4ng/L, abnormal DRE, or at end of 7y if no prior abnormality.

Results

	Finasteride	Placebo	p
Number randomised	9423	9459	–
Number participated	4368	4692	–
All tumours detected	803 (18.4%)	1147 (24.4%)	<0.001
% of above tumours=$T_{1/2}$	97.7%	98.4%	Not stated
% of above tumours=high grade (Gleason 7–10)	37.0% (280 of 757 graded tumours) *or* 6.4% of total 4,368	22.2% (237 of 1068 graded tumours) *or* 5.1% of total 4,692	<0.001 (comparison of % of all graded tumours)
End-of-study biopsies positive for malignancy	368/3,652 (10%)	576/3,820 (15%)	<0.001

Patient losses between randomisation and participation due to early study termination, death, refusal of biopsy, loss to F/U.

- PSA and cancer detection: 21.1% of the cancer-positive end-of-study biopsies were in patients with PSA 2.5–3.9ng/mL or less. 15.4% of tumours were high grade in those with PSA ≤2.5ng/mL.
- Side effects:
  - Sexual side effects (decreased ejaculate volume, erectile dysfunction, loss of libido) significantly more common in finasteride group (all $p \leq 0.001$);
  - Breast cancer incidence same in both groups (one case, ns).
  - Benign prostatic hyperplasia (BPH)/lower urinary tract symptoms more common in placebo group (all $p \leq 0.001$, except for urinary incontinence).

Discussion

Administration of finasteride resulted in a 24.8% reduction in the prevalance of prostate cancer over the F/U period; however, it was associated with a greater number of sexual side effects and an increased risk of developing higher-grade disease (more likely to undergo clinical progression). This was proposed as being due to lower levels of dihydrotestosterone. Clinically significant tumours were common in patients with both normal and elevated PSA levels.

Problems

- No trial entry prostate biopsies; these would have been useful given the high incidence of positive end-of-trial biopsies.
- Higher rates of cancer detection in the placebo group (24.4%) than previously quoted lifetime incidence (16.7%). The authors suggest this was due to overdiagnosis of disease.

Prostate cancer: radiotherapy and androgen suppression

> **EORTC (European Organisation for Research and Treatment of Cancer) study:** Long-term results with immediate androgen suppression and external irradiation with locally advanced prostate cancer.
>
> **AUTHORS:** Bolla M, Collette L, Blank L et al.
> **REFERENCE:** Lancet (2002) 360, 103–8.
> **STUDY DESIGN:** RCT
> **EVIDENCE LEVEL:** 1b

Key message
Immediate androgen suppression with a luteinising hormone releasing hormone (LHRH) analogue given during and for 3y after radiotherapy (RT) improves disease-free and overall survival in patients with locally advanced prostate cancer.

Impact
This regime has become standard practice for this group of patients.

Aims
Long-term outcomes for locally advanced prostate cancer after RT were poor. One approach to improve this involved use of an increased RT dose to the prostate, with 3-dimensional conformal RT to target the treatment more accurately. Studies, including an earlier EORTC trial, had found survival benefits when irradiaton was combined with androgen suppression to destroy hormone-dependent micrometastases outside the treatment volume. This phase III trial aimed to assess the long-term impact of adding hormone therapy (LHRH analogue) to radiation, on disease-free and overall survival in patients with locally advanced prostate cancer.

Methods
Patients: 415 patients from multiple European and Canadian centres.

Inclusion criteria:
- Age <80y old, with newly diagnosed prostatic adenocarcinoma;
- T_{1-2} cancer with World Health Organization histological grade 3 or T_{3-4} cancer of any grade;
- N0 or N1 disease.

Exclusion criteria
- Previous other malignancy of any kind (except basal cell carcinoma (BCC) of the skin);
- Evidence of distal metastases; involvement of common iliac/para-aortic lymph nodes.

Groups:
- RT alone: 50 Gray to the pelvis over 5wk, and 20 Gray as boost to the prostate over 2wk (n=208);

- Combined RT with hormonal treatment: RT as above, plus LHRH analogue, goserelin) for 3y (period chosen empirically) (n=207).

Primary endpoint: Disease-free survival at 5y.

Secondary endpoints: Overall and biochemical disease-free survival.

Follow-up: Assessment by PSA measurement: 2 months after irradiation, then every 3 months for 3y, then every 6 months. Median F/U=66 months (range 1–126).

Results

	RT (n=208)	Combined (n=207)	p
Clinical progression			
Any	90 (43%)	27 (13%)	Not stated
Loco-regional (5y cumulative incidence)	16.4%	1.7%	<0.0001
Distant (5y cumulative incidence)	29.2%	9.8%	<0.0001
Primary endpoint			
Disease-free survival at 5y	40%	74%	<0.0001
Secondary endpoints			
5y survival	62%	78%	<0.0002
5y disease-specific survival	79%	94%	<0.0001
Biochemical disease-free survival at 5y	45%	76%	<0.0001

- Similar results when patients stratified by tumour stage (T_{1-2} vs T_{3-4})

Discussion

Three years of androgen suppression with external beam RT improved 5y survival in patients with locally advanced prostate cancer, vs RT alone. These significant benefits of combined hormone and radiation therapy have been proposed as being additive and resulting from the induction of apoptosis, leading to elimination of occult systemic disease. Other studies have also shown survival benefit from hormonal therapy after radical prostatectomy *(N Engl J Med* (1999) 341, 1781–88). The side effects of androgen deprivation need to be considered, and include hot flushes, fatigue, and sexual dysfunction as well as others. These resulted in 10% of those receiving LHRH stopping hormonal treatment early.

Problems

- No mention of Gleason scores.
- 3y hormonal treatment duration was empirical. Trials to determine whether shorter durations are suitable are currently in progress.
- The impact of nodal status unclear due to only a small number of patients with N1 disease
- RT technique used in the trial may not have been optimal and the role of chemotherapy was not investigated.

Prostate cancer: brachytherapy

10year disease free survival after transperineal sonography-guided iodine-125 brachytherapy with or without 45 Gray external beam irradiation in the treatment of patients with clinically localised, low to high Gleason grade prostate carcinoma.

AUTHORS: Ragde H, Elgamal A, Snow P *et al.*
REFERENCE: Cancer (1998) 83, 989–1001.
STUDY DESIGN: Non-randomised, prospective, cohort
EVIDENCE LEVEL: 2b

Key message
Brachytherapy offers 10y actuarial survival rates comparable to radical prostatectomy and external beam radiotherapy.

Impact
This study has led to brachytherapy increasingly becoming a mainstream treatment option.

Aims
Increased use of prostate specific antigen (PSA)-based screening has led to the detection of an increasing number of organ-confined prostate carcinomas, the management of which have been widely debated. Early data had shown brachytherapy to have comparable outcomes to external beam radiotherapy (EBRT) and radical prostatectomy. This study aimed to report the 10y outcomes of patients with clinically organ-confined prostate cancer who received brachytherapy.

Methods
Patients: 152 patients at 1 centre in the USA.

Inclusion criteria: Patients undergoing brachytherapy for localised prostate carcinoma between January 1987 and June 1988.

Exclusion criteria: 10 patients excluded due to high clinical stage, palladium treatment, and prior hormonal treatment, or radiation failure.

Groups: Consecutively recruited into two groups:
- 1: Brachytherapy: iodine-125 implants (160 Gray) (n=98; 64%);
- 2: Brachytherapy and EBRT ('high risk'): iodine-125 implants (120 Gray) and EBRT (45 Gray) (n=54; 36%).

Follow-up:
- First year: digital rectal examination (DRE) and PSA testing every 3–6 months, then annually. PSA threshold ≥0.5ng/mL;
- Annual prostate biopsy (3–8 cores) for 5y;
- Recurrence classified as positive biopsy, radiological evidence of metastases, or both;
- Median F/U=110; 12.5 patients lost to F/U.

Results

- Baseline: Median age=70y. Palpable lesions in 82% (124/152). Variable Gleason grade (median 5) and disease range T_{1-3} (median T_2). Average PSA=8.5ng/mL (brachytherapy), 15.6ng/mL (brachytherapy and EBRT), PSA 11.0ng/mL (combined). 26.6% had PSA >10ng/mL.
- Outcomes: 97 patients (64%) clinically and biochemically disease-free at 10y (average PSA=0.18ng/mL). In this group, it took an average of 42 months to reach a PSA of 0.5ng/mL, with PSA <1.0ng/mL at 2y. No statistical differences in PSA, stage, and Gleason grade observed between the groups post-treatment. 6% developed bone metastasis.
- Post-operative biopsy (average time=55 months post-implant): 56% negative, 15% positive (of which 3 patients had PSA of 0.3–0.6ng/mL), 29% unavailable.
- Survival: 53 patients died over the 10y (3 due to prostate carcinoma). 65% overall survival, 71% survival for successfully treated patients, and 98% disease-specific survival at 10y (no difference between groups).

Discussion

Brachytherapy shows long-term outcomes comparable to radical prostatectomy and may even be superior to EBRT. Other studies have confirmed its significantly lower morbidity. Serum PSA <1.0ng/mL has been reported as the most important predictor of disease-free survival (p=0.005). The authors compare the study with Adolfsson J et al. (Urology (1997) 50, 722–6) who reported a series of 122 patients with low-grade prostate cancer managed by deferred treatment. They reported a median age of 68 (younger than the present study), with a 10y overall and disease-specific survival of 52% and 90%, respectively. 26% had detectable skeletal metastases. The use of EBRT for high-risk patients needs further study, but may represent optimal treatment.

Problems

- Although this study reported a high level of F/U biopsies (71%), negative results could be due to sampling error. In addition, data is unknown for 29% of cases.
- Long-term complications were not discussed (e.g. seed migration, dysuria, erectile dysfunction, incontinence, stricture, fistula formation, etc.).

Prostate cancer: high intensity focused ultrasound

5year experience of transrectal high intensity focused ultrasound using the Sonablate device in the treatment of localised prostate cancer.

AUTHORS: Uchida T, Ohkusa H, Yamashita H et al.
REFERENCE: BJU Int (2006) 13, 228–33.
STUDY DESIGN: Prospective, Cohort
EVIDENCE LEVEL: 2b

Key message

High intensity focused ultrasound (HIFU), a relatively new minimally invasive treatment option for patients with localised prostate cancer, appears to have comparable safety to other techniques.

Impact

The benefit of HIFU is still debated. Although not yet established as first-line therapy, it is a promising option for patients with localised cancers.

Aims

Conventional surgical treatments for prostate cancer, such as radical pros-tatectomy, are associated with significant morbidity. HIFU, a novel non-invasive technique for thermally ablating the prostate, works by focusing pulses of high energy ultrasound waves at the target tissue in order to induce heat destruction and coagulative necrosis. This study reported the first long-term outcomes of HIFU.

Methods

Patients: 181 consecutive patients at 1 centre in Japan.

Inclusion criteria: Histological (Gleason graded) prostatic carcinoma:
- Clinical stage $T_{1c-2b} N_0 M_0$ (i.e. localised disease);
- Gland volumes ≤40mL (limited focal length of HIFU).

Exclusion criteria:
- Adjuvant hormonal or chemotherapy;
- Gland calcification >1cm;
- Anal stricture.

Groups: Classified according to the number of risk factors (0, 1, and 2, respectively) for prostate specific antigen (PSA) >10ng/mL, Gleason score >7, and stage T_{2b}):
- Low risk (n= 52);
- Intermediate risk (n=81);
- High risk (n=48).

Protocol: Epidural/spinal anaesthesia used. Rectal HIFU probe inserted, and prostate resected layer by layer (each=10mm), as per transrectal ultrasound (TRUS) imaging. Uretheral or suprapubic catheter left in situ.

Follow-up: At 6 monthly intervals with PSA, prostate biopsy, clinical examination, and questionnaires. '*Time to biochemical failure*'=midway between post-treatment PSA nadir and the first of 3 consecutive PSA rises. '*Biochemical recurrence*'=3 consecutive PSA rises after a nadir had been reached, classified according to the American Society for Therapeutic Oncology and Radiology (ASTRO). Mean F/U=21.1 months.

Results

- Baseline: Median age=70y. Stage: T1c (n=92), T2a (n=63), T2b (n=26). Gleason score: 2–4 (n=23), 5–7 (n=134), 8–9 (n=24). Mean pre-treatment PSA=9.76ng/mL (range 3.39–89.6).
- Treatment: Average=1.2 sessions (range 1–3). n=95 (52%) had neo-adjuvant hormones, for an average of 6 months.
- Biochemical disease-free survival rates:
  - 84% (1y), 80% (3y), 78% (5y).
  - 92% (low risk), 75% (intermediate risk), 64% (high risk).
- 3y biochemical disease-free survival by PSA levels:
  - 94% (<10ng/mL), 75% (10–20ng/mL), 35% (>20ng/mL)=$p<0.0001$.
  - Other factors (grade, stage, or neoadjuvant hormone use)=ns.
- Gland volume: decrease from 24.3mL to 12.8mL=$p<0.0001$.
- Mean operative time: 152min.
- Main complications: 22%=urethral strictures, 20%=erectile dysfunction (not on anti-androgens), 6%=epididymitis, 1%=recto-urethral fistula, 0.6%=stress incontinence, 0.6%=prolonged urinary retention.

Discussion

Early studies (*e.g. Endourol* (2003) 17, 673–7) had shown HIFU to be a safe and efficacious primary procedure for localised prostate cancer. This study provided the first long-term F/U data with the newer Sonablate® machine, demonstrating improved outcomes and lower complication rates compared with those reported for other devices such as the Ablatherm. 5y biochemical disease-free rates and morbidities associated with HIFU appeared comparable to those quoted for other modalities such as brachytherapy and radical prostatectomy, without the associated surgical risks and complications. Pre-treatment PSA was shown to be an independent predictor of relapse. However, procedure times appeared long, many patients required more than one session, and the use of HIFU was limited to gland volumes of 40mL, due to limited focal length.

Problems

- The mean F/U was stated as 21.1 months, hence the 3 and 5y data may be underpowered.

Erectile dysfunction: sildenafil

Oral sildenafil in the treatment of erectile dysfunction.

AUTHORS: Goldstein I, Lue T, Padma-Nathan H *et al.*
REFERENCE: N Engl J Med (1998) 338, 1397–404.
STUDY DESIGN: RCT
EVIDENCE LEVEL: 1b

Key message
Oral sildenafil is effective in the treatment of erectile dysfunction (ED).

Impact
Sildenafil (Viagra®) became the first mainline pharmacological therapy for ED.

Aims
No effective oral treatment for ED was available at the time of this study. Sildenafil, a selective inhibitor of cyclic GMP specific phosphodiesterase type 5, assists with erections in response to sexual stimulation. It is effective for 3–5h and is absorbed to maximum plasma levels within 1h. This study aimed to evaluate the safety and efficacy of sildenafil with variable dosing regimes.

Methods
Patients: 532 patients from 37 centres in the USA.

Inclusion criteria:
- Men aged ≥18y;
- ED of organic, psychogenic, or mixed cause.

Exclusion criteria:
- Penile anatomical defects or spinal cord injury;
- Primary diagnosis of another sexual disorder;
- Major psychiatric disorder or alcohol/drug abuse;
- Poorly controlled diabetes mellitus;
- Active peptic ulcer;
- Myocardial infarction (MI)/stroke in the past 6 months, or ongoing nitrate use.

Groups:
- Placebo;
- Oral sildenafil (dose of 25, 50, or 100mg);
- Grouped as above, for two sequential, double-blind studies:
  - 1st=24wk dose response study (n=216 placebo, 316 sildenafil);
  - 2nd=12wk flexible dose escalation study (n=166 placebo, 163 sildenafil).

Primary endpoint: Efficacy assessed using the International Index of Erectile Function (IIEF) and event log at regular intervals, assessing the ability to achieve and maintain an erection sufficient for intercourse.

Follow-up: Regular F/U throughout duration of 24wk study, including 15-question IIEF questionnaire: 1 (never/poor) to 5 (always/good) scale.

Results

	Dose response		Dose escalation	
	Placebo (n=216)	**Sildenafil (n=316)**	**Placebo (n=166)**	**Sildenafil (n=163)**
Mean age (y) (range)	57 (20–79)	58 (24–87)	59 (31–81)	60 (26–79)
ED, mean duration (y)	3.2	3.2	4.7	5.0
ED, organic causes (n)	77	78	63	55
Completed study	180 (83%)	285 (90%)	153 (92%)	154 (94%)
Stopped due to side effects	1 (<1%)	1 (1%)	–	1 (<1%)
Stopped due to poor response	11 (5%)	5 (2%)	–	1 (<1%)
Improvement in frequency of penetration (all men)	5%	25mg=60% 50mg=84% 100mg=100%	10%	95%
Improvement in maintenance of erection post-intercourse	24%	25mg=121% 50mg=133% 100mg=130%	13%	140%
Completion dose	–	–	–	25mg=2% 50mg=23% 100mg=74%

- 92% (n=207) in the dose escalation study completed an additional 32wk of sildenafil, with only 2% (n=4) withdrawing due to side effects.

Discussion

Sildenafil was safe, well tolerated, and increasingly effective with higher doses (improved frequency of penetration and maintenance of erection) irrespective of the underlying cause of ED. The main side effects were transient headache, flushing, dyspepsia, and rhinitis. Visual disturbances (PDE-6 related) were transient, dose-related, lasting up to a few hours.

Problems

- The study relied on patient self-reporting of successful sexual function, prone to an element of subjective bias.
- Drug company funded study; however, unclear if this had any bearing on the results.

Vascular surgery

Introduction

Over the last two decades, Vascular surgery has transformed into a new speciality incorporating endovascular therapies. The field of vascular and endovascular therapy covers an extensive range of conditions and disorders of the arteries and veins.

Lower limb ischaemia

Bypass surgery for lower limb ischaemia owes much of its success to the pioneering work of Alexis Carrel in 1902, who described a reliable technique for vascular anastomosis. It was over 60 years later when an endovascular alternative, percutaneous transluminal angioplasty, was described by Dotter and Judkins. It was not until 1971 when the pioneering work of Gruntzig led to the introduction of balloon angioplasty in the treatment of arterial stenoses and occlusions.

Abdominal aortic aneurysm (AAA)

Conventional repair of AAA remains largely similar to the technique described by Dubost in 1951. However, outcomes have improved through better understanding and management of their peri-operative, anaesthetic, intensive care, and transfusion requirements. In 1991, Volodos and Parodi described a novel, less invasive technique for repairing AAAs by placing a stent graft from within the vessel. Since then, endovascular aneurysm repair (EVAR) has progressed enormously from the initial custom built devices—with design faults that led to late device failures—to the modular 'off the shelf' variety, which are proving more durable.

Carotid disease

Eastcott et al. first described carotid endarterectomy in 1954, and it was not long before it was considered the standard of care for those patients with carotid artery disease. Carotid revascularisation with balloon angioplasty began in the early 1980s, and a stent was first used in 1989 to treat an intimal flap after angioplasty. Since the initial deployment of the first carotid stent in 1989, technological advances have improved the durability and safety of this device and technique.

Varicose veins

The treatment of varicose veins has also seen major developments: traditional thoughts would still advocate surgical ligation and 'stripping' of incompetent truncal veins. However, minimally invasive techniques such as endovenous laser ablation and radiofrequency ablation have been introduced widely as first-line therapy.

Carotid artery stenosis: asymptomatic endarterectomy

ACST (Asymptomatic Carotid Surgery Trial): Prevention of disabling and fatal strokes by successful carotid endarterectomy in patients without recent neurological symptoms.

AUTHORS: Asymptomatic Carotid Surgery Trial Collaborative Group.
REFERENCE: Lancet (2004) 363, 1491–502.
STUDY DESIGN: RCT
EVIDENCE LEVEL: 1b

Key message
Younger patients with asymptomatic carotid stenosis >70% benefit from a small but significant long-term reduction in the risk of stroke following carotid endarterectomy (CEA), provided that the peri-operative stroke and mortality rate is low (<3.0%).

Impact
Following the publication of this trial, the number of CEAs performed in Europe for asymptomatic stenosis increased (doubled in Scandinavia and the UK, and increased by 25% in mainland European countries). Younger patients (<75y old) with asymptomatic significant stenosis >70% are now considered for CEA.

Aims
Asymptomatic carotid stenoses are common and present a small risk of future stroke. The benefit of CEA in this group of patients was previously unclear. This study aimed to determine the balance of surgical risks and long-term benefits following CEA in patients with significant carotid artery stenosis, but no recent neurological symptoms.

Methods
Patients: 3120 patients from 126 centres in 30 countries (mainly Europe).

Inclusion criteria:
- Severe unilateral or bilateral carotid stenoses (>60% on ultrasound);
- No neurological symptoms for the previous 6 months.

Exclusion criteria:
- Previous ipsilateral CEA;
- Poor surgical risk, especially significant coronary artery disease;
- Poor life expectancy which precluded long-term F/U;
- Potential cardiac source of emboli.

Groups:
- Surgical treatment: 'immediate' CEA and best medical treatment (n=1560);
- Medical arm: best medical treatment only (unless became symptomatic during the F/U period at which point they underwent 'deferred' CEA) (n=1560).

Primary endpoints:
- Any peri-operative morbidity and mortality—stroke and myocardial infarction (MI);
- Any non-peri-operative stroke.

Follow-up: At 4 and 12 months, and yearly thereafter (mean F/U=3.4y).

Results

	Surgical (Immediate CEA)	Medical (Deferred CEA)	Net gain	p
Any stroke	6.4%	11.8%	5.4%	<0.0001
Fatal or disabling stroke	3.5%	6.1%	2.5%	<0.004
Any non-peri-operative stroke	3.8%	11%	7.2%	<0.0001
Fatal stroke	2.1%	4.2%	2.1%	<0.006
Non-peri-operative carotid territory ischaemic stroke	2.7%.	9.5%	6.8%	<0.0001

Kaplan–Meier life table methods to assess the 5y stroke risk.

- 30d peri-operative stroke and mortality rate=3.1%.
- Subgroup analysis found no significant heterogeneity in peri-operative hazards or post-operative benefits. These benefits were separately significant for men and women, for about 70%, 80%, and 90% carotid artery stenosis and for entry age less than 75y.
- No significant benefit found for older patients (>75y).

Discussion

One in 8 patients with asymptomatic severe carotid artery stenosis (>70% on ultrasound) have a stroke within 5y. This risk could be halved (1 in 16) with CEA. The 10y F/U results are not yet published, but provisional data indicate that the benefit of surgery over best medical therapy increases with time. The results from this trial reinforced the findings of a similar trial from the USA, ACAS (*JAMA* (1995) 273, 1421–8), which demonstrated a significant reduction in major ipsilateral stroke or any major peri-operative stroke or death in patients undergoing CEA for asymptomatic carotid stenoses.

Problems

- While there was a relative reduction of 50% in favour of surgery, this correlated to an absolute risk reduction of only 1% per year.
- To maximise the benefits of CEA, the patient needs to be young and to have a reasonably long life expectancy (at least 5y).
- This benefit is present only if the peri-operative stroke rate is low (e.g. 3% in this study).

Carotid artery stenosis: symptomatic endarterectomy (1)

ECST (European Carotid Surgery Trial): Randomised trial of end-arterectomy for recently symptomatic carotid stenosis.

AUTHORS: European Carotid Surgery Trialists' collaborative group.
REFERENCE: Lancet (1991) 351, 1379–87.
STUDY DESIGN: RCT
EVIDENCE LEVEL: 1b

Key message
Carotid endarterectomy (CEA) reduces the incidence of strokes in patients with symptomatic ipsilateral high-grade carotid stenosis (70 to 99%).

Impact
The findings of this and the NASCET trial have led to CEA becoming an integral part of the management strategy for stroke prevention. CEA should be considered for every patient who has suffered a recent transient ischaemic attack (TIA) or non-disabling ischaemic stroke with a significant ipsilateral carotid stenosis.

Aims
Carotid stenoses may be responsible for 20–30% of ischaemic strokes. However, the precise degree of carotid stenosis at which CEA is beneficial was previously unclear. This study aimed to establish whether CEA improved stroke-free life expectancy in patients with symptomatic carotid stenoses.

Methods
Patients: 3024 patients from 96 centres in 12 European countries and 1 centre in Australia.

Inclusion criteria: Patients of any age with:
- Recent TIA or mild stroke in the distribution of the carotid artery (within the previous 6 months);
- Internal carotid artery (ICA) stenosis identified by arteriogram and considered responsible for the patient's symptom.

Exclusion criteria:
- Cardiac conditions likely to cause embolic events;
- More severe disease of the distal rather than proximal ICA.

Groups:
- Medical treatment: best medical treatment only (smoking cessation advice, hypertension treatment, and antiplatelets) (n=1213=40%);
- Surgical treatment: CEA as soon as possible, in addition to best medical treatment (n=1811=60%).

Primary endpoint: Major stroke or death (from randomisation to study end).

Secondary outcomes:
- Surgical events (death or major stroke within 30d of CEA);
- Risk of ipsilateral major ischaemic stroke following uncomplicated surgery;
- Risk of ipsilateral major ischaemic stroke in control patients;
- Estimated gain in stroke-free life expectancy.

Follow-up: At 4 and 12 months; then annually. Mean F/U=6.1y.

Results

- Baseline: 72% patients in each group=male.

	80–99% stenosis	
	Surgery	Control
Major stroke/death at 30d	4.8%	0%
Ipsilateral major stroke, excluding peri-operative*	2.0%	20.6%
	Absolute difference=18.6, p<0.0001	
Major ipsilateral ischaemic stroke, including peri-operative*	6.8%	20.6%
	Absolute difference=13.8, p<0.0001	
Any major stroke or death*	14.9%	26.5%
	Absolute difference=11.6, p=0.001	

* Kaplan–Meier estimates at 3y

- The overall 30d major stroke or death rate following surgery was 7%, and the risk did not vary substantially with the severity of stenosis.
- Control group: risk of stroke related to stenosis severity, particularly >80%. Number needed to treat (NNT) to prevent 1 stroke at 3y=9.
- No overall benefit for CEA over best medical treatment with respect to the combined outcomes of adverse surgical events and other disabling strokes in patients with carotid stenoses <70%.

Discussion

For patients with symptomatic carotid stenosis >80%, CEA conferred a significant benefit over medical treatment alone.

Problems

- This trial strengthened the findings from the equivalent North American study, NASCET, although the measurement of carotid stenoses between these two trials was different; a 70% stenosis measured using NASCET criteria was equivalent to an 80% stenosis by ECST.
- Medical therapy was not specified in ECST (unlike in NASCET) and was left to the discretion of the clinicians.
- Furthermore, unlike NASCET, clinicians were allowed to select patients whom they felt should be randomised in this study and to exclude those that they considered should have CEA. This calls into question the randomised nature of this study.

Carotid artery stenosis: symptomatic endarterectomy (2)

> **NASCET** (**N**orth **A**merican **S**ymptomatic **C**arotid **E**ndarterectomy **T**rial): Beneficial effect of carotid endarterectomy in symptomatic patients with high-grade carotid stenosis.
>
> **AUTHORS:** NASCET Collaborators.
> **REFERENCE:** N Engl J Med (1991) 325, 445–53.
> **STUDY DESIGN:** RCT
> **EVIDENCE LEVEL:** 1b

Key message

Carotid endarterectomy (CEA) reduces the incidence of strokes in patients with symptomatic ipsilateral high-grade stenosis (70–99%) of the internal carotid artery (ICA).

Impact

CEA has became an integral part of the management strategy for stroke prevention, and should be considered for every patient that has suffered a recent transient ischaemic attack (TIA) or non-disabling ischaemic stroke with an ipsilateral significant carotid stenosis ≥70%.

Aims

Despite the lack of good evidence of benefit, the number of CEAs performed in the USA for stroke prevention increased dramatically until the mid-1980s, then declined. This study aimed to correlate the relationship between the degree of carotid stenosis with outcome from either medical or surgical treatment.

Methods

Patients: 659 patients from 50 clinical centres in the USA and Canada.

Inclusion criteria:
- Hemispheric or retinal TIA, or non-disabling stroke within 120d;
- 70–99% stenosis in the symptomatic ICA measured by two-plane selective angiography.

Exclusion criteria:
- Severe intracranial atherosclerotic stenosis;
- Organ failure or cancer with poor life expectancy;
- Disabling stroke;
- Cardiac valvular or rhythm disorder likely to cause embolic symptoms;
- Uncontrolled hypertension, unstable angina, recent (previous 6 months) myocardial infarction (MI), or recent major surgery (previous 30d).

Groups:
- Medical treatment: aspirin plus a combination of anti-lipid, anti-hypertensive and anti-diabetic therapy as indicated (n=331);
- Surgical treatment: CEA plus best medical treatment (n=328).

Primary endpoints:
- Fatal and non-fatal ipsilateral stroke;
- Any stroke or death.

Follow-up: At 1, 3, 6, 9, and 12 months, and then every 4 months by neurologists. CT brain and carotid duplex performed for every new suspected cerebrovascular event.

Results

Adverse events at 2y F/U*	Medical patients	Surgical patients	Absolute difference	Relative risk reduction
Ipsilateral stroke	61 (26.0%)	26 (9.0%)	17.0±3.5%	65%
Major or fatal ipsilateral stroke	29 (13.1%)	8 (2.5%)	10.6±2.6%	81%
Any stroke or death	73 (32.3%)	41 (15.8%)	16.5±4.2%	51%

* Kaplan–Meier estimates.

- The peri-operative stroke and death rate was 5.8%, reduced to 2.1% if only major strokes were considered.
- The Data and Safety Monitoring Board prematurely stopped the enrolment of patients with 70–99% stenoses, and the National Institute of Health issued a 'clinical alert' informing physicians of the results of this study. Patients in the medical arm of the study with high-grade stenoses were subsequently offered surgery.

Discussion

Among symptomatic patients with high-grade stenosis (70–99%), those who underwent surgery benefited from an absolute reduction of 17% in the risk of ipsilateral stroke at 2y, representing a 65% relative risk reduction. Although, this study is over 15y old, it still remains the cornerstone of evidence behind the need for carotid surgery.

Problems

- The surgical results of the vascular surgeons or neurosurgeons in NASCET were reviewed by the surgical committee before each centre was certified as acceptable, and morbidity and mortality rates had to be ≤5%.
- Whilst inclusion criteria were based on angiography, NASCET's ultrasound/angiography findings were subject to an error of approximately 15%.
- Currently, carotid stenoses are measured on the basis of duplex ultrasound and not angiography.

Carotid artery stenosis: stenting vs endarterectomy (1)

> **SAPPHIRE (Stenting and Angioplasty with Protection in Patients HIgh Risk for Endarterectomy):** Protected carotid artery stenting vs endarterectomy in high-risk patients.
>
> **AUTHORS:** SAPPHIRE Investigators.
> **REFERENCE:** N Engl J Med (2004) 351, 1493–501.
> **STUDY DESIGN:** RCT
> **EVIDENCE LEVEL:** 1b

Key message
Carotid stenting, with the use of a cerebral protection device, is not inferior to conventional carotid endarterectomy (CEA) in patients with severe carotid artery stenosis and coexisting conditions that potentially increase their risk for CEA.

Impact
There is a stronger argument in favour of carotid stenting with cerebral protection in high-risk patients.

Aims
Carotid stenting is a less invasive approach for the treatment of carotid stenosis. However, surgery has been demonstrated to yield very good results, with a low risk of major stroke or death. This study was designed to determine whether carotid stenting with cerebral protection devices was superior or inferior to CEA.

Methods
Patients: 334 patients at 29 centres in the USA.

Inclusion criteria:
- Symptomatic stenosis >50% of the luminal diameter or asymptomatic stenosis of ≥80% of the luminal diameter;
- High risk (at least one factor): significant cardiac disease, severe pulmonary disease, contralateral carotid occlusion, 'hostile' neck (radiotherapy, previous surgery including CEA), age >80y.

Exclusion criteria:
- Ischaemic stroke within previous 48h;
- Intraluminal thrombus or total occlusion of the target vessel;
- Ostial lesion of common carotid or brachiocephalic artery;
- Life expectancy <1y.

Groups:
- Endarterectomy group (n=167);
- Stent group (n=167).

Primary endpoint: Cumulative incidence of major cardiovascular event (death, stroke, MI) at 30d or death from neurological causes within 1y.

Secondary endpoints:
- Target vessel revascularisation at 1y;
- Cranial nerve injury;
- Complications at surgical or vascular access site.

Results

Cumulative adverse events at 1y*	Stent	CEA	*p*
Death	7.4%	13.5%	0.08
Stroke	6.2%	7.9%	0.6
MI	3.0%	7.5%	0.07
Cranial nerve palsy	0	4.9%	0.004
Target vessel revascularisation	0.6%	4.3%	0.04
Peri-procedural adverse events (stroke/MI/death at 30d)	4.8%	9.8%	0.09
Primary endpoint	12.2%	20.1%	0.05
Conventional endpoint (stroke/death at 30d and ipsilateral stroke/death from neurological causes within 1y)	5.5%	8.4%	0.4

* Kaplan–Meier method; data based on intention-to-treat.

- Among the subgroup of symptomatic patients, the peri-procedural cumulative incidence of adverse events (death, stroke, and MI) was 2.1% (stent-treated) and 9.3% (CEA-treated) (*p*=0.2).
- Among the subgroup of asymptomatic patients, the incidence of peri-procedural adverse events was 5.4% (stent) and 10.2% (CEA).
- This trial was terminated early because of a sudden slowdown of enrolment when several smaller stent registries were set up.

Discussion

Carotid artery stenting with the use of an embolic protection device was not inferior to CEA for the prevention of stroke, death, or MI in high-risk patients. The early termination of the trial prevented analysis of a larger sample, which might have provided proof of the superiority of stenting over CEA in this group of patients.

Problems

- Selection bias: 747 patients were initially enrolled in the study, but only 334 were randomised. All the remaining (excluding 7) underwent stenting.
- Selection bias: most trial authors acknowledged some financial support from the company that manufactured the cerebral protection device.
- Over 70% of patients in both groups underwent treatment for asymptomatic carotid disease. The cumulative peri-procedural adverse event rates in this trial were excessively high in both treatment groups. This was justified by the authors on account of selection of high-risk patients.

Carotid artery stenosis: stenting vs endarterectomy (2)

EVA-3S (**E**ndarterectomy **V**s **A**ngioplasty in patients with **S**ymptomatic **S**evere carotid **S**tenosis): Endarterectomy vs stenting in patients with symptomatic severe carotid stenosis.

AUTHORS: EVA-3S Investigators.
REFERENCE: N Engl J Med (2006) 355, 1660–71.
STUDY DESIGN: RCT
EVIDENCE LEVEL: 1b

Key message
Among patients with symptomatic >60% critical carotid stenosis, carotid endarterectomy (CEA) is safer than carotid stenting.

Impact
CEA remains the gold standard treatment for symptomatic carotid stenosis. Stenting has a limited role.

Aims
Carotid artery stenting is less invasive than CEA. However, it was previously unclear whether it was safe in patients with symptomatic carotid artery stenosis. This study aimed to determine whether carotid stenting was comparable to carotid endoarterectomy (CEA) in patients with symptomatic critical internal carotid artery (ICA) stenosis.

Methods
Patients: 520 patients from 30 vascular centres in France.

Inclusion criteria:
- Transient ischaemic attack (TIA) or non-disabling stroke within 120d from enrolment in the trial;
- 60–99% stenosis in the symptomatic ICA confirmed by catheter angiography or magnetic resonance angiography (MRA).

Exclusion criteria:
- Disabling stroke (≥3 on Rankin score);
- Severe tandem lesions (proximal common carotid, intracranial);
- Previous ipsilateral carotid surgery;
- Bleeding disorders or contraindications to heparin or clopidogrel;
- Uncontrolled hypertension or diabetes, unstable angina, and other comorbidities leading to a less than 2y life expectancy.

Groups: Treatment within 2wk from randomisation:
- CEA (n=259);
- Stenting (n=261).

Primary endpoints: 30d incidence of any stroke or death.

Secondary endpoints:
- Composite any stroke or death from treatment to end of F/U;
- MI, TIA, local complications, cranial nerve injury.

Follow-up: Neurologist review at 48h, and 6 months after treatment, and every 6 months thereafter.

Results

	Endarterectomy	Stenting	Relative risk	*p*
30d incidence of stroke or death	3.9%	9.6%	2.5	0.01
30d incidence of disabling stroke or death	1.5%	3.4%	2.2	0.3
Any stroke or death at 6 months	6.1%	11.7%	1.9	0.02
Local complications	1.2%	3.1%	2.6	0.2
Cranial nerve injury	7.7%	1.1%	0.15	<0.001

- One additional stroke or death resulted when 17 patients underwent stenting rather than endarterectomy (absolute risk increase of 5.7%).

Discussion

The trial was stopped early for reasons of both safety and futility. The risk of peri-operative stroke or death was significantly higher after stenting than after CEA.

Problems

- The incidence of stroke after stenting was 9.2%. This was significantly higher than that reported in the SAPPHIRE study or in other stent registries.
- Different stents and cerebral protection devices were used by the various participating centres in this study.
- Furthermore, there was no specified antiplatelet regime proposed for patients who had a carotid stent.

Abdominal aortic aneurysm: screening

MASS (**M**ulticentre **A**neurysm **S**creening **S**tudy): The MASS into the effect of abdominal aortic aneurysm screening on mortality in men.

AUTHORS: Multicentre Aneurysm Screening Study Group.
REFERENCE: Lancet (2002) 360, 1531–9.
STUDY DESIGN: RCT
EVIDENCE LEVEL: 1b

Key message

Large-scale population screening of 65y old men for abdominal aortic aneurysm (AAA) significantly reduces aneurysm-related deaths.

Impact

In the UK, the Department of Health has recently approved a national screening programme.

Aims

In men older than 65y, ruptured AAA is responsible for 2–3% of all deaths. Ultrasound had been routinely utilised as a very sensitive and specific test to detect AAA. This study aimed to assess whether ultrasound screening for AAAs was beneficial in terms of mortality, morbidity, and quality of life.

Methods

Patients: 67,800 men from 4 centres in the UK.

Inclusion criteria:
- Males, aged 65–74y;
- Resident in any trial centre area (Oxford, Winchester, Southampton, Portsmouth).

Exclusion criteria:
- Critical illness or serious health problems preventing screening test;
- Previous aortic surgery.

Groups:
- Invited group: Invited via general practitioner to attend for an abdominal ultrasound scan (n=33,839).
- Control group: Not invited (n=33,961).

Primary endpoints: Aneurysm-related mortality.

Secondary endpoints:
- All-cause mortality;
- Frequency of ruptured AAA;
- Quality of life.

Follow-up: Mean F/U=4.1y.
- <5.5cm aneurysm: Received surveillance scans;
- Rapidly expanding, symptomatic or ≥5.5cm aneurysm: Referred to a vascular surgeon and considered for surgery.

Results

- 80% of 'invited for screening' population accepted and were scanned.
- Aneurysm detected in 4.9% of the men scanned.
- The screened aneurysms were distributed as the following:
  - 3.0–4.4cm AAA: 71%
  - 4.5–5.4cm AAA: 17%
  - ≥5.5cm AAA: 12%

	Control (n=33961)	Invited (n=33839)	HR/p
Total AAA-related deaths	113 (0.3%)	65 (0.2%)	HR 0.58 p=0.0002
	Relative risk reduction of 42% in the invited group and 53% in those who attended the ultrasound scan		
Ruptured AAA	140 (0.4%)	82 (0.2%)	HR 0.59 p=0.00006
Elective AAA repair mortality	9 (10%)	15 (5%)	p=0.1
Emergency AAA repair mortality	22 (41%)	8 (30%)	p=0.3

- More individuals in the invited group (n=322, 1%) had elective operations than in the control group (n=92, 0.3%).
- There were fewer emergency operations done in the invited group (n=27, 0.08%) than in the control group (n=54, 0.1%).
- 30d mortality was 6% for elective repair and 37% for emergency operations; no significant differences between the two groups.
- No difference in all-cause mortality between groups (11% died in each group by the end of the trial).

Discussion

Screening significantly reduced mortality rates associated with AAA. There was no significant reduction in all-cause mortality between the two groups. This was to be expected as AAA only accounted for 2–3% of all deaths. There was a good acceptance rate in the invited group for ultrasound screening.

Problems

- Mortality data was based on death certification provided by the Office of National Statistics. Many patients are certified without postmortem, and hence the accuracy of this data is uncertain. The coding used to establish AAA-related deaths could have included patients with ruptured thoracic aortic aneurysms.
- Many of the deaths within the invited group were in patients who failed to attend their screening ultrasound, did not comply with a subsequent surveillance programme, or were deemed unfit for surgery.
- The incidence of ruptured AAA in the invited group who did not attend reduces the benefit for screening overall.

Abdominal aortic aneurysm: small aortic aneurysms

UK Small Aneurysm Trial: Long-term outcomes of immediate repair compared with surveillance of small abdominal aortic aneurysms.

AUTHORS: United Kingdom Small Aneurysm Trial Participants.
REFERENCE: N Engl J Med (2002) 346, 1445–52.
STUDY DESIGN: RCT
EVIDENCE LEVEL: 1b

Key message
There is no survival benefit associated with the elective open repair of abdominal aortic aneurysms (AAAs) smaller than 5.5cm.

Impact
Elective repair is considered for patients with AAAs greater than 5.5cm in diameter.

Aims
AAAs are common, with a prevalence of around 6% in 65y old males. Ruptured AAA is associated with a high mortality rate. However, more patients die from other conditions with their aneurysm intact. This study aimed to determine whether early open repair of small AAAs (≤5.5cm in maximum diameter) was beneficial, or whether a policy of active surveillance was acceptable.

Methods
Patients: 1090 patients from 93 centres in the UK.

Inclusion criteria:
- Age 60–76y;
- Asymptomatic infrarenal AAA of 4.0–5.5cm in diameter;
- Fit for open AAA repair.

Groups:
- Surgical arm: Early elective aneurysm repair (n=593);
- Surveillance arm: Remained on ultrasound surveillance and had surgical repair if the aneurysm became symptomatic or expanded by more than 1cm per year, or exceeded 5.5cm (n=527).

Primary endpoints: All-cause mortality.

Secondary endpoints:
- Aneurysm-related mortality;
- 30d mortality.

Follow-up: Mean F/U=8y (range 6–10y).

Results

	Surveillance (n=527)	Surgery (n=593)	Hazard Ratio/p
All-cause mortality	254 (8.3 patients/100 patients years)	242 (7.1 patients/100 patients years)	0.83 ($p=0.05$)
30d mortality	28/389 (7.2%)	29/526 (5.5%)	$p=0.3$
Mean years of survival	6.5y	6.7y	$p=0.3$

- By the end of the study, 321 (62%) patients in the surveillance group had undergone AAA repair, along with 38 (7%) patients outside trial protocol.
- In the surgical group, 520 (92%) patients had open AAA repair. 34 patients either refused or were subsequently deemed unfit. 9 patients died before their contemplated surgery.
- Elective mortality for elective repair was 5.4%. Women had a higher risk of aneurysm rupture than men (hazard ratio 4.0, $p<0.001$).

Discussion

Early repair of small AAA did not result in a survival benefit at 5y, over active surveillance. However, at 8y, there was a small reduction in mortality in the early surgery group. This was interpreted as the result of a change in lifestyle among those patients, many of whom stopped smoking. By the end of the trial, three quarters of patients in the surveillance group eventually underwent AAA repair. The results of this trial were similar to those of the ADAM trial (*N Engl J Med* (2002) 346, 1437–44), a similar RCT conducted in the USA.

Problems

- This study was not designed to specify the size at which AAA should be treated. It used a threshold of 5.5cm for both men and women. 17% of patients in this trial were women, for whom this threshold may have been too high.
- Subgroup analysis demonstrated a benefit for early surgery in younger patients (<72y) with larger AAA (>4.5cm). However, as the study was not powered to assess this group, it does not influence current practice for the majority of clinicians.

Abdominal aortic aneurysm: endovascular vs open repair in 'fit' patients

EVAR 1 (EndoVascular Aneurysm Repair): EVAR vs open repair in patients with abdominal aortic aneurysm.

AUTHORS: The EVAR trial participants.
REFERENCE: Lancet (2005) 365, 2179–86.
STUDY DESIGN: RCT
EVIDENCE LEVEL: 1b

Key message

Endovascular aneurysm repair (EVAR) reduces aneurysm-related mortality by 3% when compared to open surgery at 4y. However, it offers no advantage with respect to all-cause mortality and health-related quality of life (HRQL). It is more expensive, and involves significantly more re-interventions.

Impact

The role of EVAR in patients fit for open surgical repair remains an area of debate.

Aims

While short-term data had suggested EVAR to have reduced morbidity and mortality compared to conventional surgery, its durability had remained a concern, with high re-intervention rates. This study aimed to compare EVAR with conventional open repair for abdominal aortic aneurysm (AAA).

Methods

Patients: 1082 patients from 34 centres in the UK.

Inclusion criteria:
- Aged ≥60y;
- Asymptomatic AAA of at least 5.5cm in diameter;
- Aneurysm morphology suitable for EVAR;
- Patient fit for open repair.

Primary endpoint: All-cause mortality.

Secondary endpoints:
- Aneurysm-related mortality;
- HRQL;
- Post-operative complications;
- Hospital costs.

Groups:
- EVAR (n=543);
- Open repair (n=539).

Results

	Open repair	EVAR	*p*
30d mortality	4.7%	1.7%	0.009
All-cause mortality*	29%	26%	0.5
Aneurysm-related mortality*	7%	4%	0.04
Post-operative complications	9%	41%	<0.0001
Re-interventions*	6%	20%	<0.0001

* Kaplan–Meier endpoint estimates at 4y.

- Although the open repair group had a diminished HRQL at 3 months, it had recovered by 12 months. 12–24 months after randomisation, there was no difference between groups.
- The total cost per patient was calculated at 4y. The EVAR was estimated (UK costs) at £13,257 and the open repair at £9946—a difference of £3311 per patient.

Discussion

EVAR conferred a 3% 30d operative mortality benefit over open aneurysm repair. However, there was no significant difference in all-cause mortality at 4y, although the 3% aneurysm-related mortality benefit remained. In view of late complications within the EVAR group, there remains a demand for long-term surveillance (predominately using CT scans). This has implications on costs.

Problems

- Not all aneurysms are suitable for EVAR, with many institutions reporting only approximately 50% being anatomically suitable.
- Interpretation of this study would have been very different if the primary endpoint was aneurysm-related mortality and not all-cause mortality.
- It is now felt that EVAR followed by an aggressive approach to treating cardiovascular risk factors would improve all-cause mortality rate.

Abdominal aortic aneurysm: endovascular repair in 'unfit' patients

> **EVAR 2** (**E**ndo**V**ascular **A**neurysm **R**epair): EVAR in patients unfit for open repair.
>
> **AUTHORS:** The EVAR Trial Participants.
> **REFERENCE:** Lancet (2005) 365, 2187–92.
> **STUDY DESIGN:** RCT
> **EVIDENCE LEVEL:** 1b

Key message
Among patients considered too unfit for open surgical repair, the focus of treatment should be on improving fitness rather than on early endovascular aneurysm repair (EVAR).

Impact
EVAR in patients unfit for open repair remains controversial.

Aims
Endovascular repair of AAAs was initially considered ideal for those patients deemed unfit for major surgery. However, many of these unfit patients die of causes unrelated to their aneurysm. This study aimed to compare EVAR of AAAs with best medical treatment, in patients unfit for open repair.

Methods
Patients: 338 patients at 31 centres in the UK.

Inclusion criteria:
- Age >60y;
- Asymptomatic AAA of at least 5.5cm in diameter;
- Aneurysm morphology suitable for EVAR;
- Patients unfit for open repair according to each unit's own guidelines (MI in the previous 3 months, unstable angina, significant arrhythmia, uncontrolled congestive cardiac failure, severe valve disease, $FEV_1<1.0L$, $PaO_2<8kPa$, $PaCO_2>6.5kPa$, serum creatinine >200micromol/L).

Exclusion criteria:
- Patients with 'hostile' abdomen anatomically unsuitable for an open repair, but anaesthetically fit enough for an open repair.

Groups:
- EVAR (n=166);
- Best medical treatment (n=172).

Primary endpoints: All-cause mortality.

Secondary endpoints:
- Aneurysm-related mortality;
- Health-related quality of life (HRQL);
- Post-operative complications;
- Hospital costs.

Follow-up: Median F/U=3.3y.

Results

	EVAR (n=166)	No intervention (n=172)	Hazard Ratio
Death from all causes	74	68	1.21 (95%CI 0.87 to 1.69)
Aneurysm-related death	20	22	1.01 (95%CI 0.55 to 1.84)
30d mortality	9%	9%	
Mean hospital cost at 4y	£13,632	£4,983	

- Estimated overall mortality at 4y was 64% (Kaplan–Meier);
- Three quarters of patients had symptomatic cardiac disease;
- No differences in HRQL between the two groups;
- 1 in 4 EVAR patients required at least one re-intervention by the end of the fourth year of F/U.

Discussion

The trial demonstrated no survival benefit from EVAR in patients unfit for open repair. EVAR was more expensive than medical therapy alone, did not affect HRQL, and required continual surveillance and often re-intervention. Therefore, improving fitness should be the main target for this group of patients.

Problems

- Nearly 50% of aneurysm-related death in the EVAR group occurred before surgery, while patients were waiting for treatment (median delay of >3 months from time of randomisation).
- 27% of patients randomised into no intervention arm subsequently underwent treatment (35 EVAR and 12 open repair).
- Only 39% of patients in the EVAR group were on statins and more than 40% were not taking any antiplatelets.

Peripheral arterial disease: surgery vs angioplasty

> **BASIL** (<u>B</u>ypass vs <u>A</u>ngioplasty in <u>S</u>evere <u>I</u>schaemia of the <u>L</u>eg)
>
> **AUTHORS:** BASIL trial participants.
> **REFERENCE:** Lancet (2005) 366, 1925–34.
> **STUDY DESIGN:** RCT
> **EVIDENCE LEVEL:** 1b

Key message

Both bypass surgery and balloon angioplasty are equally effective first-line treatments for severe ischaemia of the leg due to infra-inguinal disease. A surgery-first approach is more costly than an angioplasty-first approach, but durability is significantly better at 2y F/U.

Impact

Fitter, younger patients with severe lower limb ischaemia are probably better off having surgery as the first approach. Those patients with severe comorbidities may be best advised towards angioplasty as a first-line treatment.

Aims

The treatment of critical limb ischaemia remains controversial, with advocates for surgical or endovascular therapies basing their decision to treat on personal preferences. This study aimed to compare the outcomes of a surgery-first strategy with an angioplasty-first strategy, in patients with severe limb ischaemia.

Methods

Patients: 452 patients from 27 centres in the UK.

Inclusion criteria:
- Severe limb ischaemia (rest pain or tissue loss for >2wk);
- Infra-inguinal disease amenable to both types of treatment.

Groups:
- Surgery-first strategy (n=228 randomised; n=195 (86%) underwent attempted intervention);
- Angioplasty-first strategy (n=224 randomised; n=216 (96%) underwent the intervention).

Primary endpoints: Amputation-free survival (alive with trial leg intact).

Secondary endpoints:
- All-cause mortality;
- 30d morbidity and mortality;
- Re-interventions;
- Health-related quality of life (HRQL);
- Use of hospital resources.

Results

Primary endpoints	Angioplasty (n=224)	Bypass (n=228)
Amputation-free survival at 1y	71%	68%
Amputation-free survival at 3y	52%	57%
Secondary endpoints		
30d mortality	3%	5%
30d morbidity	41%	57%
Re-intervention rate	26%	18%
Inpatient annual treatment cost (per person)	£17,419	£23,322

NB Kaplan–Meier methods used to construct survival curves.

- At the end of the F/U, 37% of patients had died (equal distribution between the two treatment groups).
- There were no significant differences in HRQL between the two groups, and an overall recorded improvement by 3 months was largely sustained during F/U.
- By 12 months, 50% patients that had angioplasty had resulted in clinical failure; more than half of these patients went on to have a second intervention, which, in most instances, was surgery.

Discussion

Patients presenting with severe limb ischaemia due to infra-inguinal occlusive disease treatable by angioplasty or surgery had broadly similar outcomes in terms of amputation-free survival. Angioplasty seemed to provide a less durable result, but was otherwise cheaper than surgery, and was associated with less peri-procedural complications. For this reason, angioplasty is often considered first choice for patients with significant comorbidities and short life expectancy. Surgery provided a more durable result and may be more appropriate for healthier younger individuals. However, failed endovascular procedures did not preclude a subsequent surgical bypass.

Problems

- Patients suitable for the trial represented only a small fraction of the total people who suffer from the condition. Only 30% of eligible patients were recruited into the trial. Approximately one third of patients in the major recruiting centres refused to join the study.
- One third of patients were not receiving antiplatelet therapy and only one third were taking statins.

Peripheral arterial disease: angioplasty vs stenting

Balloon angioplasty vs implantation of nitinol stents in the superficial femoral artery.

AUTHORS: Schillinger M, Sabeti S, Loewe C et al.
REFERENCE: N Engl J Med (2006) 354, 1879–88.
STUDY DESIGN: RCT
EVIDENCE LEVEL: 1b

Key message
Treatment of superficial femoral artery (SFA) disease using self-expanding nitinol (nickel-titanium) stents is associated with superior anatomical and clinical results in the intermediate term.

Impact
These findings have the potential to change the endovascular treatment of SFA disease.

Aims
Restenosis, particularly in long segments, is a major problem in the endo-vascular treatment of the SFA. Stainless steel stents have not been shown to be any more beneficial than angioplasty (*J Vasc Interv Radiol* (2001) 12, 935–42). This study aimed to compare the anatomical and clinical outcomes of newer, self-expanding nitinol stents with conventional balloon angioplasty.

Methods
Patients: 104 patients at 1 centre in Austria.

Inclusion criteria:
- Clinically severe claudication or chronic limb ischaemia due to stenosis or occlusion of the SFA;
- Anatomically (based on angiography at the time of intervention) >50% stenosis or occlusion length >30mm;
- At least one patent runoff vessel.

Exclusion criteria:
- Acute critical limb ischaemia;
- Previous bypass surgery or stenting;
- Untreated iliac artery disease;
- Known intolerance to medications or contrast.

Groups:
- Primary nitinol stent implantation (n=51);
- Angioplasty (n=53).

Primary endpoint: Restenosis of >50% of the treated segment's diameter on angiogram at 6 months.

Secondary endpoints: Anatomically: restenosis >50% (Ultrasound (US) scan or angiogram at any time). *Clinically:* Rutherford stage and the maximal walking capacity on the treadmill. *Haemodynamically:* resting ankle–brachial pressure index (ABPI).

Follow-up: Clinical review at 24h, 3 and 6 months, and 1y. Duplex US scan at 3 and 6 months, and 1y. Angiogram (digital subtraction or CT) at 6 months. Data evaluated by two independent observers.

Results

Restenosis rate	Stenting (n=51)	Angioplasty (n=53)*	*p*
6 months	24%	37%	0.05
1y	43%	63%	0.01

* 17 underwent secondary stenting, mostly due to a suboptimal angioplasty result.

- At both 6 months and 1y, patients in the stenting group were able to cover a greater distance on a treadmill compared to the angioplasty group.

Discussion

At 1y, there was a benefit from primary stenting compared with angioplasty. This may be explained by nitinol's improved radial strength, the ability to recover from being crushed, and reduced foreshortening allowing precise placement. Bypass surgery with venous grafts remains the gold standard treatment of chronic limb ischaemia. However, this study suggests that nitinol stents may be an effective alternative for longer lesions in patients who are poor candidates for surgery or do not have a harvestable saphenous vein. This depends upon a low complication rate and ensuring the surgical target zone remains unaffected in case a subsequent bypass is required. Both of these requirements were fulfilled in this study.

Problems

- Only 1y F/U; longer-term data is needed.
- The primary endpoint was assessed by a combination of CT angiography (CTA) and digital subtraction angiography (DSA). However, the use of CTA vs DSA in stent stenosis has not yet been validated.

Varicose veins: surgical technique

Stripping of the long saphenous vein reduces the rate of reoperation for recurrent varicose veins: Five-year results of a randomised trial.

AUTHORS: Dwerryhouse S, Davies B, Harradine K *et al.*
REFERENCE: J Vasc Surg (1999) 29, 589–92.
STUDY DESIGN: RCT
EVIDENCE LEVEL: 1b

Key message
Venous stripping should be performed for the treatment of primary long saphenous varicose veins.

Impact
Stripping of the long saphenous vein at the sapheno-femoral junction and ligation is now the standard treatment for primary varicose veins.

Aims
Recurrence is common after primary long saphenous vein surgery, with recurrence rates of up to 40% being reported at 5y. This study aimed to investigate the possible long-term clinical advantages of stripping the long saphenous vein during routine primary varicose vein surgery.

Methods
Patients: 100 patients (133 legs) from a single UK centre.

Inclusion criteria: Primary uncomplicated long saphenous varicose veins, with incompetence of the sapheno-femoral junction (SFJ) diagnosed on handheld Doppler (HHD).

Groups:
- SFJ ligation only (n=50; 69 legs);
- SFJ ligation plus long saphenous stripping to the knee level (n=50; 64 legs).

Primary endpoint: Varicose vein recurrence.

Follow-up: At 5y, with clinical and duplex assessment.

Results

	Stripping	Ligation	Relative risk	p
Patients needing surgery for SFJ incompetence at 5y	6%	21%	0.28	0.02
Significant recurrent varicose veins	21%	14%	1.54	0.3
Trivial recurrent varicose veins	13%	26%	0.87	0.1
Groin neovascularisation causing recurrent SFJ incompetence	23%	52%	0.45	0.002
Recurrent SFJ incompetence on F/U duplex	29%	71%	0.41	0.0001
Patient satisfied at F/U	90%	77%	1.17	0.1

Discussion

Although there was no significant difference in the rate of significant or trivial varicose vein recurrence, the number of patients that needed reoperation was considerably greater in the group who only had SFJ ligation. This was probably related to the more frequent groin neo-vascularisation observed among the ligation alone group. Stripping reduced the risk of reoperation for recurrent varicose vein by two thirds after 5y.

Problems

• While this study reported a significant reduction in reoperations for recurrent varicose veins in patients who had their long saphenous vein stripped, it is widely known that the reasons for varicose vein surgery are complex and not always related to symptomatic recurrences. In this study, patients themselves requested reoperation, particularly around the time of the F/U scans.

Venous ulcers: surgery vs compression

ESCHAR (Effect of Surgery and Compression on venous ulcers Healing And Recurrence) study: Comparison of surgery and compression with compression alone in chronic venous ulceration.

AUTHORS: Barwell J, Davies C, Deacon J et al.
REFERENCE: Lancet (2004) 363, 1854–9.
STUDY DESIGN: RCT
EVIDENCE LEVEL: 1b

Key message
Surgical correction of superficial venous reflux reduces ulcer recurrence at 12 months.

Impact
In addition to elastic compression therapy, superficial venous surgery is now considered in most patients with chronic venous ulcers related to superficial venous insufficiency.

Aims
Chronic venous ulcers cause significant morbidity. They have a protracted course of healing, with a high probability of future recurrences. This study aimed to assess the effect of surgery and compression on the healing and recurrence of venous ulcers.

Methods
Patients: 500 patients from 3 vascular centres in the UK.

Inclusion criteria: Pure venous leg ulcerations:
- Open or recently healed (within the preceding 6 months) ulceration, for longer than 4wk, between the ankle and the malleoli;
- Ankle–brachial pressure index (ABPI) >0.85;
- Evidence of superficial venous reflux alone or mixed superficial and deep venous reflux (on duplex imaging).

Exclusion criteria:
- Complete occlusion of deep veins on duplex imaging;
- Unfit for surgery;
- Malignant ulcers.

Groups:
- Compression group: multilayer compression bandaging until ulcer healed, and class 2 elastic compression stockings thereafter (n=242);
- Surgery group: long or short saphenous disconnection, stripping and avulsion, in addition to compression hosiery therapy (n=258).

Primary endpoints:
- 24wk healing rate;
- 12 months ulcer recurrence rate.

Results

	Compression and surgery	Compression alone	*p*
24wk healing rate	65%	65%	0.9
12 months ulcer recurrence rate	12%	28%	<0.0001

- Subgroup analysis by venous reflux pattern (incompetent superficial system only, incompetent superficial and deep system) showed no significant difference in ulcer healing or ulcer recurrence rate.

Discussion

Ulcer healing was not enhanced by superficial venous surgery and could be achieved by multilayer compression bandaging alone. The main benefit of surgery was in reducing ulcer recurrence. In patients receiving surgery, the ulcer recurrence rates were reduced by 20% (about 5 operations would be necessary to prevent 1 ulcer recurrence at 1y).

Problems

- There was poor compliance with surgical treatment, with 24% of patients randomised to surgery refusing to attend for their operation.
- Patients waited a median of 7wk for their operation, and therefore may not have achieved an immediate benefit.
- Furthermore, there was no assessment of compliance for the use of compression stockings.

Index

Glossary

Quick-reference glossary of statistical terms

- **Absolute risk:** The probability of an event in a population under study.
- **Confidence interval (CI):** A measure of how precise the results are. A narrow confidence interval implies precision, a wide confidence interval, imprecision. A 95% CI is the range in which 95% of the 'true' values lie.
- **Exposure:** The factor suspected to alter disease risk.
- **Hazard ratio (HR):** Probability of a hazard at time 't' in the treatment group vs time 't' in the control group. Sometimes referred to as the 'relative risk'.
- **Likelihood ratio (LR):** Estimate of how much a test result will change the odds of having a disease. For a positive result (LR+), it is how much the odds of the disease increase when a test is positive. For a negative result (LR–), it is how much the odds of the disease decrease when a test is negative.
- **Negative predictive value (NPV):** Proportion of people with a negative test who do not have the disorder.
- **Number needed to treat (NNT):** Number of patients who need to be treated with the intervention in order to prevent one additional adverse outcome.
- **Odds ratio (OR):** Ratio between the odds of disease in one group compared with another. Odds are used to approximate risk.
- ***p* value (*p*):** Probability that observed difference is due to chance. Usually, $p<0.05$ is considered statistically significant.
- **Positive predictive value (PPV):** Proportion of people with a positive test who actually have the disorder.
- **Relative risk (RR):** Risk of an event in one group divided by the risk of the event in another (usually control) group.
- **Sensitivity:** Proportion of people with a disorder that are correctly diagnosed as positive by the test.
- **Specificity:** Proportion of people without the disorder that are correctly excluded as negative by the test.

(For a detailed examination of these terms see pp. 40–43)